Recent Advances in

Pathology-1

Recent Advances in Pathology-1

Editor

Pranab Dey

MBBS MD MIAC FRCPath

Currently: Director of Pathology and Transfusion Medicine
National Institute of Medical Science (NIMS)
Jaipur, Rajasthan, India
Ex-Professor
Department of Cytology and Gynecologic Pathology
Postgraduate Institute of Medical Education and Research
Chandigarh, India

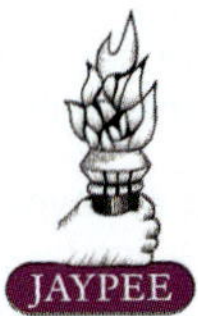

JAYPEE BROTHERS MEDICAL PUBLISHERS

The Health Sciences Publisher

New Delhi I London

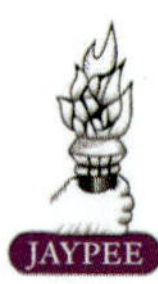

JAYPEE **Jaypee Brothers Medical Publishers (P) Ltd**

Headquarters
Jaypee Brothers Medical Publishers (P) Ltd
23/23-B, Ansari Road, Daryaganj
New Delhi110 002, India
Phone:+91-11-23272143, +91-11-23272703
+91-11-23282021, +91-11-23245672
E-mail: jaypee@jaypeebrothers.com

Corporate Office
Jaypee Brothers Medical Publishers (P) Ltd.
4838/24, Ansari Road, Daryaganj
New Delhi 110 002, India
Phone: +91-11-43574357
Fax: +91-11-43574314
E-mail: jaypee@jaypeebrothers.com

Overseas Office
JP Medical Ltd
83 Victoria Street, London
SW1H 0HW (UK)
Phone: +44 20 3170 8910
E-mail: info@jpmedpub.com

EU GPSR Authorised Representative
Logos Europe, 9 rue Nicolas Poussin
17000, La Rochelle, France
Phone: +33 (0) 6 67 93 73 78
E-mail: Contact@logoseurope.eu

Website: www.jaypeebrothers.com
Website: www.jaypeedigital.com

Inquiries for bulk sales may be solicited at: jaypee@jaypeebrothers.com

Recent Advances in Pathology-1* / *Pranab Dey

First Edition: **2025**

Reprint : **2026**

ISBN: 978-93-6616-098-6

Printed at: Sterling Graphics Pvt. Ltd.

Dedicated to

Shree Shree Satyananda Giri,
Shree Shree Paramahansa Yogananda
And
My wife Rini and daughter Madhumanti

Contributors

Akriti Jindal MD
Senior Resident
Department of Pathology
All India Institute of Medical Sciences (AIIMS)
Bathinda, Punjab, India

Alka Bhatia MD
Professor
Department of Experimental Medicine and Biotechnology
Postgraduate Institute of Medical Education and Research (PGIMER)
Chandigarh, India

Arghya Bandyopadhyay MD(Pathology)
Fellowship in Genetic Diagnostics(AIIMS, New Delhi)
Associate Professor
Department of Pathology
NRS Medical College
Kolkata, West Bengal, India

Debajyoti Chatterjee MD
Assistant Professor
Department of Histopathology
Postgraduate Institute of Medical Education and Research (PGIMER)
Chandigarh, India

Debasis Gochhait MD
Additional Professor
Department of Pathology
Jawaharlal Institute of Postgraduate Medical Education and Research (JIPMER)
Puducherry, India

Dipanwita Biswas MD DNB
Senior Resident
Department of Histopathology
Postgraduate Institute of Medical Education and Research (PGIMER)
Chandigarh, India

Divya Midha MD
Professor
TATA Medical Center
Kolkata, West Bengal, India

Gargi Kapatia MD DNB PDCC
Assistant Professor
Department of Pathology
All India Institute of Medical Sciences (AIIMS)
Bathinda, Punjab, India

Laxmi Kumari PhD
Student
Department of Experimental Medicine and Biotechnology
Postgraduate Institute of Medical Education and Research (PGIMER)
Chandigarh, India

Nalini Gupta MD DNB
Professor
Department of Cytology and Gynecologic Pathology
Postgraduate Institute of Medical Education and Research (PGIMER)
Chandigarh, India

Niraj Kumari MD DNB
Professor and Head
Department of Pathology
All India Institute of Medical Sciences (AIIMS)
Raebareli, Uttar Pradesh, India

Nishtha Ahuja MD
Consultant of Pathology
Homi Bhabha Cancer Hospital and Research Centre
Mullanpur, Punjab, India

Nivetha Ambalavanan DM
Student
Department of Histopathology
Postgraduate Institute of Medical Education and Research (PGIMER)
Chandigarh, India

Nupur Pradhan MBBS MD(Pathology) DNB(Pathology)
Senior Resident
Department of Pathology
Postgraduate Institute of Medical Education and Research (PGIMER)
Chandigarh, India

Parikshaa Gupta MD DNB MIAC
Associate Professor
Department of Cytology and Gynecologic Pathology
Postgraduate Institute of Medical Education and Research (PGIMER)
Chandigarh, India

Pranab Dey MBBS MD MIAC FRCPath
Currently: Director of Pathology and Transfusion Medicine
National Institute of Medical Science (NIMS)
Jaipur, Rajasthan, India
Ex-Professor
Department of Cytology and Gynecologic Pathology
Postgraduate Institute of Medical Education and Research
Chandigarh, India

Prasenjit Das MD
Professors of Pathology
All India Institute of Medical Sciences (AIIMS)
New Delhi, India

Praveen Sharma MBBS MD
Assistant Professor
Department of Hematology
Postgraduate Institute of Medical Education and Research (PGIMER)
Chandigarh, India

Sananda Kumar MBBS MD
Senior Resident
Department of Pathology
Postgraduate Institute of Medical Education and Research (PGIMER)
Chandigarh, India

Sankalp Sancheti MD
Professor of Pathology
Homi Bhabha Cancer Hospital and Research Centre
Mullanpur, Punjab, India

Shruti Gupta MD
Associate Professor
Department of Pathology
All India Institute of Medical Sciences (AIIMS)
Raebareli, Uttar Pradesh, India

Soundarya Ravi MD
Senior Resident
Department of Pathology
Jawaharlal Institute of Postgraduate Medical Education and Research (JIPMER)
Puducherry, India

Suvendu Purkait MD PhD
Additional Professor
Department of Pathology and Lab Medicine
All India Institute of Medical Sciences (AIIMS)
Bhubaneswar, Odisha, India

Suvradeep Mitra MD DM(Histopathology)
Assistant Professor
Department of Histopathology
Postgraduate Institute of Medical Education and Research (PGIMER)
Chandigarh, India

Yashwant Kumar MD
Professor
Department of Immunopathology
Postgraduate Institute of Medical Education and Research (PGIMER)
Chandigarh, India

Preface

Pathology is a rapidly advancing area and with the application of various recent technologies, the subject has gained high development momentum. Molecular techniques and computerization have brought significant changes in pathology. The book *"Recent Advances in Pathology-1"* describes the different molecular techniques, computerization, and recent developments in histopathology of the various lesions. The chapters of this book are written by eminent pathologists from the various prestigious institutes of India. The chapters are short, simple, and updated. Each chapter is equipped with multiple tables and figures to illustrate the text. I firmly believe that this book will help the postgraduate students and also the practicing pathologists to understand the frontiers of pathology.

Pranab Dey

Acknowledgments

I am thankful to Mr Jitendar P Vij and Ms Chetna Malhotra of Jaypee Brothers Medical Publishers, who offered me the opportunity to edit this book.

The chapters of this book are contributed by various eminent pathologists. They have enriched the book with their vast knowledge and experiences. I am thankful to them. I wish to express my heartiest thanks to my wife Rini and my daughter Madhumanti for their continuous cooperation and patience toward me.

Last, I wish to express my gratitude to Almighty God; without His support, nothing is possible.

Pranab Dey

Contents

1

CHAPTER

Updates in Liver Pathology

Suvradeep Mitra

INTRODUCTION

Liver pathology is a growing branch and numerous advances and clarifications in the concept and the criteria have been made in the last decade. This branch of histopathology surpasses the realm of histomorphology alone and encompasses various immunohistochemistry, molecular methods, in silico analysis, and recently artificial intelligence. The advent of different molecular techniques, machine learning, and artificial intelligence caused a paradigm shift from invasive biopsy procedures to relatively noninvasive/minimally invasive techniques. However, histopathological evaluation remains the gold standard. We aim to briefly mention and discuss the salient changes and advances in the current concepts and practices in various branches of liver pathology though a detailed discussion on each topic is beyond the ambit of this chapter. These branches of liver pathology include both non-neoplastic hepatocellular changes as well as hepatic neoplasms. We have retained the older terminology in the subheading for the benefit of the readers especially in situations where a change in the nomenclature is recommended/considered.

UPDATES IN NONALCOHOLIC FATTY LIVER DISEASE

Historically alcoholism is considered to be the major reason behind the accumulation of neutral fat within the hepatocytes. Accumulation of neutral fat within the hepatocytes in causes other than alcoholism is known under the rubric of nonalcoholic fatty liver disease (NAFLD). The classic form of NAFLD is associated with metabolic syndrome and affects nearly a quarter of the population.[1,2] The hepatic fat is not innocuous, as historically perceived and can lead to both reversible and irreversible hepatocellular damage portending to cirrhosis/advanced-stage chronic liver disease (aCLD). Though there are various causes of fatty liver disease other than alcoholism, metabolic syndrome/metabolic dysfunction-associated fatty liver disease needs to be distinguished from all other causes due to its prevalence among the general population including pediatric age groups. Thus, an attempt has been made to change the nomenclature of NAFLD, an umbrella term encompassing metabolic syndrome, drug/toxin/chemotherapy-associated fatty liver, and miscellaneous other causes. Thus, a consensus panel proposed the terminology of metabolic-associated fatty liver disease (MAFLD) considering metabolic dysfunction to be the critical pivot of this disease rather than an exclusionary terminology of NAFLD.[1,2] Although the absence of significant alcohol intake is considered to be a crucial criterion for the diagnosis of a "pure" MAFLD, the disease is caused by metabolic dysfunction and can coexist with alcoholic liver disease. MAFLD recognizes the primary driving force/association of the disease rather than merely excluding alcoholism as the cause. This consensus statement recognizes the heterogeneity of MAFLD, its association with other CLDs including alcoholism, and recognizes this disease to be a modern epidemic.

A more recent Delphi consensus had further modified the MAFLD terminology to metabolic dysfunction-associated steatotic liver disease (MASLD) as "fatty" was considered to be stigmatizing for individual patients.[3] The reasons for the change in the nomenclature are depicted in **Table 1**.

The diagnostic criteria of MASLD have also been modified **(Table 2)**.

The MAFLD criteria recognize any patient with fatty liver who is obese, has type 2 diabetes mellitus, or has any two of the seven metabolic risk factors. These risk factors include central obesity, hypertension, prediabetes, and four laboratory features including hypertriglyceridemia, low high-density lipoprotein (HDL), elevated high-sensitivity C-reactive protein (hs-CRP), and insulin resistance assessed by homeostatic model assessment for insulin resistance (HOMA-IR).[4,5] The MAFLD criteria in contrast to the latest MASLD criteria had a few drawbacks including (1) failure to identify the cases of lean NAFLD and (2) difficult-to-follow parameters like hs-CRP or HOMA-IR.[4,5] The latest Delphi consensus also redefined and renamed other causes of steatotic liver diseases (SLD) **(Flowchart 1)**.

Broadly, there are five major causes of SLD. This includes alcohol-associated/alcohol-related liver disease (ALD), MASLD, a combination of both where an individual with MASLD has increased alcohol intake (MetALD), specific-etiology SLD, and cryptogenic SLD. Insignificant alcohol intake to diagnose "pure" MASLD requires an average daily alcohol intake of <20 g/day for females and <30 g/day for males [weekly alcohol intake < 140 g/week (females)/

TABLE 1: Reason for the change in nomenclature from nonalcoholic fatty liver disease (NAFLD) to metabolic dysfunction-associated steatotic liver disease (MASLD).[3]

Old terminology	New terminology	Reason for change
Nonalcoholic	Metabolic dysfunction-associated	• The nonalcoholic is an exclusionary term and merely states the absence of lack of association of significant alcohol intake. However, it does not highlight the salient background cause in the form of metabolic dysfunction/metabolic syndrome. • New terminology highlights the fundamental pathogenesis of the disease instead of the exclusion of significant alcohol intake
Fatty liver disease	Steatotic liver disease	"Fatty" is believed to be stigmatizing for individuals

TABLE 2: Diagnostic criteria of metabolic dysfunction-associated steatotic liver disease (MASLD).[3]

Diagnostic criteria	• Presence of hepatic steatosis proven by biopsy/imaging • Exclusion of other known causes of hepatic steatosis (alcohol, drug, toxin, and others) • Presence of at least one (out of five) cardiometabolic criteria	
	Adult cardiometabolic criteria	**Pediatric cardiometabolic criteria**
Body mass index (BMI)	BMI ≥ 25 kg/m^2 (23 kg/m^2 for Asians) or waist circumference > 94 cm (male)/80 cm (female) or ethnicity adjusted values	BMI ≥ 85th percentile for age/sex (BMI z-score ≥ +1) or waist circumference > 95th percentile or ethnicity adjusted values
Glucose	Fasting serum glucose ≥ 100 mg/dL OR 2-hour postload glucose level ≥ 140 mg/dL or HbA1c ≥ 5.7% or type 2 diabetes mellitus (without on treatment)	Fasting serum glucose ≥ 100 mg/dL or serum glucose ≥ 200 mg/dL or 2-hour postload glucose level ≥ 140 mg/dL or HbA1c ≥ 5.7% or type 2 diabetes mellitus (without on treatment)
Blood pressure	Blood pressure ≥ 130/85 mm Hg or on antihypertensive treatment	*For ≥13 years*: Blood pressure ≥ 130/85 mm Hg or on antihypertensive treatment *For <13 years*: Blood pressure ≥ 130/85 mm Hg or blood pressure ≥ 95th percentile (whichever is lower)
Plasma triglycerides	Plasma triglycerides ≥ 150 mg/dL or on lipid-lowering agent treatment	*For ≥10 years*: Plasma triglycerides ≥ 150 mg/dL or on lipid-lowering agent treatment *For <10 years*: Plasma triglycerides ≥ 100 mg/dL
Plasma HDL-cholesterol	Plasma HDL-cholesterol ≤ 40 mg/dL (male)/50 mg/dL (female) OR on lipid-lowering agent treatment	Plasma HDL cholesterol ≤ 40 mg/dL or on lipid-lowering agent treatment

Note: Red highlights are differences between the adult and pediatric cardiometabolic criteria.
(HbA1c: glycated hemoglobin; HDL: high-density lipoprotein)

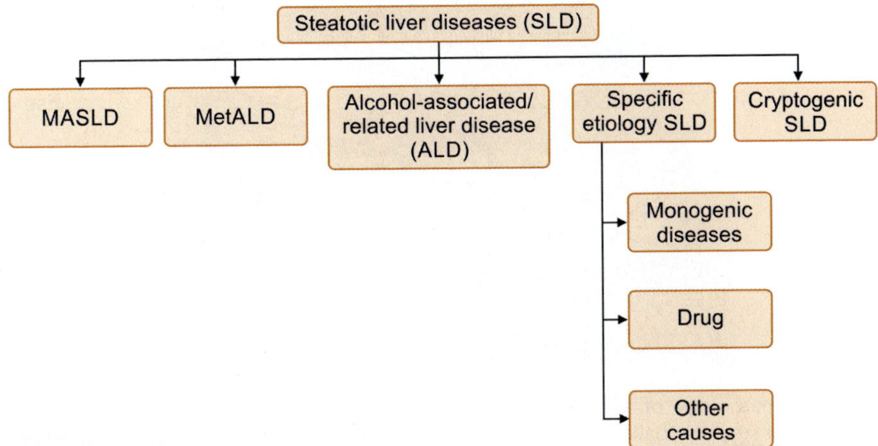

FLOWCHART 1: A schematic diagram depicting different causes of steatotic liver diseases.[3]

<210 g/week (males)]. An average daily alcohol intake of 20–50 g/day for females (140–350 g/week) and 30–60 g/day (210–420 g/week) for males along with metabolic dysfunction qualifies for MetALD, a combination of metabolic dysfunction and ALD. Different specific diseases are responsible for SLD, including many drugs causing drug-induced liver injury (DILI), monogenic diseases such as Wilson disease, liposomal acid lipase deficiency, and other inborn errors of metabolism, and miscellaneous causes such as chronic hepatic C, celiac hepatopathy, and malnutrition. Cryptogenic SLD is the preferred terminology if no specific cause of SLD is identified.[3]

The recent recommendations also highlight the role of genetic testing in the evaluation/management of MASLD. While the single nucleotide polymorphism p.I148M variant (rs738409) in the *PNPLA3* gene is one of the most well-validated drivers of hepatic steatosis, other variants involving *GCKR, TM6SF2, MBOAT7, APOE*, and *GPAM* also affect MASLD. In contrast, a few other genetic variants involving *HSD17B13* and *CIDEB* may be protective for MASLD.[6]

Histologically, NAFLD/MASLD is identified by zonal macrovesicular steatosis in >5% of the liver parenchyma. The macrovesicular steatosis in adult MASLD and a subset of pediatric MASLD affect zone 3 (centrizonal) hepatocytes while pediatric MASLD can also affect zone 1 (periportal) hepatocytes. The steatosis can be associated with lobular inflammation in NAFL/MASL. The diagnosis of steatohepatitis, a more active form of NAFL/MASL requires the unequivocal presence of ballooned hepatocytes in zone 3 (adult/occasional pediatric MASLD) or in zone 1 (subset of pediatric MASLD) with/without the presence of intrahepatocytic Mallory hyaline **(Fig. 1)**.

The identification of nonalcoholic steatohepatitis/metabolic dysfunction-associated steatohepatitis (NASH/MASH) is crucial as this form progresses to aCLD/cirrhosis/hepatocellular carcinoma (HCC). NASH CRN (NASH clinical research network) histologic scoring system/SAF (steatosis, activity, and fibrosis) scores are the reliable histologic scores to assess the activity of NASH/MASH **(Table 3)**.[7,8]

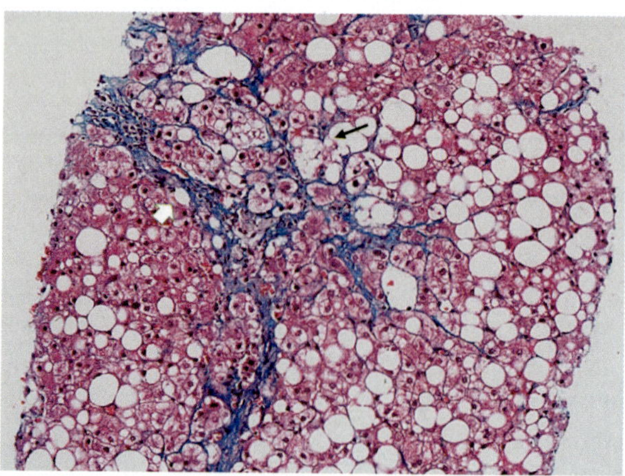

FIG. 1: Histopathology of a case of metabolic dysfunction-associated steatohepatitis with macrovesicular steatosis, ballooned hepatocyte (black arrow), and perivenular/pericellular fibrosis (white arrow) (Masson trichrome stain, 200×).

TABLE 3: A schematic diagram depicting the components of NASH CRN score and SAF score.[7,8]

NASH CRN score: NAS (NAFLD activity score) and fibrosis score			
Steatosis: • 0: <5% • 1: 5–33% • 2: 34–66% • 3: >67%	*Lobular Inflammation*: • 0: None • 1: <2 foci/20× optical field • 2: 2–4 foci/20× optical field • 3: >4 foci/20× optical filed	*Ballooning*: • 0: None • 1: Mild, few • 2: Moderate, marked, many	*Fibrosis (F)*: • 0: None • 1a: Mild (delicate) zone 3 perisinusoidal fibrosis • 1b: Moderate (dense) zone 3 perisinusoidal fibrosis • 1c: Portal/periportal fibrosis only • 2: Zone 3 perisinusoidal with portal/periportal fibrosis • 3: Bridging fibrosis • 4: Cirrhosis
SAF Score: Steatosis, Activity (lobular inflammation and ballooning) and Fibrosis			
Steatosis (S): Quantities of large or medium-sized lipid droplets, but not foamy microvesicles: • S0: <5% • S1: 5–33%, mild • S2: 34–66%, moderate • S3: >67%, marked	*Activity (A) (0-4)*: Unweighted addition of ballooning and lobular inflammation A1: mild, A2: moderate, A3,4: Severe *Ballooning*: • 0: Normal hepatocytes with cuboidal shape and pink eosinophilic cytoplasm • 1: Presence of clusters of hepatocytes with a rounded shape and pale cytoplasm usually reticulated. Size similar to that of normal hepatocytes, shape different • 2: Same as grade 2 with some enlarged hepatocytes, at least twofold that of normal cells	*Lobular Inflammation*: Focus of two or more inflammatory cells within the lobule counted at ×20 magnification: • 0: None • 1: 2 foci/×20 • 2: >2 foci/×20	*Fibrosis (F)*: • Stage 0 (F0): None • Stage 1 (F1): Zone 3 perisinusoidal (1a or 1b) or portal (1c) fibrosis • Stage 2 (F2): Perisinusoidal and periportal fibrosis without bridging • Stage 3 (F3): Bridging fibrosis • Stage 4 (F4): Cirrhosis

(CRN: clinical research network; NAFLD: Nonalcoholic fatty liver disease; NASH: nonalcoholic steatohepatitis; SAF: steatosis, activity, and fibrosis)

However, these existing staging and grading systems are not without fallacies and though simple and easy to apply in day-to-day practice, these systems do not provide accurate weightage to individual features, are subject to inter- and intraobserver variabilities, and ignore multiple important histopathological parameters.[9-11] Therefore, an expanded NAFLD activity score (NAS) including Mallory Denk bodies, portal inflammation, an alternate calculation of lobular inflammation, and ballooned hepatocytes is proposed.[11]

The fibrosis in MASLD and most other liver diseases is a reliable indicator of disease progression. It is a dynamic process and the existing fibrosis staging system falls short of commenting on the type of fibrosis (progressive or regressive) and quantitating it. Thus, many morphometry-based methods are employed to characterize the type and quantitate the amount of fibrosis in various liver diseases including MASLD. Measurement of collagen proportionate area (CPA), second harmonic generation (SHG) microscopy, two-photon excitation filter (TPEF) microscopy, and automated computational algorithm tools like qFIBS shows reliable results and even outperform hepatopathologists.[12,13] Various noninvasive radiology-based methods are also tested for accurate prediction of the disease activity and disease progression and form the basis of artificial intelligence-based predictions. These methods are operator-independent and algorithm-based and reduce the interobserver and intraobserver variability, reduce the time, and need of skilled/trained pathologists in interpreting the liver biopsies and predict the course of the disease more accurately.[12,13]

The management of MASLD depends on lifestyle changes, dietary modification, exercise, and pharmacotherapy. INASL guidelines recommend the use of vitamin E, pioglitazone, and saroglitazar in MASLD-MASH.[14] Vitamin E and pioglitazone are recommended by various international societies in biopsy-proven NASH/MASH. While vitamin E should be used in individuals without diabetes, pioglitazone can be used in both diabetics and nondiabetics. Saroglitazar is approved by the drug controller general of India for use in NAFLD/MASLD with comorbidities and NASH/MASH with F1-F3 fibrosis.[14] Various other drugs are also under various clinical trials and some of them appear to show promising pharmacotherapeutic results including farnesoid-X-receptor (FXR) agonists such as obeticholic acid and tropifexor, GLP-1 agonist such as semaglutide, and peroxisome proliferation-associated receptor (PPAR) agonist such as elafibranor to name a few.[15] These drugs along with the antioxidants, anti-inflammatory agents, and immunomodulators are expected to unravel a new horizon of effective pharmacotherapy in the near future.[15]

UPDATES IN IDIOPATHIC NONCIRRHOTIC PORTAL HYPERTENSION

Idiopathic noncirrhotic portal hypertension (INCPH) is traditionally characterized by the presence of clinical features of portal hypertension in the absence of cirrhosis of the liver or any underlying CLD that may explain the portal hypertension. The patency of portal and hepatic veins is also required for the diagnosis of INCPH. INCPH has many monikers including noncirrhotic portal fibrosis (NCPF), idiopathic portal hypertension, hepatoportal sclerosis, and benign intrahepatic portal hypertension to name a few.[16,17] Despite the knowledge and acceptance of the presence of INCPH for more than a few decades, a unified terminology, definition, and descriptions are lacking. Therefore, the clinical as well as histopathological diagnosis of INCPH remains variable and individualistic. Besides, the pathogenesis also remains poorly understood owing to the variability of the definitions.

The vascular liver disease interest group (VALDIG) proposed a novel nomenclature in 2019 to circumvent these issues. Thus, the term porto-sinusoidal vascular disease (PSVD) has been introduced by the VALDIG.[18,19] The VALDIG has recognized several limitations to the previous definition of INCPH—(1) the exclusion of all individuals without portal hypertension also excludes individuals with preportal hypertension/subclinical portal hypertension, (2) the exclusion of all cases of portal venous thrombosis (PVT) also excludes cases of INCPH diagnosed after the development of PVT, as PVT is a complication of INCPH, and (3) the definition of INCPH excludes all causes associated with the development of portal hypertension thereby refuting the possibility of coexisting INCPH with another liver disease.[18,19]

The new term "porto-sinusoidal vascular disease" has been coined to encompass the whole spectrum keeping in mind that all pathology about this entity essentially involves the portal venules and/or the sinusoids. The diagnosis of PSVD does not require portal hypertension, but a characteristic histomorphology in the absence of cirrhosis in a given clinical scenario suffices for the diagnosis. The presence of risk factors for parenchymal liver diseases does not negate a diagnosis of PSVD if the histopathology is supportive. The definition and the diagnostic criteria of PSVD are depicted in **Table 4**.

Though inclusive of multiple entities causing CLD, the definition of PSVD excludes various entities such as Budd–Chiari syndrome and other causes of hepatic venous outflow tract obstruction, Abernathy syndrome, hereditary hemorrhagic telangiectasia, history of bone marrow transplantation, cardiac failure, congenital hepatic fibrosis, sarcoidosis, etc.

The detailed discussion of the hepatic histomorphology of the specific and nonspecific features of PSVD is beyond the scope of this chapter. However, obliterative portal venopathy (OPV) is characterized by the thickening of the wall and fibrosis of the portal venous radicles with obliteration and loss of the venous radicles. The nodules of nodular regenerative hyperplasia (NRH) show hyperplastic hepatocytes with the double-cord pattern at the center of the nodule while the periphery of the nodule shows atrophic hepatocytes with reticulin stretching in the absence of any fibrous septa. Delicate fibrous septa emanating from a portal tract and blindly ending into the hepatic lobule without any connection with another portal tract or central vein denote incomplete septal fibrosis/cirrhosis **(Figs. 2A and B)**.

The proposal of PSVD has received many flaks from experts in recent times, despite its simplicity and easy applicability. The too-simplistic approach of PSVD fails to address the complexity and heterogeneity of the disease. Some

TABLE 4: Definition and criteria of porto-sinusoidal vascular disease (PSVD).[18,19]

	Clinical	Histopathological
Specific features	Gastric, esophageal, or ectopic varices	Obliterative portal venopathy
	Portal hypertensive bleeding	Nodular regenerative hyperplasia
	Imaging: Portosystemic collaterals	Incomplete septal fibrosis/cirrhosis
Nonspecific features	Ascites	Architectural changes (irregular distribution of portal tracts and central veins)
	Platelet count < 1,50,000/μL	
	Spleen size ≥ 13 cm in its largest axis	Lobular changes (nonzonal sinusoidal dilatation, megasinusoids, perisinusoidal fibrosis, and central vein abnormalities)
		Portal tract changes (multiplication, arterial dilatation, arterialization of portal veins, periportal shunting vessels, herniated portal vein, aberrant vessels, and portal tract remnant)
Diagnosis of PSVD (requires a liver biopsy ≥ 20 mm without cirrhosis)	• One specific clinical sign • One nonspecific clinical sign	• One specific histopathological feature • One nonspecific histopathological feature

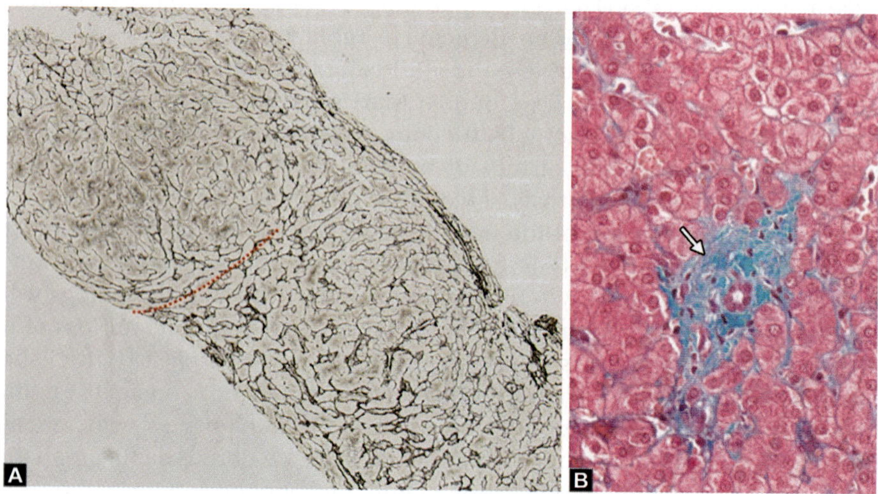

FIGS. 2A AND B: Histopathology highlighting specific histopathological signs of PSVD: (A) Nodules of nodular regenerative hyperplasia (Reticulin stain, 100×) (the margin of a nodule marked with red dotted line); (B) Obliterated portal vein (white arrow) in a portal tract (Masson trichrome stain, 400×).

cases diagnosed as PSVD may be a CLD evolving into a precirrhotic/cirrhotic disease. The specific histopathological signs of PSVD can be associated with "aging", trauma, cholecystectomy, hemochromatosis, dialysis, or various other causes unrelated to INCPH and thus lack in their specificity. A subset of individuals diagnosed based on only histopathological signs of PSVD without any clinical signs of PSVD fail to develop portal hypertension on an extended follow-up period. Thus, the concept of preportal hypertensive phase of PSVD does not appear true for all cases.[18,19] In short, the new moniker "PSVD" appears lucrative in terms of simplicity and increases the sensitivity of diagnosis. However, it lacks specificity, needs to address multiple questions, and requires revision for uniform worldwide acceptance.

UPDATES IN AUTOIMMUNE HEPATITIS

Autoimmune hepatitis (AIH) is a relatively uncommon cause of CLD although it is increasingly recognized globally. A hepatitic form of autoimmune liver disease, AIH is characterized by an immune/inflammatory injury to the hepatocytes dominantly attributed to T cell-mediated injury along with autoantibody production.[20,21] The diagnosis of AIH depends on the clinical features, biochemical parameters (increase in serum transaminases), serology (autoantibody positivity and hypergammaglobulinemia), histopathology, and often response to immunosuppression. However, seronegativity in AIH is seen in early acute, severe, and fulminant forms (10–40% of cases).[22,23] Normal serum gamma globulin can be seen in 25–47% of cases.[22,23] Thus, histopathological evaluation of AIH often becomes crucial in the diagnosis of AIH.

The histopathological features of AIH are portal/periportal-based inflammation/fibroinflammation including interface hepatitis, the inflammatory milieu comprising lymphocytes, and plasma cells. Besides, hepatocellular rosettes and emperipolesis are considered important histopathological features. These traditional histopathological features essentially depict chronic AIH although the portal-based inflammation can be less reliable in acute AIH which may show lobulocentric inflammation. Therefore, consensus criteria using a modified Delphi panel approach were proposed for a uniform histological diagnosis of both acute and chronic AIH.[24] In brief, the consensus recommends histopathology to be the standard of AIH diagnosis.

A portal hepatitis is considered "likely AIH" when portal lymphoplasmacytic infiltrate is associated with (1) more than mild interface activity and/or (2) more than mild lobular inflammation in the absence of histological features of another liver disease. Any lobular hepatitis with/without centrilobular necroinflammation is considered "likely AIH" when more than mild lobular hepatitis (with/without centrilobular necroinflammation) is associated with either (1) portal-based fibrosis, or (2) lymphoplasmacytic infiltrate, or (3) interface hepatitis in the absence of histological features of another liver disease **(Fig. 3)**.[24]

Diagnostic criteria for possible AIH and unlikely AIH had also been proposed **(Table 5)**.[24]

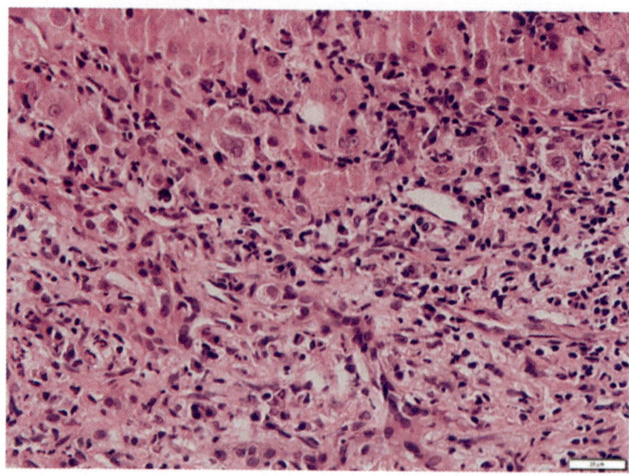

FIG. 3: Histopathology of a case of autoimmune hepatitis depicting moderate portal lymphoplasmacytic inflammation, marked interface activity, and foci of lobular inflammation (Hematoxylin and eosin, 400×) (scale bar attached).

TABLE 5: Diagnostic histopathological criteria for autoimmune hepatitis (AIH).[24]

	Portal hepatitis	**Lobular hepatitis**
Likely AIH	Portal lymphoplasmacytic infiltrate + one/both of the following: • More than mild interface hepatitis • More than mild lobular inflammation Absence of features of other liver disease	More than mild lobular inflammation ± centrilobular necroinflammation + at least one of the following: • Lymphoplasmacytic infiltrate • Interface hepatitis • Portal-based fibrosis Absence of features of other liver disease
Possible AIH	*Portal lymphoplasmacytic infiltrate*: • Without either of the "likely" features • Absence of features of other liver disease OR • With one/both of the "likely" features • Presence of features of other liver disease	More than mild lobular inflammation ± centrilobular necroinflammation • Without either of the "likely" features • Absence of features of other liver disease OR • With any of the "likely" features • Presence of features of other liver disease
Unlikely AIH	Portal hepatitis • Without either of the "likely" features • Presence of features of other liver disease	Any lobular hepatitis • Without either of the "likely" features • Presence of features of other liver disease

This consensus also disregards emperipolesis or hepatocellular rosettes to be the specific features of AIH.[24] Thus, these features are considered histopathological features of AIH but not pathognomonic of AIH.

The conceptual acceptance and recognition of acute AIH led to the clinical terminologies in relation to AIH causing acute liver failure (ALF).[22,25] Thus, AIH presenting within ≤26 weeks without any evidence of preexisting liver disease is clinically divided into (1) acute icteric AIH (icteric, no coagulopathy, and no encephalopathy), (2) acute severe AIH (AS-AIH) [icteric and coagulopathy (INR ≥ 1.5), no encephalopathy], and (3) AS-AIH with ALF [icteric, coagulopathy (INR ≥ 1.5), and encephalopathy].[22]

UPDATES IN INFECTIOUS HEPATITIS (COVID-19 AND OTHER UNCOMMON INFECTIOUS FORMS)

Various forms of hepatotropic and nonhepatotropic organisms especially viruses affect the hepatic parenchyma manifesting as minor elevations in the serum transaminases to fatal and fulminant hepatic failure. The hepatotropic viruses including hepatitis A, hepatitis E, hepatitis B, hepatitis C, and hepatitis D are well known to cause hepatocellular damage. However, there is growing evidence of hepatic injury caused by the nonhepatotropic viruses. The non-hepatotropic viruses often inflict injury in the immunocompromised individuals although immunocompetent individuals can also be affected.

Severe acute respiratory syndrome-related coronavirus 2 (SARS-CoV-2) has emerged as a viral agent affecting multiple systems including the liver during COVID-19 (Coronavirus disease 2019) pandemic. Dominantly, it affects the lungs causing diffuse alveolar damage although hepatic manifestations are not uncommon.

The hepatic manifestations of COVID-19 occur through both direct and indirect pathways. Direct hepatotoxicity occurs following the direct entry of the SARS-CoV-2 virus within the cholangiocyte and hepatocyte through the angiotensin-converting enzyme 2 (ACE2) and transmembrane serine protease 2 (TMPRSS2) receptors, the cholangiocytes being the primary cells of injury.[26] The indirect modes of hepatic injury occur due to immune overactivation and hypercytokinemia, systemic inflammatory drive, hypoxic ischemic hepatitis with/without reperfusion injury especially in the setting of respiratory failure, endothelial damage due to endothelial dysfunction, DILI, and also vaccine-induced liver injury.[26-28] Direct or indirect viral-mediated injury and vaccine-induced liver injury are often overwhelmingly diagnosed while the possibility of DILI should not be overlooked.[29]

The most common form of derangement in the liver function test occurs in the form of hypoalbuminemia, elevated levels of gamma-glutamyl transferase (GGT), aspartate transaminase (AST), and alanine transaminase (ALT), and hyperbilirubinemia in nearly 61%, 28%, 23%, 23%, and 11% of the individuals.[27] This data was obtained from the meta-analysis of 128 studies. The most common histopathological change in COVID-19 infection is macrovesicular steatosis (75%) followed by mild portal and lobular inflammation (50% each), and variable porto-sinusoidal vascular pathology including dilatation of the portal venous radicles, portal venous and sinusoidal thrombi, focal to multifocal phlebosclerosis, and other minor changes. Portal fibrosis and incomplete fibrous septa, cholestasis, and hepatocellular swelling are also observed **(Fig. 4)**.[26,30-32]

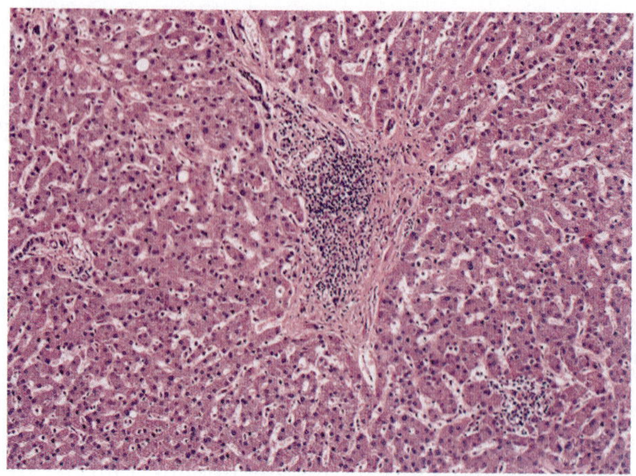

FIG. 4: Histopathology of a case of COVID-19 hepatitis depicting mild portal and periportal fibrosis along with mild lymphocytic porto-lobular inflammation (hematoxylin and eosin, 200×).

Electron microscopy and viral immunostains usually fail to demonstrate the viral particles in the liver though an expansion of the endoplasmic reticulum and edematous mitochondria with disruption of the cristae can be documented by transmission electron microscopy.[31]

Several other uncommon nonhepatotropic viruses have gained recognition for causing hepatic injury in recent times. An epidemic of adenoviral hepatitis has occurred among the pediatric population in 2021–2022 causing significant morbidity and mortality.[33] While the reason for the severity of adenoviral hepatitis, usually a mild disease, is debatable, the histopathology uniformly mimics AIH and is characterized by marked portal mixed inflammatory infiltrate, portal plasmacytosis with/without plasma cell clustering, more than mild interface hepatitis, and milder lobular inflammation.[33] The liver tissue usually does not show any viral inclusion although serological evidence of adenoviral infection remains strong.[33]

Epstein–Barr virus (EBV), a nonhepatotropic virus, causes infectious mononucleosis characterized by fever, diarrhea, lymphadenopathy, and hepatosplenomegaly. Infectious mononucleosis is usually associated with a mild form of hepatitis. EBV-associated ALF comprises 0.21% of all ALF cases according to the US ALF study group.[34] Usually, a disease of immunocompromised individuals, a fatal form of infectious mononucleosis-associated acute hepatitis can affect the immunocompetent individuals.[35] The disease is usually caused by hypercytokinemia where the innocent hepatocytes are killed by the immune insult inflicted by the cytotoxic-T-lymphocytes against the viral-infected B cells as collateral damage. The characteristic histomorphology of EBV-hepatitis includes dense portal-based mixed inflammation comprising of T-lymphocytes and plasma cells along with eosinophils, portal-based lymphoid aggregate/periductal lymphoid cuffing, an intrasinusoidal linear array of lymphocytes in a string-of-beads appearance, and abundant hemophagocytosis, especially erythrophagocytic figures. Endotheliitis, bile duct damage, and epithelioid/fibrin-ring granuloma can also be seen **(Figs. 5A to C)**.[35,36]

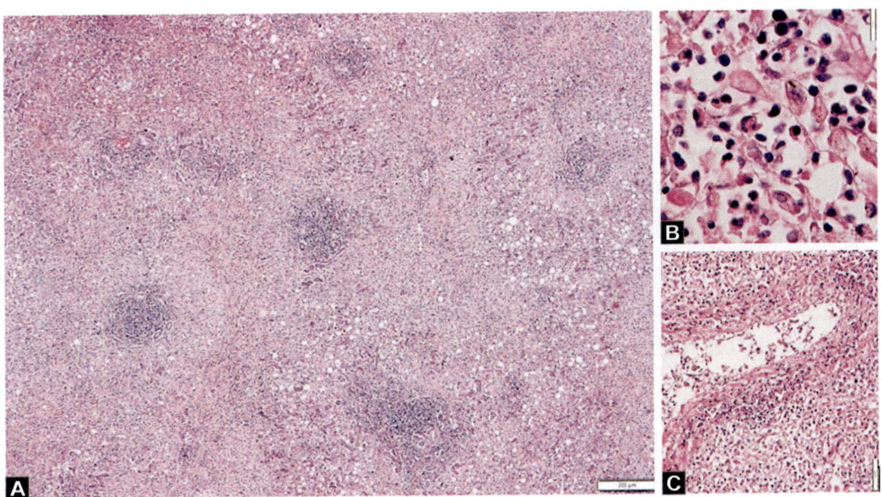

FIGS. 5A TO C: Histopathology of a case of EBV-associated hepatitis depicting panacinar multiacinar confluent hepatocellular necrosis with focal periportal hepatocyte preservation and dense portal-based lymphocytic infiltrate (A), multiple hemophagocytic figures (B), and central vein endotheliitis (C) (hematoxylin and eosin) (scale bars attached).

Epstein–Barr virus-DNA detection by serology and occasional EBV-encoded-RNA-in situ hybridization (EBER-ISH) positive B-lymphocytes in the tissue (liver) confirms the diagnosis of EBV-associated acute hepatitis in such cases.

Among the hepatotropic viruses, the morphological spectrum of hepatitis E has recently been reexplored. Although hepatitis E usually causes acute hepatitis with a high mortality rate among pregnant individuals, a chronic variant is also discovered owing to the rampant use of immunosuppressants and an increased rate of solid organ transplants.[37] The histomorphology of chronic hepatitis E is similar to other chronic viral hepatitis though the occurrence of florid nondestructive cholangitis along with neutrophilic infiltration and immunohistochemical demonstration of hepatitis E open-reading frame (ORF) distinguishes this entity from other chronic viral hepatitis.[38] The histomorphological feature of hepatitis E also depends on the patient's immune status and the preexisting liver disease. While a subset of individuals shows only the features of preexisting liver disease, the immunocompetent individuals display florid hepatitis, and the immunocompromised individuals show a smoldering hepatitis.[39]

Different other atypical forms of liver injury associated with many other organisms have various clinical, histopathological, immunohistochemical, and serological features which are beyond the scope of this chapter.

UPDATES IN DRUG-INDUCED LIVER INJURY

Drug-induced liver injury is not a new disease rather variable drugs causing hepatic injury are well known. It is partly because the majority of the drugs administered through oral routes reach the liver through enterohepatic circulation and a substantial proportion of these drugs are partly or completely metabolized and/or detoxified in the liver. Different drugs administered through nonoral routes also reach the liver to a variable extent and can cause hepatic injury.

Traditionally, antitubercular drugs and paracetamol are the two drugs that cause DILI. These drugs along with many other antibiotics continue to cause DILI in the modern-day practice. In addition, multiple newer drugs especially immune checkpoint inhibitors (ICIs), antifibrotic agents, chemotherapeutic agents, and monoclonal antibodies have emerged as the known offenders. Besides, variable dietary habits including consumption of complementary and alternative medicines (CAM), green tea, herbs, and dietary supplements (HDS) are important offenders to cause DILI/herb-induced liver injury (HILI). Numerous patterns of hepatic injury associated with different drugs are beyond the ambit of this chapter hence we will limit our discussion to the patterns of injury associated with ICIs and antifibrotic agents. In short, the most common patterns identified by drug-induced liver injury network (DILIN) are cholestatic hepatitis (29%) followed by acute (21%) and chronic hepatitis (14%), and acute (9%) and chronic cholestasis (10%).[40] Other patterns include steatotic/steatohepatitic injury, microvesicular steatosis, vascular injury, granulomatous reaction, etc. **(Table 6)**. DILI caused by multiple agents has also become more prevalent in the modern era (nearly 30% in DILIN data).[40]

Immune checkpoint inhibitors acting against cytotoxic-T-lymphocyte-associated antigen 4 (CTLA-4), programmed cell death-1 (PD-1), and programmed

TABLE 6: Various patterns of drug-induced liver injury (DILI).[40]

Patterns of injury	Possible incriminating drugs
Acute hepatitis	Ciprofloxacin, isoniazid
Chronic hepatitis	Isoniazid, nitrofurantoin, minocycline
Acute cholestasis	Anabolic steroids
Chronic cholestasis	Amoxicillin-clavulanate
Cholestatic hepatitis	Duloxetine
Granulomatous changes	Atenolol
Macrovesicular steatosis	Steroid
Microvesicular steatosis	Erythromycin, valproate
Steatohepatitis	Methotrexate, amiodarone
Coagulative/confluent hepatic necrosis	Paracetamol, isoniazid
Massive/submassive necrosis	Paracetamol
Vascular injury	Oral contraceptives, arsenic, chemotherapeutics
Hepatocellular alteration	Phenytoin, cyanamide
Pigment deposition	Gold, thorotrast
Nodular regenerative hyperplasia	Azathioprine
Minimal nonspecific changes	Miscellaneous drugs
Absolutely normal	Miscellaneous drugs
Mixed/otherwise unclassifiable injury	Miscellaneous drugs, multiple drugs
Neoplastic	Anabolic steroids, thorotrast

cell death ligand-1 (PD-L1) are increasingly utilized in various malignancies. These agents cause various immune-mediated injuries known as immune-related adverse events (iRAEs). The liver is also a target organ in iRAE and can show panlobular hepatitis, isolated centrizonal necrosis, granulomatous hepatitis, sclerosing cholangitis, and miscellaneous forms of injury (NRH, steatosis, and lymphocytic cholangitis) in decreasing order of frequency. A CD8+ CD3+ cytotoxic-T-cell mediated lymphocyte phenotype is usual.[41-43]

Antifibrotic agents such as pirfenidone and nintedanib are used for the treatment of idiopathic pulmonary fibrosis (IPF) and they are also evaluated to prevent/reverse liver fibrosis. They are usually safe drugs although various instances of DILI are reported. Both nintedanib and pirfenidone usually cause a centrizonal necrosis pattern along with mild portal-based inflammation comprising lymphocytes and occasional eosinophils.[29,44]

UPDATES IN GENETIC FORMS OF NEONATAL/INFANTILE/ PEDIATRIC CHOLESTATIC LIVER DISEASES

Pediatric cholestatic disorders comprise a vast array of cholestatic illnesses with variable disease-defining genetic alterations, histomorphology, and clinical presentations. The spectrum of pediatric cholestatic liver disease is expanding due to the advent of advanced molecular genetic testing. The most common cause of neonatal/infantile cholestasis is biliary atresia (BA), a fibroinflammatory disease of the extrahepatic as well as intrahepatic biliary tree that if left uncorrected leads to progressive liver fibrosis and failure. BA has typical clinical features in the form of high-GGT cholestasis from the beginning of life, the passage of pale stools, and abortive/small gallbladder. The hepatic histomorphology shows an obstructive cholangiopathy pattern in the form of variable degrees of portal expansion due to fibrosis and edema, ductal proliferation, ductular cholestasis, occasional ductal plate malformation, and lobular cholestasis.[45,46] An intraoperative cholangiogram highlighting an absence of the passage of the dye into the proximal part of the biliary tree is usually diagnostic of the disease. The pathogenesis of BA remains unexplored to date and it is considered to be the terminal manifestation of variable perinatal insults to the cholangiocytes and/or biliary tree. The proposed etiological factors include viral infection, genetic predisposition, ciliopathy, etc.[47] However, a few uncommon genetic cholangiopathies can give rise to the obstructive cholangiopathy pattern in the absence of BA (patent biliary tree). These diseases include isolated neonatal sclerosing cholangitis, neonatal ichthyosis-sclerosing cholangitis syndrome (*CLDN1* mutation and *DCDC2* mutation), Kabuki syndrome, and *KIF12*-mutated cholestasis syndrome to name a few.[48-51]

The most salient advances in recent years occurred in the classification of progressive familial intrahepatic cholestasis (PFIC), a conglomerate of genetic diseases with the common feature of intrahepatic cholestasis and progressive liver disease. Three subtypes of PFIC are the most prevalent namely (1) PFIC 1 (caused by the mutation of *ATP8B1* gene encoding FIC1 protein), (2) PFIC 2 (caused by the mutation of *ABCB11* gene encoding BSEP protein), and (3) PFIC 3

TABLE 7: Different subtypes of progressive familial intrahepatic cholestasis (PFIC) according to the mutations (OMIM library).

PFIC subtype	Mutation	Chromosomal location
PFIC 1	*ATPB81*	*18q21.31*
PFIC 2	*ABCB11*	*2q31.1*
PFIC 3	*ABCB4*	*7q21.12*
PFIC 4	*TJP2*	*9q21.11*
PFIC 5	*NR1H4*	*12q23.1*
PFIC 6	*SLC51A*	*3q29*
PFIC 7	*USP53*	*4q26*
PFIC 8	*KIF12*	*9q32*
PFIC 9	*ZFYVE19*	*15q15.1*
PFIC 10	*MYO5B*	*18q21.1*
PFIC 11	*SEMA7A*	*15q24.1*
PFIC 12	*VPS33B*	*15q26.1*

(caused by the mutation of *ABCB4* gene encoding MDR3 protein).[52,53] These subtypes show different clinical features, biochemical parameters, prognosis, histomorphology, immunohistochemistry, and molecular alterations although considerable overlapping features exist.

The newer PFIC subtypes include PFIC 4 (caused by the mutation of the *TJP2* gene encoding zonula occludens-2 protein) and PFIC 5 (caused by the mutation of the *NR1H4* gene encoding FXR protein).[54,55] The Online Mendelian Inheritance in Man (OMIM) library has assigned numbers to each mutation discovered thereby dividing PFIC into 12 varieties from PFIC 1 to PFIC 12 **(Table 7)**. The clinical and histological features of PFIC 1–PFIC 5 are depicted in **Table 8**.

UPDATES IN TRANSPLANT LIVER PATHOLOGY

Liver transplant has emerged as a lifesaving modality in patients with aCLD/cirrhosis and a subset of HCC (stage T2).[56] The global frequency of liver transplants sees a 20% increase from 2015 to 2021 with an increasing rate of demand.[53] Nevertheless, a transplant is not the end of the plight and is the beginning of a complex theranostic journey. Therefore, the histopathologists play a pivotal role in the diagnosis and decision-making of the transplanted liver.

Two major changes have occurred in the role of transplant pathologists and liver pathologists in the past few years. These changes include (1) the assessment of large droplet fat (LDF) in the donor liver and (2) the concept of antibody-mediated rejection (AMR) in the liver.

The assessment of macrovesicular steatosis of the donor liver by frozen section is an established pretransplant protocol. This is performed as severe

TABLE 8: Comparison of clinical and pathological feature of progressive familial intrahepatic (PFIC) cholestasis subtypes (1-5).[54]

	PFIC 1	PFIC 2	PFIC 3	PFIC 4	PFIC 5
Mutated protein/gene/ chromosome	FIC1/*ATP8B1/18q*	BSEP/*ABCB11/2q*	MDR3/*ABCB4/7q*	ZO-2/*TJP2/9q*	FXR/*NR1H4/12q*
Clinical features	Cholestasis, pruritus, deficiency of fat-soluble vitamin	Cholestasis, pruritus, deficiency of fat-soluble vitamin	Cholestasis, pruritus, deficiency of fat-soluble vitamin	Cholestasis, pruritus, hepatomegaly, deficiency of fat-soluble vitamin	Rapidly progressive cholestasis, pruritus, hepatomegaly, deficiency of fat-soluble vitamin
Extrahepatic manifestations	Sensorineural deafness, pancreatitis, cholecystitis, delayed sexual development	–	–	Deafness, respiratory symptoms, neurological features	–
Serum GGT	Low-normal	Low-normal	Elevated	Normal/mild elevation	Normal
Histopathology	Bland cholestasis, small hepatocytes, nil—moderate portal fibrosis	Giant cell transformation, hepatocellular necrosis cirrhosis	Ductular reaction, chronic cholestasis, variable fibrosis	Giant cell transformation, hepatocellular necrosis, and cirrhosis	Diffuse giant cell transformation and cirrhosis
BSEP/MDR3 immunohistochemistry	Retained/retained	Loss/retained	Retained/loss	Retained/retained	Loss/retained
Specific immunohistochemistry	Loss of canalicular FIC1 expression	Loss of canalicular BSEP expression	Loss of canalicular MDR3 expression	Loss of canalicular claudin-1/TJP2 expression	Loss of nuclear FXR expression
Progression	Mild-moderate	Rapid	Mild-moderate	Rapid	Very rapid
Complications	Post-transplant marked graft steatosis, and diarrhea	Hepatocellular carcinoma	Gall stone disease, mild increase in risk of hepatocellular carcinoma	Hepatocellular carcinoma	Post-transplant graft steatosis
Treatment	Medical management and partial external biliary diversion, liver transplant in late stage	Liver transplant	Medical management, liver transplant	Medical management, some role of biliary diversion, liver transplant	Liver transplant

(BSEP: bile salt export pump; GGT: gamma-glutamyl transferase; MDR3: multidrug-resistance protein 3)

macrovesicular steatosis of the donor liver can lead to early allograft dysfunction, primary nonfunction, and reperfusion syndrome making the donor liver not suitable for the transplant.[57] The pathologists aid in the crucial decision-making by examining the donor liver. However, there was no consensus criteria or any algorithmic approach regarding steatosis to maintain a uniformity of reporting. The 15th Banff Conference on Allograft Pathology in September 2019 defined the LDF, the risk factor of graft dysfunction as a single fat droplet that enlarges the hepatocyte to make it larger than the adjacent asteatotic hepatocyte. The consensus also defined the algorithmic approach of estimating LDF as the multiplication percentage between the low-magnification approximate estimate of the surface area involved by the fat and the high-magnification estimation of LDF within the fatty area.[57] This consensus aids in the uniformity in the global reporting of the pretransplant donor liver specimens though a safety cut-off of steatosis is not defined which remains institution-specific.

The liver is an immune-privileged organ and rarely suffers from AMR. The true incidence of AMR is estimated to be 1% of all liver transplants compared to renal transplants (20–50% of all renal transplants).[58] Besides, the coexistence/presence of recurrent viral hepatitis especially hepatitis C, AIH, and T cell-mediated rejection make the diagnosis of AMR challenging. However, there is a recent shift in focus to diagnose cases of subclinical AMR to prevent long-term graft dysfunction/loss. These issues were addressed in the 2016 Banff working group meeting on allograft pathology therefore setting a guideline for the diagnosis of acute and chronic AMR **(Table 9)**.[58,59] Though the classical cases require histopathological, immunohistochemical (C4d positivity), and serological [donor-specific antibody (DSA) positivity] confirmation with the exclusion of other related causes, the majority of the cases show slight deviation from the criteria. Besides, the treatment protocol is not yet well-defined and robust follow-up data on subclinical AMR is lacking.

UPDATES IN THE NEOPLASTIC DISEASES OF THE LIVER

The classification of the hepatic neoplasms, a vast array of benign, and malignant primary tumors of the liver has undergone multiple refinements. The hepatocellular neoplasms include intrahepatic space-occupying lesions with reactive/neoplastic nature and encompass epithelial tumors of hepatocellular, cholangiocellular, neuroendocrine, or combined hepatocellular-cholangiocellular origin, mesenchymal tumors, germ cell tumors, hematolymphoid tumors, metastatic tumors, tumors of miscellaneous origin/differentiation, and other tumor-like lesions. While there is an increase in the recognition and diagnosis of various uncommon tumors and/or their variants, the main refinements occurred in the form of molecular identities of the hepatocellular neoplasms.[60-64] Besides, intrahepatic cholangiocarcinoma (iCCA) is divided into small-duct and large-duct types due to their clinical, histopathological, molecular, and etiopathological variabilities in the WHO 5th Edition.[65]

Focal nodular hyperplasia (FNH) is not a true neoplasm and rather considered a hyperplastic response of the hepatocytes in response to a liver-limited localized alteration in the vascular flow. Thus, it is a benign reactive

TABLE 9: Diagnostic criteria of acute and chronic antibody-mediated rejection (AMR) in liver transplant.[58,59]

	Definition	Description
Acute AMR	Histopathology	• Endothelial cell hypertrophy in the portal microvasculature • Microvascular injury involving central veins • Microvasculitis/capillaritis with monocytes, eosinophils (±neutrophils) • Portal stromal edema, ductular reaction, cholestasis • RBC extravasation, fibrin deposition in the subsinusoidal region
	Diffuse C4d positivity (by immunohistochemistry)	• >50% positivity of C4d in the portal vasculature in ABO-compatible grafts • Positivity in the portal stroma in the ABO-incompatible grafts
	Elevated donor-specific antibody (DSA)	
	Exclusion of other liver diseases/ complications causative of similar injury patterns	Includes TCMR, HCV infection
Chronic AMR	Compatible histopathology	• Dense keloid-like portal fibrosis • Obliterative portal venopathy • Periductal fibrosis and ductopenia • Mild non-specific porto-lobular inflammation and mild interface hepatitis
	Focal C4d positivity (by immunohistochemistry)	>10% portal tracts
	Positive DSA within 3 months of biopsy	
	Exclusion of other liver diseases/ complications causative of similar injury-patterns	

(HCV: hepatitis C virus; RBC: red blood cell; TCMR: T-cell mediated rejection)

condition that poses as a hepatocellular neoplasm. The gross morphology of FNH shows a central scar that lodges multiple dystrophic vessels by histopathology. These dystrophic vessels are thick-walled and are unaccompanied by any bile duct although the junction of the scar and the cellular part of the lesion contains ductular reaction. The cellular part of the lesion is composed of benign hepatocytes arranged in one-cell to two-cell thick cords. Immunohistochemically, an FNH typically shows cytoplasmic staining of glutamine synthetase (GS) in a map-like pattern consequent to the activation of β-catenin without any *CTNNB1* mutation. The lesions that simulate FNH without fulfilling all the necessary criteria are variably labeled as FNH-like lesion/nodules. In a recent study, FNH-like nodules (morphologically FNH without map-like pattern of GS immunohistochemistry) occurring in the setting of chronic hepatic vascular disorders showed *CTNNB1* mutation with diffuse homogeneous/diffuse heterogeneous pattern of GS staining, occasional focal reticulin loss, and variable nuclear β-catenin staining in occasional cases. This proves that a small subset of FNH lesions occurring in the setting of chronic hepatic vascular disorders can be clonal with the propensity of malignant transformation though the large majority of the FNH lesions are polyclonal and reactive in nature.[66]

Hepatocellular adenoma (HCA) has been classified according to their molecular alterations into *HNF1A*-inactivated HCA (H-HCA), inflammatory-HCA (I-HCA), β-catenin-activated HCA (β-HCA), and β-catenin-activated inflammatory HCA (β-IHCA). The IHCA occurs due to the activating mutations in the interleukin-6/Janus kinase/signal transducer and activator of transcription (IL-6/JAK/STAT) pathway. These variants have different clinical presentations, histopathology, immunohistochemical expression, and prognosis in terms of complications and propensity for malignant transformation. Therefore, the recognition of these subgroups is crucial in the decision-making and management of these benign hepatocellular neoplasms. However, approximately 10% of HCAs remain unclassified. Recently, a new subgroup representing approximately 4% of all HCAs has been recognized.[67] This subgroup shows activation of sonic hedgehog signaling due to the fusion of the promoter of the *INHBE* (inhibin β E) gene with *GLI1* and is associated with obesity and bleeding (shHCA).[67] Histologically, this variant of HCA shows foci of hemorrhage and steatosis of the background liver. Immunohistochemistry highlights prostaglandin D2 synthetase positivity in the tumor cells of shHCA.[67] The uncommon histopathological variants of HCA are also increasingly identified. In different recent studies, a myxoid variant of HCA is recognized that shows deposition of abundant extracellular mucinous material in the space of Disse separating the cords of neoplastic hepatocytes. This uncommon variant shows *HNF1A* inactivation at the molecular level with/without additional mutations in the genes of/genes that are regulators of the PKA pathway. Consequently, these tumors show a high risk of malignant transformation and occur in older individuals (>60 years of age). This is in contrast to the other H-HCAs that show low risk of malignant transformation and occur below 40 years of age.[68,69]

WHO 5th Edition recognizes eight subtypes of HCC, the primary malignancy of the liver with hepatocellular differentiation. Approximately 35% of all HCCs can be classified into these subtypes.[65,70] These subtypes are distinguished by their molecular pathogenesis, histomorphology, and prognosis. **Table 10** highlights these subtypes of HCC with their characteristic molecular and histopathological features **(Figs. 6A to D)**.

Various other morphological types such as sarcomatoid HCC and undifferentiated carcinoma are well-recognized and different uncommon molecular alterations with their molecular counterparts are also being documented in the

TABLE 10: Hepatocellular carcinoma (HCC) subtypes with their molecular and histopathological features (modified from WHO 5th edition).[65]

Subtype of HCC	Molecular alterations	Histopathological features
Steatohepatitic	IL-6/JAK/STAT activation	Intratumoral steatohepatitis (macrovesicular steatosis, inflammatory cells, ballooning with/without Mallory Denk bodies)
Clear cell	Unknown	>80% tumor cells showing abundant glycogen-rich tumor cells (PAS positive diastase sensitive) with/without a few steatotic tumor cells. No focal nuclear anaplasia
Macrotrabecular massive	*FGF19* amplification/*TP53* mutation	>50% tumor cells show macrotrabecular (≥10 cells thick) pattern
Scirrhous	*TSC1/2* mutations/TGF-β activation	>50% tumor cells show intratumoral fibrous bands mimicking cholangiocarcinoma
Chromophobe	ALT (alternative lengthening of telomeres)	Chromophobe cytoplasm, abrupt focal nuclear anaplasia in the background of bland small round nuclei without nucleolar prominence, pseudocyst
Fibrolamellar	*DNAJB1-PRKACA* fusion	• Dense intratumoral bands of fibrosis, large tumor cells with voluminous eosinophilic cytoplasm, and prominent nucleoli • Immunostain showing diffuse membranocytoplasmic positivity for Heppar-1, CK7, and CD68
Neutrophil-rich	G-CSF producing tumor	Diffuse intratumoral infiltration by neutrophils, usually poorly-differentiated tumor cells including sarcomatoid areas
Lymphocyte-rich	Unknown	Numerous intratumoral lymphocytes at places obscuring the tumor cells

(G-CSF: granulocyte colony-stimulating factor; IL-6: interleukin-6; JAK: Janus kinase; PAS: periodic acid–Schiff stain; STAT: signal transducer and activator of transcription)

literature.[71,72] A homogeneous group of HCC with mixed histological features of fibrolamellar and conventional HCC has been recognized. This uncommon variant shows *BAP1* inactivating mutation causing PKA activation and is morphologically recognized by abundant fibrous stroma, intratumoral steatosis, abundant intratumoral lymphocytes, and a higher propensity for biliary tract and perineural invasion than any conventional HCC.[72] An integrative molecular and pathological classification divides the HCC into a poor-prognostic proliferation class and a better-prognostic nonproliferation class. While the proliferation class usually shows stem cell/macrotrabecular-massive pattern, chromosome instability, and *TP53* mutation, the nonproliferation class shows steatohepatitic/microtrabecular pattern, chromosome stability, and *CTNNB1/TERT* promoter mutation.[73]

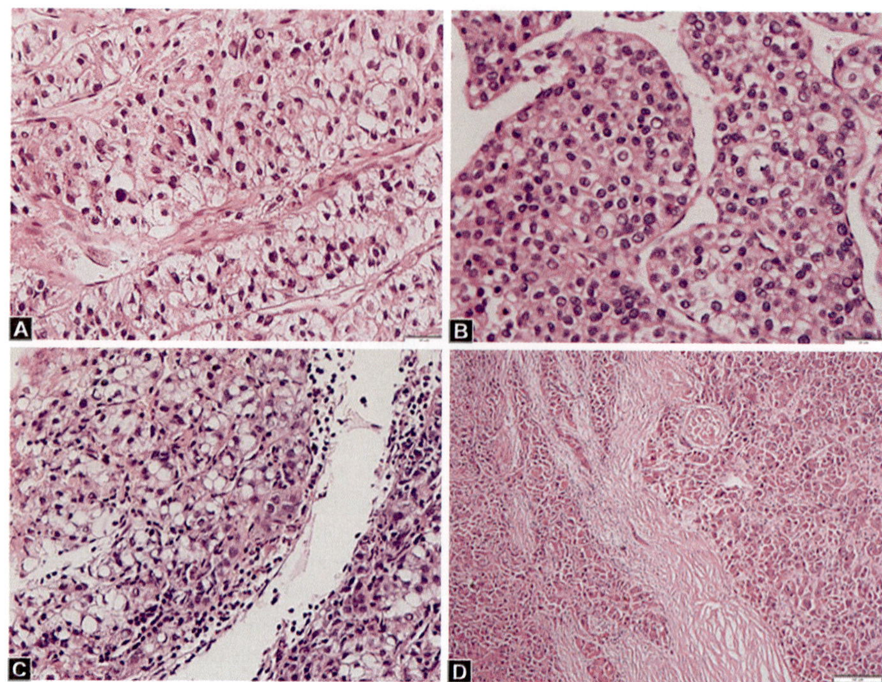

FIGS. 6A TO D: Histopathology of different morphological subtypes of hepatocellular carcinoma (HCC): Clear cell HCC (A), Macrotrabecular-massive HCC (B), Steatohepatitic HCC (C), Fibrolamellar HCC (D) (hematoxylin and eosin) (scale bars attached).

The iCCA is subclassified into small-duct and large-duct types based on the characteristic histomorphology, immunophenotype, and molecular alterations. The small-duct type iCCA shows a mass-forming lesion comprising of nonmucin-secreting small irregular glands, has a cirrhotic etiopathogenesis, and *IDH1/2* mutation. In contrast, the large-duct type iCCA shows a peripherally infiltrating mass comprising of mucin-secreting glands, has a ductal pathogenesis, and *KRAS* mutation.[65]

The molecular paradigm of many other liver tumors is unraveled changing the morphomolecular landscape of these tumors. However, a detailed discussion of each such entity is beyond the scope of this chapter.

CONCLUSION

Medical science is a constantly growing field. The advent of advanced molecular techniques, awareness of the entities among the general population, clinicians, radiologists, surgeons, and pathologists, and the application of artificial intelligence and machine learning have caused a paradigm shift in liver pathology. Therefore, there is a constant endeavor to classify the entities in a more objective, globally acknowledged, and universally reproducible fashion. Besides, such updates aid in the personalized treatment of individuals and are the future of modern medicine.

REFERENCES

1. Eslam M, Newsome PN, Sarin SK, Anstee QM, Targher G, Romero-Gomez M, et al. A new definition for metabolic dysfunction-associated fatty liver disease: An international expert consensus statement. J Hepatol. 2020;73:202-9.
2. Eslam M, Sanyal AJ, George J; International Consensus Panel. MAFLD: A Consensus-Driven Proposed Nomenclature for Metabolic Associated Fatty Liver Disease. Gastroenterology. 2020;158:1999-2014.e1.
3. Rinella ME, Lazarus JV, Ratziu V, Francque SM, Sanyal AJ, Kanwal F, et al; NAFLD Nomenclature consensus group. A multisociety Delphi consensus statement on new fatty liver disease nomenclature. Hepatology. 2023;78:1966-86.
4. De A, Bhagat N, Mehta M, Taneja S, Duseja A. Metabolic dysfunction-associated steatotic liver disease (MASLD) definition is better than MAFLD criteria for lean patients with NAFLD. J Hepatol. 2024;80:e61-2.
5. De A, Mehta M, Singh P, Bhagat N, Mitra S, Das A, et al. Lean Indian patients with non-alcoholic fatty liver disease (NAFLD) have less metabolic risk factors but similar liver disease severity as non-lean patients with NAFLD. Int J Obes (Lond). 2023;47:986-92.
6. Konkwo C, Chowdhury S, Vilarinho S. Genetics of liver disease in adults. Hepatol Commun. 2024;8(4):e0408.
7. Brunt EM, Kleiner DE, Wilson LA, Belt P, Neuschwander-Tetri BA; NASH Clinical Research Network (CRN). Nonalcoholic fatty liver disease (NAFLD) activity score and the histo-pathologic diagnosis in NAFLD: Distinct clinicopathologic meanings. Hepatology. 2011;53: 810-20.
8. Bedossa P, Poitou C, Veyrie N, Bouillot JL, Basdevant A, Paradis V, et al. Histopathological algorithm and scoring system for evaluation of liver lesions in morbidly obese patients. Hepatology. 2012;56:1751-9.
9. Brunt EM, Clouston AD, Goodman Z, Guy C, Kleiner DE, Lackner C, et al. Complexity of ballooned hepatocyte feature recognition: Defining a training atlas for artificial intelligence-based imaging in NAFLD. J Hepatol. 2022;76:1030-41.
10. Brunt EM, Kleiner DE, Carpenter DH, Rinella M, Harrison SA, Loomba R, et al; American Association for the Study of Liver Diseases NASH Task Force. NAFLD: Reporting Histologic Findings in Clinical Practice. Hepatology. 2021;73:2028-38.
11. Pai RK, Jairath V, Hogan M, Zou G, Adeyi OA, Anstee QM, et al. Reliability of histologic assessment for NAFLD and development of an expanded NAFLD activity score. Hepatology. 2022;76:1150-63.
12. Chang PE, Goh GBB, Leow WQ, Shen L, Lim KH, Tan CK. Second harmonic generation microscopy provides accurate automated staging of liver fibrosis in patients with non-alcoholic fatty liver disease. PLoS One. 2018;13:e0199166.
13. Ting Soon GS, Wee A. Liver biopsy in the quantitative assessment of liver fibrosis in nonalcoholic fatty liver disease. Indian J Pathol Microbiol. 2021;64(Supplement): S104-11.
14. Duseja A, Singh SP, De A, Madan K, Rao PN, Shukla A, et al. Indian National Association for Study of the Liver (INASL) Guidance Paper on Nomenclature, Diagnosis and Treatment of Nonalcoholic Fatty Liver Disease (NAFLD). J Clin Exp Hepatol. 2023;13:273-302.
15. Albhaisi SAM, Sanyal AJ. New drugs for NASH. Liver Int. 2021;41(Suppl 1):112-8.
16. Dhiman RK, Chawla Y, Vasishta RK, Kakkar N, Dilawari JB, Trehan MS, et al. Non-cirrhotic portal fibrosis (idiopathic portal hypertension): experience with 151 patients and a review of the literature. J Gastroenterol Hepatol. 2002;17:6-16.
17. Rajekar H, Vasishta RK, Chawla YK, Dhiman RK. Noncirrhotic portal hypertension. J Clin Exp Hepatol. 2011;1:94-108.
18. De Gottardi A, Rautou PE, Schouten J, Rubbia-Brandt L, Leebeek F, Trebicka J, et al; VALDIG group. Porto-sinusoidal vascular disease: proposal and description of a novel entity. Lancet Gastroenterol Hepatol. 2019;4:399-411.

19. Kmeid M, Liu X, Ballentine S, Lee H. Idiopathic non-cirrhotic portal hypertension and porto-sinusoidal vascular disease: Review of current data. Gastroenterology Res. 2021;14: 49-65.
20. Mitra S, Anand S, Das A, Thapa B, Chawla YK, Minz RW. A molecular marker of disease activity in autoimmune liver diseases with histopathological correlation; FoXp3/RORγt ratio. APMIS. 2015;123(11):935-44.
21. Mitra S, Minz RW. Autoantibodies in autoimmune liver diseases-methods of detection and interpretation: An update for the reporting pathologist. Int J Surg Pathol. 2016;24(7): 576-85.
22. Rahim MN, Miquel R, Heneghan MA. Approach to the patient with acute severe auto-immune hepatitis. JHEP Rep. 2020;2(6):100149.
23. Taneja S, Mehtani R, De A, Mitra S, Rathi S, Verma N, et al. Spectrum of autoimmune liver disease and real-world treatment experience from a tertiary care hospital. J Clin Exp Hepatol. 2023;13(2):241-51.
24. Lohse AW, Sebode M, Bhathal PS, Clouston AD, Dienes HP, Jain D, et al. Consensus recommendations for histological criteria of autoimmune hepatitis from the International AIH Pathology Group: Results of a workshop on AIH histology hosted by the European Reference Network on Hepatological Diseases and the European Society of Pathology: Results of a workshop on AIH histology hosted by the European Reference Network on Hepatological Diseases and the European Society of Pathology. Liver Int. 2022;42(5): 1058-69.
25. Taneja S, Kumar P, Mitra S, Duseja A, Minz R, Das A, et al. Acute exacerbation to autoimmune hepatitis mimicking acute viral hepatitis-a case series and review of literature. J Clin Exp Hepatol. 2018;8(1):98-103.
26. Hu WS, Jiang FY, Shu W, Zhao R, Cao JM, Wang DP. Liver injury in COVID-19: A minireview. World J Gastroenterol. 2022;28(47):6716-31.
27. Kumar MP, Mishra S, Jha DK, Shukla J, Choudhury A, Mohindra R, et al. Coronavirus disease (COVID-19) and the liver: a comprehensive systematic review and meta-analysis. Hepatol Int. 2020;14(5):711-22.
28. Bangash MN, Patel J, Parekh D. COVID-19 and the liver: little cause for concern. Lancet Gastroenterol Hepatol. 2020;5(6):529-30.
29. Jena A, Aggarwal T, Mitra S, Singh AK. Nintedanib-induced liver injury: Not every liver injury is virus or vaccine-induced in the era of COVID-19. Liver Int. 2022;42(5):1210-1.
30. Lagana SM, Kudose S, Iuga AC, Lee MJ, Fazlollahi L, Remotti HE, et al. Hepatic pathology in patients dying of COVID-19: a series of 40 cases including clinical, histologic, and virologic data. Mod Pathol. 2020;33(11):2147-55.
31. Chu H, Peng L, Hu L, Zhu Y, Zhao J, Su H, et al. Liver Histopathological Analysis of 24 Post-mortem Findings of Patients With COVID-19 in China. Front Med (Lausanne). 2021;8: 749318.
32. Sonzogni A, Previtali G, Seghezzi M, Grazia Alessio M, Gianatti A, Licini L, et al. Liver histopathology in severe COVID 19 respiratory failure is suggestive of vascular alterations. Liver Int. 2020;40(9):2110-6.
33. Liang J, Kelly DR, Pai A, Gillis LA, Sanchez LHG, Shiau HH, et al. Clinicopathologic Features of Severe Acute Hepatitis Associated With Adenovirus Infection in Children. Am J Surg Pathol. 2023;47(9):977-89.
34. Mellinger JL, Rossaro L, Naugler WE, Nadig SN, Appelman H, Lee WM, et al. Epstein-Barr virus (EBV) related acute liver failure: a case series from the US Acute Liver Failure Study Group. Dig Dis Sci. 2014;59:1630-7.
35. Mitra S, Hanumanthappa MK, Sarkar S, Bhalla A, Minz R, Ratho RK. Epstein Barr virus-related acute liver failure and hemophagocytosis in an immunocompetent individual: An autopsy report. Int J Surg Pathol. 2024;32(4):838-44.
36. Schechter S, Lamps L. Epstein-Barr virus hepatitis: A review of clinicopathologic features and differential diagnosis. Arch Pathol Lab Med. 2018;142:1191-5.

37. Ma Z, de Man RA, Kamar N, Pan Q. Chronic hepatitis E: Advancing research and patient care. J Hepatol. 2022;77(4):1109-23.
38. Beer A, Holzmann H, Pischke S, Behrendt P, Wrba F, Schlue J, et al. Chronic Hepatitis E is associated with cholangitis. Liver Int. 2019;39(10):1876-83.
39. Lenggenhager D, Pawel S, Honcharova-Biletska H, Evert K, Wenzel JJ, Montani M, et al. The histologic presentation of hepatitis E reflects patients' immune status and pre-existing liver condition. Mod Pathol. 2021;34(1):233-48.
40. Kleiner DE, Chalasani NP, Lee WM, Fontana RJ, Bonkovsky HL, Watkins PB, et al; Drug-Induced Liver Injury Network (DILIN). Hepatic histological findings in suspected drug-induced liver injury: Systematic evaluation and clinical associations. Hepatology. 2014;59(2):661-70.
41. Zen Y, Yeh MM. Hepatotoxicity of immune checkpoint inhibitors: a histology study of seven cases in comparison with autoimmune hepatitis and idiosyncratic drug-induced liver injury. Mod Pathol. 2018;31(6):965-73.
42. Zen Y, Yeh MM. Checkpoint inhibitor-induced liver injury: A novel form of liver disease emerging in the era of cancer immunotherapy. Semin Diagn Pathol. 2019;36(6):434-40.
43. Patil PA, Zhang X. Pathologic manifestations of gastrointestinal and hepatobiliary injury in immune checkpoint inhibitor therapy. Arch Pathol Lab Med. 2021;145(5):571-82.
44. Verma N, Kumar P, Mitra S, Taneja S, Dhooria S, Das A, et al. Drug idiosyncrasy due to pirfenidone presenting as acute liver failure: Case report and mini-review of the literature. Hepatol Commun. 2017;2(2):142-7.
45. Ayyanar P, Mahalik SK, Haldar S, Purkait S, Patra S, Mitra S. Expression of CD56 is not limited to biliary atresia and correlates with the degree of fibrosis in pediatric cholestatic diseases. Fetal Pediatr Pathol. 2022;41(1):87-97.
46. Biswal S, Biswas D, Mahalik SK, Purkait S, Mitra S. Assessment of matrix metalloprotease-7 (MMP7) immunohistochemistry in biliary atresia and other pediatric cholestatic liver diseases. Fetal Pediatr Pathol. 2023:1-10.
47. Mitra S, Ayyanar P, Mahalik SK, Patra S, Purkait S, Satapathy AK. Diminution of the primary cilia from the intrahepatic cholangiocytes in a pediatric choledochal cyst. Appl Immunohistochem Mol Morphol. 2021;29(10):773-80.
48. Grammatikopoulos T, Sambrotta M, Strautnieks S, Foskett P, Knisely AS, Wagner B, et al; University of Washington Center for Mendelian Genomics; Bull L, Thompson RJ. Mutations in DCDC2 (doublecortin domain containing protein 2) in neonatal sclerosing cholangitis. J Hepatol. 2016;65(6):1179-87.
49. Boniel S, Szymańska K, Śmigiel R, Szczałuba K. Kabuki syndrome-clinical review with molecular aspects. Genes (Basel). 2021;12(4):468.
50. Samanta A, Sarma MS, Srivastava A, Poddar U. Cholestatic liver disease in a child with KIF12 mutation. Indian J Pediatr. 2024;91(7):733-6.
51. Ünlüsoy Aksu A, Das SK, Nelson-Williams C, Jain D, Özbay Hoşnut F, Evirgen Şahin G, et al. Recessive Mutations in *KIF12* Cause High Gamma-Glutamyltransferase Cholestasis. Hepatol Commun. 2019;3(4):471-7.
52. Mitra S, Das A, Thapa B, Kumar Vasishta R. Phenotype-genotype correlation of North Indian progressive familial intrahepatic cholestasis type2 children shows p.Val444Ala and p.Asn591Ser variants and retained BSEP expression. Fetal Pediatr Pathol. 2020;39(2): 107-23.
53. Srivastava A. Progressive familial intrahepatic cholestasis. J Clin Exp Hepatol. 2014;4(1): 25-36.
54. Vinayagamoorthy V, Srivastava A, Sarma MS. Newer variants of progressive familial intrahepatic cholestasis. World J Hepatol. 2021;13(12):2024-38.
55. Amirneni S, Haep N, Gad MA, Soto-Gutierrez A, Squires JE, Florentino RM. Molecular overview of progressive familial intrahepatic cholestasis. World J Gastroenterol. 2020;26(47): 7470-84.
56. Terrault NA, Francoz C, Berenguer M, Charlton M, Heimbach J. Liver transplantation 2023: Status report, current and future challenges. Clin Gastroenterol Hepatol. 2023;21(8): 2150-66.

57. Neil DAH, Minervini M, Smith ML, Hubscher SG, Brunt EM, Demetris AJ. Banff consensus recommendations for steatosis assessment in donor livers. Hepatology. 2022;75(4):1014-25.
58. Lee BT, Fiel MI, Schiano TD. Antibody-mediated rejection of the liver allograft: An update and a clinico-pathological perspective. J Hepatol. 2021;75(5):1203-16.
59. Demetris AJ, Bellamy C, Hübscher SG, O'Leary J, Randhawa PS, Feng S, et al. 2016 Comprehensive update of the Banff Working Group on liver allograft pathology: Introduction of antibody-mediated rejection. Am J Transplant. 2016;16(10):2816-35.
60. Mitra S, Rathi S, Debi U, Dhiman RK, Das A. Primary hepatic leiomyosarcoma: Histopathologist's perspective of a rare case. J Clin Exp Hepatol. 2018;8(3):321-6.
61. Panigrahi C, Nayak HK, Patra S, Mitra S. Hepatic follicular dendritic cell sarcoma with epithelioid morphology: Histopathologist's perspective. J Clin Exp Hepatol. 2022;12(2):677-85.
62. Bhardwaj N, Parkhi M, Kumar M, Kaman L, Mitra S. Adult diffuse hepatic hemangiomatosis. Autops Case Rep. 2022;12:e2021401.
63. Parkhi M, Joshi R, Kumar M, Sharma A, Mitra S, Kaman L. Biliary adenofibroma: A precursor lesion of intrahepatic cholangiocarcinoma. Autops Case Rep. 2023;13:e2023453.
64. Ahuja N, Mitra S, Bal A, Das A, Tandup C, Krishnaraju VS. Multiple Biliary Adenofibromas with Adenocarcinoma of Gallbladder: Histopathological Conundrum. J Gastrointest Cancer. 2023;54(3):986-8.
65. WHO Classification of Tumours Editorial Board. Digestive System Tumours, 5th edition. Lyon (France): International Agency for Research on Cancer; 2019.
66. Umetsu SE, Joseph NM, Cho SJ, Morotti R, Deshpande V, Jain D, et al. Focal nodular hyperplasia-like nodules arising in the setting of hepatic vascular disorders with portosystemic shunting show β-catenin activation. Hum Pathol. 2023;142:20-6.
67. Nault JC, Couchy G, Balabaud C, Morcrette G, Caruso S, Blanc JF, et al. Molecular classification of hepatocellular adenoma associates with risk factors, bleeding, and malignant transformation. Gastroenterology. 2017;152(4):880-94.e6.
68. Rowan DJ, Yasir S, Chen ZE, Mounajjed T, Erdogan Damgard S, Cummins L, et al. Morphologic and molecular findings in myxoid hepatic adenomas. Am J Surg Pathol. 2021;45(8):1098-107.
69. Yasir S, Chen ZE, Jain D, Kakar S, Wu TT, Yeh MM, et al. Hepatic adenomas in patients 60 and older are enriched for HNF1A inactivation and malignant transformation. Am J Surg Pathol. 2022;46(6):786-92.
70. Loy LM, Low HM, Choi JY, Rhee H, Wong CF, Tan CH. Variant Hepatocellular Carcinoma Subtypes According to the 2019 WHO Classification: An Imaging-Focused Review. AJR Am J Roentgenol. 2022;219(2):212-23.
71. Mitra S, Gupta S, Dahiya D, Saikia UN. A Rare case of primary sarcomatous hepatocellular carcinoma without previous anticancer therapy. J Clin Exp Hepatol. 2017;7(4):378-84.
72. Hirsch TZ, Negulescu A, Gupta B, Caruso S, Noblet B, Couchy G, et al. BAP1 mutations define a homogeneous subgroup of hepatocellular carcinoma with fibrolamellar-like features and activated PKA. J Hepatol. 2020;72(5):924-36.
73. Rebouissou S, Nault JC. Advances in molecular classification and precision oncology in hepatocellular carcinoma. J Hepatol. 2020;72(2):215-29.

2

CHAPTER

Advances in Lung Cancer Classification and Molecular Characterization

Shruti Gupta, Nalini Gupta

INTRODUCTION

Lung cancer accounts for approximately 1.8 million deaths among both men and women.[1] The Indian subcontinent observes age standardized incidence rate of 6.9 per 100,000 population and 8.1% of cancer-related deaths in the country are associated with lung cancer.[2] The definite epidemiologic link with tobacco smoking with all histologic forms of carcinoma lung has been established centuries back, with reference to multifold increased risk with amount of tobacco usage and duration of exposure. However, techniques as next-generation sequencing (NGS) and The Cancer Genome Atlas (TCGA) project have cracked the code for molecular subtyping of various histological forms of lung cancer with huge impact on therapeutic regimens and prognostication. Diverse samples including fine-needle aspirates, cell blocks, small tissue biopsies, and liquid biopsies can be utilized for molecular characterization. The era of integrated diagnosis of lung cancer with reference to definite histological classification, molecular subtyping, and sensitivity to immunotherapy makes the way for an algorithmic stepwise diagnosis of lung cancer.

A major shift has been witnessed in classification and treatment of lung cancer over the last decade with improved chances of survival. The 5th edition of the World Health Organization (WHO) classification of thoracic tumors, released in 2021, has taken into account the recent advances in the tumor evolution pathway of lung cancer and has integrated the genetic testing along with the immunohistochemistry (IHC) and morphology. The major changes in the latest classification have been compiled in **Box 1**.

Cytological findings have been included, in acknowledgement of the importance of fine-needle aspiration (FNA) and other cytology specimens as a diagnostic modality in unresectable lesions.[3]

The 2015 classification discussed histological and molecular correlation primarily among lung adenocarcinomas. The 5th edition has extrapolated the molecular coordinates and molecular testing has been advised for various lung cancer types.

BOX 1 Major changes in 5th edition of the World Health Organization (WHO) classification.[3]

- Workflow and characterization of cytology and small diagnostic biopsies
- Classification of precursor glandular lesions as a separate entity
- Inclusion of percentage of specific growth pattern in lung adenocarcinomas for their prognostic value
- Three tier grading for lung adenocarcinomas
- Recognition of tumor cell spread through air spaces (STAS) as a mode of spread
- Subclassification of large cell pulmonary neuroendocrine tumors with corresponding molecular characteristics
- Inclusion of newer entities as bronchiolar adenoma/ciliated muconodular papillary tumor (BA/CMPT) and SMARCA4 deficient undifferentiated tumors

The NGS data has tempted WHO to evolve the understanding of pulmonary neuroendocrine tumors (NETs). Newer entities as SMARCA4 deficient undifferentiated tumors have been added based on immunohistochemical and genetic characteristics.

ADVANCES IN CLASSIFICATION

Majority of lung malignancies are detected at late stages and are usually unresectable, prompting the need of accurate subtyping on cytology and small biopsies. Specimens from FNA, bronchial washings, sputum, bronchoalveolar lavage (BAL), and transbronchial needle aspiration (TBNA) can be effectively utilized for morphological subtyping. The availability of biomarkers and targeted therapy necessitates the need of utilizing the tiniest of specimens for tissue diagnosis. The inclusion of special stains for mucin, IHC, and molecular techniques has aided in the specific diagnosis of cytology and small biopsies from lung, leaving less space for non-small cell lung carcinoma, not otherwise specified (NSCLC, NOS). Emphasis has been given to specify adenocarcinoma and squamous cell carcinoma (SqCC), wherever possible. The terms such as non-SqCC and large cell carcinoma are discouraged. The suspicion of neuroendocrine cytological features should prompt the use of IHC.

The tumor heterogeneity can generate various limitations in morphological diagnoses in tiny biopsies and cytological specimens and must be kept in mind. An algorithmic approach of guidelines for terminologies defined in the latest WHO classification is illustrated in **Flowchart 1**.

Majority of peripherally located lung masses are adenocarcinomas. The premalignant lesions are not amenable to diagnosis on cytological samples and small biopsies. The differentiation between atypical adenomatous hyperplasia (AAH) of the lung, described as <5 mm localized proliferation and adenocarcinoma in situ (AIS) requires a resection specimen. A close evaluation of radiological and pathological findings needs to be done when designating a diagnosis of AIS. Similarly, the diagnosis of minimally invasive adenocarcinoma (MIA) requires a resection specimen. A cut-off of size <30 mm and foci of invasion <5 mm invasion measured using a ruler are essential diagnostic criteria

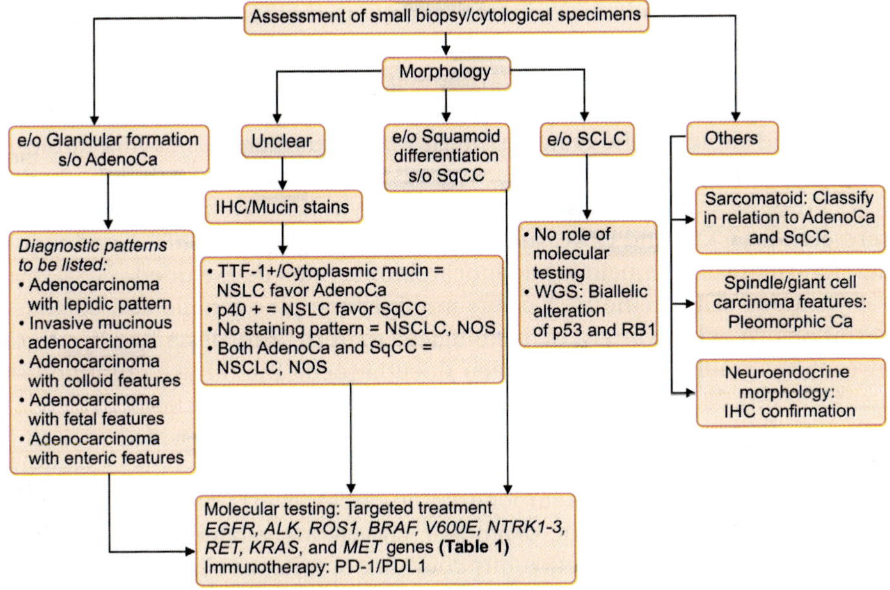

FLOWCHART 1: Diagnostic algorithm for non-small cell lung carcinoma.[3]

(AdenoCa: adenocarcinoma; e/o: evidence of; IHC: immunohistochemistry; NOS: not otherwise specified; NSCLC: non-small cell lung carcinoma; s/o: suggestive of; SqCC: squamous cell carcinoma; SCLC: small cell lung carcinoma; TTF-1: transcription factor-1)

for MIA. Any evidence of lymphovascular invasion, tumor necrosis, and spread through air spaces (STAS) should be excluded by meticulous examination. The improved prognostic and disease-free survival of patients with AAH, AIS, and MIA as evaluated in multiple studies makes it crucial that accurate diagnosis must be done.

The morphological distinction between invasive nonmucinous adenocarcinoma (INMA) and invasive mucinous adenocarcinoma (IMA) has been done based on presence of columnar cells with intracytoplasmic mucin and/or goblet cells. The radiological appearance, immunohistochemical features, and discrete molecular profiles make the distinction clinically and prognostically relevant. The various architectural patterns of INMA—lepidic, acinar, papillary, micropapillary, and pure solid pattern have described with prognostic implications. Clear cell and signet ring features among the various patterns can be noted. The micropapillary pattern includes a filigree pattern which consists of delicate lace-like narrow stacks of more than three tumor cells. A three-tiered grading has been proposed based on predominant histological pattern. The lepidic predominant pattern (<20% high grade features) has been designated as well differentiated with best prognosis as opposed to solid and micropapillary predominant (>20% high grade features) designated as poorly differentiated with worst prognosis. The solid pattern is diagnosed in conjunction with IHC using transcription factor-1 (TTF-1) and napsin positivity or evidence of intracellular mucin in more than five tumor cells. In view of the prognostic significance, the percentage of the various patterns must be recorded.

The tumor STAS is adenocarcinoma represents another important indicator of tumor spread and has been shown to be associated with worse outcome. STAS is not included in the total tumor size while staging of tumors.[3]

Invasive mucinous adenocarcinomas are less common lung adenocarcinomas and show lepidic growth pattern with columnar cells having intracytoplasmic mucin and/or goblet cells. No grading systems have been described for IMAs. IMAs have characteristic immunopositivity for CK7 and show focal co-expression for CK20 and CDX2 and are immune-negative for TTF-1 and napsin. Therefore, metastatic mucinous adenocarcinoma must be excluded.

Squamous cell carcinoma harbors multiple complex genetic and epigenetic aberrations. A wide variety of histological patterns are described for SqCC; however, no grading system has been documented. The diffuse immunohistochemical expression of p40 is the most specific marker for lung SqCC.

The neuroendocrine neoplasms of the lung NETs are classified as a single group of tumors with diagnostic criteria to classify each entity—carcinoid, atypical carcinoid, large cell neuroendocrine carcinoma (LCNEC), and small cell carcinoma **(Flowchart 2)**. The diagnostic criteria are established for resection specimens and advocates meticulous counting of mitoses per 2 mm^2. The term carcinoid, NOS can be used in setting of small scant biopsies. The small biopsies and metastatic foci need additional IHC using Ki-67 to distinguish carcinoids, LCNEC, small cell lung carcinoma (SCLC), and metastatic lesions. A Ki-67 > 30% is more likely to be higher grade lesion as opposed to Ki-67 < 5% which corresponds to lower end of the spectrum.

Bronchiolar adenoma/ciliated muconodular papillary tumor (BA/CMPT) and SMARCA4-deficient undifferentiated tumor (SMAR-CA4-UT) are the new entities introduced in the latest classification.

The BA/CMPT is benign lesion with characteristic BRAFV600E driver mutations and morphologically comprises of circumscribed peribronchiolar lung nodule with bilayered proliferation of luminal epithelial cells and basal cells

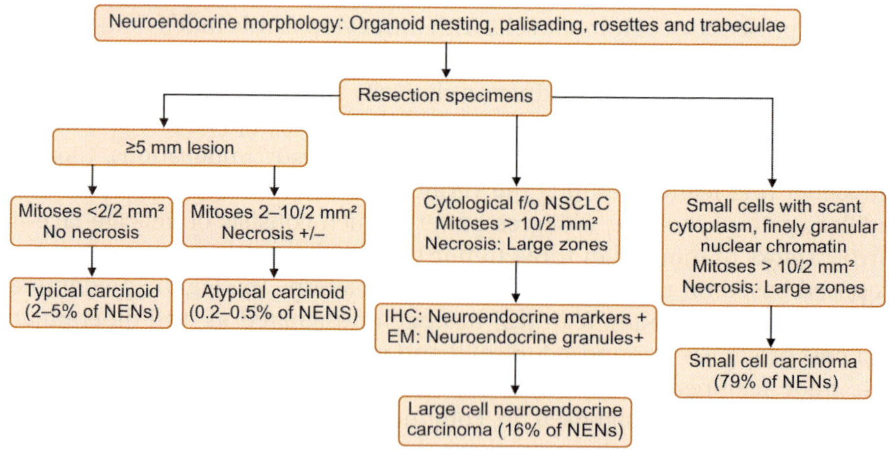

FLOWCHART 2: Diagnostic algorithm for lung neuroendocrine carcinomas.[3]

(EM: electron microscopy; IHC: immunohistochemistry; NENs: neuroendocrine neoplasms; NSCLC: non-small cell lung carcinoma)

in papillary/flat arrangement. The most important differential diagnosis is well-differentiated adenocarcinoma. Immunohistochemical markers for basal layer expressing p40 and CK5/6 can be used for diagnosis.

SMAR-CA4-UT are highly aggressive and high grade undifferentiated tumors with complete loss of SMARCA4 on IHC and presence of SMARCA4 mutation on sequencing.

MOLECULAR CHARACTERIZATION

The advances in understanding of genetic profiling of lung cancer through large scale genomic work-up have aided to devise a molecular classification. A wide variety of methodologies including real-time polymerase chain reaction (PCR), Sanger sequencing, NGS, and microarray-based studies have been done to accomplish the feat of classification of lung tumors for targeted treatment. Molecular diagnostics are a mandatory aid in cases where morphological and immunophenotypical features are inconclusive.

Lindeman et al. have discussed College of American Pathologists (CAP), International Association for the Study of Lung Cancer (IASLC), and Association for Molecular Pathology (AMP) guidelines for clinical practice and treatment of lung cancer and advocate the classification as well as molecular testing in lung cancers.[4]

A layered reporting of lung cancer diagnosis including cytological/histopathological diagnosis, immunohistochemical, and mucin staining character along with details of molecular testing is encouraged, wherever possible. **Table 1**

TABLE 1: Spectrum of oncogenic drivers in subtypes of lung cancer.[3]

	Molecular profile	
Subtype	**Mutations**	**Fusions**
Invasive non-mucinous adenocarcinoma (INMA)	• EGFR (40–55%) • KRAS (8–10%) • HER2 (2–3%) • BRAF (0.5–1%)	• ALK (3–5%) • ROS (2–3%) • RET (1–2%)
Invasive mucinous adenocarcinoma (IMA)	• KRAS (62%) • BRAF (2%) • ERRB2 (1%) • EGFR (1%) • PIK3CA (1%)	• NTRK1 (1%) • RET (1%) • ERBB2/4 (1%) • ALK (2%) • NRG (7%)
Squamous cell carcinoma (SqCC)	• EGFR • ALK	
Large cell neuroendocrine carcinoma (LCNEC)	• TP53 • STK11 • KEAP1 • RB1	
Small cell carcinoma (SCC)	• TP53 • RB1	

illustrates the spectrum of oncogenic drivers of clinical and therapeutic relevance associated with various histological subtypes of lung cancers. Among all the targetable mutations, epidermal growth factor receptor (EGFR) mutations are the most common mutations in NSCLCs. INMAs harbor EGFR mutations more commonly than IMAs, where KRAS are more common in IMAs.

The Cancer Genome Atlas project has gathered evidences based on genomic alterations, creating a roadmap for molecularly targeted therapies for various malignancies, including lung cancers.[5] The TGCA included lung adenocarcinomas, SqCCs, and mesotheliomas and postulated that adenocarcinomas harbor higher rate of mutations. **Table 2** discusses the impact of TCGA in the molecular characterization of lung cancers. In the genomic project, the most frequently mutated genes among SqCC were found to be TP53, CDKN2A, PTEN, PIK3CA, and KEAP1 while among adenocarcinoma were TP53, KRAS, EGFR, and BRAF.

Based on messenger ribonucleic acid (mRNA) profiling, lung adenocarcinomas are classified as proximal proliferative, proximal inflammatory, and terminal respiratory unit. On the basis of deoxyribonucleic acid (DNA) methylation profiling adenocarcinoma are divided into CpG island methylator phenotypes. The CIMP-high phenotype has a poor prognosis as compared to CIMP-low phenotype.[6]

The role of micro ribonucleic acid (miRNA) has been utilized widely for prognostication of lung adenocarcinoma. Nadal et al. has accomplished clustering of lung adenocarcinoma based on miRNA profiling and three clusters with histological correlation were done.[7] The various subtypes of adenocarcinoma based on RNA, DNA, and miRNA profiling are given in **Table 3**.

The Cancer Genome Atlas has postulated that among SqCC, TP53 is altered in 90% of cases and 72% cases showed CDKN2A inactivation. Frequent alterations in SOX2/TP63/NOTCH1, PI3K/AKT, and NFE2L2/KEAP1/CUL3 pathways are also noted.[8] Four subtypes of SqCC are described based on mRNA profiling namely classical, basal, secretory, and primitive. These subtypes and their genetic profile have been given in **Table 4**.

TABLE 2: The impact of The Cancer Genome Atlas (TCGA) in the molecular characterization of lung cancers.[5]

	Squamous cell carcinoma	Adenocarcinoma
Most frequently mutated genes	*TP53, CDKN2A* *PTEN, PIK3CA, KEAP1*	*TP53, KRAS, EGFR* *BRAF*
Notable amplifications	SOX2, TP63, Chr3q	• NKX2-1, TERT • MDM2, KRAS • EGFR, MET
Disease progression markers	• IR-A and IR-B • ARHGDIB and HOXD3 • PIAS3 expression • Gene fusions • BCAR-1	• Intra-tumor signaling entropy • 8-miRNA prognostic signature • miR-31 • Gene fusions • BCAR-1

TABLE 3: Molecular subtyping in lung adenocarcinomas.[6,7]

Adenocarcinoma lung	Subtypes		
mRNA profiling	Proximal proliferative	Proximal inflammatory	Terminal respiratory unit
DNA methylation profiling	CIMP-high	CIMP-intermediate	CIMP-low
miRNA profiling	• *Cluster 1*: Lepidic or mucinous • Invasive adenocarcinomas	*Cluster 2*: Acinar	*Cluster 3*: Solid tumors

(DNA: deoxyribonucleic acid; miRNA: micro ribonucleic acid; mRNA: messenger ribonucleic acid)

TABLE 4: Squamous cell carcinoma subtypes based on messenger ribonucleic acid (mRNA) profiling.[5]

Squamous cell carcinoma subtype	Genetic characterization
Classical	*KEAP1*, *NFE2L2*, and *PTEN* genes, hypermethylation and chromosome instability
Basal	NF1 mutations
Secretory	TP53 and RB1 activation
Primitive	RB1 and PTEN mutations

The WHO classification of lung tumors does not discuss any molecular testing for carcinoid tumors. In fact, the carcinoids arising from lung are usually clinically indolent and harbor low mutational burden.

Neuroendocrine carcinomas and small cell carcinomas have higher mutation rates including biallelic inactivation of TP53 and RB1. Andrew et al. have postulated that transcriptomic studies have categorized LCNECs into two major and one minor groups. The first major group resembles the molecular features of non-small cell carcinomas and show biallelic alterations in TP53, SKT11, and KRAS, while the other group has mutational profile of small cell carcinomas such as RB1 alterations and TP53 inactivation.[9]

Among all lung cancers, small cell carcinomas show strongest association with smoking and have an extremely poor prognosis. A molecular classification devised by Rudin et al. based on differential expression of transcription regulators has four categories namely SCLC-A, SCLC-N, SCLC-P, and SCLC-Y. The categories are defined based on the expression of transcription factors ASCL1, NeuroD1, POU2F3, and YAP1, respectively.[10] **Table 5** illustrates the salient features of the proposed molecular subtypes of small cell carcinoma.

Sivakumar et al. analyzed recurrent genetic abnormalities in 3,600 SCLC cases and have discussed three genomic subtypes. Based on the molecular findings, the authors proposed three genomic subtypes.[11] **Table 6** has compiled the salient features of the proposed molecular subtypes of small cell carcinoma based on recurrent molecular alterations.

The technological advancement in the field of detection methods have made the classification and targeted therapy possible. These technologies have different

TABLE 5: Proposed molecular subtypes of small cell carcinoma.[10]

Small cell carcinoma proposed molecular subtype	Salient features
SCLC-A	• Most common subtype of SCLC (70% of all cases) • Neuroendocrine phenotype • High expression of ASCL1, MYC, and thyroid transcription factor-1 (TTF-1) • Low expression of NeuroD1 • *Targeted therapy*: Inhibitors of DLL3 and BCL2
SCLC-N	• High expression of NeuroD1 and DLL3 • Low expression of ASCL1 • *Targeted therapy*: Inhibitors of Aurora kinase and WEE-1
SCLC-P	• Non-neuroendocrine, squamous cell carcinoma-like phenotype • High expression of POU2F3 • Low expression of ASCL1 and NeuroD1 • High expression of genes involved in squamous cell differentiation • *Targeted therapy*: Inhibitors of IGF1R
SCLC-Y	• Least common subtype • Mesenchymal phenotype • High expression of *YAP1* gene • Low expression of ASCL1 and NeuroD1 • Resistance to chemotherapy

(SCLC: small cell lung carcinoma)

TABLE 6: Proposed molecular subtypes of small cell carcinoma.[11]

Small cell carcinoma proposed molecular subtype	Salient features
Tumors without alterations of TP53/RB1	• Lowest tumor mutational burden • *MDM2 amplifications*: Mutually exclusive with inactivation of TP53 • *RB1 inactivation*: Mutually exclusive with inactivating alteration of CDKN2A • Possible HPV association
Tumors with STK11 mutations	• Higher tumor mutational burden • Reduced percentage of RB1 losses • KRAS and KEAP1 mutation
Tumors with oncogenic driver mutations associated with NSCLC	Subclonal evolution from EGFR-mutant clonal population

(EGFR: epidermal growth factor receptor; HPV: human papillomavirus; NSCLC: non-small cell lung carcinoma)

abilities, specificities, sensitivities, and pitfalls to detect the molecular alterations. The biomarker testing platform needs to be chosen in view of loco-regional factors, cost-effectivity, and the tools available. A vast majority of low-income countries

TABLE 7: Methodologies for biomarker detection in non-small cell lung carcinoma (NSCLC).

Target	Testing methodology with higher sensitivity	Testing methodologies available
EGFR	Digital PCR and qPCR	PCR, direct sequencing, NGS
ALK	FISH	IHC clones [D5F3/5A4], FISH, RT-PCR, NGS
ROS1	FISH (gold standard)	IHC clones [SP384/1A1]
BRAF	NGS	• *Tissue*: Allele specific PCR, NGS • *Liquid*: ddPCR, qPCR
NTRK fusions	RNA-NGS	• FISH, qPCR, FISH • IHC clones [EPR1734/A7H6R]
RET fusion	FISH	NGS, qPCR
MET exon 14 skipping	RNA-NGS	• *Tissue*: NGS, FISH, IHC, qPCR • *Liquid biopsy*: ctDNA-NGS
KRAS		PCR, NGS
HER2 mutations	NGS	Sanger sequencing, ARMS-PCR
HER2 amplifications	FISH	NGS, qPCR
HER2 overexpression	IHC	
NRG1	RNA-NGS	FISH, DNA-NGS

neither have access to expensive testing assays nor to targeted drugs for treatment. IASLC, CAP, and AMP have discussed the guidelines and recommendations for various molecular tests and the commercially available platforms in the market. The various methodologies available are given in **Table 7**.

Based on the availability of resources and targeted drugs, the guidelines for biomarker testing have been devised. **Flowchart 3** illustrates an algorithmic approach based on the Indian consensus guidelines for biomarker testing in India.[12]

Next-generation sequencing is being widely used for biomarker detection in NSCLC as it can detect the four most commonly occurring oncogenic driver mutations (ALK, ROS1, NTRK, and RET) and their specific variants.[13]

EPIDERMAL GROWTH FACTOR RECEPTOR MUTATION

Epidermal growth factor receptor mutation is the most frequent mutation found among the lung adenocarcinomas with most common molecular alterations noted in the exon 18-21. The most frequently detected mutations are exon 19 deletion and L858R point mutation in exon 21.[14] Various uncommon mutations are also described in literature such as L861X in exon 21 and S768I in exon 20.[15] The lung adenocarcinomas with EGFR mutations have shown improved prognosis and overall survival.[14] The occurrence of EGFR mutations in NSCLC patients shows distinct geographic variation. Specific gender predilection for younger, never-smoker, and female patients is well documented.[16] A recent meta-analysis by Melosky et al. have discussed the highest prevalence of EGFR mutations in

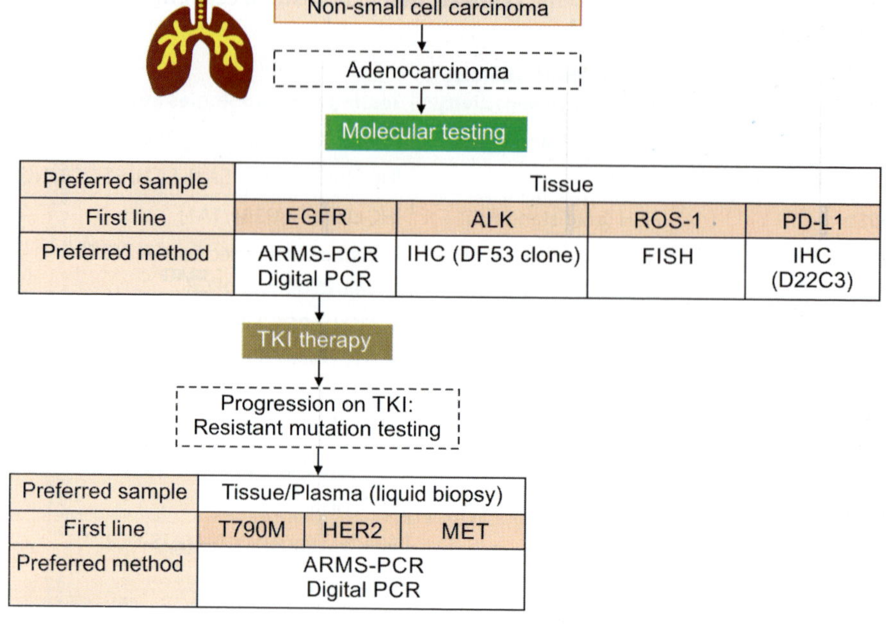

FLOWCHART 3: Algorithm devised from expert panel recommendation for biomarker testing in non-small cell lung carcinoma (NSCLC) in India.[12]

(ALK: anaplastic lymphoma kinase; ARMS: amplification-refractory mutation system; EGFR: epidermal growth factor receptor; FISH: fluorescence in situ hybridization; IHC: immunohistochemistry; NSCLC: non-small cell lung carcinoma; PCR: polymerase chain reaction; PD-L1: programmed death-ligand 1; TKI: tyrosine kinase inhibitor)

Asian NSCLC patients.[17] Quantitative real-time PCR (qPCR) is the method of choice for EGFR mutations detection. Mutation specific EGFR IHC against L858R and del19 has been tried with limited sensitivity.

Various studies done across the Indian subcontinent have shown that NSCLCs have EGFR mutation rates ranging from 22 to 45%. The most frequent mutation among Indians is deletion of exon 19, noted in 26–79% of cases followed by L858R point mutation, noted in 13–47% cases.[18]

Recent studies have demonstrated EGFR mutation in SqCCs along with adenocarcinomas.[19]

The targeted therapy using tyrosine kinase inhibitors (TKIs) has been actively utilized with improved progression free survival for NSCLCs with EGFR activating mutations. Multiple clinical trials have investigated the role of TKIs. The first-generation TKIs are reversible inhibitors, include erlotinib and gefitinib while the second-generation TKIs are irreversible inhibitors and include afatinib and dacomitinib. The third-generation TKI, osimertinib, was developed for patients with metastatic NSCLC and T790M mutation.[20] Osimertinib selectively inhibits both EGFR-TKI sensitizing and EGFR T790M resistance mutations and is effective in NSCLC with brain metastases.[21] Overall, osimertinib was found to superior to first- and second-generation TKIs.[22] Resistance to TKIs is an emerging challenge for the oncologists. The major mechanisms of resistance for TKI are also extensively studied. The osimertinib resistance can be due to three major mechanisms:

"On-target", "off-target/bypass", and histologic transformation. A hoard of unknown mechanisms is also being investigated.[23] **Table 8** depicts the various resistance and mechanisms of targeted therapy available for EGFR mutant NSCLC.

ANAPLASTIC LYMPHOMA KINASE MUTATIONS

Anaplastic lymphoma kinase (ALK) gene encodes a tyrosine kinase receptor of the same name. Similar to other tyrosine kinase receptors, various mutations, amplifications, and rearrangements are being attributed to carcinogenesis. Genetic variations in ALK are seen in 1.9–6.8% cases of NSCLCs. In NSCLCs, *EML4-ALK* fusion gene occurs due to the inversion between *EML4* and *ALK* genes on chromosome 2. ALK fusions are usually found in young, nonsmokers, patients who do not smoke, or smoke infrequently. Both CAP and IASCLC guidelines advocate testing for *ALK* gene rearrangements in NSCLC patients. The detection of ALK mutations can be done using IHC using D5F3/5A4 clone, fluorescence in situ hybridization (FISH), reverse transcriptase-polymerase chain reaction (RT-PCR) and NGS. FISH is the gold standard method for detection of *ALK* gene-rearranged NSCLC. ALK testing using IHC is associated with higher positivity owing to the fact IHC detects ALK protein expression. The first generation of ALK inhibitors, i.e., crizotinib, is validated to be beneficial for ALK rearranged NSCLCs. Crizotinib targets ALK, ROS, and MET oncogene and is considered as first-line therapy. The second- and third-generation include ceritinib, alectinib, brigatinib, ensartinib, and lorlatinib, respectively.[24] TKI resistance in ALK positive NSCLCs is another challenge and resistance mechanisms are elaborated in **Table 8.**[13]

ROS MUTATIONS

ROS proto-oncogene 1 (ROS1) is a receptor tyrosine kinase, located on chromosome 6. ROS1 rearrangement is seen in 0.9–2.6% of NSCLCs, with a significantly higher rate in younger women and nonsmokers.[25] For ROS1 testing, IHC is the recommended screening test and FISH, RT-PCR, and NGS can be done for confirmation. Specific antibody clones are available for ROS1 testing including D4D6, SP384, and 1A1 and specificity is dependent on the clone used.[26] Crizotinib and entrectinib, which are multikinase inhibitors, have been approved as first-line treatment for ROS1 mutated NSCLCs. The resistance mechanisms for TKIs are similar to those of ALK mutated NSCLCs.[25]

PD-1/PD-L1

Programmed cell death protein 1 (PD-1)/programmed death-ligand 1 (PD-L1) immune checkpoint are known to play a crucial role in evasion of tumor immunity.[26] In view of increasing benefits of immunotherapy for cancer management, anti-PD-1/PD-L1 agents have been approved and have shown beneficial effects in advanced NSCLC. The Food and Drug Administration (FDA)-approved biomarker for immune checkpoint inhibitors in lung cancer is PD-L1 expression, which can be detected by IHC.[27,28] The FDA has approved four assays listed in **Table 9** for detection of PD-L1 expression.[29]

TABLE 8: TKI resistance and mechanisms.[13,23]

Mechanism of resistance	On-target resistance			Off-target resistance		
	Gate-keeper mutation	Solvent front mutation	Others	Histomorphological transformation	Downstream signaling pathway abnormalities	Bypass signaling pathway abnormalities
EGFR mutant NSCLC	• EGFR T790M • ALK L1196M • RET V804M	• NTRK G595R • ALK G1202R	• Compound mutations • DFG motif	SCLC transformation	MAPK/PI3K pathway	• MET amplification • FGFR1 amplification
EML-ALK and NSCL			• Compound mutations • Oncogene amplification • Oncogene loss • ALK-exon 23 mutation		• KRAS exon 3 mutation • MET amplification • MEK activation • IGF-1R activation • KRAS G12C mutation • RET fusion • AKT pathway MAPK pathway • TP53 mutation PI3K-JAK-STAT pathway • SRC activation • YAP activation • EGFR activation • KIT activation • HER family activation	

(ALK: anaplastic lymphoma kinase; EGFR: epidermal growth factor receptor; EML: echinoderm microtubule associated protein-like 4; NSCLC: non-small cell lung carcinoma; TKI: tyrosine kinase inhibitor)

TABLE 9: Targeted drugs and IHC clones for PD-L1 expression.[29]

PD-L1 clone	Targeted immunotherapeutic drug
SP142	Atezolizumab
28-8	Nivolumab
22C3	Pembrolizumab
SP263	Durvalumab

(IHC: immunohistochemistry; PD-L1: programmed death-ligand 1)

However, the interpretation of PD-L1 expression on IHC is not straightforward. The variable intensity and pattern of expression of PD-L1 makes it challenging for the pathologist. In addition, the temporal and spatial heterogeneity of PD-L1 expression makes it difficult to be analyzed and interpreted on tiny biopsies and cytological specimens and guidelines for sample adequacy and analysis are important considerations. In NSCLC, tumor proportion score (TPS) is assessed in at least 100 viable, nonoverlapping tumor cells (excluding macrophages and inflammatory cells) and all staining-membranous or cytoplasmic, is counted as positive. The scores range from 1 to ≥50% of positively stained tumor cells in a sample.[30] Fixed guidelines for assessment of PD-L1 expression needs to be formulated for uniform and accurate immunohistochemical assessment.

ROLE OF LIQUID BIOPSY

Owing to the invasiveness of specimen collection of lung cancer diagnosis and recurrence detection, the tissue and cytological samples are often insufficient for molecular tests. The developments in the field of liquid biopsy (LB) genomics have made it as an emerging technique of choice for comprehensive tumor genotyping and metastases detection. Analysis of blood and body fluids for circulating tumor cells (CTCs), circulating tumor DNA (ctDNA), and exosomes are the most commonly employed methods and analysis is performed using PCR-based assays and NGS-based technologies. PCR-based assays have variable sensitivity and can perform single gene testing as opposed to NGS-based assays which have higher sensitivity and can be used for detection of gene rearrangements and amplifications.[31]

The ctDNA refers to the tumor DNA shed by tumor cells in the bloodstream, making peripheral blood, a real-time tumor biomarker. The usage of ctDNA from the peripheral blood for EGFR mutation testing was first approved for patients with advanced NSCLCs. Since then, LB has been used for various stages in NSCLCs. For early-stage NSCLCs, LBs can be used for early detection and for assessment of minimal residual disease, while for advanced and metastatic NSCLCs, LB is being used for diagnosis of recurrent disease, for monitoring response to therapy, and for detection of resistance for TKIs.[32]

Paturu et al. worked on a cohort of 110 treatment naïve NSCLC patients and has postulated that concurrent tissue and blood samples for LB for EGFR mutations is beneficial than tissue alone as LB can pick the missed mutations, if any.[33]

TABLE 10: The Food and Drug Administration (FDA) approved drugs for targeted treatment.[34]

Target	FDA approved drugs
EGFR	Afatinib, entrectinib, erlotinib, gefitinib, and osimertinib
ALK and ROS1	Alectinib, brigatinib, ceritinib, lorlatinib, crizotinib, and entrectinib
KRAS G12C mutations	Sotorasib
NTRK fusions	Larotrectinib
BRAFV600E mutations	Dabrafenib and trametinib
MET exon 14 skipping	Capmatinib and tepotinib
RET fusion	Pralsetinib and selpercatinib
VEGF	Bevacizumab
PD-1 pathway	Atezolizumab, nivolumab, and pembrolizumab
CTLA-4 pathway	Ipilimumab

(ALK: anaplastic lymphoma kinase; EGFR: epidermal growth factor receptor; PD-1: Programmed cell death protein 1; VEGF: vascular endothelial growth factor)

MOLECULAR MARKERS AND TARGETED THERAPY

As discussed, the molecular classification of lung cancer aids to understand the pathogenesis and is crucial for the targeted and personalized treatment. The most effective therapy can be implemented by identification and detection of the genetic profile of the tumor. The FDA has approved drugs for treatment in NSCLCs that target EGFR, ALK, ROS1, KRAS, NTRK fusions, BRAFV600E mutations, RET fusions, and MET exon 14. The implications of immune environment of the tumors have been utilized for the therapeutic potential. The FDA has approved drugs that target vascular endothelial growth factor (VEGF), PD-1 and CTLA-4 pathway. **Table 10** illustrates the list of the FDA approved drugs for treatment of lung cancer.[34]

Figures 1 to 3 represent cytomorphological features along with immunochemistry performed on cell blocks of lung adenocarcinoma, SqCC, and small cell carcinoma, respectively.

Pathologists are pivotal in lung cancer diagnosis, especially with limited tissue samples. Techniques such as fine-needle aspiration cytology (FNAC), Bronchoalveolar lavage (BAL), endobronchial ultrasound-guided transbronchial needle aspiration (EBUS-TBNA), and small biopsies provide sufficient material for comprehensive analysis. Advances in lung cancer molecular testing and targeted therapy have significantly transformed diagnostics and treatment. Techniques such as real-time PCR and NGS enable precise identification of genetic mutations such as EGFR, BRAF, ALK, ROS1, and PD-L1. PD-L1 testing has facilitated the rise of immunotherapies, with pembrolizumab and nivolumab significantly benefiting patients with high PD-L1 expression. The pathologists maximize diagnostic information from minimal tissue, ensuring precise molecular profiling crucial for effective lung cancer targeted therapies. Ongoing research and technological advancements continue to enhance the precision and effectiveness of lung cancer treatments, offering improved survival rates and quality of life.

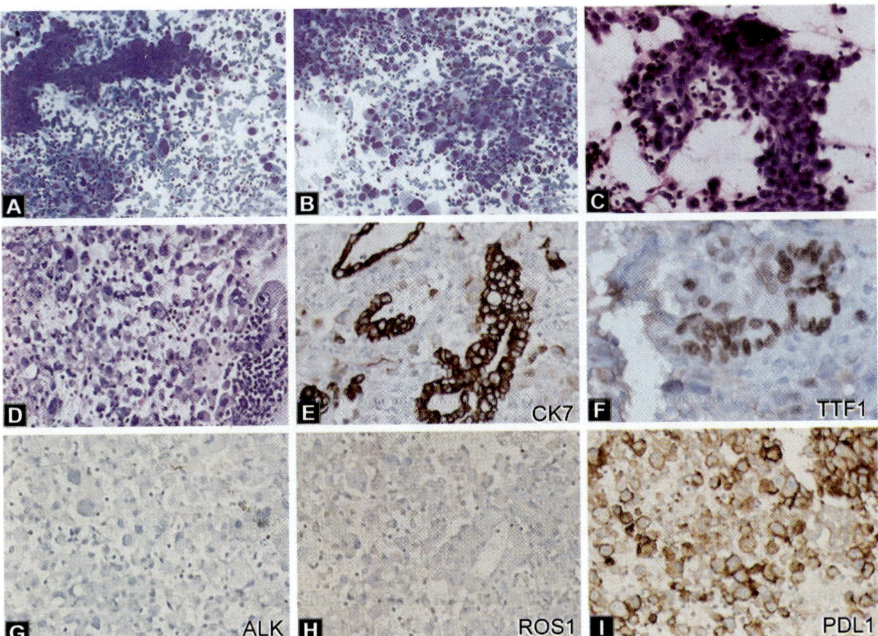

FIGS. 1A TO I: A panel of microphotographs of pulmonary adenocarcinoma. (A to C) Cytology smears showing clusters and singly scattered malignant cells [A and B: MGG ×200; C: hematoxylin and eosin (H&E) ×200]; (D) Cell block showing the same tumor (H&E ×400); (E) Tumor cells are positive for CK7 (ICC ×400); (F) Tumor cells show nuclear positivity for transcription factor-1 (TTF-1) [immunohistochemistry (IHC) ×400]; (G and H) Tumor cells are negative for anaplastic lymphoma kinase (ALK) and ROS1 (IHC ×400); (I) More than 90% tumor cells showing membranous positivity for programmed death-ligand 1 (PD-L1) (IPOX).

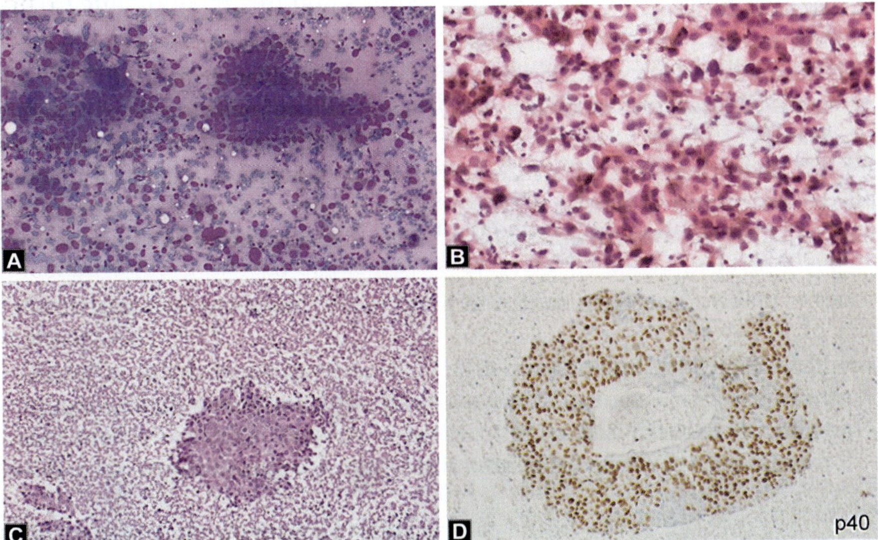

FIGS. 2A TO D: A panel of microphotographs of pulmonary squamous cell carcinoma. (A and B) Cytology smears showing clusters and singly scattered malignant cells [A: MGG ×200; B: hematoxylin and eosin (H&E) ×200]; (C) Cell block showing the same tumor (H&E ×200); (D) Tumor cells show nuclear positivity for p40 [immunohistochemistry (IHC) ×400].

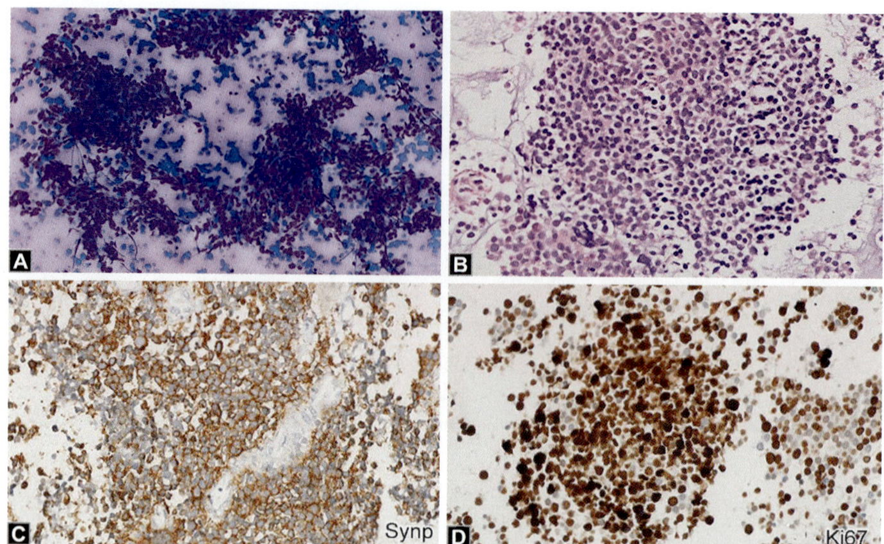

FIGS. 3A TO D: A panel of microphotographs of pulmonary small cell carcinoma. (A) Cytology smear showing predominantly singly scattered small-sized malignant cells showing nuclear molding (A: MGG ×200); (B) Cell block showing the same tumor [hematoxylin and eosin (H&E) ×200]; (C) Tumor cells show cytoplasmic positivity for synaptophysin [immunohistochemistry (IHC) ×200]; (D): Strong nuclear positivity for Ki67 with >95% Ki67 score (IHC ×400).

CONCLUSION

Lung cancer remains a leading cause of death of thoracic tumors and has significantly changed the scenario for diagnosis and treatment of lung cancers. The usage of diverse samples and the latest molecular techniques has paved the way for early accurate diagnosis and targeted therapy for lung cancer. The Cancer Genome Atlas has played a pivotal role in molecular characterization and subtypes are proposed based on the genome alterations. The chapter summarizes the key updates of the 5th edition of the WHO classification of thoracic tumors with special emphasis to algorithmic approach and tabulation of relevant oncogenic drivers. The chapter further discusses the latest trends in the molecular characterization of lung tumors and targeted treatment in detail.

REFERENCES

1. Sung H, Ferlay J, Siegel RL, Laversanne M, Soerjomataram I, Jemal A, et al. Cancer statistics 2020: GLOBOCAN estimates of Incidence and mortality worldwide for 36 cancers in 185 countries. CA Cancer J Clin. 2021;71:209-49.
2. Parikh PM, Ranade AA, Govind B, Ghadyalpatil N, Singh R, Bharath R, et al. Lung cancer in India: Current status and promising strategies. South Asian J Cancer. 2016;5:93-5.
3. World Health Organization. Thoracic Tumours. WHO Classification of Tumours, 5th Edition. Geneva, Switzerland: Geneva, Switzerland; 2021.
4. Lindeman NI, Cagle PT, Aisner DL, Arcila ME, Beasley MB, Bernicker EH, et al. Updated molecular testing guideline for the selection of lung cancer patients for treatment with targeted tyrosine kinase inhibitors: Guideline from the College of American Pathologists,

the International Association for the Study of Lung Cancer, and the Association for Molecular Pathology. J Mol Diagn. 2018;20:129-59.

5. Chang JT, Lee YM, Huang RS. The impact of the Cancer Genome Atlas on lung cancer. Transl Res. 2015;166:568-85.
6. Yoshizawa A, Motoi N, Riely GJ, Sima CS, Gerald WL, Kris MG, et al. Impact of proposed IASLC/ATS/ERS classification of lung adenocarcinoma: prognostic subgroups and implications for further revision of staging based on analysis of 514 stage I cases. Mod Pathol. 2011;24:653-64.
7. Nadal E, Zhong J, Lin J, Reddy RM, Ramnath N, Orringer MB, et al. A microRNA cluster at 14q32 drives aggressive lung adenocarcinoma. Clin Cancer Res. 2014;20:3107-17.
8. The Cancer Genome Atlas Research Network. Comprehensive genomic characterization of squamous cell lung cancers. Nature. 2012;489:519-25.
9. Nicholson AG, Tsao MS, Beasley MB, Borczuk AC, Brambilla E, Cooper WA, et al. The 2021 WHO classification of lung tumors: Impact of advances since 2015. J Thorac Oncol. 2022;17:362-87.
10. Rudin CM, Poirier JT, Byers LA, Dive C, Dowlati A, George J, et al. Molecular subtypes of small cell lung cancer: a synthesis of human and mouse model data. Nat Rev Cancer. 2019;19:289-97.
11. Sivakumar S, Moore JA, Montesion M, Sharaf R, Lin DI, Colón CI, et al. Integrative analysis of a large real-world cohort of small cell lung cancer identifies distinct genetic subtypes and insights into histologic transformation. Cancer Discov. 2023;13:1572-91.
12. Prabhash K, Advani SH, Batra U, Biswas B, Chougule A, Ghosh M, et al. Biomarkers in non-small cell lung cancers: Indian Consensus Guidelines for molecular testing. Adv Ther. 2019;36:766-85.
13. Elshatlawy M, Sampson J, Clarke K, Bayliss R. EML4-ALK biology and drug resistance in non-small cell lung cancer: a new phase of discoveries. Mol Oncol. 2023;17:950-63.
14. Maturu VN, Singh N, Bal A, Gupta N, Das A, Behera D. Relationship of epidermal growth factor receptor activating mutations with histologic subtyping according to International Association for the Study of Lung Cancer/American Thoracic Society/European Respiratory Society 2011 adenocarcinoma classification and their impact on overall survival. Lung India. 2016;33:257-66.
15. John T, Taylor A, Wang H, Eichinger C, Freeman C, Ahn MJ. Uncommon EGFR mutations in non-small-cell lung cancer: a systematic literature review of prevalence and clinical outcomes. Cancer Epidemiol. 2022;76:102080.
16. Midha A, Dearden S, McCormack R. EGFR mutation incidence in non-small-cell lung cancer of adenocarcinoma histology: a systematic review and global map by ethnicity (mutMapII). Am J Cancer Res. 2015;5:2892-911.
17. Melosky B, Kambartel K, Häntschel M, Bennetts M, Nickens DJ, Brinkmann J, et al. Worldwide prevalence of epidermal growth factor receptor mutations in non-small cell lung cancer: A meta-analysis. Mol Diagn Ther. 2022;26:7-18.
18. Nayanar SK, Mohan A, Shenoy P, Saravanan M, Gopinath V, Deepak Roshan VG. Frequency of EGFR mutations in lung adenocarcinoma patients- A study from tertiary cancer center of South India. J Can Res Ther. 2023;19:S712-8.
19. Kumari N, Singh S, Haloi D, Mishra SK, Krishnani N, Nath A, et al. Epidermal growth factor receptor mutation frequency in squamous cell carcinoma and its diagnostic performance in cytological samples: A molecular and immunohistochemical study. World J Oncol. 2019;10:142-50.
20. Batra U, Biswas B, Prabhash K, Krishna MV. Differential clinicopathological features, treatments and outcomes in patients with Exon 19 deletion and Exon 21 L858R EGFR mutation-positive adenocarcinoma non-small cell lung cancer. BMJ Open Resp Res. 2023;10:e001492.
21. Wu YL, Tsuboi M, He J, John T, Grohe C, Majem M, et al. Osimertinib in resected EGFR-mutated non-small-cell lung cancer. N Engl J Med. 2020;383:1711-23.
22. Wu J, Lin Z. Non-small cell lung cancer targeted therapy: Drugs and mechanisms of drug resistance. Int J Mol Sci. 2022;23:15056.

23. Xiao Y, Liu P, Wei J, Zhang X, Guo J, Lin Y. Recent progress in targeted therapy for non-small cell lung cancer. Front Pharmacol. 2023;14:1125547.
24. Rachagiri S, Gupta P, Gupta N, Rohilla M, Singh N, Rajwanshi A. Detection of ALK gene rearrangements in non-small cell lung cancer by immunocytochemistry and fluorescence in-situ hybridization on cytologic samples. Turk Patoloji Derg. 2022;38:16-24.
25. Gendarme S, Bylicki O, Chouaid C, Guisier F. ROS-1 fusions in non-small cell lung cancer: Evidence to date. Curr Oncol. 2022;29:641-58.
26. Remon J, Pignataro D, Novello S, Passiglia F. Current treatment and future challenges in ROS1- and ALK-rearranged advanced non-small cell lung cancer. Cancer Treat Rev. 2021;95:102178.
27. Vathiotis IA, Gomatou G, Stravopodis DJ, Syrigos N. Programmed death-ligand 1 as a regulator of tumor progression and metastasis. Int J Mol Sci. 2021;22:5383.
28. Schoenfeld AJ, Rizvi H, Bandlamudi C, Sauter JL, Travis WD, Rekhtman N, et al. Clinical and molecular correlates of PD-L1 expression in patients with lung adenocarcinomas. Ann Oncol. 2020;31:599-608.
29. Brody R, Zhang Y, Ballas M, Siddiqui MK, Gupta P, Barker C, et al. PD-L1 expression in advanced NSCLC: Insights into risk stratification and treatment selection from a systematic literature review. Lung Cancer. 2017;112:200-15.
30. Jöhrens K, Rüschoff J. The Challenge to the Pathologist of PD-L1 Expression in tumor cells of non-small cell lung cancer- An overview. Curr Oncol. 2021;28:5227-39.
31. Ghosh RK, Pandey T, Dey P. Liquid biopsy: A new avenue in Pathology. Cytopathology. 2019;30:138-43.
32. Rolfo C, Mack P, Scagliotti GV, Aggarwal C, Arcila ME, Barlesi F, et al. Liquid biopsy for advanced NSCLC: A consensus statement from the International Association for the Study of Lung Cancer. J Thorac Oncol. 2021;16:1647-62.
33. Paturu R, Lingaiah R, Kumari N, Singh S, Krishnani N, Srivastava S, et al. Non-small cell lung cancer: Targetable variants in concurrent tissue and liquid biopsy testing in a North Indian cohort. Asian Pac J Cancer Prev. 2023;24:3467-75.
34. Alduais Y, Zhang H, Fan F, Chen J, Chen B. Non-small cell lung cancer (NSCLC): A review of risk factors, diagnosis, and treatment. Medicine (Baltimore). 2023;102:e32899.

3

CHAPTER

Artificial Intelligence in Pathology: Challenges and Opportunities

Pranab Dey

INTRODUCTION

In the year 1956, a bunch of computer scientists first time proposed the concept of artificial intelligence (AI).[1] AI is a field that simulates human intelligence and is helpful in the diagnosis, classification, and future prediction of diseases. Machine learning (ML) and deep learning (DL) are based on artificial neural networks (ANNs). They are the specific methods to reach the target of AI. In the past decades, AI was mainly used to make different complex mathematical models. However, currently, there is significant progress in the applications of AI in the field of pathology.[2] This progress is due to the rapid improvement of the hardware of computers, cheaper storage of data, faster networks, improved operation protocol, and the introduction of whole slide imaging (WSI). AI in pathology has immense potential such as reducing turnaround time, replacing manual work with automation, modernization of the workflow, and most importantly patient-based treatment. Pathologists are the main end users of AI. Despite the significant progress in AI, unfortunately, to date, the routine applications of AI are restricted, and pathologists are unaware of its potential. Moreover, AI faces several roadblocks that need to be removed from its path.

TERMINOLOGIES

Several terminologies are used in the field of AI. **Table 1** explains the terminology. The most commonly used terminology is AI. AI is the simulation of human intelligence with the help of the computer **(Fig. 1)**. An ANN is a computer model that simulates the biological neurons of the human brain. ML is a branch of AI. It utilizes the algorithmic software program of the computer to do the specific task without any external interference. DL or deep neural network (DNN) is a subset of ML. The convolutional network (CNN) is a subset of DL that deals with images. The name convolutional indicates that a single or multiple filter is used here to do multiple convolutions. It reduces the dimension of the images.

TABLE 1: Terminologies used in artificial intelligence.

Terminologies	Definition
Artificial intelligence (AI)	AI is a part of computer science that helps to simulate human intelligent behavior with the help of machine
Machine learning (ML)	ML is a branch of AI that utilizes the commuter algorithmic software and learns from the data to perform the specific tasks. The ML can solve the specific problems without any external interference
Artificial neural network (ANN)	ANN is the computer model that simulates the biological neurons in the brain. It is composed of well-structured multiple layers that consists of input layer, hidden layer, and output layer
Deep learning (DL)	DL is a subset of ML that trains the software to perform specific task. It can handle large amount of data and widely used in image classification and diagnosis
Convolutional network (CNN)	CNN is a subset of DL that deals with images. Here the filter is used to convolute the image. After multiple convolutions, the dimension of the images is reduced
Generative AI	Generative AI means to use the AI to generate text, images, videos, etc

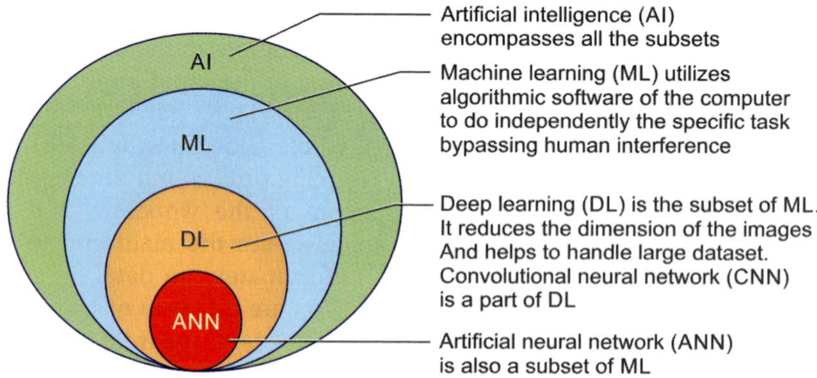

FIG. 1: Relation between the different terminologies of AI.

ARTIFICIAL NEURAL NETWORK AT A GLANCE

Artificial neural network is a computer program that simulates the human brain.[2,3] Just like a biological neuron in the brain, ANN is composed of nodes. The node receives the input signal, processes the entire collected signal, and then transmits the signal to the next node **(Fig. 2)**.

Depending on the intensity of the final summed signals, the node may or may not fire the next node **(Fig. 2)**. ANN consists of three parts: Input layer, hidden layer, and output layer. The input layer receives the signals from the outer environment which means the dataset. These signals are transmitted to the next level of ANN known as the hidden layer (also known as black box). There are

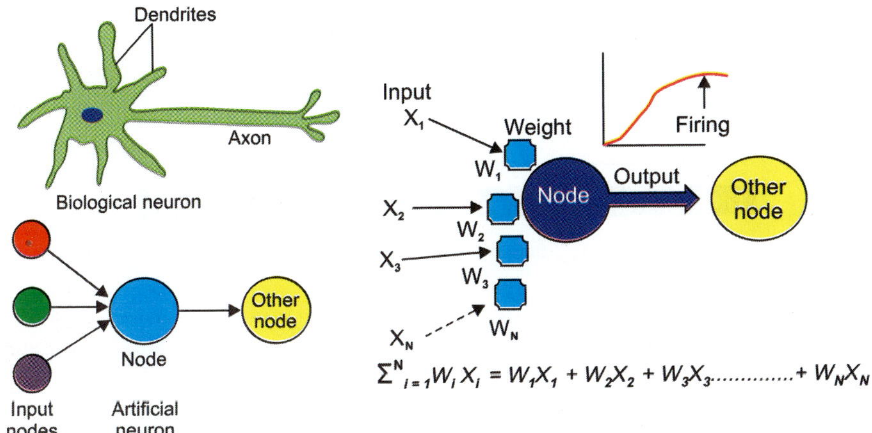

FIG. 2: The comparison of biological neuron and node in artificial neural network is shown. Firing of the next node is also shown.

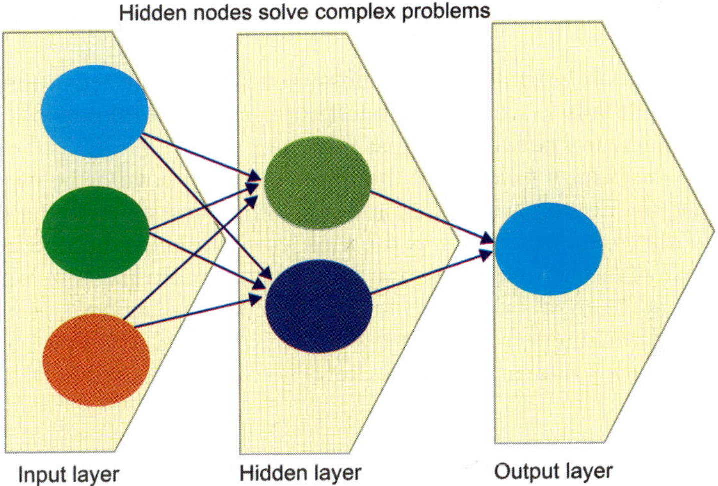

FIG. 3: The architecture of artificial intelligence (AI) is shown.

always multiple hidden layers. The hidden layer gives the capability of ANN to handle complex data. Finally, the signals from the input layer reach the output layer and the result comes out **(Fig. 3)**. A single-layer ANN contains one input, hidden, and output layer with the minimum capability to solve the complex problem. Multiple hidden layers help to solve complex problems. So multilayer perceptron is commonly used in building an ANN model.

ACTIVATION FUNCTIONS

A neural network starts the processing of data by activation functions. Several types of activation functions are used: Linear activation function, threshold

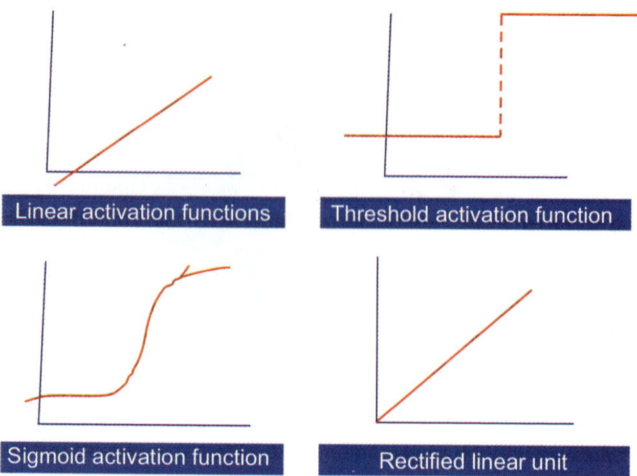

FIG. 4: The different type of activation function.

activation function, sigmoid activation function, and rectified linear unit (ReLU) function **(Fig. 4)**.

- *Linear activation function*: It is not possible to use linear activation function in the ANN. It fails to work in the backpropagation neural network as all the layers of the neural network collapse into one.
- *Threshold activation function*: If the input value is above or below a certain threshold, the neuron is activated and sends the same signal to the next layer.
- *Sigmoid activation function*: It is the most commonly used function in ANN. In the case of the sigmoid activation function, a smooth gradient is generated that prevents "jumps" in output values and a clear prediction is possible.
- *ReLU*: Here the function returns 0 if it receives any negative input, but for any positive value x it returns that value. ReLU is commonly used in DL.

LEARNING

Artificial neural network learns from experiences. The learning experiences come from either an example or the training data. During learning the connection between the neurons is strengthened and it is stored as weight-value. Each iteration of learning changes the connection weights till it reaches a value that gives minimum error in the system. So learning is a continuous process of evaluation of output, adopting weight, and incorporating new input.

The ANN learns by supervised learning, unsupervised learning, and reinforcement learning.

Supervised Learning

In this learning mode, the labeled data with well-defined output is provided to the network. So in each iteration, the ANN gets direct feedback. Supervised learning is mainly applied to predict the future outcome and classification of diseases.

Unsupervised Learning

In the case of the unsupervised learning method, no help is available from the outside, no training data is provided, and no information is available regarding the desired output. So the ANN learns by doing. The unsupervised learning method is used to cluster the data and also to reduce the dimension.

Reinforcement Learning

Here, the random weight is distributed between the neurons and the performance score is measured. According to the performance score, the weight is again shuffled. Overall, it is a slow process of learning and is not encouraged to use in ANN.

DIFFERENT TYPES OF NEURAL NETWORK

The vast categories of ANN are used in the field of pathology. Each category of ANN contains specific advantages and disadvantages.

Convolutional Neural Network

Convolutional neural network (CNN) is widely used in histopathology for classification and diagnosis of malignancy.[4] The steps of CNN are **(Fig. 5)**:

- *Convolution*: Here, the filter with small matrix is superimposed on the image and the convolution operation is done. The convolution operation reduces the dimension of the image.
- *Activation by ReLU*: The nonlinear ReLU operation is done for the activation function.
- *Pooling of images*: The image dimension is further reduced by the pooling of the pixels of the image.

  The convolution, ReLU, and pooling operations are repeated several times to reduce the image dimension significantly.
- *Fully connected network*: Finally fully connected ANN is made which is just like a multilayer perceptron.

Feedforward Neural Networks

In feedforward neural network (FNN), the information flows only in one direction which means from the input layer to the hidden layer to the output layer. As the data moves only in the forward direction it is known as feedforward neural network. FNN is the common type of ANN. It is comprised of three layers which are input, hidden, and output. Each layer is made of neurons or nodes and the node of one layer is connected by all the nodes of the subsequent layer. FNN is trained by the supervised learning process. FNN is commonly used in prediction and classification.

Recurrent Neural Network

Here, the signals are moved in both directions, and weights are regulated both by the current and last time step. Recurrent neural network (RNN) generally

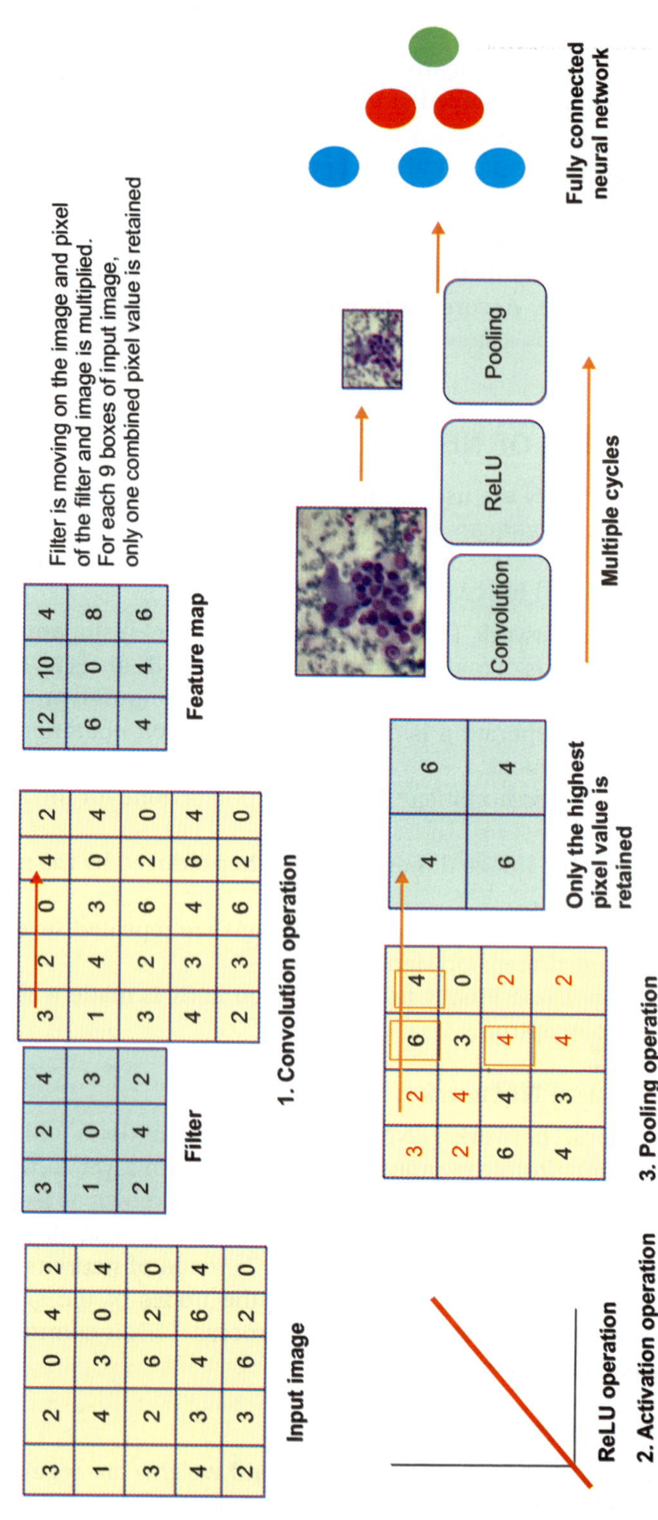

FIG. 5: The steps of convolutional neural network are highlighted.
(ReLU: rectified linear unit)

deals with sequential data and at each point of time, the current data is affected by the previous data because recurrent connections help to pass the information from the previous steps to the next step. RNN retains a hidden state vector that behaves as a form of memory. This hidden state is altered based on the present input and the previous hidden state. RNN is mainly used in time series prediction, natural language processing, and sequence generation such as text generation and music composition.

Recursive Neural Network

Recursive neural networks (ReNNs) work on hierarchical structures and the input nodes may be of variable sizes. ReNN recursively applies the same set of weights to the input. ReNN demonstrates the hierarchical relationship between the inputs data. It is mainly used for the natural language processing.

Hopfield Network

It is a variant of RNN developed by John Hopfield in the year 1982. The Hopfield network can retain and recall patterns and is therefore used in pattern recognition.[5] This network is composed of a single layer of neurons connected with every other neurons. Hopfield network is trained by the Hebbian learning process.

Generative Adversarial Network

Generative adversarial network (GAN) is introduced in the year 2014 by Ian Goodfellow.[6] Here two models are trained simultaneously a generative model (G) and a discriminative model (D). The G model captures the data distribution and D model estimates the probability that the data is real and coming from training data instead of G. Both these models are trained simultaneously by backpropagation. At certain point of training the discriminator cannot distinguish the fake from real data. GAN is applied to produce synthetic data that looks like real data. So synthetic histopathology images can be produced with the help of GAN. GAN can be used to fill the gap in the dataset. It also may help in to augment the limited data to make it robust.

Autoencoders

Autoencoders are used to reduce the dimension of the data. The unsupervised learning technique is used to train the autoencoders. There are two components of autoencoders: Encoder and decoder. The encoder reduces the dimension of the original data and it picks up the most important features of the original data or the pattern of image. The decoder transforms the encoded image back to the original image by reconstructing the compressed image or data. Autoencoders are commonly used for feature extraction from histopathology images and molecular genetic data. It may also help to extract the significant features from the unlabeled data.

APPLICATIONS OF ARTIFICIAL INTELLIGENCE IN PATHOLOGY

Artificial intelligence is applied in large variety of areas such as screening of malignancy, identification of tumor tissue, additional diagnostic information, automated quantification, prognosis prediction, training, and education of pathology **(Flowchart 1)**.

Diagnostic Application of Artificial Intelligence

Large amount of slides are now freely available in The Cancer Genome Atlas (TCGA).[7] These data can be used for training and validation and to make ANN models by the researchers. The ANN is made to identify metastatic carcinoma of breast in the sentinel lymph node in CAMELYON dataset.[8] The CNN with supervised learning was used to make the ANN model. In case of prostatic carcinoma, the Gleason grading was done successfully in PANDA challenge.[9] AI algorithm showed an almost equal confidence interval (CI) (0.862) in comparison to CI of the trained pathologist (0.868). A DL model was made in case of lung carcinoma that can classify the adenocarcinoma from squamous cell carcinomas with sensitivity and specificity of 89% and 93%.[10] In another study, a CNN model identified the tumor area and different histological types of adenocarcinoma of lung such as acinar, lepidic, papillary, micropapillary, and solid.[11] The ANN model and the pathologist's performance were excellent (within 95% CI). In case of colonic cancer,[12] the colonic and gastric adenoma and adenocarcinoma were successfully identified by ANN model. The area under the receiver operating curve was >0.96 in both colonic and gastric tumors.[13]

The various diagnostic algorithms can be incorporated into the digital reporting system. The AI algorithm can tell us the diagnosis from WSI without any external input from the pathologist. The pathologists can verify the initial diagnosis offered by the AI.

Currently, WSI enables to store large number of digital slides. The effective storage may be a free source of vast numbers of histopathology images. Immediate retrieval of these images is possible by AI. AI has the unique power of retrieve similar type of images from a large pathology database. This is known as content-based image retrieval (CBIR). The CBIR is helpful for the pathologist to diagnose rare and difficult cases.[14]

Additional Tools for Diagnosis

The AI algorithms can identify the tumor grade, type, extent, and micrometastasis. Trained pathologists can diagnose tumor metastasis with confidence. However, the assistance of an AI model can help to identify the metastasis more easily and accurately. It has been shown that the pathologist with AI assistance have high sensitivity (91%), compared to pathologist without AI assistance (82%).[15]

Automated Quantification Immunohistochemistry

Automated quantification of the various immunological markers draws attention because it reduces the work time of the pathologists and also provides

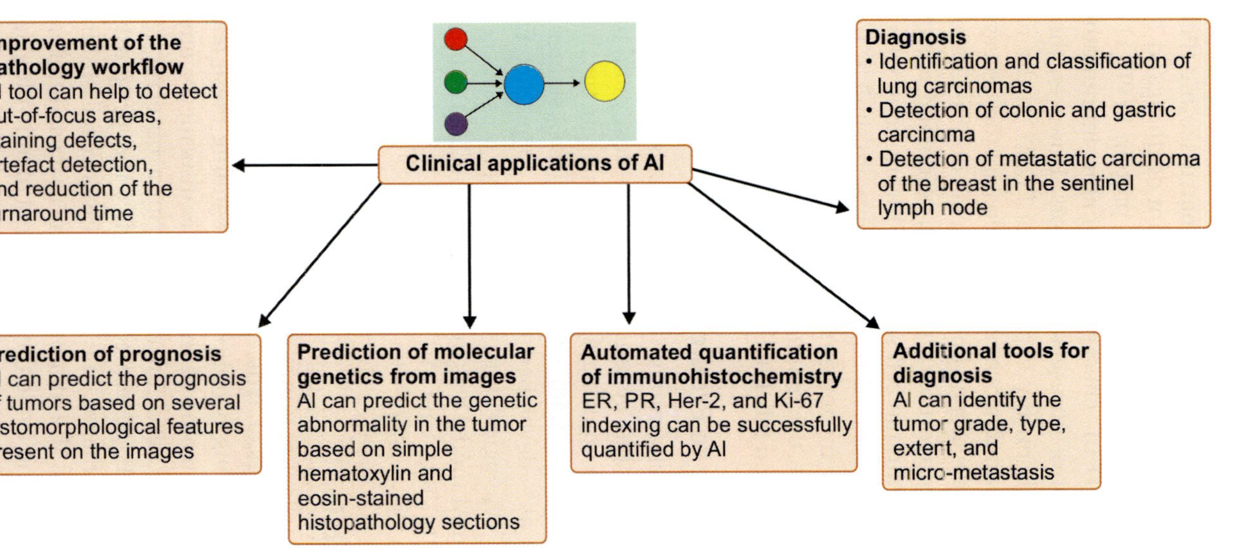

FLOWCHART 1: Clinical applications of artificial intelligence (AI).

objectivity. The various markers of carcinoma of breast such as estrogen receptor (ER), progesterone receptor (PR), human epidermal growth factor receptor-2 (HER2), and Ki-67 indexing can be successfully quantified by AI mode.[16] AutoIHC-Analyzer and ImmunoMembrane software give similar HER2 score between the expert pathologists and the automated scoring (Pearson's correlation coefficient are 0.9448 vs. 0.8521).[17] Program death-ligand 1 (PD-L1) of the tumor cells binds with programmed cell death protein 1 (PD-1) of the cytotoxic T lymphocytes. The PD-L1 checkpoint inhibitor immunotherapy is often helpful in the treatment of unresectable tumors. However, the success of the immunotherapy depends on the expression of PD-L1 in the tumor cells, and PD-L1 scoring on immunohistochemistry helps in the assessment of PD-L1 expression. Puladi et al. developed and AI model to do PD-L1 scoring.[18] All three scoring such as tumor proportion score (TPS), combined positive score (CPS), and tumor-infiltrating immune cell score (ICS) were done with the help of DL software. Both the manual and AI-based scoring were similar. The deep-earning AI model was also used in non-small cell lung carcinomas. The automated scoring matches well with the manual scoring. AI-based automated scoring is objective, reproducible, and reliable.[19]

Artificial Intelligence to Predict Molecular Genetics

The knowledge of the genetic mutation in carcinoma is effective in the treatment. However, tests to demonstrate genetic mutation are costly and time-consuming. Currently, researchers are applying AI to predict the genetic abnormality in the tumor based on a simple hematoxylin and eosin (H&E) stained histopathology section.[20,21] Ishii et al.[21] developed an AI model to predict EGFR and KRAS mutation from the cytological images. This model was successful with high prediction (0.95). An AI model was developed to predict the mutation of STK11, EGFR, FAT1, SETBP1, KRAS, and TP53 with relatively high accuracy [area under the curve (AUC) is 0.733–0.856].[10,22]

Prognosis Prediction

The prognosis of a malignant tumor depends on the several histomorphological features such as histological type, grade, lymphovascular invasion, stromal architecture, and infiltrating lymphocytes. Integrating these features and then predicting the clinical outcome of the tumor is difficult for any human being. There may be subjective variation and inter/intra observer reproducibility.[23] The DL-based model was generated to predict the prognosis of the tumor from the histopathology images. The AI model was successful in the prediction from the graphical images. The AI model is novel as it can interpret and integrate all the different features and avoid the assessment of individual features.

Yuan et al.[24] showed that the spatial distribution of the lymphocytes within a tumor is related with the prognosis of triple negative breast carcinomas. Saltz et al.[25] developed an AI model from the digitized H&E stained images and did computational staining of tumor-infiltrating lymphocytes (TILs). The AI model successfully correlates the TIL maps with the survival, tumor subtypes, and immune profiles of the patient. Wang et al. generated an AI model to predict the prognosis of non-small cell carcinoma of lung from the H&E stained images of tissue microarray slides. Nuclear features of the tumor cells were extracted by the model and predicted the treatment response of nivolumab immunotherapy.[26] In a meta-analysis study by Wessels F et al.[27] the prognostic prediction of prostate and renal cell carcinoma was assessed by AI model. The most of the studies successfully predicted the risk of recurrence and metastasis. However, the studies were mostly early pilot study and there is a need of more elaborative studies.

Overall, the AI model is promising to predict the tumor prognosis from the H&E stained images of the tumor.

Artificial Intelligence to Improve Pathology Workflow

The integration of the AI model with the laboratory information management system, and WSI imaging system may help to improve the overall workflow of the pathology laboratory. The AI tool can help to detect out-of-focus areas, staining defects, artefact detection, and reduction of the turnaround time.[28] AI may help in automated requests for further investigations such as immunohistochemistry or any other special stains in certain cases. Some cases should be reported urgently. AI model can flag such cases so that pathologists report them on a priority basis. Moreover, the AI model may be helpful in screening for malignancy and even primary diagnosis. These may reduce the reporting time of the pathologists.

INTEGRATION OF HISTOPATHOLOGY, MOLECULAR PATHOLOGY, AND ONCOLOGY DATA

The data from next-generation sequencing (NGS) provides significant information such as detection of disease, prognostic prediction, and novel drug discovery. AI models have been developed to identify precise information in individual tumors.[29] The extraction of NGS data by AI is difficult.

The integration of the AI model with the imaging may have immense potential.[30] However, the data of NGS is huge, and mainly in text format. The NGS data may be in gigabytes or terabytes. So it may be difficult to integrate the two systems. Particularly validation and training of the AI will be challenging.

CHALLENGES TO IMPLEMENT ARTIFICIAL INTELLIGENCE

Despite considerable success, AI encounters several roadblocks for its implementation **(Fig. 6)**.

- *Quality of data*: The successful performance of AI depends on the high-quality input data. The input data should be cleaned, well-curated, and high signal-to-noise ratio. Moreover, the data should be huge and comprehensive. The resolution of the images to use as input data is important. The resolution at 20 magnification provides a better result than 40 magnification. Doyle S et al.[31] have shown the decreased performance of AI in prostatic carcinomas when the images are in higher resolution. They noted a stepwise decrease of AUC from 0.84, 0.83, and 0.76 in lower, intermediate, and higher resolution

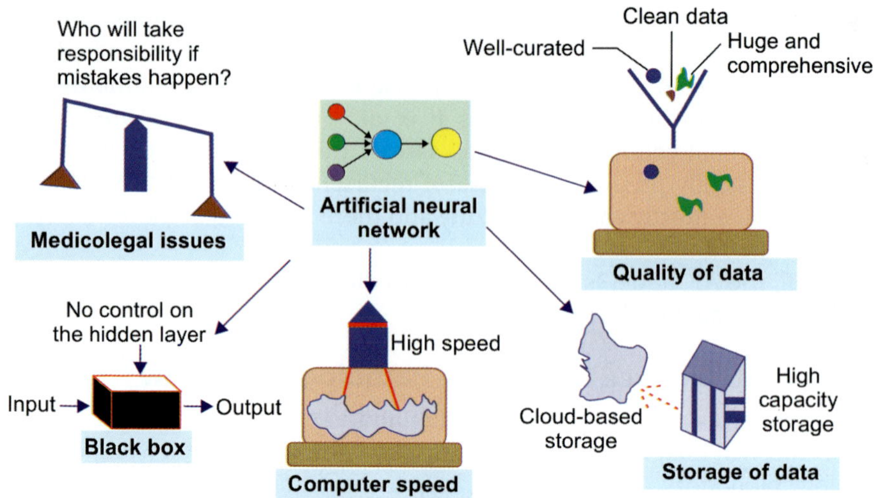

FIG. 6: Challenges to implement artificial intelligence.

of images. In addition to a huge well-curated dataset, it may be necessary to have annoted tumor areas and at time the region of special interest such as mitotic figures or lymphovascular invasion.

- *Data storage*: AI deals with huge data that needs a proper storage capacity of the tumor. Cloud-based storage may be a solution of this problem.
- *Computer speed*: As AI uses CNN and lot of graphical images so the speed of the computer should be high. The huge data processing needs a faster computer.
- *Black box*: The pathologists have no control on the hidden layer or so called "black box". This is a relatively discredit as the black box is a mystery.
- *Data protection*: AI uses data from different individual from different laboratories. Every patient has the right to protect his or her data from misuse. The data should be properly protected so that the commercial company should not use the data.
- *Medicolegal issues*: The diagnosis or management prediction given by AI may not always be right. If AI makes a mistake then who will take the responsibility.

CONCLUSION

In brief, AI is a rapidly growing branch with huge potential in diagnosis, classification, and disease management. Till date, AI has not moved from the research laboratory to a routine clinical laboratory. The implementation of AI in clinical laboratories needs full cooperation between pathologists, oncologists, computer scientists, and bioinformatics. Currently, AI faces several challenges such as data storage, quality of data, computer speed, and medicolegal issues. It is expected that AI will overcome all these problems.

REFERENCES

1. Moor J. The Dartmouth College Artificial intelligence conference: the next fifty years. AI Mag. 2006;27:87-91.
2. Dey P. Artificial neural network in diagnostic cytology. Cytojournal. 2022;19:27.
3. Dey P, Dey R. Artificial neural network—mechanism and application in pathology. Indian J Pathol Microbiol. 2002;45(3):371-4.
4. Dey P. The emerging role of deep learning in cytology. Cytopathology. 2021;32(2):154-60.
5. Massini G. Hopfield Neural Network. Subset Use Misuse. 1998;33(2):481-8.
6. Goodfellow IJ, Mirza M, Xu B, Ozair S, Courville A, Bengio Y. Generative Adversarial Networks. [online] Available from https://arxiv.org/pdf/1406.2661 [Last accessed November, 2024].
7. Cancer Genome Atlas Research Network; Weinstein JN, Collisson EA, Mills GB, Shaw KR, Ozenberger BA, Ellrott K, et al. The Cancer Genome Atlas Pan-Cancer analysis project. Nat Genet. 2013;45(10):1113-20.
8. Litjens G, Bandi P, Ehteshami Bejnordi B, Geessink O, Balkenhol M, Bult P, et al. 1399 H&E-stained sentinel lymph node sections of breast cancer patients: the CAMELYON dataset. Gigascience. 2018;7(6):giy065.
9. Bulten W, Kartasalo K, Chen PC, Ström P, Pinckaers H, Nagpal K, et al.; PANDA challenge consortium. Artificial intelligence for diagnosis and Gleason grading of prostate cancer: the PANDA challenge. Nat Med. 2022;28(1):154-63.
10. Coudray N, Ocampo PS, Sakellaropoulos T, Narula N, Snuderl M, Fenyö D, et al. Classification and mutation prediction from non-small cell lung cancer histopathology images using deep learning. Nat Med. 2018;24(10):1559-67.
11. Wei JW, Tafe LJ, Linnik YA, Vaickus LJ, Tomita N, Hassanpour S. Pathologist-level classification of histologic patterns on resected lung adenocarcinoma slides with deep neural networks. Sci Rep. 2019;9(1):3358.
12. Gertych A, Swiderska-Chadaj Z, Ma Z, Ing N, Markiewicz T, Cierniak S, et al. Convolutional neural networks can accurately distinguish four histologic growth patterns of lung adenocarcinoma in digital slides. Sci Rep. 2019;9(1):1483.
13. Iizuka O, Kanavati F, Kato K, Rambeau M, Arihiro K, Tsuneki M. Deep Learning Models for Histopathological Classification of Gastric and Colonic Epithelial Tumors. Sci Rep. 2020;10(1):1504.
14. Agrawal S, Chowdhary A, Agarwala S, Mayya V, Kamath SS. Content-based medical image retrieval system for lung diseases using deep CNNs. Int J Inf Technol. 2022;14(7):3619-27.
15. Steiner DF, MacDonald R, Liu Y, Truszkowski P, Hipp JD, Gammage C, et al. Impact of Deep Learning Assistance on the Histopathologic Review of Lymph Nodes for Metastatic Breast Cancer. Am J Surg Pathol. 2018;42(12):1636-46.
16. Mungle T, Tewary S, Das DK, Arun I, Basak B, Agarwal S, et al. MRF-ANN: a machine learning approach for automated ER scoring of breast cancer immunohistochemical images. J Microsc. 2017;267(2):117-29.
17. Tewary S, Arun I, Ahmed R, Chatterjee S, Mukhopadhyay S. AutoIHC-Analyzer: computer-assisted microscopy for automated membrane extraction/scoring in HER2 molecular markers. J Microsc. 2021;281(1):87-96.
18. Puladi B, Ooms M, Kintsler S, Houschyar KS, Steib F, Modabber A, et al. Automated PD-L1 Scoring Using Artificial Intelligence in Head and Neck Squamous Cell Carcinoma. Cancers (Basel). 2021;13(17):4409.
19. Kapil A, Meier A, Zuraw A, Steele KE, Rebelatto MC, Schmidt G, et al. Deep Semi supervised generative learning for automated tumor proportion scoring on NSCLC tissue needle biopsies. Sci Rep. 2018;8:17343.
20. Ninomiya H, Hiramatsu M, Inamura K, Nomura K, Okui M, Miyoshi T, et al. Correlation between morphology and EGFR mutations in lung adenocarcinomas Significance of the micropapillary pattern and the hobnail cell type. Lung Cancer. 2009;63(2):235-40.

21. Ishii S, Takamatsu M, Ninomiya H, Inamura K, Horai T, Iyoda A, et al. Machine learning-based gene alteration prediction model for primary lung cancer using cytologic images. Cancer Cytopathol. 2022;130(10):812-23.
22. Unger M, Kather JN. Deep learning in cancer genomics and histopathology. Genome Med. 2024;16(1):44.
23. Wulczyn E, Steiner DF, Xu Z, Sadhwani A, Wang H, Flament-Auvigne I, et al. Deep learning-based survival prediction for multiple cancer types using histopathology images. PLoS One. 2020;15(6):e0233678.
24. Yuan Y. Modelling the spatial heterogeneity and molecular correlates of lymphocytic infiltration in triple-negative breast cancer. J R Soc Interface. 2015;12(103):20141153.
25. Saltz J, Gupta R, Hou L, Kurc T, Singh P, Nguyen V, et al. Spatial Organization and Molecular Correlation of Tumor-Infiltrating Lymphocytes Using Deep Learning on Pathology Images. Cell Rep. 2018;23(1):181-93.e7.
26. Wang X, Barrera C, Velu P, Bera K, Prasanna P, Khunger M, et al. Computer extracted features of cancer nuclei from H&E stained tissues of tumor predicts response to nivolumab in non-small cell lung cancer. J Clin Oncol. 2018;36(15_suppl):12061.
27. Wessels F, Kuntz S, Krieghoff-Henning E, Schmitt M, Braun V, Worst TS, et al. Artificial intelligence to predict oncological outcome directly from hematoxylin and eosin-stained slides in urology. Minerva Urol Nephrol. 2022;74(5):538-50.
28. Kohlberger T, Liu Y, Moran M, Chen PC, Brown T, Hipp JD, et al. Whole-Slide Image Focus Quality: Automatic Assessment and Impact on AI Cancer Detection. J Pathol Inform. 2019;10:39.
29. Richesson RL, Sun J, Pathak J, Kho AN, Denny JC. Clinical phenotyping in selected national networks: demonstrating the need for high-throughput, portable, and computational methods. Artif Intell Med. 2016;71:57-61.
30. Dlamini Z, Francies FZ, Hull R, Marima R. Artificial intelligence (AI) and big data in cancer and precision oncology. Comput Struct Biotechnol J. 2020;18:2300-11.
31. Doyle S, Feldman M, Tomaszewski J, Madabhushi A. A boosted Bayesian multiresolution classifier for prostate cancer detection from digitized needle biopsies. IEEE Trans Biomed Eng. 2012;59(5):1205-18.

4

CHAPTER

Molecular Mechanism of Metastasis in Cancer

Gargi Kapatia, Akriti Jindal

INTRODUCTION

Metastasis can be defined as the development of secondary tumors distant from the primary site and may occur within or distant from the organ of origin.[1,2] It is the leading cause of treatment failure in cancer patients and results in death in over 90% of patients.[3] A large number of cancer cells enter the bloodstream daily in patients, however, only <0.1% of these cells successfully metastasize.[1] For metastasis to occur, cancer cells should undergo a cascade of upregulation and downregulation of various complex mechanisms, e.g., disengagement of few cancer cells from the primary site, travel to target organs through the circulation, adapt to new microenvironment at secondary locations, and evade the immune system[1] **(Flowchart 1)**. Invasion of adjacent tissues and establishment of tumor cells at distant sites to form metastases is characteristic of malignant tumors.[1,2] The time from initial diagnosis to metastasis varies widely among different types of malignant tumors.[2] This variability depends on factors such as the type of cancer, its aggressiveness, genetic mutations, and individual patient characteristics. For instance, breast cancers can show a delayed metastatic relapse, while lung cancers often metastasize within the first year of diagnosis[2] **(Box 1)**. Moreover, cancers tend to spread to specific organs depending on its type, a phenomenon known as tumor-type-specific organ tropism.[2] These variations in timing and location of metastasis suggest that specific mechanisms play a vital role in the metastatic processes.[2] Understanding the dynamics of metastasis can help in identifying molecular therapy targets to halt or potentially reverse cancer growth and metastasis.[1]

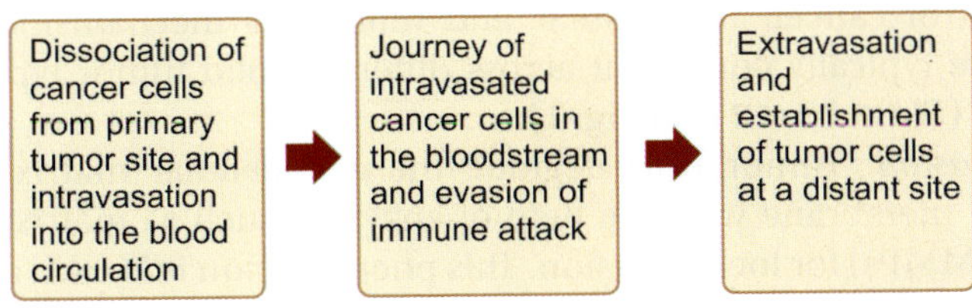

FLOWCHART 1: Key steps in metastasis of malignant tumors to distant sites.

BOX 1 Examples of time variation in metastasis of different cancers.

- *Breast cancer*: Some types, like triple-negative breast cancer, tend to metastasize more quickly than others, like hormone receptor-positive breast cancer
- *Prostate cancer*: This can be slow-growing, with some patients living for many years without metastasis, while other more aggressive forms can spread faster
- *Lung cancer*: Small-cell lung cancer often metastasizes quickly, while non-small-cell lung cancer might have a slower progression
- *Melanoma*: This skin cancer can vary greatly; some forms spread rapidly, while others may take years to metastasize
- *Colorectal cancer*: The progression can be variable, with some cases metastasizing quickly and others remaining localized for a longer time

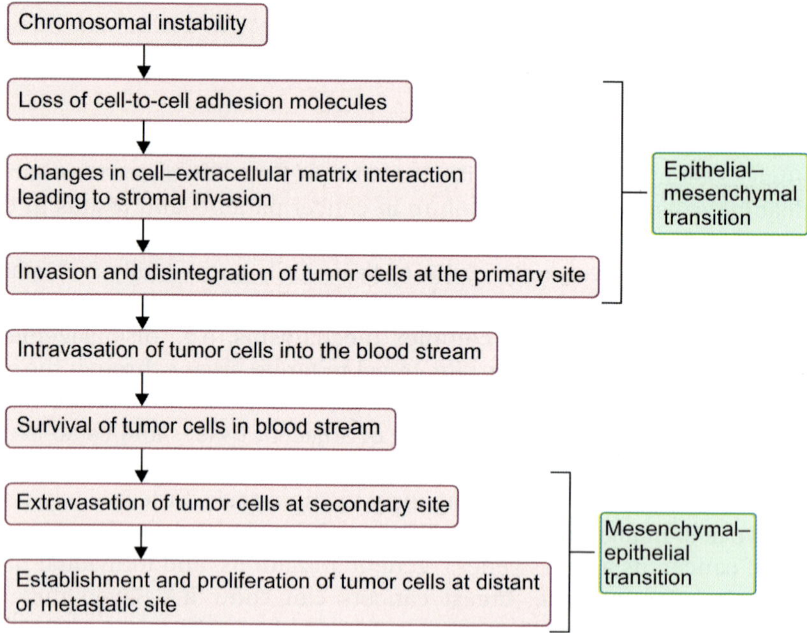

FLOWCHART 2: Cascade of events occurring in metastasis of malignant tumors.

MOLECULAR MECHANISM OF METASTASIS OF CANCER CELLS

While the genetic factors driving tumor formation can differ significantly between various types of cancer, the cellular and molecular mechanisms underlying metastasis are typically consistent across different solid tumor types.[4-14] These steps include **(Flowchart 2 and Fig. 1)**:

1. *Local invasion:* Tumor cells degrade the extracellular matrix (ECM) and basement membrane with the help of enzymes such as matrix metalloproteinases (MMPs) for local invasion. This phenomenon is known as epithelial–mesenchymal transition (EMT).

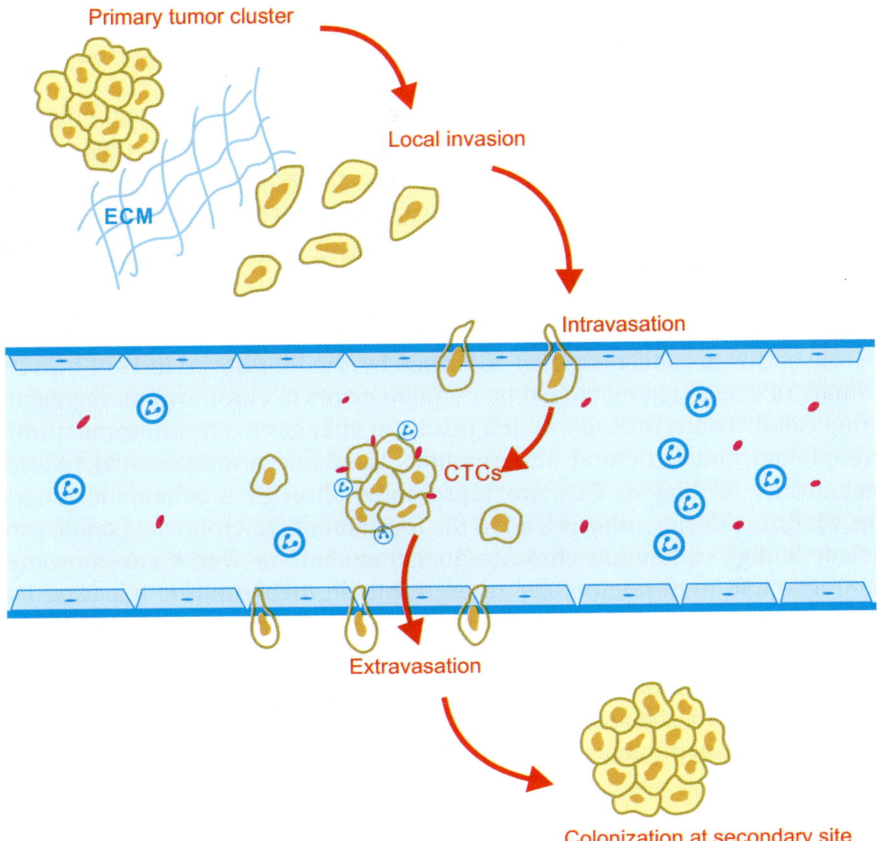

FIG. 1: Step-by-step path of tumor cells from their primary site of origin to metastatic site. (CTCs: circulating tumor cells; ECM: extracellular matrix)

2. *Intravasation:* After degradation of ECM and basement membrane; the tumor cells move into blood circulation or lymphatic system. This involves breaching the wall of blood vessels or lymphatic vessels, often facilitated by changes in cell adhesion molecules like E-cadherin.
3. *Survival in circulation:* Tumor cells must survive the shear forces and immune surveillance in the blood circulation or lymphatic system. They often do this by forming clusters with platelets or other cells, which can help protect them.
4. *Extravasation*: Tumor cells exit the blood circulation or lymphatic system at their target organ. This process is like intravasation and involves interaction with the endothelial cells lining the blood vessels.
5. *Colonization*: After extravasation, tumor cells must adjust to the new microenvironment of target organ and begin to proliferate. This step is often the most challenging, as the new environment may be inhospitable to the tumor cells initially.

6. *Angiogenesis*: To support growth at the new site, cancer cells often induce the formation of new blood vessels. This is typically mediated by signaling molecules such as vascular endothelial growth factor (VEGF).

These steps are regulated by a complex interplay of genetic and epigenetic changes, signaling pathways, and interactions with the tumor microenvironment. Despite the differences in the genetic drivers of various cancers, the general process of metastasis tends to follow these common steps.

STEP 1: CHROMOSOMAL INSTABILITY

The initial trigger of metastasis of tumor cells begins with chromosomal instability.[1] The role of CIN in cancer was first described by Theodor Boveri in 1914.[5] CIN is a hallmark of cancer characterized by frequent errors in chromosome segregation during cell division (mitosis), which results in changes in chromosome number (aneuploidy) and structural abnormalities (genomic arrangements).[6] Various mechanisms leading to CIN are represented through a schematic diagram **(Fig. 2)**. Errors during mitosis lead to the formation of micronuclei (small, extra-nuclear bodies containing chromosomal fragments or whole chromosomes). The fragile nature of micronuclei often results in their rupture, releasing DNA into the cell cytoplasm. This activates the cGAS-STING (cyclic GMP–AMP synthase-stimulator of interferon genes) pathway, a DNA-sensing mechanism present in cell cytoplasm, and subsequently triggers noncanonical nuclear factor-κB (NF-κB) signaling downstream, which is involved in inflammatory responses and can influence cancer progression.[5,7]

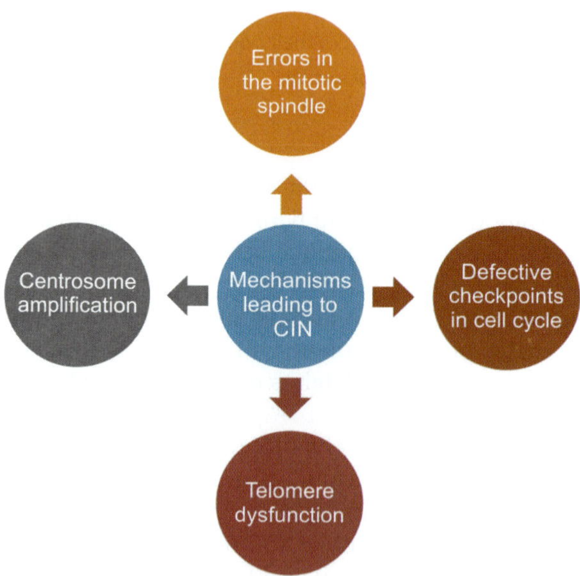

FIG. 2: Mechanisms leading to chromosomal instability (CIN).

Role of Chromosomal Instability in Cancer

- It is observed in many cancers and is associated with poor prognosis and resistance to treatment.
- Tumors with high CIN often show increased aggressiveness and the ability to adapt to different environment, aiding in metastasis.
- CIN can generate novel mutations that provide a selective advantage to cancer cells under various conditions, including treatment pressures.

Therapeutic Implications

- Targeting the mechanisms underlying CIN, such as stabilizing the mitotic spindle or enhancing checkpoint function, could provide therapeutic avenues.
- Exploiting the high level of stress and DNA damage in CIN-positive cancer cells, e.g., by using drugs that further increase DNA damage, may selectively kill these cells.
- *Targeting cGAS-STING pathway*: Modulating this pathway could provide therapeutic benefits by enhancing antitumor immunity or reducing inflammation-driven cancer progression.
- *NF-κB inhibition*: Inhibiting noncanonical NF-κB signaling might reduce cancer-related inflammation and tumor growth.

STEP 2: EPITHELIAL–MESENCHYMAL TRANSITION

During both normal tissue homeostasis and malignant transformation, there is dynamic interplay between epithelial cells or tumor cells and their surrounding microenvironment, including fibroblasts, endothelial cells and the ECM. In the context of cancer, these interactions become deregulated, but they still play a crucial role in tumor progression.[6]

Epithelial–mesenchymal transition is highly complex reversible cellular process by which epithelial cells, which are normally stationary and tightly interconnected to each other as well as their surrounding ECM, undergo biochemical changes (loss of apical–basal polarity, loss of intercellular junctions, and adherence to basement membrane) to acquire a mesenchymal phenotype, enabling them to migrate, invade, and spread to distant sites.[1,8] The role of EMT was first described for the cell growth and differentiation in early embryonic development.[9]

The epithelial cells have some inherent properties, which include maintained apical basal polarity, cell–cell interactions via adhesion molecules (such as E-cadherin and cytokeratin) within various types of intercellular junctions such as tight junctions (TJ), adherens junctions (AJ), gap junctions (GJ), and desmosomes.[9]

For both the epithelial cells (during homeostasis) and cancer cells to migrate, they must undergo the following changes:[9]

- *Activate genes for differentiation*: Initiate pathways necessary for transitioning to a more motile state.
- *Slow down proliferation*: Reduce cell division rates to focus on migration.

- *Activate anti-apoptotic mechanisms*: Prevent cell death since differentiation can trigger pathways of apoptosis.
- *Alteration of cellular characteristics*: Transition from their epithelial phenotype to mesenchymal state.
- *Downregulate cell-to-cell attachment receptors*: Reduce receptors that maintain strong cell-to-cell adhesion (i.e., loss of epithelial markers like E-cadherin, occludin, claudin, cytokeratin, and increased expression of mesenchymal markers like vimentin, N-cadherin, EMT transcription factors).
- *Degrade cell-to-cell junctions*: Break down junctions to allow detachment and migration.
- *Activate surface proteases*: Utilize enzymes for the degradation of ECM for easier movement.

Epithelial–mesenchymal transition is a biological process classified into three types:[10]

- *Type 1 EMT*: Related with embryogenesis, supporting processes such as pro-intestinal formation, neural crest stratification, mesodermal formation, and endocardial morphogenesis.
- *Type 2 EMT*: Involved in tissue regeneration, playing a key role in wound healing and inflammation by restoring epithelial and endothelial integrity.
- *Type 3 EMT*: Linked to cancer progression, contributing to tumor invasion and metastasis.

Each type of EMT serves distinct functions, from developmental processes to healing and pathological conditions like cancer.[10]

In addition to EMT, various other mechanisms are also operating in parallel fashion resulting in cell migration and distant metastasis, e.g., passive shedding of tumor cells, intratumoral vascular migration of tumor cells, etc.[8]

The major limitation of EMT lies in the fact that it is a transient, dynamic, multidimensional and reversible phenomenon, thus making it difficult to demonstrate in vitro by various methods.[8] Different cancer cell populations exhibit unique epigenetic patterns that drive these changes, each with distinct clinical implications. The complexity of EMT and metastasis is due to cancer cells heterogeneity—not all tumor cells undergo EMT simultaneously, and not all cells that have undergone EMT will successfully metastasize.[9]

The EMT transition is regulated by multiple transcription factors, noncoding RNAs, epigenetic regulators, various growth factors, and signaling pathways, thus making it a complex mechanism to understand.[1,8] Till date the exact mechanism of EMT is still not completely elucidated.

Mechanism of Epithelial–Mesenchymal Transition (Flowchart 3)

Loss of Cellular Junctions (Fig. 3)

The intercellular junctions span from the apical surface to the basal membrane of the cells and includes TJ, AJ, GJ, desmosomes, and integrins.[11]

- In cancer cells, several pathways gets activated due to hypoxia (hypoxia inducing factor pathway, NOTCH pathway) and release of growth factors due

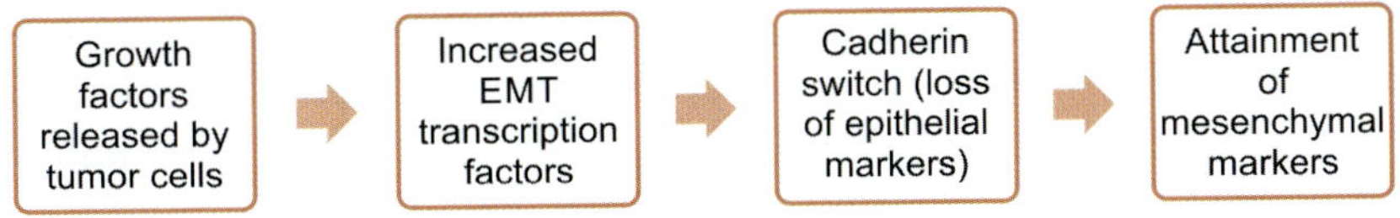

FLOWCHART 3: Steps involved in epithelial–mesenchymal transition.

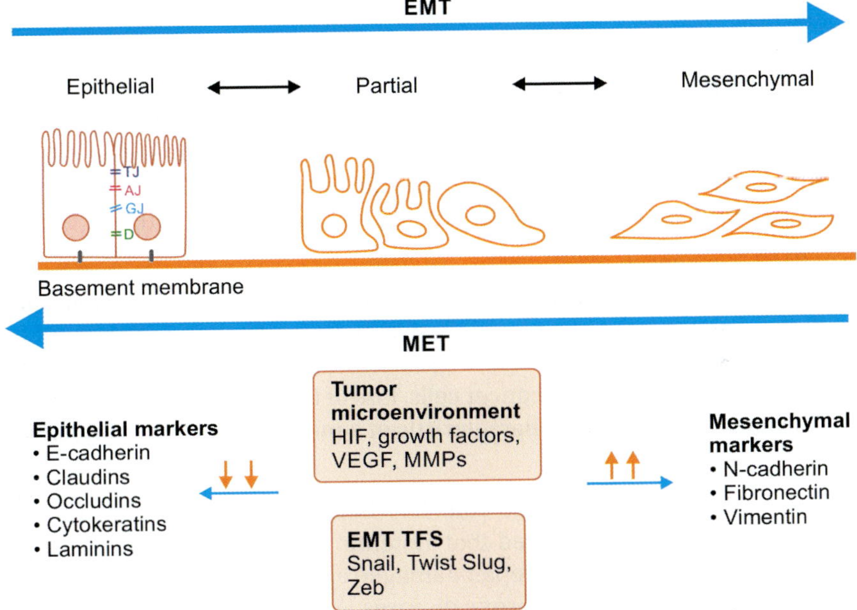

FIG. 3: Phenotypic changes in cancer cells during epithelial–mesenchymal transition (EMT) and mesenchymal–epithelial transition (MET) and the associated factors present in tumor microenvironment involved in these transitions.

(AJ: adherens junction; D: desmosomes; GJ: gap junction; HIF: hypoxia-induced factor; MMPs: matrix metalloproteinases; TJ: tight junction; VEGF: vascular endothelial growth factor)

to inflammation [hepatocyte growth factor (HGF), epidermal growth factor (EGF), transforming growth factor beta (TGF-β), NF-κB].[9]

- It causes upregulation of various transcription factors of EMT in the tumor microenvironment like SNAIL, ZEB1, TWIST, and Slug.[6,11]
- SNAIL family includes SNAIL1, SNAIL2, and SNAIL3, which downregulate epithelial-related genes and upregulate mesenchymal-related genes.
- *BHLH family*: TWIST1 and TWIST2 also play roles in the repression of epithelial-related genes and activation of mesenchymal-related genes.
- *ZEB family*: ZEB1 and ZEB2 bind to E-box sequences in gene promoters potentially either activating or repressing transcription.
- *MicroRNAs (miRNAs)*: These noncoding RNAs can bind to target messenger RNAs (mRNAs), resulting in their degradation or inhibition of translation, thereby regulating gene expression post-transcriptionally.

- *It further induces "cadherin switch"*: Epigenetic silencing of epithelial cell junction proteins through hypermethylation and histone deacetylation leading to suppression of E-cadherin, claudins, occludins, ZO-1 (epithelial phenotypic markers) on the cell surface and escalated expression of N-cadherin, fibronectin, vimentin on the cell surface (mesenchymal phenotypic markers).[9,11]
- It helps the cancer cells to attain more motility, thus helping in migration and metastasis.

Bone Morphogenetic Protein 7

It is a member of TGF-β superfamily, which plays a significant role in regulating EMT processes. As discussed above TGF-β is involved in EMT of tumor cells, thus facilitating metastasis. However, on the contrary, BMP-7 has been seen to reverse the EMT by upregulating E-cadherin protein, a key epithelial marker.[11]

Role of BMP-7 in cancer:

- *Breast cancer*: Reduced expression of BMP-7 in breast carcinoma is associated with the development of a more invasive mesenchymal phenotype and bone metastasis.[11]
- *Prostate cancer*: In prostate cancer cells, loss of BMP-7 is linked with increased invasiveness and motility, characteristic of a mesenchymal phenotype.[11]

Therapeutic potential of BMP-7:

- *Renal fibrosis*: Its therapeutic role has been demonstrated in mice with severe renal fibrosis. It showed that systemic administration of recombinant BMP-7 can reverse EMT and repair damaged epithelial structures, highlighting its therapeutic potential in fibrotic diseases.[11]

Role of Matrix Metalloproteinases in Epithelial–Mesenchymal Transition

The ECM is a network of macromolecules that shapes the characteristics of cells, impacting their propensity to grow and move.[1] ECM-degrading enzymes remodel the ECM to maintain tissue homeostasis in response to physiological and pathological triggers. MMPs are a group of zinc-dependent endopeptidases that play a role in breaking down ECM components, facilitating the invasion of migratory cells into surrounding stroma.[1] In addition to invasion, MMPs are crucial in cell proliferation, cell survival, immune responses, and angiogenesis. Here are key aspects of MMPs involvement in tumor metastasis:

- *Degradation of ECM and basement membrane*: MMPs degrade various components of the ECM and basement membrane, facilitating tumor cells to invade into surrounding tissues and enter the blood circulation or lymphatic system. Disintegration of E-cadherin by MMPs generates a fragment, sE-cad, which helps in tissue dissociation and EMT.[9]
- *Tumor cell migration*: By breaking down ECM barriers, MMPs create pathways that allow tumor cells to migrate from the primary tumor site to distant organs.

- *Angiogenesis*: MMPs contribute to angiogenesis by releasing ECM-bound growth factors and creating space for new vessels to grow. This supports tumor growth and provides a channel for metastatic cells to enter the circulation.
- *Modulation of cell-cell and cell-ECM interactions*: MMPs alter cell-cell and cell-ECM interactions, aiding in the detachment of tumor cells from one another and promoting their invasion into surrounding tissues.
- *Evasion of immune surveillance*: MMPs can modulate the immune response by degrading cytokines and chemokines, helping tumor cells evade immune surveillance and destruction.
- *Creation of pre-metastatic niche*: MMPs are involved in the development of pre-metastatic niche, which is microenvironment in the metastatic organ that is supportive of the survival and growth of metastatic tumor cells.

STEP 3: INTRAVASATION

Intravasation is defined as the access of cells in the blood vessels or lymphatic channels **(Fig. 1)**. It can be physiological or pathological. Physiological example includes entry of dendritic cells into the circulation from skin or mucous membranes in cases of adaptive immune responses.[12] Pathological examples of intravasation includes passage of tumor cells into the blood circulation, which results in the formation of circulating tumor cells (CTCs) in the vascular and lymphatic spaces.[12] These cells have the potential to form metastatic deposits at distant sites, depending on their number. For example, studies have shown that metastatic breast cancer patients with a CTC count above 5 CTCs per 7.5 mL of blood tend to have worse clinical outcomes.[12] This suggests that higher numbers of CTCs are linked with more aggressive disease and poorer prognosis.[12]

Tumor cell intravasation into lymphatic vessels occurs more readily as compared to blood vessels because of the following reasons:

- Lymphatic vessels lack the firm inter endothelial junctions as found in blood vessels.
- Lymph flow is slower compared to blood circulation.

During the process of intravasation, several changes occur within the tumor cells to overcome several physical and biological barriers, including the basement membrane, ECM, and the endothelial cell layer of blood vessels:

- *Changes in cytoskeletal activity*: Tumor cells undergo alterations in their cytoskeletal activity in response to chemoattractant gradients. This means that they reorganize the structure of their cytoskeleton, which is the network of protein filaments that gives the cell its shape, provides mechanical support, and facilitates movement.[13]
- *Upregulation of integrins and adhesion molecules*: There is evidence showing that tumor cells upregulate integrins and other adhesion molecules, which help tumor cells to better attach to endothelial cells lining the vascular channels or lymphatics. This enhanced adhesion is critical for the tumor cells to breach the vessel walls and enter the circulation.[13]

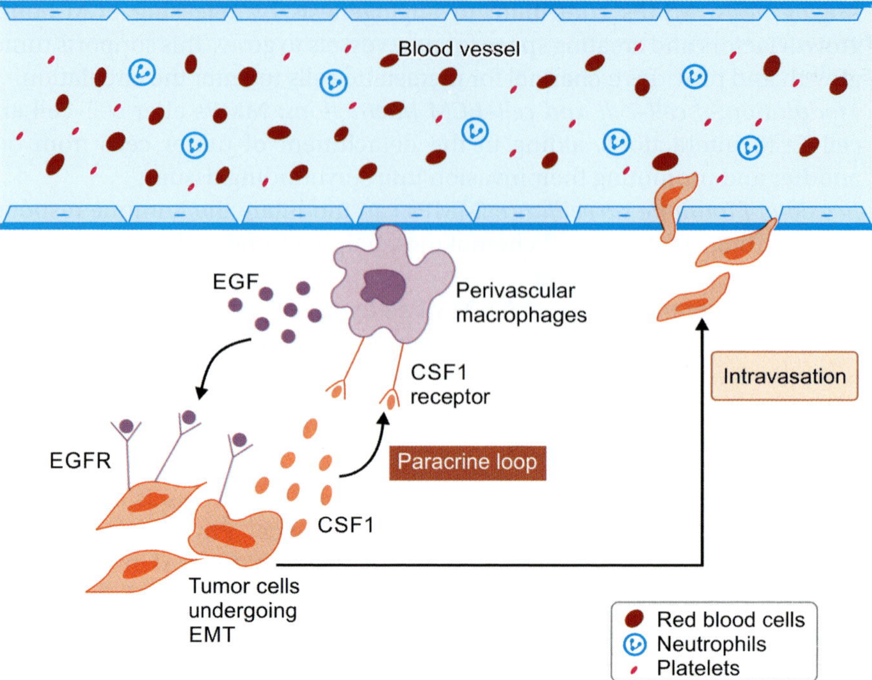

FIG. 4: Process of intravasation of tumor cells, which involves the formation of paracrine loop between tumor cells and perivascular macrophages.

(CSF1: colony-stimulating factor; EGF: epidermal growth factor; EGFR: epidermal growth factor receptor; EMT: epithelial–mesenchymal transition)

These changes enable tumor cells to move through the ECM toward blood or lymphatic vessels, adhere to endothelial cells, and eventually invade into the vasculature to initiate the process of metastasis.[13]

Mechanism of Intravasation of Tumor Cells into the Vascular/Lymphatic Channels

The migration of tumor cells toward blood vessels involves tumor-associated macrophages located in perivascular regions. Using the murine breast cancer model, it was demonstrated that perivascular macrophages secrete EGF, the receptor of which is located on the tumor cells undergoing EMT, thus acting as a chemoattractant for the tumor cells. In response, these tumor cells secrete colony-stimulating factor 1 (CSF1), the receptor of which is located on perivascular macrophages. CSF1 stimulates the macrophages to release more EGF, thus completing this paracrine loop **(Fig. 4)**. Wyckoff et al. reported that intravasation of tumor cells could be prevented by drugs, which inhibit epidermal growth factor receptor (EGFR) signaling, thus supressing intravasation described earlier. Increased expression of CSF1 by tumor cells and EGF by macrophages serves as an independent prognostic marker and is linked to poorer prognosis.[12]

One of the key mechanisms involved in intravasation is the physical deformation or "nuclear squeezing" of tumor cells to pass through all the barriers. It is aided by EMT, which has been described in detail earlier in this chapter.[1]

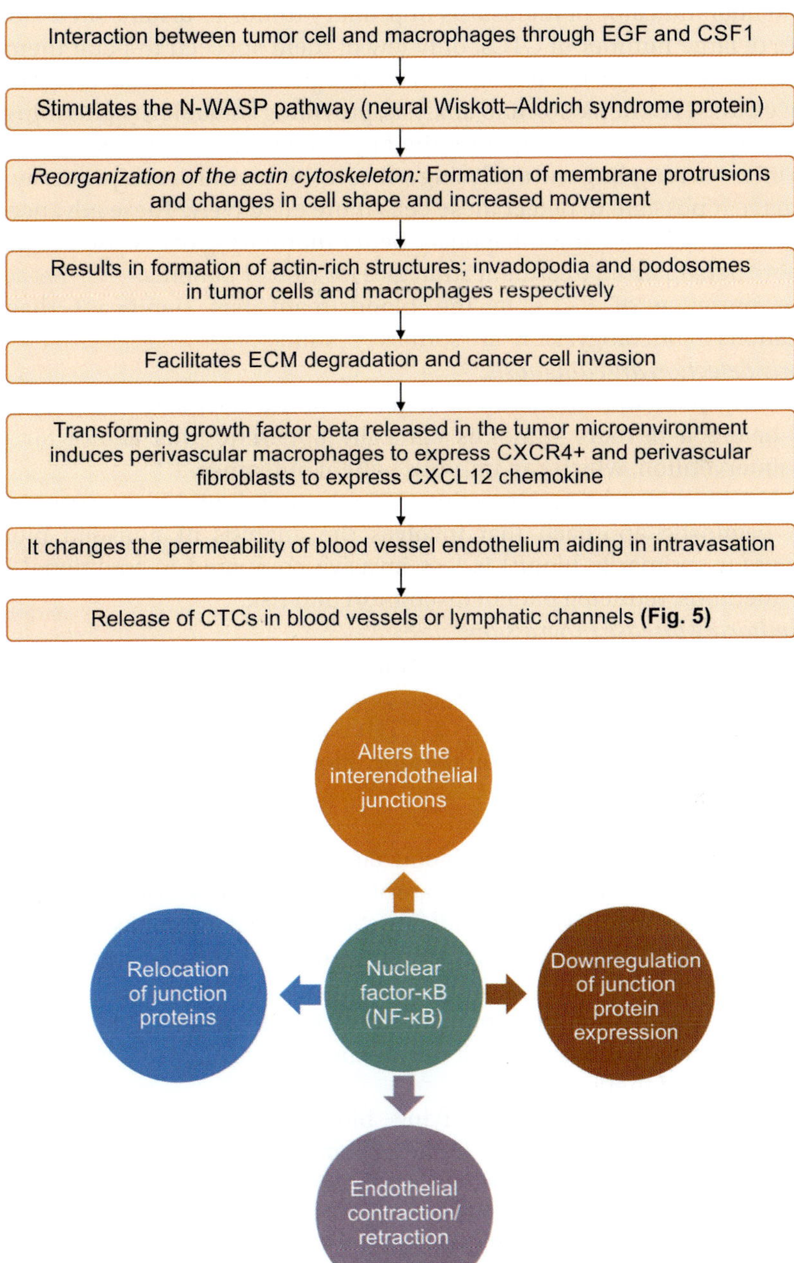

FIG. 5: Mechanism of increased endothelial cell permeability by factors secreted from circulating tumor cells (CTCs).

Circulating Tumor Cells

Once carcinoma cells intravasate into the bloodstream, they can travel throughout the body via the venous and arterial systems.[14] The presence of CTCs in the blood is a potential indicator of metastasis of primary tumor to distant sites. However, in spite of large number of CTCs, only few of them succeed to plant themselves at other sites to form metastasis.[15] Technological advances have significantly improved the CTCs detection and analysis, providing valuable insights into cancer progression and potential targets for therapy.[14] Techniques such as liquid biopsy, which involves sampling and analyzing nonsolid biological tissue, primarily blood, have made it possible to detect these cells more effectively. These advancements offer the potential for earlier diagnosis, better monitoring of disease progression, and more personalized treatment strategies for cancer patients.

The presence of CTCs in the bloodstream has significant diagnostic implications in oncology. Here are some key points:

- *Early detection and diagnosis*:[16]
  - Early detection: CTCs can be detected in the early stages of cancer, even before a primary tumor is clinically apparent. This allows for earlier intervention, which can improve patient outcomes.
  - Noninvasive testing: Detecting CTCs through liquid biopsy (noninvasive diagnostic approach that involves the analysis of nonsolid biological tissue, primarily blood) is less invasive compared to traditional biopsy methods, reducing patient discomfort and risk.
- *Monitoring disease progression*:[17]
  - Real-time monitoring: Regular monitoring of CTC levels can provide real-time data on disease progression or response to treatment.
  - Treatment efficacy: Changes in CTC count can indicate how well a patient is responding to a particular therapy, allowing for adjustments in treatment plans.
- *Prognostic value*:[18]
  - Prognosis: CTCs count in blood circulation can serve as a prognostic marker. Higher counts of CTCs are often correlated with a poorer prognosis.
  - Metastasis risk: CTCs can indicate the potential for metastasis, providing valuable information for risk assessment and management strategies.
- *Personalized medicine*:[16]
  - Molecular characterization: Analyzing CTCs can reveal specific genetic and molecular characteristics of a patient's cancer, aiding in the selection of targeted therapies.
  - Therapeutic targets: Identifying biomarkers on CTCs can help in developing personalized treatment plans, enhancing the efficacy of targeted treatments. Developing strategies to disrupt CTC clusters could also reduce metastatic potential.
- *Minimal residual disease (MRD)*:[19]
  - Detection of residual disease: After treatment, the presence of CTCs can indicate MRD, which is the minor quantities of cancer cells that persist in the body and could potentially cause a relapse.
  - Post-treatment surveillance: Monitoring CTCs post-treatment can help detect recurrence at an early stage, allowing for prompt intervention.

- *Research and development*:
  - Biological insights: Studying CTCs provides insights into the biology of tumor evolution and metastasis, contributing to cancer research and the development of new therapeutic strategies.
  - Clinical trials: CTC detection and analysis are increasingly used in clinical trials to evaluate the efficacy of new treatments and understand their mechanisms of action.

Overall, the diagnostic implications of CTCs are vast and hold great promise for improving cancer diagnosis, monitoring, and treatment, ultimately leading to better patient outcomes.

STEP 4: SURVIVAL IN THE CIRCULATION

Circulating tumor cells face significant challenges in surviving within the bloodstream. Hemodynamic shear forces and the innate immune system, particularly natural killer (NK) cells, pose substantial threats to these cells. However, carcinoma cells have developed a mechanism to overcome these obstacles by exploiting normal blood coagulation processes.[14,20]

Mechanism of Survival of Circulating Tumor Cells in Blood

- *Platelet coating*: CTCs can recruit platelets to form an embolus with platelets shielding them from shear forces and immune detection. It is facilitated by the expression of tissue factor and/or L- and P-selectins on the surface of the tumor cells. The platelets coat the tumor cells, shielding them from damage and immune attack.[14,21] This platelet-mediated protection allows the tumor cells to survive longer in the circulation and increases the likelihood of arresting at distant tissue sites.[14,20]
- *Role of neutrophils*: Neutrophils tend to slow down the neutrophil-associated tumor clusters due to direct interaction with endothelial cells with the help of selectins and integrins. Beta 2 integrins of neutrophils (LFA1, MAC1) bind with their receptor intercellular adhesion molecule 1 (ICAM-1) present on the endothelium to form firm attachment with the endothelial cells. Neutrophils also facilitate the extravasation of tumor cells through endothelium due to their primary function as immune cells.[15] It has been seen that cases in which neutrophil-associated CTC clusters are found, show more aggressive clinical course with lower rates of progression free survival.[15] The detailed molecular analysis showed that in these cases there is upregulation of several genes, which promotes cellular growth. One of the important mutations occur as inactivating mutation of *TLE1* gene (transcriptional repressor), which leads to increased response to inflammation and stimulates formation of inflammation induced tumor clusters. Neutrophil extracellular traps (NETs), cytokines like interleukin 6 (IL-6), IL-1b along with granulocyte–macrophage colony-stimulating factor (GM-CSF) also play a notable role in the interaction of CTCs with neutrophils.
- *EMT*: EMT enhances the ability of CTCs to invade tissues and resist apoptosis (programmed cell death). It also confers stem cell-like properties to CTCs, increasing their ability to survive in the bloodstream and initiate new tumors at distant sites.[22]

- *Expression of immune evasion molecules*: Some CTCs express programmed death ligand 1 (PD-L1) and binds with programmed cell death 1 (PD-1) present on immune cells, thereby inhibiting their activity and allowing CTCs to evade immune destruction.
- *Formation of clusters*: CTCs can travel as clusters rather than individual cells, enhancing their survival, as clusters have increased resistance to apoptosis and immune attack compared to single CTCs.[23]
- *Metabolic adaptations*: CTCs can undergo metabolic reprogramming to survive in the nutrient-limited conditions of the bloodstream.

STEP 5: EXTRAVASATION OF TUMOR CELLS

When CTCs in the vascular or lymphatic channels reach their target organ, they undergoe the next step of extravasation. It involves invasion and proliferation of tumor cells in the target organ to develop a full-blown metastatic deposit.

For the process of extravasation, tumor cells must adhere to endothelial cells at the secondary site to cross the barrier formed by endothelial cells. Extravasation through venules is comparatively easier as compared to arterioles due to higher permeability and leakiness of endothelial cells.[15] The following main steps are involved in the process of extravasation of tumor cells **(Flowchart 4)**:

1. Margination (deviation of cells from the mainstream to the periphery of vessels)
2. Rolling (tumor cells come in contact with the endothelial cells, which reduces the speed of cells)
3. Extravasation through the blood vessel at target site

Abovementioned steps are also seen in case of extravasation of leukocytes in cases of inflammation with the help of selectins and integrins. However, tumor cells may or may not use the same molecules for extravasation.[15]

Tumor cells may opt for the following mechanism for the process of extravasation:[24]

- *Adhesion to the endothelium*: Tumor cells in the bloodstream must first adhere to the endothelial cells lining the blood vessels of the target organ. This adhesion is mediated by selectins (help in the initial weak interaction of tumor cells with endothelium), integrins (facilitate stronger adhesion between tumor cells and endothelium), cell adhesion molecules [molecules like ICAM-1 and vascular cell adhesion molecule 1 (VCAM-1) on endothelial cells interact with their corresponding ligands on tumor cells, aiding in firm adhesion].
- *Transendothelial migration*: Once adhered, tumor cells undergo transendothelial migration, also known as diapedesis. This involves cytoskeletal remodeling, i.e., tumor cells and endothelial cells undergo cytoskeletal changes to allow tumor cells to squeeze through the endothelial junctions.

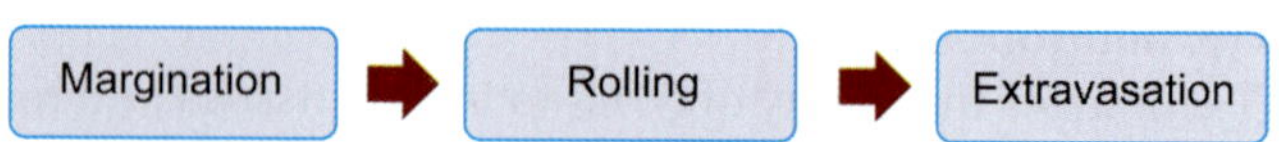

FLOWCHART 4: Key steps involved in the extravasation of tumor cells.

- *Basement membrane degradation*: After passing through the endothelium, tumor cells encounter the basement membrane. To penetrate this barrier, tumor cells secrete proteolytic enzymes, such as MMPs (degrade components of the basement membrane and ECM, facilitating invasion by tumor cells).
- *Survival and proliferation in the target organ*: For successful metastasis, tumor cells must adapt to the new microenvironment of the target organ. This involves angiogenesis (mediated by VEGF), immune evasion (mediated by TGF-β), and interaction with stromal cells.

Organotropism

The metastatic process of cancer is a highly complex phenomenon. While it was once believed that metastases primarily occurred in the first capillary bed encountered due to mechanical trapping of CTCs, this explanation does not fully account for the observed patterns of all the metastasis. For instance, the frequent occurrence of bone metastases in prostate cancer suggests that additional factors help in the selective homing of tumor cells to specific organs.[25] According to the "seed and soil" hypothesis, which was first proposed by Stephen Paget in 1889, metastases only develop at those sites (the "soil") where the tumor cells (the "seeds") are suitably adapted for survival and proliferation. This idea emphasizes that not all organs are equally conducive to metastatic growth and that both the conditions—characteristics of tumor cells as well as the microenvironment of the potential metastatic site play crucial roles in the establishment and growth of secondary tumors.[26]

This selective homing can be attributed to various factors, including:

- *Organ-specific microenvironment*: Certain organs provide a conducive environment for tumor cells to thrive. For instance, bone marrow provides a niche that supports the proliferation of prostate cancer cells.[27]
- *Chemokines and receptors*: Chemokines are signaling proteins that can attract cancer cells to specific sites. Cancer cells often express receptors for these chemokines, which guide them to organs where these chemokines are abundant.[28] For example, tumor cells of breast carcinoma commonly demonstrate the chemokine receptor CXCR4, which binds to its ligand CXCL12, abundantly produced in organs like the lungs, liver, and bone marrow.
- *Adhesion molecules*: Tumor cells express specific adhesion molecules that allow them to attach more easily to the endothelial cells of certain organs.[28] For example, the interaction between selectins on endothelial cells and their ligands on tumor cells can promote metastasis to the liver and other organs.
- *Growth factors*: Some organs produce growth factors that promote the survival and proliferation of metastatic cancer cells. For example, bone tissue produces growth factors that support the prostate cancer cells proliferation.[28]
- *Immune evasion*: Certain organs may offer a more favorable environment for tumor cells to overcome immune attack.[28]

Understanding these factors can shed light on the mechanisms of metastasis and might pave the way for creating targeted treatments to prevent or treat metastatic disease.

Examples of organotropism:
- *Breast cancer*: It frequently metastasize to bones, lungs, liver, and brain.
- *Prostate cancer*: It tends to metastasize to bones.
- *Lung cancer*: It often spreads to the brain, bones, liver, and adrenal glands.
- *Colorectal cancer*: It commonly metastasizes to the liver and lungs.

STEP 6: SEEDING AND PROLIFERATION OF TUMOR CELLS IN THE TARGET ORGAN AT DISTANT SITE

Following extravasation, tumor cells must acclimatize to the foreign micro-environment of target metastatic organ and escape from immune responses to form a metastatic deposit.[14] According to some authors, tumor cells establish a premetastatic niche at the metastatic site.[29] A premetastatic niche is a specific environment in distant organs or tissues that has been altered to become conducive to the growth and survival of metastatic tumor cells even before those cells arrive. This concept suggests that primary tumors can send signals like cytokines, growth factors, and extracellular vesicles to distant sites in the body to support cancer cell adhesion, immune evasion, angiogenesis, and remodeling of the ECM.[30,31] After the tumor cells reach their target organ, they start attaining the epithelial phenotype and lose their mesenchymal phenotype **(Fig. 3)**. This phenomenon is known as mesenchymal–epithelial transition (MET) and is a pivotal step in the terminating stages of development of metastasis.[15] All the steps described above for the EMT process occur in reverse direction for MET with re-expression of E-cadherin being the hallmark of MET.[15]

CONCLUSION

The molecular mechanisms involved in tumor metastasis are intricate and multifaceted, comprising of a series of coordinated steps that enable tumor cells to spread from the primary site to distant sites. Key processes such as chromosomal instability, EMT, and the cellular heterogeneity of tumors contribute to the complexity of metastasis. Not all tumor cells undergo simultaneous EMT, and even those that do may not always successfully establish secondary tumors. Furthermore, the potential of cancer cells to evade immune attack, survive in circulation, and colonize new environments adds additional layers of complexity. Despite significant progress in our understanding, many aspects of metastasis remain elusive. Future research should aim to dissect these processes at a deeper level, identify biomarkers for early detection, and develop targeted therapies to inhibit metastatic spread. Advancing our knowledge in these areas is essential for improving prognosis and treatment strategies for cancer patients, ultimately leading to better clinical outcomes and prolonged survival.

REFERENCES

1. Fares J, Fares MY, Khachfe HH, Salhab HA, Fares Y. Molecular principles of metastasis: a hallmark of cancer revisited. Signal Transduct Target Ther. 2020;5(1):28.
2. Khan SU, Fatima K, Malik F, Kalkavan H, Wani A. Cancer metastasis: Molecular mechanisms and clinical perspectives. Pharmacol Ther. 2023;250:108522.
3. Hanahan D, Weinberg RA. The hallmarks of cancer. Cell. 2000;100(1):57-70.
4. Woodhouse EC, Chuaqui RF, Liotta LA. General mechanisms of metastasis. Cancer. 1997;80(S8):1529-37.
5. Bakhoum SF, Ngo B, Laughney AM, Cavallo JA, Murphy CJ, Ly P, et al. Chromosomal instability drives metastasis through a cytosolic DNA response. Nature. 2018;553(7689):467-72.
6. Hsu MY, Meier F, Herlyn M. Melanoma development and progression: a conspiracy between tumor and host. Differentiation. 2002;70(9-10):522-36.
7. Coquel F, Silva MJ, Técher H, Zadorozhny K, Sharma S, Nieminuszczy J, et al. SAMHD1 acts at stalled replication forks to prevent interferon induction. Nature. 2018;557(7703):57-61.
8. Mittal V. Epithelial Mesenchymal Transition in Tumor Metastasis. Annu Rev Pathol. 2018;13:395-412.
9. Heerboth S, Housman G, Leary M, Longacre M, Byler S, Lapinska K, et al. EMT and tumor metastasis. Clin Transl Med. 2015;26;4:6.
10. Huang Y, Hong W, Wei X. The molecular mechanisms and therapeutic strategies of EMT in tumor progression and metastasis. J Hematol Oncol. 2022;15(1):129.
11. Martin TA, Ye L, Sanders AJ, Lane J, Jiang WG. Cancer invasion and metastasis: molecular and cellular perspective. Madame Curie Bioscience Database. Austin: Landes Bioscience. 2000-2013.
12. Zavyalova MV, Denisov EV, Tashireva LA, Savelieva OE, Kaigorodova EV, Krakhmal NV, et al. Intravasation as a Key Step in Cancer Metastasis. Biochemistry (Mosc). 2019;84(7):762-72.
13. Chiang SP, Cabrera RM, Segall JE. Tumor cell intravasation. Am J Physiol Cell Physiol. 2016;311(1):C1-C14.
14. Valastyan S, Weinberg RA. Tumor metastasis: molecular insights and evolving paradigms. Cell. 2011;147(2):275-92.
15. Di Russo S, Liberati FR, Riva A, Di Fonzo F, Macone A, Giardina G, et al. Beyond the barrier: the immune-inspired pathways of tumor extravasation. Cell Commun Signal. 2024;22(1):104.
16. Alix-Panabières C, Pantel K. Clinical Applications of Circulating Tumor Cells and Circulating Tumor DNA as Liquid Biopsy. Cancer Discov. 2016;4(6):650-61.
17. Pantel K, Alix-Panabières C. Circulating Tumor Cells in Cancer Patients: Challenges and Perspectives. Trends Mol Med. 2010;16(9):398-406.
18. Cristofanilli M, Budd GT, Ellis MJ, Stopeck A, Matera J, Miller MC, et al. Circulating Tumor Cells, Disease Progression, and Survival in Metastatic Breast Cancer. N Engl J Med. 2004;351:781-91.
19. Zhu L, Xu R, Yang L, Shi W, Zhang Y, Liu J, et al. Minimal residual disease (MRD) detection in solid tumors using circulating tumor DNA: a systematic review. Front Genet. 2023;14:1172108.
20. Joyce JA, Pollard JW. Microenvironmental regulation of metastasis. Nat Rev Cancer. 2009;9(4):239-52.
21. Gay LJ, Felding-Habermann B. Contribution of platelets to tumour metastasis. Nat Rev Cancer. 2011;11(2):123-34.
22. Alizadeh AM, Shiri S, Farsinejad S. Metastasis review: from bench to bedside. Tumour Biol. 2014;35(9):8483-523.

23. Sarioglu AF, Aceto N, Kojic N, Donaldson MC, Zeinali M, Hamza B, et al. A microfluidic device for label-free, physical capture of circulating tumor cell clusters. Nat Methods. 2015;12(7):685-91.
24. Reymond N, d'Água BB, Ridley AJ. Crossing the endothelial barrier during metastasis. Nat Rev Cancer. 2013;13(12):858-70.
25. Bogenrieder T, Herlyn M. Axis of evil: molecular mechanisms of cancer metastasis. Oncogene. 2003;22(42):6524-36.
26. Paget S. The distribution of secondary growths in cancer of the breast. Lancet. 1889;133(3421):571-3.
27. Chambers AF, Groom AC, MacDonald IC. Dissemination and growth of cancer cells in metastatic sites. Nat Rev Cancer. 2002;2(8):563-72.
28. Müller A, Homey B, Soto H, Ge N, Catron D, Buchanan ME, et al. Involvement of chemokine receptors in breast cancer metastasis. Nature. 2001;410(6824):50-6.
29. Psaila B, Lyden D. The metastatic niche: adapting the foreign soil. Nat Rev Cancer. 2009; 9(4):285-93.
30. Peinado H, Zhang H, Matei IR, Costa-Silva B, Hoshino A, Rodrigues G, et al. Pre-metastatic niches: organ-specific homes for metastases. Nat Rev Cancer. 2017;17(5):302-17.
31. Sceneay J, Smyth MJ, Möller A. The pre-metastatic niche: finding common ground. Cancer Metastasis Rev. 2013;32(3-4):449-64.

5

CHAPTER

Pan-Cancer Biomarkers

Pranab Dey

INTRODUCTION

The vast information obtained from next-generation sequencing (NGS) in all tumors, has led us to the detection of various molecular markers that are common between multiple types of tumors. These common molecular markers are shared in different tumors and genotype-directed therapies are available in those cases. These common sharing molecular alterations are known as pan-cancer biomarkers. These pan-cancer biomarkers may show alteration of DNA sequence, copy number changes, and gene rearrangement. The identification of pan-cancer biomarkers is important in early diagnosis, selection of specific treatment, and prediction of prognosis.

Recently, Food and Drug Administration (FDA) has approved specific targeted therapy based on molecular alterations irrespective of the histopathological diagnosis of the primary site; e.g., neurotrophic receptor kinase (*NTRK*) inhibitor mutation is seen in secretory carcinoma of the breast, infantile fibrosarcoma, non-small-cell carcinoma, and so on. FDA has approved larotrectinib and entrectinib tyrosine kinase inhibitors in *NTRK* gene fusion irrespective of the primary histopathological diagnosis.[1,2]

Similarly, microsatellite instability (MSI) is noted in endometrioid carcinoma of the uterus, pancreatic cancer, and gastroesophageal cancer. Pembrolizumab is approved by FDA in case of MSI.[3]

Therefore, the actionable mutational changes can be treated by an FDA-approved specific drug. According to this current strategy, the identification of different molecular markers is important and the laboratory should find out all the clinically important genes in the different cancers. NGS is the preferred method to detect pan-cancer biomarkers. Besides that, other techniques such as immunohistochemistry (IHC), fluorescent in situ hybridization (FISH), reverse transcriptase polymerase chain reaction (RT-PCR), and multiplex PCR can be employed to detect these biomarkers **(Table 1)**. **Table 2** highlights the FDA-approved pan-cancer biomarkers in different tumors, drugs, and indications for treatment.

TABLE 1: Different tests to detect the pan-cancer markers.

Tests	Material requirement	Turnaround time	Sensitivity	Advantages	Disadvantages
IHC	Only one unstained slide	1 day	95%	Easy, cheap	May not be accurate, may miss genetic mutation with retained functional activity
FISH	Three unstained slides	1–3 days	High, >96%	Easy, visible detection	Knowledge of the altered genes needed
RT-PCR	10 µg RNA/10–20 unstained slides	1 week	Usually >96%	Rapid, specific	Needs to know the altered genes
DNA-NGS	50–250 ng of DNA/10–20 unstained slides	2 weeks	Variable	Provides complete panel of altered genes	Time-consuming, costly, complex procedure
RNA-NGS	200–250 ng of RNA/10–20 unstained slides	1–2 weeks	Very high	Provides a comprehensive assessment of functioning gene	Time-consuming, complex, costly

(DNA-NGS: DNA next-generation sequencing; FISH: fluorescent in situ hybridization; IHC: immunohistochemistry; RNANGS: RNA next-generation sequencing; RT-PCR: reverse transcriptase polymerase chain reaction)

FDA-APPROVED PAN-CANCER BIOMARKERS

Many pan-cancer molecular biomarkers have emerged in the last few years. However, FDA-approved pan-cancer molecular biomarkers are limited in number.

The following pan-cancer biomarkers are approved by FDA:

- MSI
- Tumor mutational burden (TMB)
- NTRK fusions
- Programmed death ligand 1/programmed cell death 1 (PD-L1/PD-1)

Microsatellite Instability

Microsatellites are short sequences of DNA consisting of 1–6 base pair units and are repeated in tandem array throughout the human genome. The length of the microsatellites may vary between individuals. Microsatellites are present both in coding and noncoding DNA regions. The mutation rate of microsatellites is higher than other genomic regions as they are prone to undergo errors in replication due to slippage by DNA polymerase. MSI is characterized by the alteration of the number and size of microsatellite sequences that are not present in the corresponding germline DNA. Normally DNA mismatch repair (MMR) proteins, MLHI, PMS2, MSH2, and MSH6 help to correct the mutational errors **(Fig. 1)**. The mutational defects in the DNA MMR system is responsible for

TABLE 2: Food and Drug Administration (FDA) approval of the drugs and diseases in pan-cancer biomarkers.

Pan-cancer biomarkers	Diseases	Approved drugs	Indications	Tests to detect
Microsatellite instability (MSI)	Colorectal carcinoma, endometrioid carcinoma of the uterus, prostate carcinoma, gastrointestinal carcinoma, pancreatic carcinoma	Pembrolizumab	Locally advanced, metastatic, or recurrent tumors	IHC, RT-PCR NGS
Tumor mutation burden (TMB)	Colorectal cancer, urothelial cancer, and many other solid tumors	Pembrolizumab	Unresectable or metastatic non-dMMR/ MSI TMB-H tumor that has progressed on prior therapy with no alternative treatment options	Whole-exome sequencing and gene-targeted sequencing by NGS
Neurotrophic receptor kinase (*NTRK*) fusions	Mammary analog secretory carcinoma of the breast fibrosarcoma, congenital mesoblastic nephroma, papillary thyroid carcinoma	larotrectinib and entrectinib	Locally advanced or metastatic cancer with *NTRK* gene fusion	IHC, FISH, DNA-NGS, RNA-NGS
Programmed death ligand 1	Non-small-cell lung carcinomas (NSCLCs), gastric carcinoma, cervical carcinomas, head–neck squamous cell carcinoma, urothelial carcinoma	Pembrolizumab, nivolumab, atezolizumab	Adjuvant treatment following resection and platinum-based chemotherapy for stage IB (T2a ≥ 4 cm), II, or IIIA NSCLC, and for the unresectable, metastatic and recurrent tumors	IHC

(dMMR: deficient mismatch repair; FISH: fluorescent in situ hybridization; IHC immunohistochemistry; NGS: next-generation sequencing; RT-PCR: reverse transcriptase polymerase chain reaction; TMB-H: high tumor mutation burden)

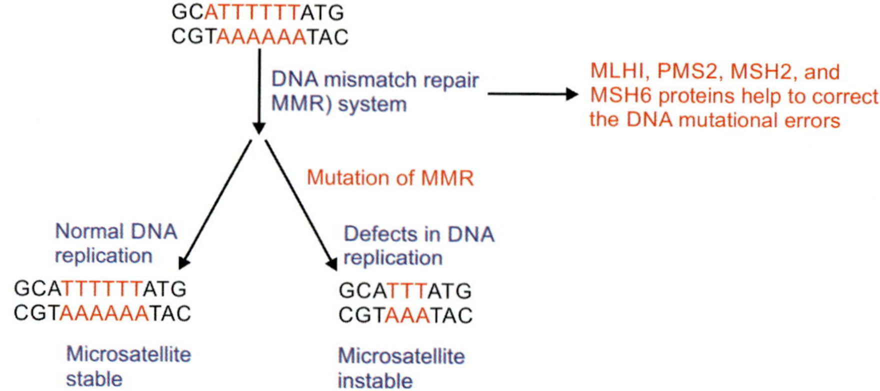

FIG. 1: Microsatellite instability and DNA mismatch repair (MMR) proteins.

MSI. In high microsatellite instability (MSI-H), there are significant number of loci of MSI. MSI-H is related with deficient MMR (dMMR) and is clinically significant. In low microsatellite instability (MSI-L) cases, MSI is infrequent and usually noted in sporadic cancer.

High microsatellite instability is noted in colorectal carcinoma and endometrioid carcinoma of the uterus. Low-frequency MSI is seen in prostate carcinoma, gastrointestinal carcinoma, pancreatic carcinoma, and many other solid tumors.[4] In the year 2017, FDA approved MSI/dMMR as the predictive molecular marker for the pembrolizumab treatment of solid tumors that are unresectable or metastatic. So, this approval of the drug for the common biomarker MSI/dMMR is irrespective of the tumor type. Tumor with dMMR also show multiple mutations of non-MSI regions.

Tests to Detect MSI/dMMR

Food and Drug Administration has approved MSI/dMMR as pan-cancer molecular biomarker but did not specify the choice of the test to detect MSI/dMMR. Currently, three different assays are available to determine MSI/MMR detection: (1) IHC, (2) PCR, and (3) NGS. Each test has its advantages and limitations.

Immunohistochemistry

The formalin-fixed paraffin-embedded (FFPE) material can be used for IHC. Every test requires normal control from the non-neoplastic FFPE tissue. IHC sees the expression of four MMR proteins: MLH1, MSH2, MSH6, and PMS2. The test is considered positive if any one or more MMR proteins show a loss of expression. MLH1 and MSH2 are obligatory proteins and MSH6 and PMS2 are secondary binding proteins. The mutational changes of the obligatory proteins are always associated with the functional loss of both types of proteins. However, the reverse is not true. Therefore, many IHC assays include only PMS2 and MSH6.

The sensitivity of IHC to detect MMR abnormality is near about 94%.[5] In certain cases, MMR proteins may have intact expression even with mutational change in *MMR* genes. This may be due to missense mutation of *MMR* gene with only functional loss of MMR proteins having intact antigenicity.

The IHC is a cheap, easy, and simple technique. It is a rapid technique and needs only 1–2 days to do. The low sensitivity and accuracy are the major limitations of IHC.

Polymerase Chain Reaction

PCR is a recognized method for detecting MSI-H. The most widely used PCR panels are: (1) Three dinucleotide repeats (D5S346, D2S123 and D17S250) which is known as Bethesda panel[6] and (2) five poly-A mononucleotide repeats (BAT-25, BAT-26, NR-21, NR-24, NR-27).[7]

Five poly-A panel is superior to Bethesda panel due to its higher sensitivity and specificity. Moreover, it does not need any corresponding normal tissue for the test control.

If any two of the biomarkers in those panels lose stability, then the tumor is identified as MSI-H.

The PCR identifies only the specific area of microsatellites, so it cannot capture the full MSI profile. Most of the clinical data on MSI is available from colorectal carcinoma. Till now there has been limited data on MSI on other cancers such as breast carcinoma, prostate carcinoma, melanoma, and other solid tumors. Therefore, even it is approved by FDA, the use of MSI as a reliable and predictive biomarker is limited.

Next-generation Sequencing

NGS is a useful test as it can target thousands of MCI loci. NGS uses cancer gene panels or whole-exome sequencing (WES).[8]

A large number of MSI can be detected by the NGS test along with many additional microsatellites with higher predictive power. It is overall a more accurate and sensitive test compared to IHC and PCR and can be used as the gold standard.

Table 3 shows the comparison of different tests to detect MSI.

TABLE 3: Comparison of different tests to detect microsatellite instability.

	Technique	Targets	Advantages	Disadvantages
IHC	Simple, easy to do	MLH1, MSH2, MSH6, PMS2	Cheap, simple and reliable	False-negative cases are known
PCR	Relatively complex	• Three dinucleotide repeats (D5S346, D2S123, and D17S250) • Five poly-A mononucleotide repeats (BAT-25, BAT-26, NR-21, NR-24, NR-27)	More sensitive and specific than IHC	Only limited and specific loci are detected
NGS	Difficult and complex; needs skill to do	Many thousands of MSI	Better than IHC and PCR with higher sensitivity and specificity	Very costly

(IHC: immunohistochemistry; MSI: microsatellite instability; NGS: next-generation sequencing; PCR: polymerase chain reaction)

Tumor Mutation Burden

Tumor mutation burden is a numeric index and is defined as the total number of nonsynonymous somatic mutations in the cancer cells per megabase of DNA.[9] High TMB is a predictive biomarker. If the TMB score is higher than a predetermined threshold, then it is considered a high TMB. This threshold is set at 20 mutations per megabase.[10] However, the cutoff value is variably expressed from 10 to 37 mutations/megabase by different studies.[11,12]

Tumor mutation burden has been approved by FDA as a predictive pan-cancer biomarker for pembrolizumab therapy in unresectable and metastatic solid tumors. Various factors may be responsible for high TMB such as ultraviolet radiation, cigarette smoking, and defective DNA damage response (*DDR*) gene.

The higher number of somatic mutations in the exonic region produces neoantigens many of which are immunogenic and responses to immunotherapy **(Fig. 2)**.[13]

Tests to Detect Tumor Mutational Burden

Tumor mutational burden is detected by WES and gene-targeted sequencing by NGS. WES is a reliable test to detect TMB and initially, it was measured from tumor tissue and corresponding normal tissue by NGS. WES provides a clear picture of most of the coding sequence. WES is difficult to do in small biopsies as the test requires a minimum 150–200 ng of genomic DNA. WES needs the examination of the corresponding normal tissue along with the tumor, which increases the cost of the test.

Gene-targeted Sequencing

An NGS panel with a good number of cancer-targeted genes can help to assess TMB. The gene panel can increase the sensitivity of the mutational detection

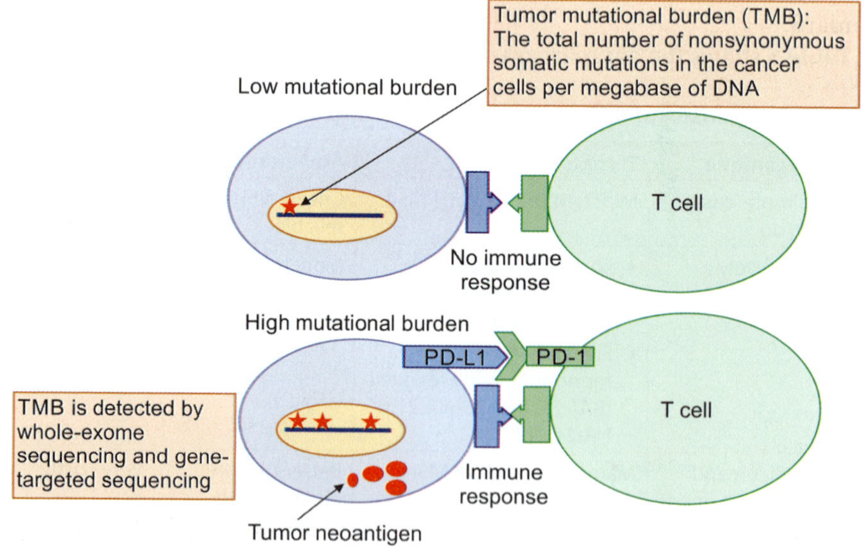

FIG. 2: Schematic diagram showing tumor mutational burden (TMB).
(PD-1: programmed cell death 1; PD-L1: programmed death ligand 1)

rate. The cost of this technique is low, with low turnover time. Moreover, small amounts of DNA and even fragmented DNA can be processed for gene-targeting sequencing. To calculate TMB, it was suggested that the specimen must contain at least 20% tumor cells and at least 50 ng of FFPE DNA.[14]

Neurotrophic Receptor Kinase Fusions

Neurotrophic receptor kinase fusions as a pan-cancer biomarker is approved by the FDA. It can predict the response to tyrosine kinase inhibitors in metastatic solid tumors. NTRK is located in chromosomes 1 (1q22), 9 (9q22), and 15 (15q25). NTRK receptor family has three members: TRKA, TRKB, and TRKC and are encoded by the three genes *NTRK1*, *NTRK2*, and *NTRK3*. NTRK is expressed in neural and smooth muscle tissue and helps in cell proliferation and survival. Mutation of *NTRK* genes causes carcinogenesis in both neural and non-neural tissues. In *NTRK* gene fusion C terminal of NTRK fuses with the 5′ N-terminal of partner genes activating the kinase domain and producing abnormal TRK fusion protein **(Fig. 3)**. Many small molecular drugs are available that successfully block the TRK activity. TRK protein is responsible for the carcinogenesis by cell proliferation, cell survival, infiltration to the surrounding tissue, and angiogenesis.

The NTRK fusion is seen in various tumors such as mammary analog secretory carcinoma of the breast (90–100%), fibrosarcoma (90–100%), congenital mesoblastic nephroma (83%), papillary thyroid carcinoma (26%), and so on.[15]

Currently, FDA approved therapy by larotrectinib and entrectinib in NTRK fusion-associated cancer treatment in 2018 and 2019. The indications of TRK inhibitor treatment are: (1) locally advanced unresectable or metastatic cancer with *NTRK* gene fusion and (2) progression of disease even after prior therapy or no good alternative therapy.

Detection of NTRK Fusion

The NTRK fusion can be detected by IHC, FISH, RT-PCR, and NGS.

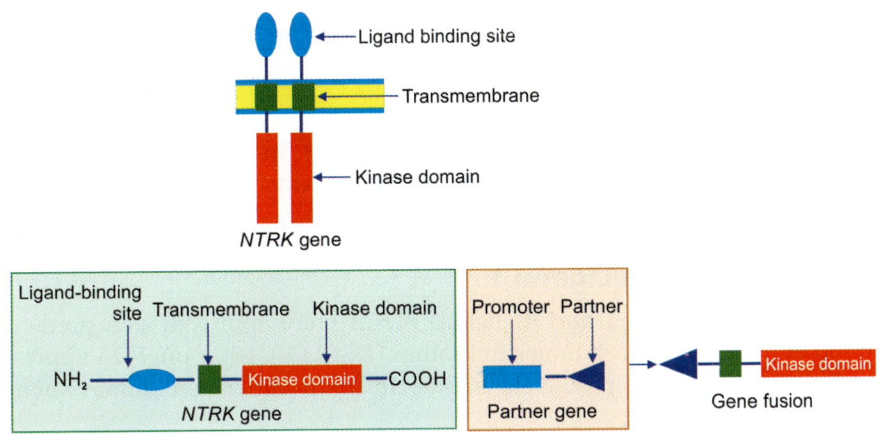

FIG. 3: *NTRK* gene and its fusion.

Immunohistochemistry

IHC is done to see the NTRK protein expression. IHC is simple, affordable, and can be done on FFPE tissue. Turnaround time of IHC is fast. The most commonly used clone of antibody is EPR17341 (Abcam and Roche/Ventana). This antibody reacts with a peptide from the C-terminus of TRKA, TRKB, and TRKC. So, it can identify any of the oncogenic *NTRK* fusions. The positive staining is labeled as at least 1% of tumor cells showing expression. IHC shows 96% sensitivity for *NTRK1* and *NTRK2*, whereas only 79% sensitivity for *NTRK3*.

Fluorescent In Situ Hybridization

Break-apart FISH can detect large structural variations in DNA.[16] *NTRK* gene commonly fuses with *ETV6*. The diagnostic test for *NTRK–ETV6* fusion is available commercially. A green signal is seen in positive cases. In the case of multiple partner fusions with *NTRK* gene, there may be missing oncogenic fusion. The sensitivity and specificity of break-apart FISH is high. However, insufficient splitting of the signals may cause false negative results. FISH can be done on one unstained glass slide and turnaround time is only 1 week.

Reverse Transcriptase Polymerase Chain Reaction

RT-PCR can detect the single fusion oncogene with known fusion partners. In the case of multiple fusion partners with break point involvement, the application of RT-PCR is limited. The turnaround time of RT-PCR is longer (1 week).

DNA-based NGS

In the case of DNA-based NGS, DNA is extracted from the FFPE tumor tissue. Some introns such as those in *NTRK3* are too long (193 KB) and therefore accurate DNA sequencing may be difficult resulting in the reduction of sensitivity.[17]

The major advantage of DNA-based NGS is that it can detect simultaneous direct assessment of many point mutations, and the assessment of TMB. There are certain disadvantages of DNA-based NGS.

When a novel structural variant is detected by NGS, it is difficult to determine whether they are functionally expressed or not. RNA-based NGS may be needed in such cases Turnaround time is significantly higher in DNA-based NGS. Moreover, the test needs more material to do compared to IHC and FISH. Increased turnaround time and the requirement of more material for the testing are the other drawbacks of DNA-based NGS.

RNA-based NGS

RNA-based NGS has high sensitivity and specificity. In this test, the introns are spliced out, so it overcomes the technical limitations of intronic coverage. In addition, the test can predict whether the fusion gene is functional or not.

Programmed Death Ligand 1

Programmed cell death 1 and its ligand PD-L1 were approved as a predictive biomarker in nonsmall-cell lung carcinomas (NSCLCs). Later on, FDA approved PD-L1 as an additional predictive marker in many other carcinomas such as

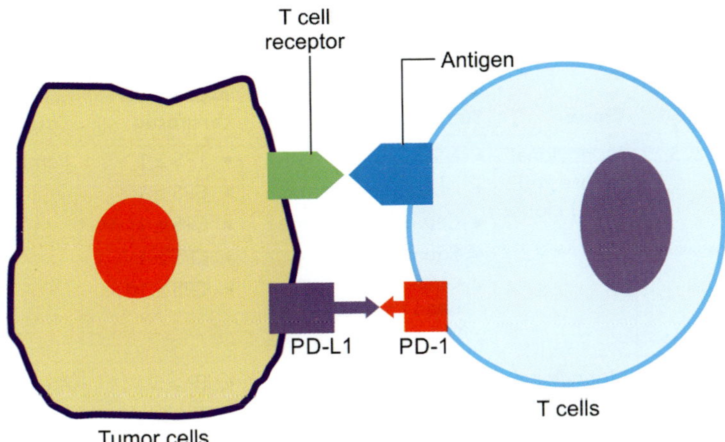

FIG. 4: Programmed death ligand 1 (PD-L1) and programmed cell death 1 (PD-1) interaction of the tumor cell and T cell.

Note: Binding of PD-1 and PD-L1 prevents killing of tumor cells by T cells.

gastric carcinoma, cervical carcinomas, head-neck squamous cell carcinoma, and urothelial carcinoma. PD-L1 is the ligand of the receptor of PD-1. PD-L1 is expressed in activated T and B lymphocytes, macrophages, and many other normal cells. PD-1 is present on the T cells. The interaction between PD-1 and PD-L1 plays an important role in immune regulation. The tumor cells often express PD-L1, which binds with PD-1 of the T cells and thereby bypass the tumor surveillance **(Fig. 4)**. Blocking the PD-L1 and PD-1 interaction by antibody helps to reactivate the action of T cells.

Programmed Death Ligand 1 Scoring

On IHC of PD-L1, two scoring methods are applied—tumor proportion score (TPS) and the combined positive score (CPS).

Tumor proportion score: TPS is calculated as PD-L1 positive tumor cells divided by viable tumor cells × 100%.

Combined positive score: CPS is calculated as PD-L1 positive tumor cells. Lymphocytes, macrophages divided by viable tumor cells × 100%.

The TPS scoring ≥1% is considered as positive and CPS scoring ≥1 is cutoff value and thresholds of ≥1, 1–9%,10–19%, and equal to or >20% are used.[18]

Programmed Death Ligand 1 Tests

The FDA approved four IHC testing methods for PD-L1 scoring. Unfortunately, these methods use different clones of monoclonal antibodies and the scoring of PD-L1 is also different with variable threshold of expression. This wide variability produces confusion in PD-L1 expression. **Table 4** shows the summary of different PD-L1 test methods.

TABLE 4: Programmed death ligand 1 (PD-L1) tests.

Testing method	Clone	Tumor type	PD-L1 expression threshold	Drugs used
PD-L1 IHC 22C3 pharmaDx	Monoclonal mouse anti-PD-L1 clone 22C3	• NSCLC • Gastric carcinoma • Cervical carcinoma • Squamous cell carcinoma of the head and neck • Urothelial carcinoma	• TPS ≥ 1 • CPS ≥ 1 • CPS ≥ 1 • CPS ≥ 1 • CPS ≥ 10	Pembrolizumab
PD-L1 IHC SP142 Ventana	Monoclonal rabbit anti-PD-L1 clone SP142	• NSCLC • Urothelial carcinoma	• TP ≥ 50 • IC ≥ 5	Atezolizumab
PD-L1 IHC SP263 Ventana	Monoclonal rabbit anti-PD-L1 clone SP263	Urothelial carcinoma	TC > 25%	Durvalumab (IMFINZI)
PD-L1 IHC 28–8 pharmaDx assay	Monoclonal rabbit anti-PD-L1 clone 28-8	• NSCLC • Gastric carcinoma • Cervical carcinoma • Squamous cell carcinoma of the head and neck • Urothelial carcinoma	TC ≥ 1%	Nivolumab

(CPS: combined positive score; IC: immune cell; NSCLC: non-small-cell lung carcinoma; TC: tumor cell; TPS: tumor proportion score)

NON-FDA-APPROVED EMERGING PAN-CANCER BIOMARKERS

Rearranged during Transfection

Rearranged during transfection (RET) is a transmembrane tyrosine kinase protein receptor and normally found in the tissues of the nervous system, thyroid, and adrenal gland. *RET* gene may be abnormally activated by mutations and fusions. *RET* fusions are the oncogenic driver mutations that are potential areas of drug targeting. *RET* is mutated in medullary carcinoma of the thyroid, and *RET* fusions are noted in papillary carcinoma of thyroid and NSCLC. Based on different clinical trials, FDA has approved selpercatinib drug therapy in *RET* fusion positive thyroid and NSCLC and *RET*-mutated positive medullary carcinoma of thyroid.[19] *RET* fusions are detected by FISH, RT-PCR, DNA-NGS, RNA-NGS, and IHC.

BRCA1: *BRC1* is a tumor suppressor gene and plays important role in DNA repair. *BRCA1* and *BRCA2* genes are often associated with homologous recombinant deficiency, which can be treated by platinum chemotherapy and small molecular inhibitors such as poly ADP ribose polymerases.[20,21]

These drugs are approved in several cancers such as breast, ovarian, prostate, and pancreatic cancer.[22]

ALK Gene

ALK gene alterations are seen in NSCLC, inflammatory myofibroblastic tumors, and anaplastic large-cell lymphomas. Till now FDA has approved multiple anaplastic lymphoma kinase (ALK) inhibitors that target the alterations, such as crizotinib, ceritinib, alectinib, brigatinib, and lorlatinib.

Fibroblast Growth Factor Receptors

Fibroblast growth factor receptors (FGFR) is a transmembrane tyrosine kinase receptor and is responsible for intracellular signaling and gene transcription. The molecular alterations of FGFR include copy number amplifications and structural rearrangements. FGFR abnormalities are seen in 7.5% of cancer. The majority of the abnormalities are copy number amplifications, followed by mutations and rearrangements. The common tumors showing FGFR abnormalities include urothelial carcinoma, intrahepatic cholangiocarcinomas, ovarian carcinomas, and adenocarcinoma of the lung.[23] In 2019, FDA approved the pan-FGFR inhibitor erdafitinib for the metastatic and locally advanced unresectable urothelial carcinoma of the bladder. In 2020, FDA approved FGFR inhibitor pemigatinib for the treatment of cholangiocarcinoma.

The FGFR fusion can be detected by DNA sequencing, RNA sequencing, FISH, and RT-PCR. NGS is superior to PCR-based studies as it detects more number of mutations than PCR.

TISSUE IS NOT THE ISSUE

Histopathology traditionally classifies cancer based on tissue morphology and the pattern of tumor cells. Accordingly, the cancer is classified as carcinoma, lymphoma, sarcoma, etc. This traditional histopathological classification of cancer is the gold standard in clinical medicine as it determines the therapy and prognosis. There is no doubt that cancer is a disease of the genome. The evolution of molecular genetics shows that various specific genetic mutations in different tumors such as *EGFR* mutations in lung cancer, *KRAS* mutations in colorectal carcinomas, BCR-ABL1 translocations in chronic myeloid leukemia, and so on. Many of these alterable mutations are treated by specific drugs that target the cancer cells at the molecular level.[24-26]

So, pathologists are mainly interested in the molecular alterations of the tumor that may confirm the diagnosis or can be treated by specific drugs approved for those mutational changes. Till now, the histopathology of the tumor is the main basis followed by the search for the mutational changes. However, the vast molecular data of the tumor, particularly obtained from the NGS, have shown that many cancers have common mutations, such as *BRAF* mutations which are shared by melanoma, lung adenocarcinoma, and colorectal adenocarcinoma. *ALK* fusions are not only seen in anaplastic large-cell adenocarcinoma but also may be noted in lung adenocarcinoma and inflammatory myofibroblastic tumors.[27,28]

Therefore, cancers with common molecular markers may be successfully treated by small molecular target drugs against the actionable mutational changes. NGS like a molecular microscope finds out all the molecular alterations that may have significance. This vast molecular data has given us new insights. FDA approval of the use of targeted therapy of the pan-cancer markers irrespective of tissue diagnosis site of origin or age of the patients has made a paradigm shift in diagnostic pathology.

CONCLUSION

Pan-cancer biomarkers have changed the landscape of molecular testing and treatment. The vast amount of molecular data gained by different molecular testing, particularly NGS, has enabled us to screen various targetable mutational changes of cancer common to different types of cancer. The number of FDA-approved drug lists is continuing to increase over time. So, awareness of the list of drugs and the specific mutation is needed. Moreover, the detection tests of the mutation are variable by different assays and need standardization. The knowledge of the pitfalls of the detection techniques is essential for the successful application of therapy. Overall, pan-cancer biomarkers are very promising and encouraging in the field of oncology and pathology.

REFERENCES

1. Hong DS, DuBois SG, Kummar S, Farago AF, Albert CM, Rohrberg KS, et al. Larotrectinib in patients with TRK fusion-positive solid tumours: a pooled analysis of three phase 1/2 clinical trials. Lancet Oncol. 2020;21(4):531-40.
2. Doebele RC, Drilon A, Paz-Ares L, Siena S, Shaw AT, Farago AF, et al.; trial investigators. Entrectinib in patients with advanced or metastatic NTRK fusion-positive solid tumours: integrated analysis of three phase 1–2 trials. Lancet Oncol. 2020;21(2):271-82.
3. Marcus L, Lemery SJ, Keegan P, Pazdur R. FDA approval summary: pembrolizumab for the treatment of microsatellite instability-high solid tumors. Clin Cancer Res. 2019;25(13): 3753-8.
4. Middha S, Zhang L, Nafa K, Jayakumaran G, Wong D, Kim HR, et al. Reliable pan-cancer microsatellite instability assessment by using targeted next-generation sequencing data. JCO Precis Oncol. 2017:2017:PO.17.00084.
5. Hechtman JF, Rana S, Middha S, Stadler ZK, Latham A, Benayed R, et al. Retained mismatch repair protein expression occurs in approximately 6% of microsatellite instability-high cancers and is associated with missense mutations in mismatch repair genes. Mod Pathol. 2020;33(5):871-9.
6. Boland CR, Thibodeau SN, Hamilton SR, Sidransky D, Eshleman JR, Burt RW, et al. A National Cancer Institute Workshop on Microsatellite Instability for Cancer Detection and Familial Predisposition: Development of International Criteria for the Determination of Microsatellite Instability in Colorectal Cancer. Cancer Res. 1998;58(22):5248-57.
7. Suraweera N, Duval A, Reperant M, Vaury C, Furlan D, Leroy K, et al. Evaluation of Tumor Microsatellite Instability Using Five Quasimonomorphic Mononucleotide Repeats and Pentaplex PCR. Gastroenterology. 2002;123(6):1804-11.
8. Hause RJ, Pritchard CC, Shendure J, Salipante SJ. Classification and Characterization of Microsatellite Instability Across 18 Cancer Types. Nat Med. 2016;22(11):1342-50.
9. Le DT, Durham JN, Smith KN, Wang H, Bartlett BR, Aulakh LK, et al. Mismatch Repair Deficiency Predicts Response of Solid Tumors to PD-1 Blockade. Science. 2017;357(6349):409-13.

10. Luchini C, Bibeau F, Ligtenberg MJL, Singh N, Nottegar A, Bosse T, et al. ESMO Recommendations on Microsatellite Instability Testing for Immunotherapy in Cancer, and Its Relationship with PD-1/PD-L1 Expression and Tumour Mutational Burden: A Systematic Review-Based Approach. Ann. Oncol. 2019;30:1232-43.
11. Marabelle A, Fakih M, Lopez J, Shah M, Shapira-Frommer R, Nakagawa K, et al. Association of Tumour Mutational Burden with Outcomes in Patients with Advanced Solid Tumours Treated with Pembrolizumab: Prospective Biomarker Analysis of the Multicohort, Open-Label, Phase 2 KEYNOTE-158 Study. Lancet Oncol. 2020;21:1353-65.
12. Schrock AB, Ouyang C, Sandhu J, Sokol E, Jin D, Ross JS, et al. Tumor Mutational Burden Is Predictive of Response to Immune Checkpoint Inhibitors in MSI-High Metastatic Colorectal Cancer. Ann Oncol. 2019;30:1096-103.
13. Kim JY, Kronbichler A, Eisenhut M, Hong SH, van der Vliet HJ, Kang J, et al. Tumor Mutational Burden and Efficacy of Immune Checkpoint Inhibitors: A Systematic Review and Meta-Analysis. Cancers (Basel). 2019;11(11):1798.
14. Chalmers ZR, Connelly CF, Fabrizio D, Gay L, Ali SM, Ennis R, et al. Analysis of 100,000 human cancer genomes reveals the landscape of tumor mutational burden. Genome Med. 2017;9(1):34.
15. Cocco E, Scaltriti M, Drilon A. NTRK fusion-positive cancers and TRK inhibitor therapy. Nat Rev Clin Oncol. 2018;15(12):731-47.
16. Solomon JP, Benayed R, Hechtman JF, Ladanyi M. Identifying patients with NTRK fusion cancer. Ann Oncol. 2019;30(Suppl_8):30.
17. Solomon JP, Benayed R, Hechtman JF, Ladanyi M. Identifying patients with NTRK fusion cancer. Ann Oncol. 2019;30(Suppl_8):viii16-viii22.
18. Burtness B, Harrington KJ, Greil R, Soulières D, Tahara M, de Castro G Jr, et al.; KEYNOTE-048 Investigators. Pembrolizumab alone or with chemotherapy versus cetuximab with chemotherapy for recurrent or metastatic squamous cell carcinoma of the head and neck (KEYNOTE-048): a randomised, open-label, phase 3 study. Lancet. 2019;394:1915-28.
19. Markham A. Selpercatinib: First approval. Drugs. 2020;80(11):1119-24.
20. Pennington KP, Walsh T, Harrell MI, Lee MK, Pennil CC, Rendi MH, et al. Germline and somatic mutations in homologous recombination genes predict platinum response and survival in ovarian, fallopian tube, and peritoneal carcinomas. Clin Cancer Res. 2014;20:764-75.
21. Nik-Zainal S, Alexandrov LB, Wedge DC, Greenman CD, Raine K, Jones D, et al.; Breast Cancer Working Group of the International Cancer Genome Consortium. Mutational processes molding the genomes of 21 breast cancers. Cell. 2012;149:979-93.
22. Kim D, Nam HJ. PARP Inhibitors: Clinical limitations and recent attempts to overcome them. Int J Mol Sci. 2022;23(15):8412.
23. Helsten T, Elkin S, Arthur E, Tomson BN, Carter J, Kurzrock R. The FGFR Landscape in Cancer: Analysis of 4,853 Tumors by Next-Generation Sequencing. Clin Cancer Res. 2016;22(1): 259-67.
24. Chang KL, Lau SK. EGFR mutations in non-small cell lung carcinomas may predict response to gefitinib: extension of an emerging paradigm. Adv Anat Pathol. 2005;12(2):47-52.
25. Kantarjian H, Sawyers C, Hochhaus A, Guilhot F, Schiffer C, Gambacorti-Passerini C, et al.; International STI571 CML Study Group. Hematologic and cytogenetic responses to imatinib mesylate in chronic myelogenous leukemia. N Engl J Med. 2002;346(9):645-52.
26. Tóthová E, Kafková A, Fricová M, Benová B, Kirschnerová G, Tóthová A. Imatinib mesylate in Philadelphia chromosome-positive, chronic-phase myeloid leukemia after failure of interferon alpha. Neoplasma. 2005;52(1):63-7.
27. Lawrence B, Perez-Atayde A, Hibbard MK, Rubin BP, Dal Cin P, Pinkus JL, et al. TPM3-ALK and TPM4-ALK oncogenes in inflammatory myofibroblastic tumors. Am J Pathol. 2000;157(2):377-84.
28. Soda M, Choi YL, Enomoto M, Takada S, Yamashita Y, Ishikawa S, et al. Identification of the transforming EML4–ALK fusion gene in non-small-cell lung cancer. Nature. 2007; 448(7153):561-6.

6
CHAPTER

Evolution of Cancer Cell Micronucleus from a Mute Spectator to an Active Player in Carcinogenesis

Laxmi Kumari, Yashwant Kumar, Alka Bhatia

EVOLVING ROLE OF MICRONUCLEUS IN CARCINOGENESIS

INTRODUCTION

Cancers are characterized by altered gene expression that leads to abnormal cell proliferation and invasion into neighboring and distant organs, thus interfering with their normal function.[1] Chromosomal instability (CIN) is an important factor implicated in the pathogenesis of malignancies. CIN is a dynamic process characterized by qualitative or quantitative changes in chromosomes during cell division to acquire a configuration favoring the evolution and progression of malignancy.[2,3] Micronuclei (MN) are considered relevant and distinguishable markers of CIN.[4] The MN or miniature nuclei have always attracted attention as they can easily be identified under the microscope as roundish chromatin bodies surrounded by a nuclear envelope (NE) with staining properties similar to the primary nucleus.[5] Many studies have outlined their role as markers of screening, diagnostic, and prognostic significance in malignancies.[6] Although several events have been held responsible, still the exact mechanisms involved in the formation of MN remain incompletely understood. Advancements in visualization techniques like time-lapse microscopy have however helped to understand some of events underlying their formation and degradation. Other studies have indicated that chromatin inside the MN can undergo processes such as transcription, replication, and repair.[7] More recent studies are especially focusing on their contents with the aim to understand what transpires inside these tiny nuclear bodies and how these events can modulate the behavior of malignancy. Identification of MN as mediators of cyclic GMP-AMP synthase-stimulator of interferon genes (cGAS-STING)-mediated immune response in tumors has rekindled the interest in MN.

Given the increasing acknowledgment of MN's role in the formation of tumors, we aim to provide a comprehensive description of MN biology and its possible clinical implications in this chapter. In addition, we will also discuss the potential application of MN as markers of the dynamic, ongoing process that defines CIN in cancer.

HISTORY OF MICRONUCLEI

In the 19th century, Von Hansemann in his pioneering work, "On pathological mitoses" advanced the concept that a chromosome lost during cell division may separate itself from the nucleus.[8] After that, Theodore Boveri in his experiment on sea urchins noticed that some of the chromosomes were not incorporated into the daughter cells. Thereafter, multipolar mitosis was reported as a frequent feature present in the malignancies.[9] The advanced understanding of chromosomes and nucleus during the early 1900s led to the first visualization of an interphase MN. At that time, it was thought that the nucleus was made up of vesicles containing the chromosomes that help preserve chromosomal uniqueness in the interphase and enable precise segregation during the ensuing mitosis.[10] Several investigations conducted in the early half of the 1900s linked MN to cytotoxic agents (radiation from X-rays) and mitotic poisons (colchicine and its equivalents).[11-14] Because of this early research, experts now recognize MN as indicators of pathologic illnesses. American scientists William Howell and Frenchman Justin Jolly recognized them as the nuclear leftovers in red cell precursors around the end of the nineteenth century.[15] Brues and Jackson (1937) found that colchicine caused individual chromosomes to expand during their examination of mitotic arrest. This procedure produced MN, whose size was correlated with the number of chromosomes it contained.[16] In his study of cellular gigantism, Schwarz (1946) postulated that the presence of chromatin particles in the cytosol during interphase is caused by chromosomal miss-egregation during the previous anaphase vesicular transformation **(Fig. 1A)**.[17] MN were identified in bone marrow red cells in 1961 by Dawson and Bury.[18] Deficiencies in vitamin B and folic acid were also related to the generation of Howell-Jolly bodies.[18] Up until the end of the 20th century, the scientific community thought that MN were miniaturized nuclei architecturally comparable to the primary nucleus. This could be attributed to poor resolution techniques used for their visualization or tools for studying their functions.[19] Between 1950 and 1970, numerous studies attempted to understand transcription in MN and its relationship to nucleolar organizing regions.[8,20,21] Contradictory findings have come from studies on MN transcription and replication as well as from those examining the capacity of MN-carrying cells to survive. The heterogeneity of observations may be attributed to the range of cell types, study periods, and methodologies employed in different studies conducted over a period of time. However, it was because of these investigations that the first evidence of chromosomal breakage or pulverization in MN was found in 1968.[22-24] This process is now understood to be the precursor of chromothripsis, the chromosomal rearrangements of complex nature.[25] Published in 1997, Kato et al. proposed the elegant theory that pulverization results from late chromosomal condensation due to damaging cytoplasmic conditions prevalent during mitosis.[22] This probably led to the hypothesis almost half a century later that the interphase chromosome in the MN exposed to the cytosolic environment due to rupture of micronuclear envelope (mNE) may trigger a sequence of oncologic events that fuel the tumor formation.[8] With the advent of next-generation sequencing (NGS) and other techniques, the past 10 years have seen a breakthrough in our comprehension of biology of MN and the ways they may impact the pathologic interaction between the cancer cells and the tumor microenvironment.

CAUSES AND MECHANISMS OF FORMATION OF MICRONUCLEI

Despite several studies on MN, their origin remains a mystery. The genesis of MN in interphase cells is proposed to be amplified DNA or nuclear blebs harboring DNA repair complexes. In the dividing cells, they may form due to lagging whole chromosomes or their fragments at the end of mitosis.[26] Various factors have been linked with the formation of MN such as exposure to genotoxic agents, ionizing radiation, free radicals, metabolite deficiency, infections, genetic diseases, and neoplasia. Typically, the MN have been used as biomarkers of genotoxicity.[27] The main mechanisms proposed for the formation of MN include defects in DNA repair machinery, cell cycle and spindle assembly checkpoints (SACs), and imperfect chromosome segregation.[28] The MN may uncommonly form in the normal cells. Certain nutrient deficiencies such as deficiency of folate and vitamin B are also known to cause MN formation.[29] MN in normal cells mostly contains X and Y chromosomes and among autosomes chromosome numbers 1, 9, and 16 are generally present.[30] In malignancies, the frequency of MN formation is much higher. Further, they may be observed in different types of cells in cancers. A study by Bochtler et al. also shows that the formation of MN is biased by chromosome size. Larger chromosomes have been reported to have a higher probability of segregation into the MN compared to small-sized chromosomes.[31]

Based on their contents, two main types of MN are identified: (1) Those containing whole chromosomes and (2) those containing acentric chromosome fragments **(Fig. 1B)**. The above two types can be distinguished by using anticentromeric/antikinetochore antibodies or centromere-specific DNA probes. The MN containing whole chromosomes are centromere and kinetochore positive whereas those with acentric fragments are centromere and kinetochore negative. Fluorescent in situ hybridization (FISH) and chromosome-specific probes also allow the detection of specific chromosomes and their fragments in MN.[32] Depending upon the ability of the genotoxic agents or anticancer drugs to generate MN with acentric fragments or whole chromosomes, they can be classified as clastogens and aneugens, respectively.

Micronuclei Bearing Acentric Chromosome or Chromatid Fragments

Multiple mechanisms lead to the generation of acentric chromosome fragments the main being the level of DNA damage beyond the capacity of the repair machinery. The unrepaired double-stranded DNA (dsDNA) breaks then lead to the formation of acentric fragments. The repair pathways such as homologous recombination and nonhomologous end joining may become dysfunctional due to mutations of key DNA repair genes such as *BRCA1* and *BRCA2*.[33] Inappropriate base insertion (e.g., uracil) or simultaneous excision repair of damaged (such as

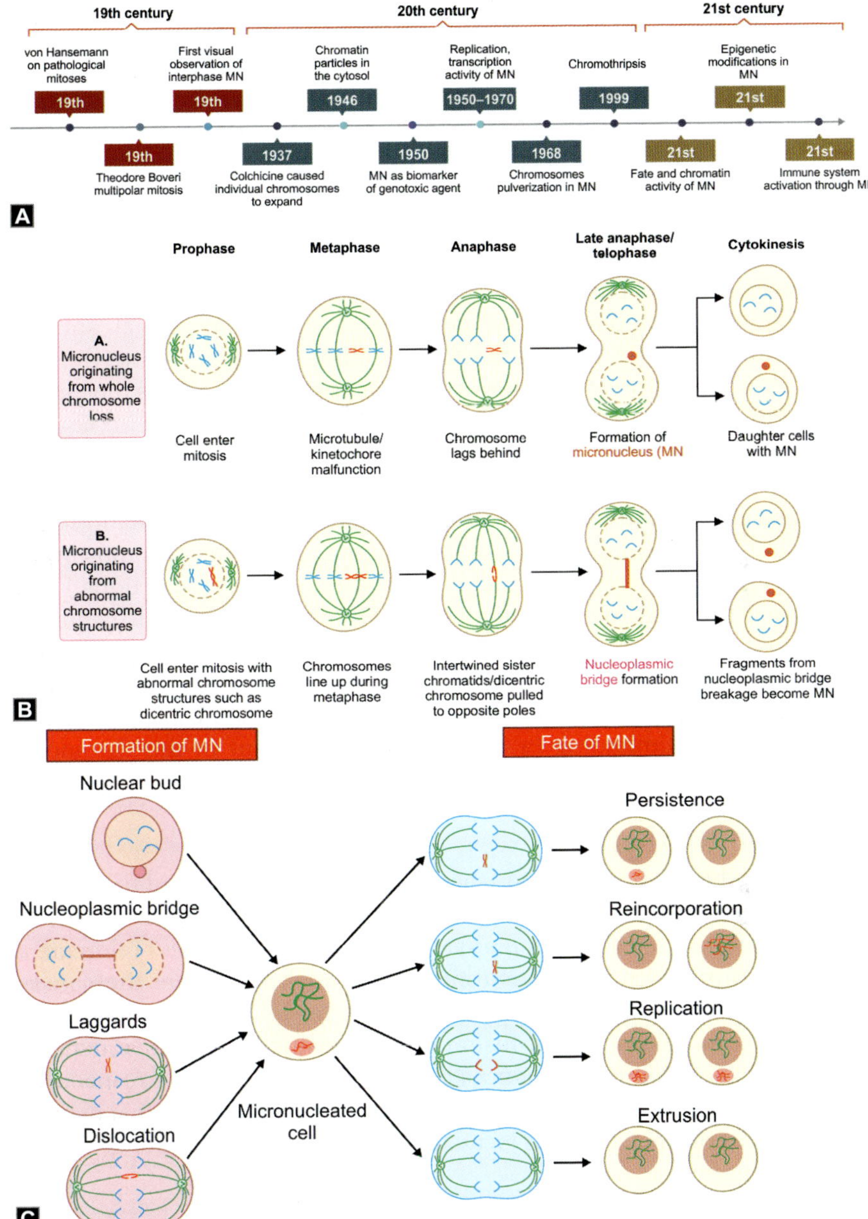

FIGS. 1A TO C: (A) Timeline of the evolution of micronuclei (MN) from passive indicator to active player in cancer pathogenesis; (B) Mechanisms of formation of MN; (C) Different abnormalities leading to the formation and possible fates of MN in cancerous cells.

8-oxo-deoxyguanosine) DNA fragments are other methods that might result in MN formation from acentric fragments. Further, stretching of a nucleoplasmic bridge (NPB) during telophase may break them to form MN with acentric fragments.[34]

Micronuclei from Missegregated Whole Chromosomes

Before a cell divides, it copies every chromosome so that each daughter cell receives an equal number during cell division. However, in case of separation machinery defects, missegregation of chromosomes generates the daughter cells with unequal numbers of chromosomes. Several mechanisms may contribute to chromosome missegregation at anaphase resulting in MN containing whole chromosome. Hypomethylation of cytosine in higher-order centromeric and pericentromeric classical satellite repeat DNA sequences, respectively, can result in faulty separation of chromosomes.[35] Such a hypomethylation is observed in immunodeficiency, centromeric instability, facial anomalies syndrome, or after DNA methyltransferase inhibitor 5-azacytidine treatment. The reduced methylation of cytosine and histones generally affects the assembly of kinetochore proteins (CENPA and CENPB) at the centromere.[36] It also leads to an increase in the pericentromeric heterochromatin region of chromosomes 1, 9, and 16. Both the above events are sufficient to promote missegregation or loss of these chromosomes as MN. The reduction in heterochromatin integrity may interfere with the attachment of the microtubule to the chromosome and correct sensing of tension from microtubule-kinetochore connections.[37] Other factors that contribute to the formation of MN include aberrant centrosome amplification, checkpoint issues during mitosis, abnormalities in the construction of the mitotic spindle, and dicentricity, resulting from the fusion of telomere tips. In the latter case, the two centromeres may be pulled by opposing forces during anaphase culminating in complete dislodgement of the chromosome from the spindle.[38]

Nucleoplasmic Bridge

Nucleoplasmic bridges are formed when the daughter nuclei and the anaphase bridge are surrounded by the NE during mitosis, and the centromeres of dicentric chromosomes are driven apart toward opposing poles. Telomere end fusions or improperly managed chromosomal break repair are the causes of NPB. NPBs, which are due to the latter event, are often telomere negative whereas those arising from telomere end fusion can be positive or negative depending upon whether the telomere sequences are well preserved or not, respectively.[39] In the first case, the NPBs may be identified using a specific probe that hybridizes to the subtelomeric area, which is located near the telomeric sequence.[34]

NUCLEAR BUD

Nuclear bud (NBUD) is another structural abnormality depicting CIN that is readily visible under the microscope. Some consider it an intermediary in MN formation due to its morphological similarity to the latter except for the presence of a pedicle attaching it to the nucleus. In line with the same, it has been claimed that exposure to ultraviolet-C might start a budding process that leads to MN formation.[40] NBUDs are believed to harbor amplified genes in cancer cells. However, despite their resemblance, the two structures may differ significantly. For example, centromeric and telomeric DNA are more common in MN (62%

and 22%, respectively) compared to NBUDs (44% and 10%, respectively), which have a higher frequency of interstitial DNA (43%) than MN (13%). Like MN, the NBUDs have also been noted in cultures grown under moderately reduced folic acid conditions; however, in that case the probability of MN and NBUDs having telomeric DNA is more.[41]

Dislocation of Chromosomes

In the normal state, the chromosomes segregate and migrate toward opposite poles during the anaphase and telophase of mitosis. However, when the chromosomes dislocate at the metaphase stage, they may decondense to form MN.[42] Also, the slower movement of a few chromosomes during segregation may result in their lagging behind at the equator during the anaphase-telophase transition. The lagged chromosomes are not incorporated into the nucleus and may decondense separately to form MN.[43]

Breakage-fusion-bridge Cycle

The breakage-fusion-bridge (BFB) cycle is a nuclear anomaly commonly seen in cancer and is believed to drive CIN in malignant cells. NPB formation is a prerequisite for the beginning of the BFB cycle. One daughter cell may have more copies of the genes if the NPBs break asymmetrically. Because of their sticky ends and absence of telomeric sequences, damaged chromosomes are likely to merge with their copy at the completion of DNA synthesis. The genes at the break or fusion point are amplified by this BFB cycle extension into the next round of cell division.[44] The extra gene copies are eventually eliminated from this abnormal chromosome by recombination mechanisms. The looped-over segments create minute chromosomes, which can proliferate or be removed via the formation of NBUDs and MN before being evacuated from the cell to make tiny cells.[45] All the above-mentioned abnormalities can lead to the formation of MN **(Fig. 1C)**.

Double Minutes

Double minutes (DMs) are self-replicating, extrachromosomal, circular, chromatin bodies without a centromere or a telomere. The amplification of specific oncogenes is primarily responsible for the malignant transformation of human cancer cells.[46] The DMs accommodate the extra copies of these genes. A decrease in DMs or the number of amplified genes can result in the reversal of malignant phenotype, reduction in proliferation, increase in cell death, and restoration of differentiated status in malignancies. Therefore, removing DMs as MN from cancer cells might offer a valid therapeutic strategy to treat cancers.[47]

STUDYING THE MICRONUCLEI

The MN have been studied in a variety of cell types such as peripheral blood lymphocytes (PBLs), malignant cells, exfoliated buccal and urothelial cells, malignant cells from patient tissues obtained by fine needle aspiration cytology or surgery as well as cell lines.[48] Although they can be seen in tissue sections, cytological specimens are better suited for their visualization as several other structures such as apoptotic bodies, small lymphocytes, phagocytosed material, and nuclear debris can be mistaken for MN in the histological slides. Different methods have been used to study the MN. Mostly the MN are identified in binucleated cells postmitotic division, however some studies have also studied them in mononucleated cells.[48] For quantitative assessment, the MN score/index can be obtained by counting them in a specific number of cells. In cultured PBLs, counting can be carried out after the introduction of binucleation by cytokinesis blocking agent cytochalasin B.[49] The cytokinesis block MN technique has now also been modified to work with a variety of cell types, including bone marrow and solid cancer cells.[50] MN in different cell types have been characterized by light microscopy after staining them with Giemsa or Pap stains. Typically, they are seen as miniaturized nuclei-like structures (approximately one-sixteenth–one-third of the mean diameter of the main nucleus), totally separate from the main nucleus.[51] Staining with more specific dyes such as 4′,6-diamidino-2-phenylindole (DAPI) and Hoechst has facilitated their visualization by fluorescent microscopy.[49] Flow cytometry has also been used as a valid method for MN scoring to gauze the genotoxicity of different types of chemicals in different cell lines in past studies by staining with fluorescent agents such as Sytox green and ethidium monoazide bromide.[52-54] The chromosomal content of the MN is studied by using FISH after staining them with specific probes.[30] Live cell imaging has been used in many studies to visualize their formation and fate.[55] Recent focus is on understanding the membrane, chromosomal contents, chromatin dynamics such as replication, transcription and repair, epigenetics, and genetics of MN by isolating them by centrifugation and studying them using other advanced techniques such as confocal microscopy and NGS **(Fig. 2)**.[56-58]

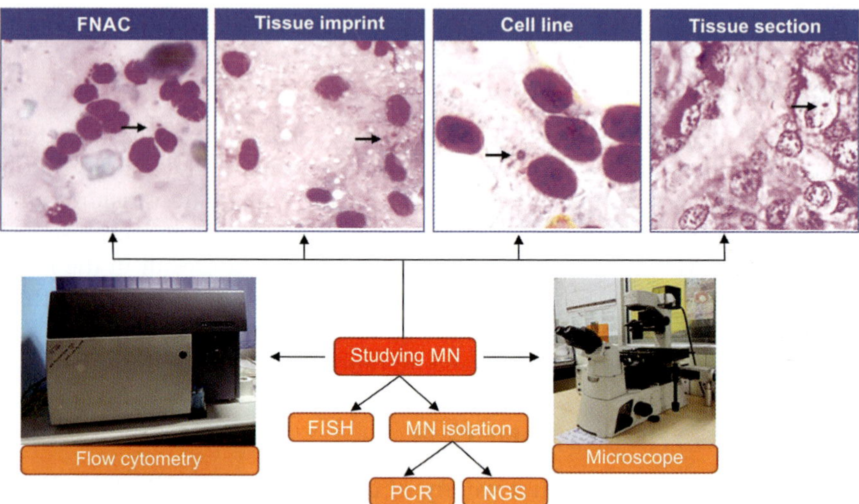

FIG. 2: Sample types and tools used for studying MN.

(FNAC: fine needle aspiration cytology; FISH: fluorescent in situ hybridization; MN: micronuclei, NGS: next-generation sequencing; PCR: polymerase chain reaction)

MICRONUCLEI AS PASSIVE BIOMARKERS OF CANCER EVOLUTION

The MN have been considered as passive indicators of cancer evolution in many past studies conducted on different types of clinical and nonclinical samples. The main reason for using them as biomarkers is their easy identification, a task that can be accomplished with little expertise and nonexpensive equipment.

Micronuclei as Biomarkers for Screening and Risk Prediction

Since MN formation is greatly enhanced in malignancies, their frequency has been used to screen high-risk populations for the development of premalignant and malignant lesions. Since in most of these studies, the MN frequency has been studied in PBLs, they can be categorized as minimally invasive biomarkers for screening large populations **(Table 1)**. The presence of a large number of MN has been found to be associated with an increased predisposition to develop pancreatic, lung, breast, gastrointestinal, urogenital, and oral cancers.[59-61] In individuals exposed to genotoxins such as nicotine-derived nitrosamine 4-(methylnitrosamino)-1-(3-pyridyl)-1-butanone, a two-fold higher risk of lung cancer was observed along with spontaneous induction of MN in the binucleated cells.[62] Pardini et al., in their work on bladder cancer, demonstrated that MN frequency in combination with genetic polymorphism in DNA repair genes may serve as a predictor of the risk of malignancy.[63] A study conducted on oral cancer showed that the frequencies of MN increased almost two-fold in the premalignant group and more than thrice in the malignant group when compared to the control. So, MN can be used for risk prediction and as the biomarkers for screening.[6,64] A meta-analysis of data involving >6,700 subjects from 20 laboratories representing 10 countries concluded that an elevated MN frequency in PBLs is predictive of increased cancer risk, especially in urogenital and gastrointestinal cancers and breast cancers.[49,65,66]

Micronuclei as Diagnostic Tools

Micronuclei assay has been proposed as an easy, simple, and reliable method to establish the diagnosis of malignancy. A meta-analysis on upper body cancers (head, neck, and breast) demonstrated a statistically significant difference in MN frequency in cancerous patients compared to the normal.[67] Another meta-analysis of 12 studies including 752 breast cancer cases and 593 controls showed an increase in MN frequency in the former category **(Table 1)**.[68] Further, increased MN frequency was observed to help in distinguishing between normal, precancerous, and cancerous lesions in cancers of endometrial, oral, breast, genitourinary, cervical, and bladder origin in different studies.[51,69-72] MN scoring has been used to diagnose some preneoplastic diseases far before any clinical symptoms appear, thus underscoring their importance as useful markers for early detection of cancer.[73] In various studies conducted on different sample types, the diagnostic accuracy of MN in different types of malignancies was reported to be 80–90% with equally good sensitivity and specificity. These studies were mainly conducted on cancers of the oral cavity, cervix, and breast.[74-77]

TABLE 1: Important studies highlighting the significance of MN as clinical biomarkers in different types of cancers.

Types of cancer	Author name (year)	Cell type, (no. of patients)	References
MN as biomarkers of cancer risk susceptibility			
Lung	El-zein et al. (2006)	PBLs, (139)	84
Different types	Bonassi et al. (2007)	PBLs, (6,718)	85
Different types	Murgia et al. (2008)	PBLs, (49)	86
Pancreatic	Chang et al. (2010)	PBLs, (346)	87
Breast	Bolognesi et al. (2014)	PBLs, (220)	88
Bladder	Pardini et al. (2017)	PBLs, (158)	80
MN as diagnostic markers of cancer			
Different types	Larmarcovai et al. (2008)	PBLs	89
Breast	Cardinale et al. (2012)	PBLs, (629)	68
Endometrium	Kiraz et al. (2016)	PBLs, (40)	72
Different types	Hovhannisyan et al. (2018)	PBLs	90
Head, neck, and breast	Bolognesi et al (2021)	PBLs, buccal cells, (1,207)	67
MN as prognostic markers of cancer			
Bladder	Pardine et al. (2017)	PBLs, (158)	80
Oral	Kiran et al. (2018)	Exfoliated cells, (60)	59
Cervical	Setayesh et al. (2020)	Cervical cells	77
Colorectal	Nikolouzakis et al. (2021)	PBLs, (55)	91
Oral, oropharyngeal	Kumar et al. (2021)	Mucosal cells, (60)	92
Role of MN in monitoring treatment			
Different types	Jagetia et al. (2001)	PBLs, (27)	93
Different types	Lee et al. (2002)	PBLs, (13)	94
Breast	Djuzenova et al. (2006)	PBLs, (50)	95
Different types	Guogyte et al. (2017)	PBLs, (5)	96
Cervical	Kobayashi et al. (2020)	Cervical cells, (7)	97

(MN: micronuclei; PBLs: peripheral blood lymphocytes)

Micronuclei as Prognostic Tools

Micronuclei frequency has been used as a prognostic tool in various cancers. The number of MN has been found to increase with the increasing grade of malignancy in several tumors. In Pap smears of cervical cancer patients, an increased frequency of MN was observed compared to low-grade tumors and normal controls **(Table 1)**.[77] Research on oral cancer by Shashikala et al. indicated a progressive rise in MN frequency from premalignant diseases to oral carcinoma and proposed a connection between this biomarker and the advancement of the malignancy. Additionally, it has been shown that MN frequency increases with an increase in the histological grade of squamous cell carcinoma.[78] Further, a significant difference has been reported in the survival time of patients with low and high MN frequency in acute nonlymphocytic leukemia.[79] Also, an increased frequency of MN is found in relapse cases compared to first-time cancer patients.[71,80,81] A meta-analysis study on pulmonary disease and lung cancer showing a significant increase in MN frequency in cancer compared to the control group concluded that MN assay can be used for prognosis of lung cancer. Further, an elevated frequency of MN has been reported to relate inflammation-induced oxidative stress to the risk of disease through genomic instability and hypoxia.[82,83]

Role of Micronuclei in Monitoring Treatment Response

Many studies have demonstrated an increase in the frequency of MN in PBLs post chemoradiotherapy (CT/RT) possibly due to treatment-induced DNA damage and genomic instability.[93,95,97,98] Some studies consider this a reflection of the surviving population of radiation-induced genetically aberrant cells.[94] Other studies however show a correlation between higher frequency of MN after in vitro irradiation of blood samples with radiosensitivity **(Table 1)**.[93,96] Additionally, other studies suggest a relationship between the frequency of MN and the appearance of acute side effects of RT.[99] In view of the above reports, the MN have been found useful as biomarkers for the prediction of response to treatment in different cancers in several past studies.[100] Another group of scientists have also emphasized the utility of MN as sensitive biomarkers to evaluate the chemotherapy-induced DNA damage in glial tumors.[101]

CONTENTS OF CANCER CELL MICRONUCLEI

The contents of MN in cancer cells have always generated interest. The MN may contain chromosomes or their fragments depending upon whether an aneugenic or a clastogenic event underlies their formation.[102] Certain chromosomes tend to be micronucleated more frequently than others. FISH studies have demonstrated that X chromosomes are more frequently micronucleated than autosomes due to their tendency to lag in anaphase.[103] Among the autosomes, chromosomes 9, 1, and 16 are most frequent in the MN.[30] Further, in malignancies such as colorectal and cervical cancer, it has been observed that the larger-sized chromosomes have more chances of segregation and entrapment into MN than the smaller ones in malignancies.[104] Apart from size, the location of chromosomes may also affect the possibility of their being present in the MN. A greater distance from the nuclear center directly increases the probability of missegregation and subsequent micronucleation in the chromosomes. In malignancies such as glioblastoma, chromosomes 1, 2, and 3 have higher chances of segregation and envelopment into the MN compared to chromosomes 18, 19, 20, etc. **(Figs. 3A to C)**.[31,104]

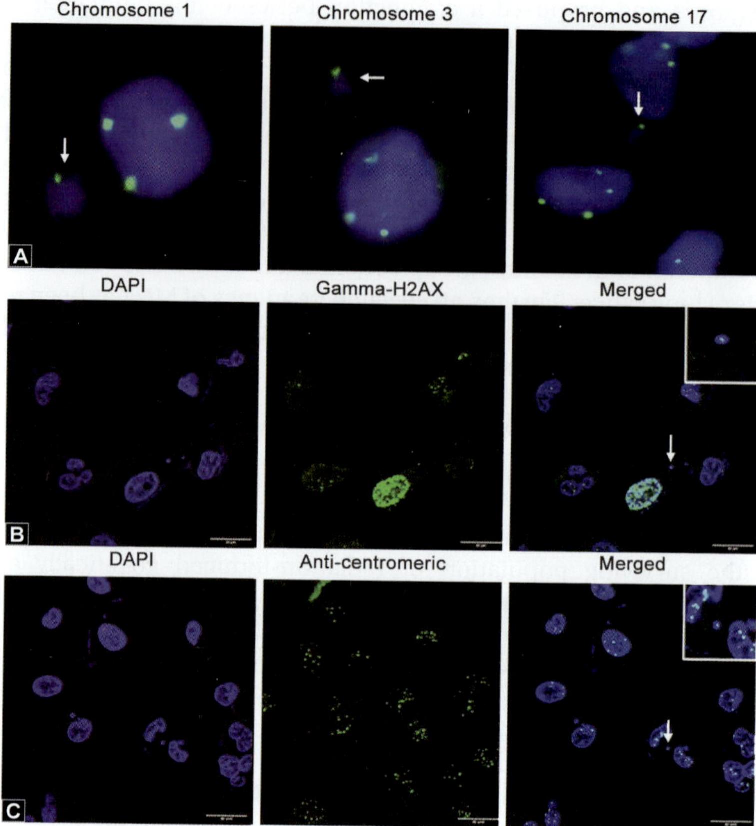

FIGS. 3A TO C: (A) FISH images depicting the presence of chromosomes 1, 3, and 17 in MCF-7 cell line (FITC-labeled pancentromeric probes, metasystem) in the MN; (B) DDR protein γH2AX-positive MN after staining with FITC-labeled anti-γH2AX antibody in MCF-7 cell line; (C) Centromere positive MN as depicted by FITC-conjugated anticentromeric antibody in MCF-7 cell line observed by FISH and confocal microscopy respectively.

(DAPI: 4′,6-diamidino-2-phenylindole; FISH: fluorescent in situ hybridization; FITC: fluorescein isothiocyanate)

BIOLOGICAL ACTIVITIES OF CHROMATIN INSIDE THE MICRONUCLEI

The chromatin that is stored inside the MN may be biologically active; however, its dynamics are not entirely clear. Still, several eventualities have been proposed depending upon the origin and contents of MN.

Micronuclei Chromatin Replication

Previous studies in different types of cancer show that chromatin in the MN is capable of replication occurring concurrently with the nuclear chromatin. However, whether or not they possess proper replication machinery is controversial.[26] Further, the replication of DNA inside the MN is believed to depend upon its genomic composition and the structure of the NE surrounding it.[105] The protein lamin B present in the MN is considered to be an important determinant of the replication process.[106] The MN in different types of cancer have also been found to exhibit differences in their chromatin condensation, e.g., the MN generated from lagging chromatids generally have more lose and those generated from chromatin bridges have more condensed chromatin compared to the main nucleus. These differences are believed to reflect different levels of replication activity.[107]

Micronuclei DNA Transcription

The cancer cell MN carrying whole chromosomes generally show transcription, whereas those containing acentric fragments do not, unless the MN are of the DM type, which are reported to be transcriptionally competent.[47] The transcriptional activity of MN is also associated with lamin B and DM-type MN are rich in it.[105] The nuclear pore complexes in mNE are also believed to play an important role in transcription as they are the only channels that allow to and fro movement of transcription-related proteins such as activated transcription factors, RNA polymerases, maturation factors, and synthesized RNA between the two cellular compartments. Inadequate MN import might also lead to faulty MN replication and transcription.[106] Different MN have been found to display heterogeneity in the distribution of nuclear pores. This provides further evidence that NPCs together with the specific MN DNA content may be the important players in determining the transcriptional activity of MN.[108]

Micronuclei DNA Damage Response

The MN induced by clastogenic agents have been found to show the accumulation of P53 in some previous studies in different types of cancers.[57] The increased expression of RAD51 and replication protein A in radiation-induced MN may indicate accumulation inside the MN with the damaged DNA and/or ongoing DNA repair **(Figs. 3A to C)**.[40] Expression of other DNA damage repair proteins such as ATM and SMAD7 has also been observed in the induced MN.[40,109] The persistence presence of these proteins may be due to stalled DNA repair activity or unresolved DNA repair. Other than that, MRE11, Rad50, and 53BP1 though found to be deposited in the main nuclei have not been reported in the MN.[110]

Epigenetics of Micronuclei

Epigenetic modifications of the contained chromatin have also been reported in the MN. The chromosome missegregation and MN formation is believed to result in significant transcriptional and epigenetic heterogeneity, favoring the enhanced growth and adaptability in tumors. Some of the common modifications include enrichment of lysine trimethylation, namely at H3K4, H3K9, and H3K27, loss of acetylation at many lysine residues on the histone H3 tail, notably H3K9Ac, H3K14Ac, and H3K27Ac. Moreover, MN chromosomes exhibit a decrease in the ubiquitination of histones H2A and H2B, which may indicate problems with a number of modifying enzymes and alterations in chromatin accessibility.[111] Compared to the main nucleus, the MN generally have a more compact chromatin structure. Still, their promoter areas include the majority of the more accessible genomic regions. The epigenetic modifications of the MN chromatin may be passed on to the next generation further accentuating the instability of the genome.[8,112]

MICRONUCLEI AS ACTIVE PLAYERS IN CARCINOGENESIS

Recognition of biological activities occurring inside the MN has led to a spurt in studies highlighting their active role in carcinogenesis. These include studies focusing on unique features and functionality of mNE, contents of MN, chromatin dynamics inside the MN and DNA damage response (DDR) machinery, epigenetic modifications, etc. that may be contributing to cancer evolution. Further, the mechanisms exploring how the MN activate the immune system leading to inflammation and ultimately cancer progression are being elucidated.

Micronuclear Envelope Dysfunction and Rupture

The mNE along with its proteins is one of the most important structures required for its structural and functional integrity as it governs the transport of molecules required for various biological processes occurring inside it. Though mNE is a derivative of NE, it may differ significantly from it in its protein composition. Different MN origins, characteristics, and physicochemical variables may contribute to the distinct features of mNE.[113] Especially the differences in the proportion of different lamin proteins have been highlighted in various studies.[114] These differences are believed to contribute to enhanced susceptibility to spontaneous rupture.[113] Lamin B1, along with lamin B2 and lamin A/C, the essential components of the nuclear lamina are often deficient in the MN **(Figs. 4A to D)**.[114] Compared to MN from laggards, the MN formed from NPBs and NBUDs are less commonly linked to lamin B. The smaller MN have a higher likelihood of being lamin B deficient than the larger MN. Further, lamin B deficiencies are more commonly observed in MN in p53-deficient cells than in p53 wild-type cells.[115]

The improperly formed NPCs may be another reason for defective mNE. The envelope of laggards-derived MN may fail to properly assemble the NPCs due to the presence of the tightly coiled spindle microtubules around them interfering with the import of lamin B1.[116-119] Chromosomes close to the spindle midzone with a high density of microtubules are more likely to generate MN with defective NPCs than the chromosomes that missegregate at the spindle poles. Consequently, peripherally generated MN are surrounded by a far more functional mNE.[117] Decreased expression of the endosomal sorting complex required for transport-III and its subunit CHMP7 that are crucial for sealing of NE in interphase may also cause rupture of the MN membrane.[120]

Furthermore, chromatins in MN may be highly compacted, normal, or decondensed, depending on the integrity of mNE. For instance, MN chromatin is very condensed when lamin B is absent. Compared to laggards, the chromatin

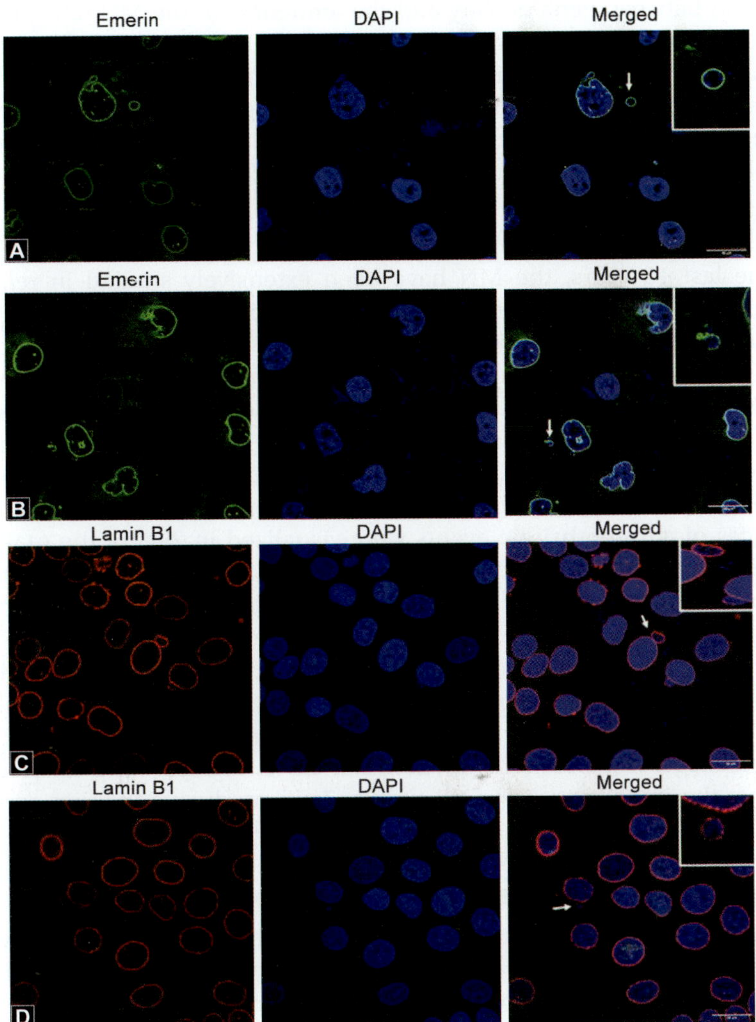

FIGS. 4A TO D: Heterogeneity in expression of mNE proteins emerin and lamin B1 in the MN in MDA-MB-231 breast cancer cells. Complete and discontinuous staining of mNE with emerin FITC-labeled antibody (A and B) and lamin B1 CY3 labeled antibody (C and D). The expression of the above proteins may determine the level of biological activity in them and the leakiness of the contained genetic material resulting in cGAS-STING-mediated immune activation.

(DAPI: 4′,6-diamidino-2-phenylindole; FITC: fluorescein isothiocyanate)

bridges form MN with condensed chromatin. Some MN undergo active DNA end processing to yield single-strand DNA (ssDNA).[11]

The mNE rupture is a critical step in the development of malignancy. While spontaneous mNE rupture is rare in young, healthy cells, it occurs often in aging (almost 40%) and tumor cells (up to 60%).[57] Innate immunity and chromothripsis are two downstream consequences of ruptured MN that are significant for inflammation, aging, and cancer.[121,122] Other studies have found a strong correlation between gene density and the tendency for the MN to rupture. This indicates that the type of chromosome encased may play an important role in deciding its fate.[57] These activities have been associated with the formation of metastases because they hasten the acquisition of genomic heterogeneity, boost immunological signaling pathways and epigenetic reprogramming, accelerate the evolution of the genome, and promote cancer cell survival.

Micronuclei as Drivers of Chromothripsis

Over the last 10 years, the MN have been extensively studied in relation to large-scale, chromosomal rearrangements called chromothripsis. The latter is a singular catastrophic shattering event involving a single chromosome partially or completely.[8,26] The chromosomal rearrangement of DNA linked to MN was first observed by Kato and Sandberg in 1968, but over the next 44 years, it was largely disregarded until Pellman's research in 2012.[22,123] After analyzing 2,658 cancer genomes, the Pan-Cancer Analysis of Whole Genome Consortium discovered that chromothripsis is quite prevalent in human cancers. High incidences of chromothriptic events were visualized in 29% of the malignancy samples with percentages for liposarcomas and osteosarcomas approaching 100% and 77%, respectively.[124] It has been shown that MN is the main site of early chromosomal breakage, followed by aberrant reassembling of the broken fragments.[125] Although the authors recognized that in unruptured MN, late replication may result in chromosomal shattering, other studies have shown a link between mNE breakdown and significant DNA damage as well as chromosome breakage. The relationship between mNE collapse and DNA damage highlights the importance of mNE rupture is in producing massive rearrangements that have a major positive selection effect.[57,120,126,127]

Micronuclei as Purveyors of Immune Response in Cancer

The role of MN as mediators of activation of innate immune pathways in cancer is relatively new. The DNA in the MN may be exposed due to improper mNE with its proneness to collapse. The nucleic acid leaked in the cytoplasm is recognized by DNA sensors such as cGAS. The cGAS catalyzes the conversion of ATP and GTP into 2′,3′-cyclic GMP-AMP (cGAMP) upon DNA binding.[128] cGAMP is the second messenger that oligomerizes and activates the endoplasmic reticulum (ER)-resident protein STING when it binds to it. The STING activates its downstream proteins and transcription factors TANK-binding kinase 1 (TBK1), interferon regulatory factor 3 (IRF3), and IκB kinase (IKK), which translocate the signal to the nucleus where the transcription factor nuclear factor kappa B (NF-κB) modifies the gene expression **(Fig. 5)**.[129] Type I IFN-stimulated genes (ISGs) are activated when the cGAS–STING system is typically engaged. This, in turn, elicits an antitumor immune response.[3,130] Remarkably, sustained activation of this system can rewire the downstream signaling, resulting in a significant reduction in type I IFN response. This occurs in tumors chromosomally unstable tumors with rupture-prone MN. Instead, cytosolic DNA from MN that causes long-term STING activation triggers an ER stress response as well as noncanonical NF-κB. This signal leads to opposite

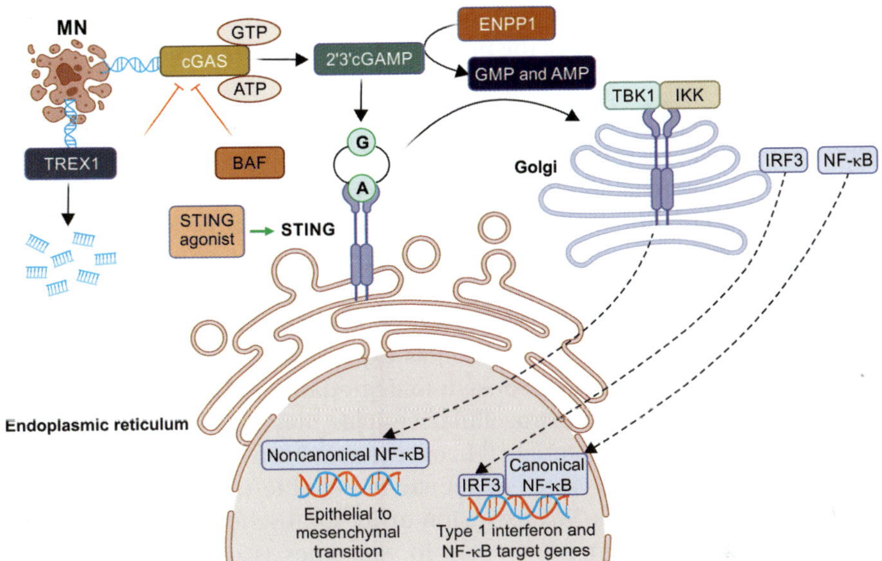

FIG. 5: Activation of cGAS-STING pathway and downstream immune response by release of genetic material from MN.

(2′3′cGAMP: 2′,3′-cyclic GMP-AMP; AMP: adenosine monophosphate; ATP: adenosine triphosphate; BAF: barrier-to-autointegration factor; cGAS-STING: cyclic guanosine monophosphate-adenosine monophosphate synthase-stimulator of interferon genes; GMP: guanosine monophosphate; GTP: guanosine triphosphate; IKK: IκB kinase; IRF3: interferon regulatory factor 3; MN: micronuclei; NF-κB: nuclear factor kappa B; TBK1: TANK-binding kinase 1; TREX1: three prime repair exonuclease 1)

effects such as immune suppression, the epithelial-to-mesenchymal transition, and distant metastatic dissemination.[131,132] Nevertheless, short-term activation of cGAS can facilitate immune surveillance through tumor-to-host cGAMP transfer and paracrine signaling that activates STING in immune and host cells.[133,134] In healthy cells tight regulation over cGAS activation by self-DNA is exhibited by the molecules like three prime repair exonuclease 1 and barrier-to-autointegration factor (BAF).[135,136] The activation of cGAS in cancer cells, however, indicates a dysregulation of the above control pathways. The antitumor immune response triggered by cGAMP export is prevented by overexpression of the ectonucleotide ENPP1, which hydrolyzes cGAMP into GMP and AMP.[14] Chromothripsis and damaged DNA inside the ruptured MN can generate mutated proteins. These potential neoantigens can also provoke a T-cell response.[137,138]

Given its increasing importance, the MN-mediated cGAS-STING pathway is being extensively investigated for pharmaceutical purposes and the induction of antitumor immunity. Especially important in this context is utilizing the modulation of the above pathway to enhance the effect of PD-1 inhibitors.

FATE OF MICRONUCLEI IN CELLS

Although the MN have been proposed to undergo different fates in the cells, several issues remain unexplained. For example, it is unclear which one is the preferred mode of MN disposal. Moreover, the factors determining its removal are poorly understood. Some of the possible fates of MN are described here.

Degradation and Extrusion of Micronuclei

Degradation of MN can occur either by enzymatic destruction of DNA or by autophagy. The latter is a catabolic process characterized by the degradation of cellular components within lysosomes. Colocalization of MN with LC3 in some studies indicates degradation in an autophagy-dependent manner.[139] Another study showed that when primary fibroblasts are treated with clastogens/aneugens, they become P53-positive over time which can be an indication of MN degradation by the nuclease.[107] Further, as explained previously, the improper structure of mNE may also predispose it to degradation **(Fig. 1C)**.[140] Also, some studies have proposed that extracellular vesicles play a role in mediating the evacuation of MN genetic material.[141] In a recent study on ovarian cancer, the MN were shown to be a major source of genetic material found in the exosomes.[142] However, whether the bulk MN extrusion or its rupture followed by transfer of contained chromatin fragments occurs in exosomes is unclear. Nevertheless, the presence of extracellular DNA and membrane blebbing favor the former phenomenon.[143] The DM-type MN are proposed to be extruded from the cells especially when not needed.[55]

Reincorporation of Micronuclei into the Main Nucleus

The MN can be reincorporated back into the primary nucleus in the next cell cycle. The evidence for this has come from some studies showing the disappearance of spontaneous and induced MN from the cells after the second mitosis, thus suggesting the possibility of their reincorporation during this cell division.[144] It is believed that about 25–50% MN are incorporated back into the primary nuclei incorporating the modifications into the genome **(Fig. 1C)**.[28] These changes include epigenetic changes, mutations, other genomic rearrangements, etc.[145,146] Although it is not clear which type of MN are incorporated back it, has been observed that those containing metacentric chromosomes are likely to be reincorporated, whereas those with subtelomeric chromosome fragments rarely do so.[147]

Persistence and Replication of Micronuclei

About 50% of MN persist in the cell due to defects in the assembly of kinetochore proteins.[28] Some studies have shown that MN may simply persist in the cytoplasm after the mitosis is complete without any change **(Fig. 1C)**.[49] Live cell imaging studies carried out on different cell lines and PBLs primary culture, reveal that some MN persist and move about freely in the cytoplasm.[48] Recent work from the Ly laboratory shows that acentric, fragmented chromosomes follow the pattern of asymmetric inheritance during mitosis. The localization of acentric portions of DNA lesions is attributed to the DDR complex CIP2A-TOPBP1, which forms clusters and leads to the segregation of lesions within the same daughter cell.[148]

MICRONUCLEI AS THERAPEUTIC TARGETS IN CANCER

From the ensuing discussion, it is clear that the MN serve as a platform for enhanced mutagenesis and act as a communication center within the tumor microenvironment. Thus, they are crucial to the development and spread of cancer. Treatments that target MN formation, rupture, and fate can be highly selective for cancer cells with unstable chromosomes. MN-mediated cGAS-STING response constitutes an important pathway that can be harnessed to generate immunity against the tumors. In line with this STING agonists have emerged as promising therapeutic agents to boost the innate immune response in cancers.[149] However, despite the promising preclinical outcomes, their therapeutic utility even in conjunction with other immunotherapies is yet to be demonstrated.[8,150] Other than that, in tumors that persistently activate cGAS to cause suppressive immunity, effective strategies can be devised to divert the immune response to antitumor immunity, thus offering an opportunity to target chromosomally unstable and drug-resistant malignancies.

Cells with collapsed MN significantly, though not always successfully, induce DDR signaling due to the absence of compartmentalization.[119] One popular cancer treatment approach is pharmacologic suppression of the DDR, which may raise DNA damage levels over the point at which cells die. Furthermore, a recent study demonstrates that MN damages DNA by activating certain pathways that are dormant in primary nuclei.[151] It is believed that RNA-DNA hybrids, or R-loops, are highly common in MN and are linked to genomic instability.[152] The adenosine deaminase acting on RNA in MN uses R-loops as a framework to change DNA and produce deoxyinosine (dI). Abasic sites are formed when alkyladenine DNA glycosylase recognizes dI, and AP-endonuclease subsequently cuts these sites. This process, which is largely absent in primary nuclei, is one of the principal causes of DNA fragmentation in MN.[153] Targeting one or more of the key actors in the above pathway can serve as an effective technique with little impact on nontransformed cells. It has been seen that when used with conventional therapy, the medications that stop MN rupture may reduce resistance development and the onset of metastatic illness. For example, recent studies suggest that MN collapse might be associated with BAF and ESCRT-III complex NE repair failure. Concentrating on these molecules to stop the mNE catastrophe is being investigated.[120,126,154] Some studies have shown that BAF inhibition raises the in vitro death rate of cancer cells. Because of ESCRT-III's role in mending plasma and NEs and decreasing pharmacologic cell death, targeting ESCRT-III subunits is also being investigated as a possible cancer treatment.[155,156]

CONCLUSION

Chromosomal instability is one of the important characteristics of malignant tumors, and MN with their contents are the most studied indicators of the above phenomenon. The MN have been used for gauzing genotoxicity and as screening, diagnostic, prognostic, and treatment response markers in malignancies. With a spurt in the studies to understand their genesis, biology, destiny, and contents, the MN have evolved from passive indicators to active players in cancer pathogenesis. The latter underscores the importance of deciphering the MN biology for targeting the MN-heavy chromosomally unstable tumors. The events such as gene rearrangement in MN including chromothripsis, epigenetic modifications, and MN collapse, persistence, or reincorporation need to be understood in greater detail for developing novel therapeutics for aggressive tumors. The MN-mediated immune responses can be harnessed to boost the therapeutic effect of immunological agents such as immune checkpoint inhibitors. The complex effects of mNE composition and structure on MN functionality are emerging as interesting areas for further research and understanding.

REFERENCES

1. Vargas-Rondón N, Villegas VE, Rondón-Lagos M. The Role of Chromosomal Instability in Cancer and Therapeutic Responses. Cancers. 2017;10(1).
2. Fenech M. Chromosomal biomarkers of genomic instability relevant to cancer. Drug Discov Today. 2002;7(22):1128-37.
3. Kumari L, Kumar Y, Bhatia A. The link between chromosomal instability and immunity in cancer. In: Rezaei N (Ed). Handbook of Cancer and Immunology. Cham: Springer International Publishing; 2022. pp. 1-20.
4. Bochtler T, Kartal-Kaess M, Granzow M, Hielscher T, Cosenza MR, Herold-Mende C, et al. Micronucleus formation in human cancer cells is biased by chromosome size. Genes, Chromosomes and Cancer. 2019;58(6):392-5.
5. Luzhna L, Kathiria P, Kovalchuk O. Micronuclei in genotoxicity assessment: from genetics to epigenetics and beyond. Front Genet. 2013;4:131.
6. Bolognesi C, Bonassi S, Knasmueller S, Fenech M, Bruzzone M, Lando C, et al. Clinical application of micronucleus test in exfoliated buccal cells: A systematic review and metanalysis. Mutat Res Rev Mutat Res. 2015;766:20-31.
7. Crasta K, Ganem NJ, Dagher R, Lantermann AB, Ivanova EV, Pan Y, et al. DNA breaks and chromosome pulverization from errors in mitosis. Nature. 2012;482(7383):53-8.
8. Di Bona M, Bakhoum SF. Micronuclei and Cancer. Cancer Discov. 2024;14(2):214-26.
9. Boveri T. Concerning the origin of malignant tumours by Theodor Boveri. Translated and annotated by Henry Harris. J Cell Sci. 2008;121(Suppl 1):1-84.
10. Lewis WH. Interphase (resting) nuclei, chromosomal vesicles and amitosis. Anat Rec. 1947;97(4):433-45.
11. Mather K, Stone LHA. The effect of X-radiation upon somatic chromosomes. J Genet. 1933;28(1):1-24.
12. Darlington CD, La Cour LF. Chromosome breakage and the nucleic acid cycle. J Genet. 1945;46(2):180-267.
13. Tennant R, Liebow AAJTYJoB, Medicine. The Actions of Colchicine and of Ethylcarbylamine on Tissue Cultures. 1940;13:39-50.4.
14. Marshak A, Bradley M. X-Ray Inhibition of Mitosis in Relation to Chromosome Number. Proc Natl Acad Sci U S A. 1944;30(9):231-7.
15. Sears DA, Udden MM. Howell-Jolly bodies: a brief historical review. Am J Med Sci. 2012;343(5):407-9.
16. Brues AM, Jackson EB. Nuclear Abnormalities Resulting from Inhibition of Mitosis by Colchicine and other Substances. Am J Cancer. 1937;30:504-11.
17. Schwarz E. Cellular gigantism and pluripolar mitosis in human hematopoiesis. Am J Anat. 1946;79:75-115.
18. Dawson DW, Bury HP. The significance of Howell-Jolly bodies and giant metamyelocytes in marrow smears. J Clin Pathol. 1961;14(4):374-80.

19. Phillips SG, Phillips DM. Sites of nucleolus production in cultured Chinese hamster cells. J Cell Biol. 1969;40(1):248-68.
20. Das NK. Synthetic capacitie of chromosome fragments correlated with their ability to maintain nucleolar material. The Journal of cell biology. 1962;15(1):121-30.
21. McLeish J. The consequences of localised chromosome breakage. Heredity. 1954;8(3): 385-407.
22. Kato H, Sandberg AA. Chromosome pulverization in human cells with micronuclei. J Natl Cancer Inst. 1968;40(1):165-79.
23. Klein G, Klein E. The viability and the average desoxypentosenucleic acid content of micronuclei-containing cells produced by colchicine treatment in the Ehrlich ascites tumor. Cancer Research. 1952;12(7):484-9.
24. Kleinfeld RG, Sisken JE. Morphological and kinetic aspects of mitotic arrest by and recovery from colcemid. J Cell Biol. 1966;31(3):369-79.
25. Crasta K, Ganem NJ, Dagher R, Lantermann AB, Ivanova EV, Pan Y, et al. DNA breaks and chromosome pulverization from errors in mitosis. Nature. 2012;482(7383):53-8.
26. Krupina K, Goginashvili A, Cleveland DW. Causes and consequences of micronuclei. Curr OpinCell Biol. 2021;70:91-9.
27. Bonassi S, Znaor A, Ceppi M, Lando C, Chang WP, Holland N, et al. An increased micronucleus frequency in peripheral blood lymphocytes predicts the risk of cancer in humans. Carcinogenesis. 2007;28(3):625-31.
28. Soto M, García-Santisteban I, Krenning L, Medema RH, Raaijmakers JA. Chromosomes trapped in micronuclei are liable to segregation errors. J Cell Sci. 2018;131(13).
29. McDorman EW, Collins BW, Allen JW. Dietary folate deficiency enhances induction of micronuclei by arsenic in mice. Environ Mol Mutagen. 2002;40(1):71-7.
30. Norppa H, Falck GC. What do human micronuclei contain? Mutagenesis. 2003;18(3):221-33.
31. Bochtler T, Kartal-Kaess M, Granzow M, Hielscher T, Cosenza MR, Herold-Mende C, et al. Micronucleus formation in human cancer cells is biased by chromosome size. Genes chromosomes Cancer. 2019;58(6):392-5.
32. Mateuca R, Lombaert N, Aka PV, Decordier I, Kirsch-Volders M. Chromosomal changes: induction, detection methods and applicability in human biomonitoring. Biochimie. 2006;88(11):1515-31.
33. Fenech M, Kirsch-Volders M, Natarajan AT, Surralles J, Crott JW, Parry J, et al. Molecular mechanisms of micronucleus, nucleoplasmic bridge and nuclear bud formation in mammalian and human cells. Mutagenesis. 2011;26(1):125-32.
34. Thomas P, Umegaki K, Fenech M. Nucleoplasmic bridges are a sensitive measure of chromosome rearrangement in the cytokinesis-block micronucleus assay. Mutagenesis. 2003;18(2):187-94.
35. Schueler MG, Sullivan BA. Structural and functional dynamics of human centromeric chromatin. Annu Rev Genomics Hum Genet. 2006;7:301-13.
36. Gieni RS, Chan GK, Hendzel MJ. Epigenetics regulate centromere formation and kinetochore function. J Cell Biochem. 2008;104(6):2027-39.
37. Heit R, Rattner JB, Chan GK, Hendzel MJ. G2 histone methylation is required for the proper segregation of chromosomes. J Cell Sci. 2009;122(Pt 16):2957-68.
38. Pampalona J, Soler D, Genescà A, Tusell L. Whole chromosome loss is promoted by telomere dysfunction in primary cells. Genes Chromosomes Cancer. 2010;49(4):368-78.
39. Fenech M. Cytokinesis-block micronucleus cytome assay. Nat Protoc. 2007;2(5):1084-104.
40. Haaf T, Raderschall E, Reddy G, Ward DC, Radding CM, Golub EI. Sequestration of mammalian Rad51-recombination protein into micronuclei. J Cell Biol. 1999;144(1):11-20.
41. Lindberg HK, Wang X, Järventaus H, Falck GC, Norppa H, Fenech M. Origin of nuclear buds and micronuclei in normal and folate-deprived human lymphocytes. Mutat Res. 2007;617 (1-2):33-45.
42. Huang Y, Fenech M, Shi Q. Micronucleus formation detected by live-cell imaging. Mutagenesis. 2011;26(1):133-8.

43. Cimini D, Fioravanti D, Salmon ED, Degrassi F. Merotelic kinetochore orientation versus chromosome mono-orientation in the origin of lagging chromosomes in human primary cells. J Cell Sci. 2002;115(Pt 3):507-15.
44. Shimizu N, Shimura T, Tanaka T. Selective elimination of acentric double minutes from cancer cells through the extrusion of micronuclei. Mutat Res. 2000;448(1):81-90.
45. Rao X, Zhang Y, Yi Q, Hou H, Xu B, Chu L, et al. Multiple origins of spontaneously arising micronuclei in HeLa cells: direct evidence from long-term live cell imaging. Mutat Res. 2008;646(1-2):41-9.
46. Shimizu N, Kanda T, Wahl GM. Selective capture of acentric fragments by micronuclei provides a rapid method for purifying extrachromosomally amplified DNA. Nat Genet. 1996;12(1):65-71.
47. Von Hoff DD, McGill JR, Forseth BJ, Davidson KK, Bradley TP, Van Devanter DR, et al. Elimination of extrachromosomally amplified MYC genes from human tumor cells reduces their tumorigenicity. Proc Natl Acad Sci U S A. 1992;89(17):8165-9.
48. Hintzsche H, Hemmann U, Poth A, Utesch D, Lott J, Stopper H. Fate of micronuclei and micronucleated cells. Mutat Res Rev Mutat Res. 2017;771:85-98.
49. Bhatia A, Kumar Y. Cancer cell micronucleus: an update on clinical and diagnostic applications. Apmis. 2013;121(7):569-81.
50. Guo X, Dai X, Wu X, Cao N, Wang X. Small but strong: Mutational and functional landscapes of micronuclei in cancer genomes. Int J Cancer. 2021;148(4):812-24.
51. Jadhav K, Gupta N, Ahmed MB. Micronuclei: An essential biomarker in oral exfoliated cells for grading of oral squamous cell carcinoma. J Cytol. 2011;28(1):7-12.
52. García-Rodríguez A, Kazantseva L, Vila L, Rubio L, Velázquez A, Ramírez MJ, et al. Micronuclei Detection by Flow Cytometry as a High-Throughput Approach for the Genotoxicity Testing of Nanomaterials. Nanomaterials (Basel, Switzerland). 2019;9(12).
53. Nicolette J, Diehl M, Sonders P, Bryce S, Blomme E. In vitro micronucleus screening of pharmaceutical candidates by flow cytometry in Chinese hamster V79 cells. Environmental and molecular mutagenesis. 2011;52(5):355-62.
54. Franz P, Bürkle A, Wick P, Hirsch C. Exploring Flow Cytometry-Based Micronucleus Scoring for Reliable Nanomaterial Genotoxicity Assessment. Chem Res Toxicol. 2020;33(10):2538-49.
55. Yasui M, Koyama N, Koizumi T, Senda-Murata K, Takashima Y, Hayashi M, et al. Live cell imaging of micronucleus formation and development. Mutat Res. 2010;692(1-2):12-8.
56. Bakhoum SF, Ngo B, Laughney AM, Cavallo J-A, Murphy CJ, Ly P, et al. Chromosomal instability drives metastasis through a cytosolic DNA response. Nature. 2018;553(7689): 467-72.
57. Hatch EM, Fischer AH, Deerinck TJ, Hetzer MW. Catastrophic nuclear envelope collapse in cancer cell micronuclei. Cell. 2013;154(1):47-60.
58. Terradas M, Martín M, Tusell L, Genescà A. Genetic activities in micronuclei: Is the DNA entrapped in micronuclei lost for the cell? Mutation Research/Reviews in Mutation Research. 2010;705(1):60-7.
59. Kiran K, Agarwal P, Kumar S, Jain K. Micronuclei as a Predictor for Oral Carcinogenesis. JCytol. 2018;35(4):233-6.
60. El-Zein RA, Lopez MS, D'Amelio AM, Jr., Liu M, Munden RF, Christiani D, et al. The cytokinesis-blocked micronucleus assay as a strong predictor of lung cancer: extension of a lung cancer risk prediction model. Cancer Epidemiol Biomarkers Prev 2014;23(11):2462-70.
61. Rothfuss A, Schütz P, Bochum S, Volm T, Eberhardt E, Kreienberg R, et al. Induced micronucleus frequencies in peripheral lymphocytes as a screening test for carriers of a BRCA1 mutation in breast cancer families. Cancer Res. 2000;60(2):390-4.
62. El-Zein RA, Schabath MB, Etzel CJ, Lopez MS, Franklin JD, Spitz MR. Cytokinesis-blocked micronucleus assay as a novel biomarker for lung cancer risk. Cancer Res. 2006;66(12): 6449-56.
63. Pardini B, Viberti C, Naccarati A, Allione A, Oderda M, Critelli R, et al. Increased micronucleus frequency in peripheral blood lymphocytes predicts the risk of bladder cancer. Br J Cancer. 2017;116(2):202-10.

64. Varga D, Hoegel J, Maier C, Jainta S, Hoehne M, Patino-Garcia B, et al. On the difference of micronucleus frequencies in peripheral blood lymphocytes between breast cancer patients and controls. Mutagenesis. 2006;21(5):313-20.
65. Hemalatha A, Suresh TN, HarendraKumar ML. Micronuclei in breast aspirates. Is scoring them helpful? J Cancer Res Ther. 2014;10(2):309-11.
66. Chang P, Li Y, Li D. Micronuclei levels in peripheral blood lymphocytes as a potential biomarker for pancreatic cancer risk. Carcinogenesis. 2011;32(2):210-5.
67. Bolognesi C, Bruzzone M, Ceppi M, Marcon F. Micronuclei and upper body cancers (head, neck, breast cancers) a systematic review and meta-analysis. Mutation research Reviews in mutation research. 2021;787:108358.
68. Cardinale F, Bruzzi P, Bolognesi C. Role of micronucleus test in predicting breast cancer susceptibility: a systematic review and meta-analysis. Br J Cancer. 2012;106(4):780-90.
69. Chatterjee S, Dhar S, Sengupta B, Ghosh A, De M, Roy S, et al. Cytogenetic monitoring in human oral cancers and other oral pathology: the micronucleus test in exfoliated buccal cells. Toxicol Mech Methods. 2009;19(6-7):427-33.
70. Gashi G, Mahovlić V, Manxhuka-Kerliu S, Podrimaj-Bytyqi A, Gashi L, Elezaj IR. The association between micronucleus, nucleoplasmic bridges, and nuclear buds frequency and the degree of uterine cervical lesions. Biomarkers. 2018;23(4):364-72.
71. Espinoza F, Cecchini L, Morote J, Marcos R, Pastor S. Micronuclei frequency in urothelial cells of bladder cancer patients, as a biomarker of prognosis. Environ Mol Mutagen. 2019;60(2):168-73.
72. Kiraz A, Açmaz G, Uysal G, Unal D, Dönmez-Altuntas H. Micronucleus testing as a cancer detector: endometrial hyperplasia to carcinoma. Arch Gynecol Obstet. 2016;293(5): 1065-71.
73. Shashikala R, Indira AP, Manjunath GS, Rao KA, Akshatha BK. Role of micronucleus in oral exfoliative cytology. J Pharm Bioallied Sci. 2015;7(Suppl 2):S409-13.
74. Elnaggar A, Madkour G, Tahoun N, Amin A, Zahran FhM. Micronuclei detection in oral cytologic smear: does it add diagnostic value? J Egypt Natl Canc Inst. 2023;35(1):31.
75. Grover S, Ahmed MB, Telagi N, Shivappa AB, Nithin KP. Evaluation of diagnostic reliability of micronuclei in potentially malignant disorders of oral cavity. CHRISMED J Health Res. 2014;1:15-20.
76. Sylvia MT, Baskaran L, Bhat RV. Micronucleus Study on Breast Cytology Aspirate Smears and its Diagnostic Utility. J Cytol. 2018;35(1):22-6.
77. Setayesh T, Kundi M, Nersesyan A, Stopper H, Fenech M, Krupitza G, et al. Use of micronucleus assays for the prediction and detection of cervical cancer: a meta-analysis. Carcinogenesis. 2020;41(10):1318-28.
78. Agarwal A, Ahuja R, Tijare M, Ghate S, Tegginamani A, Pathak S. Micronuclei: a prognostic tool. J EvolMed Dent Sci. 2014;3:11762-6.
79. Högstedt B, Gunnar Nilsson P, Mitelman F. Micronuclei in erythropoietic bone marrow cells: Relation to cytogenetic pattern and prognosis in acute nonlymphocytic leukemia. Cancer Genet Cytogenet. 1981;3(3):185-93.
80. Pardini B, Viberti C, Naccarati A, Allione A, Oderda M, Critelli R, et al. Increased micronucleus frequency in peripheral blood lymphocytes predicts the risk of bladder cancer. Br J Cancer. 2017;116(2):202-10.
81. Podrimaj-Bytyqi A, Borovečki A, Selimi Q, Manxhuka-Kerliu S, Gashi G, Elezaj IR. The frequencies of micronuclei, nucleoplasmic bridges and nuclear buds as biomarkers of genomic instability in patients with urothelial cell carcinoma. Sci Rep. 2018;8(1):17873.
82. Asanov M, Bonassi S, Proietti S, Minina VI, Tomino C, El-Zein R. Genomic instability in chronic obstructive pulmonary disease and lung cancer: A systematic review and meta-analysis of studies using the micronucleus assay. Mutat Res Rev Mutat Res. 2021;787:108344.
83. Raj SG, Rajitha V. Assessment of genotoxic instability markers in peripheral blood lymphocytes of breast cancer patients: a case control study. J Biomol Struct Dyn. 2024; 42(3):1559-63.

84. El-Zein RA, Schabath MB, Etzel CJ, Lopez MS, Franklin JD, Spitz MR. Cytokinesis-Blocked Micronucleus Assay as a Novel Biomarker for Lung Cancer Risk. Cancer Res. 2006;66(12): 6449-56.
85. Bonassi S, Znaor A, Ceppi M, Lando C, Chang WP, Holland N, et al. An increased micronucleus frequency in peripheral blood lymphocytes predicts the risk of cancer in humans. Carcinogenesis. 2007;28(3):625-31.
86. Murgia E, Ballardin M, Bonassi S, Rossi AM, Barale R. Validation of micronuclei frequency in peripheral blood lymphocytes as early cancer risk biomarker in a nested case–control study. Mutat Res-Fund Mol M. 2008;639(1):27-34.
87. Chang P, Li Y, Li D. Micronuclei levels in peripheral blood lymphocytes as a potential biomarker for pancreatic cancer risk. Carcinogenesis. 2010;32(2):210-5.
88. Bolognesi C, Bruzzi P, Gismondi V, Volpi S, Viassolo V, Pedemonte S, et al. Clinical application of micronucleus test: a case-control study on the prediction of breast cancer risk/susceptibility. PloS One. 2014;9(11):e112354.
89. Iarmarcovai G, Ceppi M, Botta A, Orsière T, Bonassi S. Micronuclei frequency in peripheral blood lymphocytes of cancer patients: A meta-analysis. Mutat Res. 2008;659(3):274-83.
90. Hovhannisyan G, Harutyunyan T, Aroutiounian R. Micronuclei and What They Can Tell Us in Cytogenetic Diagnostics. Curr Genet Med Rep. 2018;6(4):144-54.
91. Nikolouzakis TK, Vakonaki E, Stivaktakis PD, Alegakis A, Berdiaki A, Razos N, et al. Novel Prognostic Biomarkers in Metastatic and Locally Advanced Colorectal Cancer: Micronuclei Frequency and Telomerase Activity in Peripheral Blood Lymphocytes. Front Oncol. 2021;11:683605.
92. Ravi KS, Pushpa NB, Kishore S, Kaur S, Mehta V, Reddy KS. Taxation of Micronuclei Frequency as a Prognostic Marker in Oral and Oropharyngeal Carcinoma: A Cytogenetic Study. Natl J Clin Anat. 2021;10(2):57-60.
93. Jagetia GC, Jayakrishnan A, Fernandes D, Vidyasagar MS. Evaluation of micronuclei frequency in the cultured peripheral blood lymphocytes of cancer patients before and after radiation treatment. Mutat Res. 2001;491(1-2):9-16.
94. Lee TK, Allison RR, O'Brien KF, Naves JL, Karlsson UL, Wiley AL. Persistence of micronuclei in lymphocytes of cancer patients after radiotherapy. Radiat Res. 2002;157(6):678-84.
95. Djuzenova CS, Mühl B, Fehn M, Oppitz U, Müller B, Flentje M. Radiosensitivity in breast cancer assessed by the Comet and micronucleus assays. Br J Cancer. 2006;94(8):1194-203.
96. Guogytė K, Plieskienė A, Ladygienė R, Vaisiūnas Ž, Sevriukova O, Janušonis V, et al. Assessment of Correlation between Chromosomal Radiosensitivity of Peripheral Blood Lymphocytes after In vitro Irradiation and Normal Tissue Side Effects for Cancer Patients Undergoing Radiotherapy. Genome Integrity. 2017;8:1.
97. Kobayashi D, Oike T, Murata K, Irie D, Hirota Y, Sato H, et al. Induction of Micronuclei in Cervical Cancer Treated with Radiotherapy. J Pers Med. 2020;10(3):110.
98. Singh S, Datta NR, Krishnani N, Lal P, Kumar S. Radiation therapy induced micronuclei in cervical cancer—does it have a predictive value for local disease control? Gynecol Oncol. 2005;97(3):764-71.
99. Borges da Silva E, Brayner Cavalcanti M, Ferreira Da Silva CS, de Salazar EFT, Azevedo Melo J, Lucena L, et al. Micronucleus assay for predicting side effects of radiotherapy for cervical cancer. Biotech Histochem. 2020:1-7.
100. Bhatia A, Kumar Y. Cancer cell micronucleus: an update on clinical and diagnostic applications. APMIS. 2013;121(7):569-81.
101. Driessens G, Harsan L, Robaye B, Waroquier D, Browaeys P, Giannakopoulos X, et al. Micronuclei to detect in vivo chemotherapy damage in a p53 mutated solid tumour. Br J Cancer. 2003;89(4):727-9.
102. Hashimoto K, Nakajima Y, Matsumura S, Chatani F. An in vitro micronucleus assay with size-classified micronucleus counting to discriminate aneugens from clastogens. Toxicol In Vitro. 2010;24(1):208-16.
103. Tucker JD, Nath J, Hando JC. Activation status of the X chromosome in human micronucleated lymphocytes. Hum Genet. 1996;97(4):471-5.

104. Klaasen SJ, Truong MA, van Jaarsveld RH, Koprivec I, Štimac V, de Vries SG, et al. Nuclear chromosome locations dictate segregation error frequencies. Nature. 2022;607(7919): 604-9.
105. Utani K, Kohno Y, Okamoto A, Shimizu N. Emergence of micronuclei and their effects on the fate of cells under replication stress. PLoS One. 2010;5(4):e10089.
106. Okamoto A, Utani K, Shimizu N. DNA replication occurs in all lamina positive micronuclei, but never in lamina negative micronuclei. Mutagenesis. 2012;27(3):323-7.
107. Hintzsche H, Hemmann U, Poth A, Utesch D, Lott J, Stopper H. Fate of micronuclei and micronucleated cells. Mutat Res. 2017;771:85-98.
108. Terradas M, Martín M, Tusell L, Genescà A. Genetic activities in micronuclei: is the DNA entrapped in micronuclei lost for the cell? Mutat Res. 2010;705(1):60-7.
109. Wang M, Saha J, Cucinotta FA. Smad7 foci are present in micronuclei induced by heavy particle radiation. Mutation research. 2013;756(1-2):108-14.
110. Fenech M, Knasmueller S, Bolognesi C, Holland N, Bonassi S, Kirsch-Volders M. Micronuclei as biomarkers of DNA damage, aneuploidy, inducers of chromosomal hypermutation and as sources of pro-inflammatory DNA in humans. Mutat Res Rev Mutat Res. 2020;786: 108342.
111. Agustinus AS, Al-Rawi D, Dameracharla B, Raviram R, Jones BSCL, Stransky S, et al. Epigenetic dysregulation from chromosomal transit in micronuclei. Nature. 2023;619(7968):176-83.
112. Luzhna L, Kathiria P, Kovalchuk O. Micronuclei in genotoxicity assessment: from genetics to epigenetics and beyond. Front Genet. 2013;4:131.
113. Guo X, Dai X, Wu X, Zhou T, Ni J, Xue J, et al. Understanding the birth of rupture-prone and irreparable micronuclei. Chromosoma. 2020;129(3):181-200.
114. Maass KK, Rosing F, Ronchi P, Willmund KV, Devens F, Hergt M, et al. Altered nuclear envelope structure and proteasome function of micronuclei. Exp Cell Res. 2018;371(2):353-63.
115. Guscott M, Saha A, Maharaj J, McClelland SE. The multifaceted role of micronuclei in tumour progression: A whole organism perspective. Int J Biochem Cell Biol. 2022;152:106300.
116. Miyazaki K, Ichikawa Y, Saitoh N, Saitoh HJC. Three types of nuclear envelope assemblies associated with micronuclei. CellBio. 2020;9(1):14-28.
117. Liu S, Kwon M, Mannino M, Yang N, Renda F, Khodjakov A, et al. Nuclear envelope assembly defects link mitotic errors to chromothripsis. Nature. 2018;561(7724):551-5.
118. Kwon M, Leibowitz ML, Lee J-H. Small but mighty: the causes and consequences of micronucleus rupture. Exp Mol Med. 2020;52(11):1777-86.
119. Terradas M, Martín M, Hernández L, Tusell L, Genescà A. Nuclear envelope defects impede a proper response to micronuclear DNA lesions. Mut Res. 2012;729(1-2):35-40.
120. Willan J, Cleasby AJ, Flores-Rodriguez N, Stefani F, Rinaldo C, Pisciottani A, et al. ESCRT-III is necessary for the integrity of the nuclear envelope in micronuclei but is aberrant at ruptured micronuclear envelopes generating damage. Oncogenesis. 2019;8(5):29.
121. Guo X, Dai X, Wu X, Zhou T, Ni J, Xue J, et al. Understanding the birth of rupture-prone and irreparable micronuclei. Chromosoma. 2020;129(3-4):181-200.
122. Barroso-Vilares M, Macedo JC, Reis M, Warren JD, Compton D, Logarinho E. Small-molecule inhibition of aging-associated chromosomal instability delays cellular senescence. 2020;21(5):e49248.
123. Zhang CZ, Spektor A, Cornils H, Francis JM, Jackson EK, Liu S, et al. Chromothripsis from DNA damage in micronuclei. Nature. 2015;522(7555):179-84.
124. Cortés-Ciriano I, Lee JJ, Xi R, Jain D, Jung YL, Yang L, et al. Comprehensive analysis of chromothripsis in 2,658 human cancers using whole-genome sequencing. Nat Genet. 2020;52(3):331-41.
125. Maiato H, Afonso O, Matos I. A chromosome separation checkpoint: A midzone Aurora B gradient mediates a chromosome separation checkpoint that regulates the anaphase-telophase transition. BioEssays. 2015;37(3):257-66.
126. Vietri M, Schultz SW, Bellanger A, Jones CM, Petersen LI, Raiborg C, et al. Unrestrained ESCRT-III drives micronuclear catastrophe and chromosome fragmentation. Nat Cell Biol. 2020;22(7):856-67.

127. Ly P, Teitz LS, Kim DH, Shoshani O, Skaletsky H, Fachinetti D, et al. Selective Y centromere inactivation triggers chromosome shattering in micronuclei and repair by non-homologous end joining. Nat Cell Biol. 2017;19(1):68-75.
128. Ablasser A, Goldeck M, Cavlar T, Deimling T, Witte G, Röhl I, et al. cGAS produces a 2′-5′-linked cyclic dinucleotide second messenger that activates STING. Nature. 2013;498(7454): 380-4.
129. Sun L, Wu J, Du F, Chen X, Chen ZJ. Cyclic GMP-AMP synthase is a cytosolic DNA sensor that activates the type I interferon pathway. Science (New York, NY). 2013;339(6121): 786-91.
130. Wang H, Hu S, Chen X, Shi H, Chen C, Sun L, et al. cGAS is essential for the antitumor effect of immune checkpoint blockade. ProcNatl Acad Sci USA. 2017;114(7):1637-42.
131. Li J, Hubisz MJ, Earlie EM, Duran MA, Hong C, Varela AA, et al. Non-cell-autonomous cancer progression from chromosomal instability. Nature. 2023;620(7976):1080-8.
132. Bakhoum SF, Ngo B, Laughney AM, Cavallo JA, Murphy CJ, Ly P, et al. Chromosomal instability drives metastasis through a cytosolic DNA response. Nature. 2018;553(7689):467-72.
133. Glück S, Guey B, Gulen MF, Wolter K, Kang TW, Schmacke NA, et al. Innate immune sensing of cytosolic chromatin fragments through cGAS promotes senescence. Nat Cell Biol. 2017;19(9):1061-70.
134. Schadt L, Sparano C, Schweiger NA, Silina K, Cecconi V, Lucchiari G, et al. Cancer-Cell-Intrinsic cGAS Expression Mediates Tumor Immunogenicity. Cell Rep. 2019;29(5):1236-48.e7.
135. Guey B, Wischnewski M, Decout A, Makasheva K, Kaynak M, Sakar MS, et al. BAF restricts cGAS on nuclear DNA to prevent innate immune activation. Science (New York, NY). 2020;369(6505):823-8.
136. Ma H, Qian W, Bambouskova M, Collins PL, Porter SI, Byrum AK, et al. Barrier-to-Autointegration Factor 1 Protects against a Basal cGAS-STING Response. mBio. 2020;11(2).
137. Schumacher TN, Schreiber RD. Neoantigens in cancer immunotherapy. Science (New York, NY). 2015;348(6230):69-74.
138. Yarchoan M, Hopkins A, Jaffee EM. Tumor Mutational Burden and Response Rate to PD-1 Inhibition. N Engl J Med. 2017;377(25):2500-1.
139. Bartsch K, Knittler K, Borowski C, Rudnik S, Damme M, Aden K, et al. Absence of RNase H2 triggers generation of immunogenic micronuclei removed by autophagy. Human Mol Genet. 2017;26(20):3960-72.
140. Erenpreisa J, Huna A, Salmina K, Jackson TR, Cragg MS. Macroautophagy-aided elimination of chromatin: sorting of waste, sorting of fate? Autophagy. 2012;8(12):1877-81.
141. Brinkmann V, Reichard U, Goosmann C, Fauler B, Uhlemann Y, Weiss DS, et al. Neutrophil extracellular traps kill bacteria. Science (New York, NY). 2004;303(5663):1532-5.
142. Yokoi A, Villar-Prados A, Oliphint PA, Zhang J, Song X, De Hoff P, et al. Mechanisms of nuclear content loading to exosomes. Sci Adv. 2019;5(11):eaax8849.
143. Shimizu N. Extrachromosomal double minutes and chromosomal homogeneously staining regions as probes for chromosome research. Cytogenet Genome Res. 2009; 124(3-4):312-26.
144. Huang Y, Hou H, Yi Q, Zhang Y, Chen D, Jiang E, et al. The fate of micronucleated cells post X-irradiation detected by live cell imaging. DNA Repair (Amst). 2011;10(6):629-38.
145. Shoshani O, Brunner SF, Yaeger R, Ly P, Nechemia-Arbely Y, Kim DH, et al. Chromothripsis drives the evolution of gene amplification in cancer. Nature. 2021;591(7848):137-41.
146. Ly P, Brunner SF, Shoshani O, Kim DH, Lan W, Pyntikova T, et al. Chromosome segregation errors generate a diverse spectrum of simple and complex genomic rearrangements. Nat Genet. 2019;51(4):705-15.
147. Rizzoni M, Tanzarella C, Gustavino B, Degrassi F, Guarino A, Vitagliano E. Indirect mitotic nondisjunction in Vicia faba and Chinese hamster cells. Chromosoma. 1989;97(4):339-46.
148. Lin Y-F, Hu Q, Mazzagatti A, Valle-Inclán JE, Maurais EG, Dahiya R, et al. Mitotic clustering of pulverized chromosomes from micronuclei. Nature. 2023.

149. Haag SM, Gulen MF, Reymond L, Gibelin A, Abrami L, Decout A, et al. Targeting STING with covalent small-molecule inhibitors. Nature. 2018;559(7713):269-73.
150. Corrales L, Glickman LH, McWhirter SM, Kanne DB, Sivick KE, Katibah GE, et al. Direct Activation of STING in the Tumor Microenvironment Leads to Potent and Systemic Tumor Regression and Immunity. Cell Rep. 2015;11(7):1018-30.
151. Cheng B, Pan W, Xing Y, Xiao Y, Chen J, Xu Z. Recent advances in DDR (DNA damage response) inhibitors for cancer therapy. Eur J Med Chem. 2022;230:114109.
152. Aguilera A, García-Muse T. R loops: from transcription byproducts to threats to genome stability. Mol Cell. 2012;46(2):115-24.
153. Tang S, Stokasimov E, Cui Y, Pellman D. Breakage of cytoplasmic chromosomes by pathological DNA base excision repair. Nature. 2022;606(7916):930-6.
154. Halfmann CT, Sears RM, Katiyar A, Busselman BW, Aman LK, Zhang Q, et al. Repair of nuclear ruptures requires barrier-to-autointegration factor. J Cell Biol. 2019;218(7):2136-49.
155. Kim W, Lyu HN, Kwon HS, Kim YS, Lee KH, Kim DY, et al. Obtusilactone B from Machilus Thunbergii targets barrier-to-autointegration factor to treat cancer. Mol Pharmacol. 2013;83(2):367-76.
156. Liu J, Kang R, Tang D. ESCRT-III-mediated membrane repair in cell death and tumor resistance. Cancer Gene Ther. 2021;28(1-2):1-4.

7

CHAPTER

Liquid Biopsy: Research Laboratory to Clinical Applications

Pranab Dey

INTRODUCTION

In the last few decades, there has been a significant advancement in the understanding of tumorigenesis and progression of cancer. However, the failure of cancer treatment is due to tumor heterogeneity and the continuous evolution of the cancer cells.[1] Histopathological examination of the tissue obtained by incisional or excisional biopsy is the gold standard for the management of cancer. The histopathological examination often misses the tumor heterogeneity. Moreover, repeated biopsy is not possible to assess the continuous evolution of the tumor. Liquid biopsy plays a critical role in the evaluation of the tumor continuously without any invasive technology.

CONVENTIONAL BIOPSY VERSUS LIQUID BIOPSY

Conventional biopsy is traditional and cheaper. However, liquid biopsy has several advantages over histopathological examination. Liquid biopsy is non-invasive, and repeated sample collection is feasible. Even the sample can be collected after the removal of the main tumor mass. Liquid biopsy often represents tumor heterogeneity. The main limitations of liquid biopsy are the high cost and the need for validation of this sophisticated technique. **Table 1** highlights the comparison of conventional and liquid biopsies.

COMPONENTS OF LIQUID BIOPSY

The major components of liquid biopsy are as shown in **Figure 1**.

- Circulating tumor cells (CTC)
- Cell-free deoxyribonucleic acid (cfDNA)
- Circulating tumor DNA (ctDNA)
- Circulating cell-free ribonucleic acid (cfRNA)
- Extracellular vesicles

TABLE 1: Comparison of conventional and liquid biopsy.

Parameters	Conventional biopsy	Liquid biopsy
Procedure	Invasive	Noninvasive
Tumor burden	Size of the tumor predicts the tumor burden	Quantity of circulating tumor cells (CTC)/ctDNA predicts the tumor burden
Classification of tumor	It is based on histopathological features in biopsy	Molecular classification may be possible based on molecular profile in CTC/ctDNA
Tumor heterogeneity	Not possible	Possible to assess
Evolution of the tumor	Not possible in transverse sampling	Serial liquid biopsy may help to assess tumor evolution
DNA quality	DNA is retrieved from formalin-fixed tissue so artefact is common	DNA is fragmented with low-yield
Cost	Cheaper	Very costly
Technical skill	No skilled technician needed	Highly skilled technical staff is needed

(DNA: deoxyribonucleic acid; RNA: ribonucleic acid)

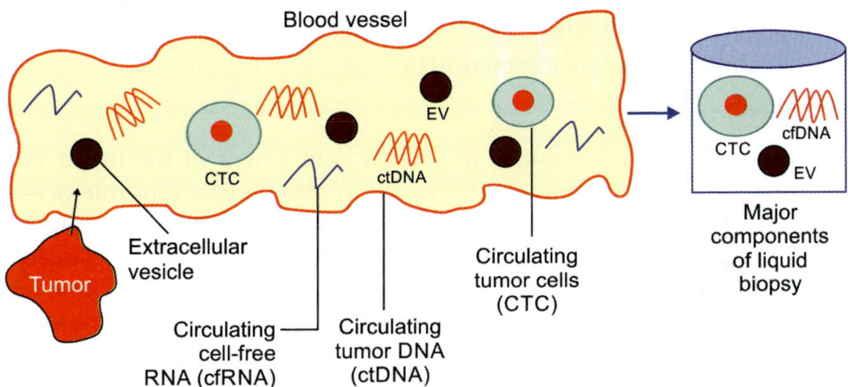

FIG. 1: Different components of liquid biopsy.

Circulating Tumor Cells

The source of CTC is the primary tumor or from the metastatic site. The life span of CTC is short as they are quickly cleared by reticuloendothelial cells of the body. They only survive for 1–2 hours. However, a small subset of CTC may survive and cause distant metastasis. The number of CTC in the blood circulation is extremely low (1 per 106 neutrophils) and it is a challenge to isolate these cells. As most of the tumors are epithelial in origin, so the CTCs are identified by the universal epithelial cell marker epithelial cell adhesion molecule (EpCAM). However, using EpCAM to identify the CTCs has its limitations as there are tumors that are negative for EpCAM or downregulation of EpCAM at the time of epithelial-mesenchymal transition (EMT). Overall, EpCAM-positive CTCs are still a reliable biomarker in the therapeutic and management decision of cancer.[2] Various other biomarkers such as prostate-specific antigen, human epidermal growth factor receptor-2 (HER-2), and estrogen receptors are also used in CTC in different cancers.

Circulating Tumor Deoxyribonucleic Acid

The sources of ctDNA are primary and metastatic tumor. (1) The entry of ctDNA in the blood is possibly from the tumor cells, (2) apoptotic or necrotic tumor cells, and (3) circulating tumor cells. The ctDNA is single or double-stranded DNA and it possesses all the molecular characteristics of cancer and therefore is thought to be generated from the tumor tissue. Both CTC and ctDNA show identical genetic mutations. The amount of ctDNA in the circulation depends on (1) tumor size and (2) tumor progression.

Cell-free Deoxyribonucleic Acid

The cfDNA is derived from normal tissue and also from tumor tissue. They are present in body fluids in three different forms: free, encapsulated, or protein-bound. There are two types of cfDNA: genomic DNA and mitochondrial cell-free DNA. In the tumor tissue cfDNA is derived from apoptotic and necrotic cells.

Circulating Cell-free Ribonucleic Acid

The cfRNA contains small RNA and mRNA.

Extracellular Vesicles

Extracellular vesicles are another important component of the liquid biopsy. These are vesicles containing exosomes, apoptotic bodies, and microvesicles. Extracellular vesicles are produced from the tumor tissue and are present in blood as well as different body fluids. The exosomes with the extracellular vesicles contain DNA, mRNA, and microRNA. Due to the peripheral lipid bilayer protection, the exosomes are not affected by enzymes and retain all the essential information.

Table 2 highlights the differences between the different components of liquid biopsy.

TABLE 2: Comparison of different components of liquid biopsy.

Features	CTC	cfDNA	Extracellular vesicles	cfRNA
Origin from viable cells	Yes	No	Yes	Yes
DNA components	Yes	Yes	Yes	No
Mutational analysis	Yes	Yes	Yes	Possibly
Copy number alterations	Yes	Yes	Yes	No
Epigenetic alteration	Yes	Yes	Yes	No
Functional assay	Yes	No	No	No
Ability to perform single cell analysis	Yes	No	No	No

(CTC: circulating tumor cells; *cfDNA:* cell-free deoxyribonucleic acid; *cfRNA:* cell-free ribonucleic acid)

CIRCULATING TUMOR CELLS ENRICHMENT TECHNOLOGIES

The constituents of the liquid biopsy are extremely low in blood and are estimated as one CTC against 106 surrounding peripheral mononuclear cells of the blood. So, the selective enrichment of the tumor cells is necessary to detect CTC and it is a challenge to isolate CTCs. CTC enrichment can be done by as shown in **Figure 2**.

Immunomagnetic Capture

- *Immunomagnetic positive enrichment*:
  - Cell search
  - Adna test
  - Mag sweeper
  - Magnetic-activated cell sorting (MACS)
  - Strep tag
- *Immunomagnetic negative enrichment*:
  - EasySep
  - Rosette Sep

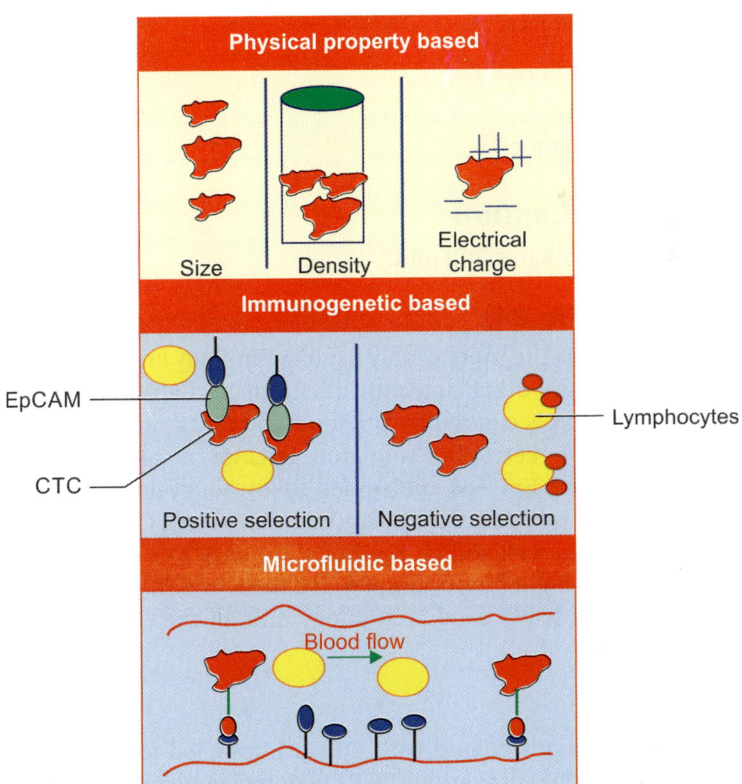

FIG. 2: Overall view of the separation of circulating tumor cells.
(CTC: circulating; EpCAM: epithelial cell adhesion molecule)

- *Microfluidic immnocapture*:
  - CTC chip
  - HB chip
  - High-throughput micro-sampling unit (HTMSU)
  - Nanovelcro
- *Biophysical property*:
  - Membrane filtration:
    - Flexible micro spring array (FMSA)
    - Screencell
    - ISET
  - Size-based microfluidics:
    - MCA
    - Clear cell FX1
    - Parsortix
    - Vortex VTX-1
  - Density-based:
    - Oncoquick
    - Accucyte
  - Dielectrophoresis:
    - Appostream
- *Combined method*:
  - CTC Chip
  - Open chip
- *In vitro*:
  - GILUPI cell collector

Immunomagnetic Capture

High-throughput micro-sampling unit.

Cell Search System (Fig. 3A)

The cell search system is the most widely used technology and can be considered as the benchmark for the other detection methods available in the market. It is the only technology that is cleared by US Food and Drug Administration (FDA). In this technology, the Ferro fluids-coated EpCAM is used to separate the cells containing surface EpCAM molecules followed by immunofluorescence imaging and detection by using CD45–, and EpCAM+, and CK8+ antibodies. The major advantages of the cell search methods are easy to use, rapid processing time, ability to process eight blood samples at a time, and in-device staining.[3,4]

This is the only clinically used technology and all the other techniques are solely for research use.

AdnaTest (Fig. 3B)

In this test magnetic beads coated with EpCAM are used followed by real-time multiplex polymerase chain reaction (PCR) to detect gene expression patterns of the specific tumor-associated markers.[5]

MACS Test (Fig. 3C)

The MACS test is an alternative method of capturing the CTC with an immunomagnetic technique. In this technique, the whole blood is first incubated with the target antibody (mainly against EpCAM) coated with superparamagnetic beads. The blood then flowed through a column that contained the ferromagnetic steel wool fibers in a magnetic field. The CTC-conjugated with EpCAM is attached in the column and later on can be released after withdrawal of the magnetic field. The MACS test is more suitable in tissue sample.[6]

Mag Sweeper Test

This is another method to capture CTC. In this technique, the blood is first incubated with EpCAM antibodies coated with magnetic beads. Then robotically controlled neodymium rod covered with nonadherent plastic sleeves is swept through blood. The nonadherent plastic sleeves allow multiple capture and subsequent release of CTC. It helps to increase the efficiency up to 70%.[7]

Strep-tag System (Fig. 3D)

In this immunomagnetic enrichment process, the magnetic beads coated with Strep-Tactin (STMB) are used. The Strep-Tactin is further conjugated with strep-tag-II derived immunoglobulin G (IgG). The whole material is undergone for magnetic enrichment. Now, simple addition of d-biotin competitively binds with Strep-Tactin and releases CTCs.[8] In addition to anti-EpCAM tagged with STMB, the technique can also use estimated glomerular filtration rate (EGFR) and HER-2 or the cocktail of all three antibodies. The capture efficiency of strep-tag technique is 79%.

Immunomagnetic Negative Enrichment

In the case of immunomagnetic negative enrichment, an antileukocyte antibody (anti-CD45) coated with magnetic beads is used. The CD45-positive cells are removed from the sample.

EasySep (Fig. 3E)

In this technology, the CD45 positive cells are separated and the supernatant residual sample contains unlabeled CTCs because no target antigen is used. The CTC recovery is variable and may be from 58% to as low as 24%.[9]

RosetteSep

RosetteSep technique uses a cocktail of multiple antibodies against the blood cell markers (CD45, CD16, CD36, CD 38, and CD2). After mixing the cocktail antibodies with the blood a rosette network is formed. Subsequently, with the help of Ficoll density gradient, the white blood cells (WBCs) and red blood cells (RBCs) are separated.

Microfluidic Immunocapture

CTC Chip

It contains a large number of micropillars coated with anti-EpCAM. The surface area of the interaction between CTC and EpCAM is significantly greater. The

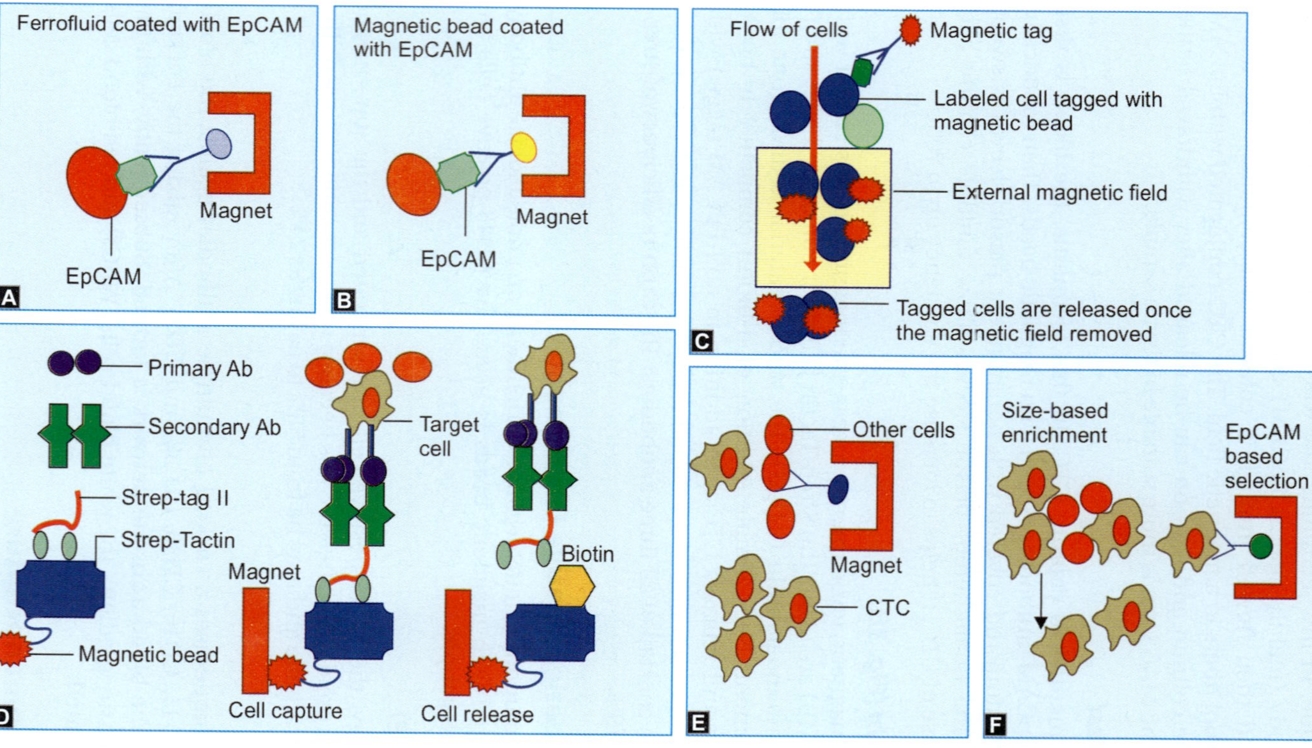

FIGS. 3A TO F: The details of the technologies to enrich circulating tumor cells. (A) Cell search; (B) AdnaTest; (C) MACS test; (D) Strep-tag system; (E) EasySep; and (F) CTC-iChip.

technique is however slow and can process 2 mL of blood per hour. The major advantage of this technique is the high recovery (98%) of viable cells.[10]

HB-Chip

It is the second generation of CTC chip. It uses eight microchannels. The upper surface of the chip has herringbone grooves that can disrupt the flow of cells for better interaction with the antibodies and cells. The inner wall of the channels contains anti-EpCAM antibodies. The HB-Chip is relatively cheap and the recovery rate is as good as CTC chip.[11]

Geometrically Enhanced Differential Immunocapture (GEDI)

The GEDI chip uses special types of microspots that are geometrically enhanced to disrupt the laminar blood flow so that the reaction between the CTC and immunoreactive chips is enhanced. There are a total 5,000 microspots coated with antibodies. The overall capture efficiency of CTC is recorded as high as 85% and compared to the cell-search system, it showed two-fold increase in the number of CTC.[12]

HTMSU

This is a simply designed HTMSU. Here, the uniqueness of the technique is the chip-single cell conductometry to count CTC and the detection of the properties of the single cell by the electrode. Thereby, the technique avoids further cell staining and manual counting by microscope. The recovery of CTC by this technique is >97%.[13]

NanoVelcro Chip

The technique uses velcro-like principle. Here, the CTC is immobilized by silicon nanowire substrate coated with anti-EpCAM on the inner wall of the chip. In addition, the chip breaks down the laminar blood flow by using a polydimethylsiloxane mixer on the roof of it. It helps to enhance the contact between the CTC and anti-EpCAM antibody. The CTC detection rate of this technique varies from 75 to 100%.[14]

Biophysical Properties

Membrane Filtration

Membrane filtration is a simple technique that uses filters with different sizes and shapes. The blood passes through the pores under pressure and the CTC is caught in the filter. The membrane filtration is rapid and easy technique.

Flexible Micro Spring Array (FMSA)

FMSA contains the filter with a pore size 8 μ diameter. The flexible microspring structures are etched into the filter. The blood passes through the filter under a pressure regulatory system. The CTC is recovered from the filter by reverse pressure. FMSA has 90% capture efficiency.[15]

ScreenCell Filter

The ScreenCell filter contains different-sized pores (7.5 and 6.5 μ) distributed randomly. The filter isolates fixed or live cells. The device needs lysis of RBCs. The capture efficiency of this technique is claimed as 100%.[16]

Isolation by Size of Tumor Cells (ISET)

The ISET consists of multiple pores of 8 μm diameter and can process 12 samples at a time. After loading the sample a gentle negative pressure is applied for steady flow. The technique is slow and there is a chance of clogging the filter. Therefore, blood must be diluted to avoid clogging of the filter.

Size-based Microfluidics

The size-based techniques are independent of the cell markers and the CTCs are detected based on the knowledge that the size of CTCs are larger than the leukocytes.

Microcavity Array (MCA)

Microcavity arrays contains the filter composed of nickel and gold. The system contains 10,000 cavities arranged in 100 × 100 arrays. Each cavity has a diameter 8–11 μm and arranged in 60 μm apart. A gentle negative pressure is used to have a steady flow of the sample. The CTC detection rate is 77%.[17]

ClearCell FX1

ClearCell FX1 system uses the principle of dean flow fractionation (DFF). When the cells flow through a curvilinear microfluidic channel they experience two types of forces, dean force and lift force. The dean force pushes the cells centrifugally. The smaller cells experience higher dean force than CTC and remain in the outer side of the channel and CTC on the inner side of the spiral channel. The label-free viable CTCs are available by this technique.[18]

Parsortix

Parsortix technique contains Parsortix GEN3 cell separation cassette for the capture of CTC. The chip contains a stepped separation structure that gradually decreases in size from 10 to 4 μm and reaches a final critical gap to capture the CTCs. This is a semiautomated technique and a relatively slower process.[19]

VTX1

Vortex technology contains chips with 16 channels and each channel contains 12 reservoirs. When the sample flows through the channels, the microvortices are produced that trap the CTCs within the microvortices. This is a fully automated system and no centrifugation is needed before processing.[20]

Density-based

The density-based separation of CTCs is the simplest technology where the CTCs are separated based on density.

OncoQuick

OncoQuick technique combines density separation along with filtration. The density gradient fluid separates the CTC from the leukocytes. CTCs are accumulated on the interface between the density gradient fluid and blood. A microfilter is placed above the top of the density gradient media to capture CTCs.[21]

AccuCyte

AccuCyte uses a separation tube that contain float. After centrifugation, the float rests in between the blood and plasma. The CTCs are trapped in the buffy coat and are retrieved subsequently.[22]

Dielectrophoresis

Dielectrophoresis technique applies the dielectrophoretic field to separate from the leukocytes.

Appostream (ApoCell)

ApoCell applies both the field flow and dielectrophoresis. At first, the Ficoll separation helps to provide buffy coat preparation. The cells in the buffy coat are then passed over a dielectrophoretic field with an alternate current that pulls the CTCs to the floor of the chamber. The recovery rate of CTCs and viability of the cells are good in ApoCell.[23]

Combined Methods

CTC-iChip (Fig. 3F)

It is the combination of immunocapture and magnetic separation of the cells. In the first step, the whole blood is incubated with EpCAM antibodies for positive enrichment of CTCs. In the next step, the cells are passed through a microfluidic channel under a magnetic field. The device has a high recovery rate and is relatively faster. Moreover, the technique provides live CTCs that can be cultured or can be used for transcriptomic analysis.[24]

OpenChip

The OpenChip technology is unique as it enriches CTC by immunocapture followed by simultaneous in situ molecular analysis using probes targeted to specific biomarkers. The other techniques perform the molecular analysis after enrichment. The major disadvantage of this technique is low recovery rate of CTCs.[25]

In Vivo Enrichment

Diagnostic Leukapheresis (DLA)

The DLA uses whole blood in vivo thereby avoiding the problem of small volume of blood. DLA does continuous flow centrifugation of blood to enrich the CTCs.[26]

Table 3 compares different enrichment techniques.

TABLE 3: Comparison of different CTC enrichment techniques.

Category	Commercially available techniques	Mode of enrichment	Capture efficiency (%)	Advantages	Disadvantages
Immunomagnetic	Cell search	Ferro fluids-coated EpCAM is used to separate the cells containing surface EpCAM molecules	40–90	FDA approved	Only EpCAM-positive CTCs are detected
	Adna test	Combination of immunomagnetic separation and multiplex PCR	47–75	Semiautomated and can process multiple samples at a time (8 samples)	Less flexible technique
	Magnetic-activated cell sorting (MACS test)	Target antibody (mainly against EpCAM) coated with superparamagnetic nanoparticles	25–90	Good detection rate	More suitable in tissue samples
	Mag Sweeper test	The blood is incubated with EpCAM antibodies coated with magnetic beads followed by passing it through a nonadherent plastic sleeve	60–70	Easy to elute CTC Multiple rounds of capture are possible to increase the capture efficiency	Only EpCAM-positive cells are recovered
	Strep-tag system	The magnetic beads coated with Strep-Tactin (STMB) are used. Strep-Tactin is further conjugated with Strep-tag-II derived IgG. The whole material is undergone magnetic enrichment	70–86	A cocktail of antibodies can be used	Only EpCAM-positive cells are recovered
Immunomagnetic negative enrichment	EasySep	CD45 positive cells are separated and the supernatant residual sample contains unlabeled CTCs	20–63	The unlabeled heterogeneous population of CTCs	Recovery rate varies
	Rosette Sep	A cocktail of multiple antibodies against the blood cell markers is used followed by the separation of of blood components by Ficoll density gradient	62	Cocktail antibodies help to enhance negative enrichment	May remove CTCs

Continued

Continued

Category	Commercially available techniques	Mode of enrichment	Capture efficiency (%)	Advantages	Disadvantages
Microfluidic immunocapture	CTC-Chip	A large number of micropillars coated with anti EpCAM are used to enhance the contact area	60	Large surface area helps in better capture of CTCs. The cells are mostly viable	Only EpCAM-positive cells are recovered
	HB-Chip	The upper surface of the chip has herringbone grooves that can disrupt the flow of cells for better interaction with the antibodies and cells	75–97	The herringbone grooves increase the contact of CTC and EpCAM	Only EpCAM-positive cells are recovered
	Geometrically enhanced differential immunocapture (GEDI chip)	Geometrically enhanced microspots are designed to disrupt the laminar blood flow so that the reaction between the CTC and immunoreactive chips is enhanced	80–90	Better capture due to the large surface area of contact	Only EpCAM-positive cells are recovered
	HTMSU	Chip-single cell conductometry is used to count CTC and the detection of the properties of the single cell is done by the electrode	97	Chip-single cell conductometry helps to count the cells	Only EpCAM-positive cells are recovered
	NanoVelcro chip	The CTC is immobilized by a silicon nanowire substrate coated with anti-EpCAM on the inner wall of the chip	95	High recovery rate	Only EpCAM-positive cells are recovered
Membrane filtration	FMSA	The filter with a pore size 8 µ diameter is used. The flexible microspring structures are etched into the filter	90	Cheap and easy to do	Clogging of the filter is common
	ScreenCell filter	It contains randomly distributed different-sized pores (7.5 and 6.5 µ)	70–90	High recovery rate, cheap, simple, easy to do	Randomly distributed pores may have a negative impact on cell recovery

Continued

Continued

Category	Commercially available techniques	Mode of enrichment	Capture efficiency (%)	Advantages	Disadvantages
Size-based microfluidics	Microcavity array (MCA)	The system contains 10,000 cavities arranged in 100 × 100 arrays. Each cavity has a diameter 8–11 µm and arranged in 60 µm apart	90	On-chip staining of CTC	Slow processing time
	Clear cell FX1	It applies the principle of dean flow fractionation (DFF). The dean force pushes the cells centrifugally. CTC remains in the central part of the flow of the sample	80	• Quick procedure • No clogging	
	Parsortix	The chip contains a stepped separation structure that gradually decreases in size from 10 to 4 µm and reaches a final critical gap to capture the CTCs	40–70	Clusters of CTC can be captured	Slow processing time
	VTX1	There are 16 channels and when blood flows through the channel microvortices are produced that trap the CTCs	70	Rapid procedure Fully automated	
Density-based	OncoQuick	It combines density separation with filtration	25–80	A heterogenous population of CTCs can be recovered	Low recovery rate
	AccuCyte	It uses a separation tube that contain float. CTCs are trapped in the buffy coat and are retrieved	90	Multiple samples can be processed	
Dielectrophoresis	Appostream (ApoCell)	Dielectrophoretic field to separate CTC	78	A heterogenous population of CTCs can be recovered	
In vivo	Diagnostic leukapheresis (DLA)	Uses whole blood in vivo	78	Recovery of heterogenous population of CTC	
Combined method	CTC-iChip	Combination of immunocapture and magnetic separation of the cells	100	Quick and highly sensitive	Only EpCAM-positive cells are enriched
	OPENchip	Immunocapture followed by simultaneous in situ molecular analysis	50	No clogging of the channel. simultaneous molecular analysis	Low recovery rate

(CTC: circulating tumor cells; EpCAM: epithelial cell adhesion molecule)

MOLECULAR TECHNIQUES TO EVALUATE ctDNA/cfDNA

The following molecular techniques are applied to evaluate ctDNA/cfDNA in liquid biopsy.

Droplet Digital Polymerase Chain Reaction

The droplet digital polymerase chain reaction (ddPCR) is highly sensitive and can detect 0.01% of ctDNA. It can identify low mutations, rare mutations, and also copy number variants.[27]

Beads, Emulsion, Amplification, and Magnetics

It is the combination of PCR and flow cytometry. Beads, emulsion, amplification, and magnetics (BEAMing) is a very sensitive and relatively cheap technique and can detect 0.01% genomic alteration.

Tagged-amplicon Deep Sequencing

It is relatively fast and highly specific and sensitive technique. It can detect DNA less than 2%. Tagged-amplicon deep sequencing (TAm-Seq) can simultaneously detect millions of DNA fragments. However, it needs previous characterization of desired sequencing.

Cancer Personalized Profiling by Deep Sequencing

Cancer personalized profiling by deep sequencing (CAPP-Seq) is an ultrasensitive next-generation sequencing-based approach that can identify multiple mutations in the same type of cancer and can assess tumor heterogeneity.

Whole Exome Sequencing

Whole exome sequencing (WES) is the widely used next generation sequencing (NGS). It sequences the protein-coding region (exomes) of the gene. It is relatively cheap with a high yield. It can characterize all known mutations. However, the sensitivity of this technique is low.[28]

Whole Genome Sequencing

It assesses the entire genome and detects various mutational changes. So it provides comprehensive knowledge of tumor mutation. Whole genome sequencing (WGS) is related to ethical and financial issues.

Whole Genome Bisulfite Sequencing

It is a very effective technique to evaluate DNA methylation analysis of single cytosine. Whole genome bisulfite sequencing (WGBS-Seq) provides important information in epigenetic studies.

CLINICAL APPLICATIONS OF LIQUID BIOPSY

The major clinical applications of liquid biopsy are described here **(Fig. 4)**.

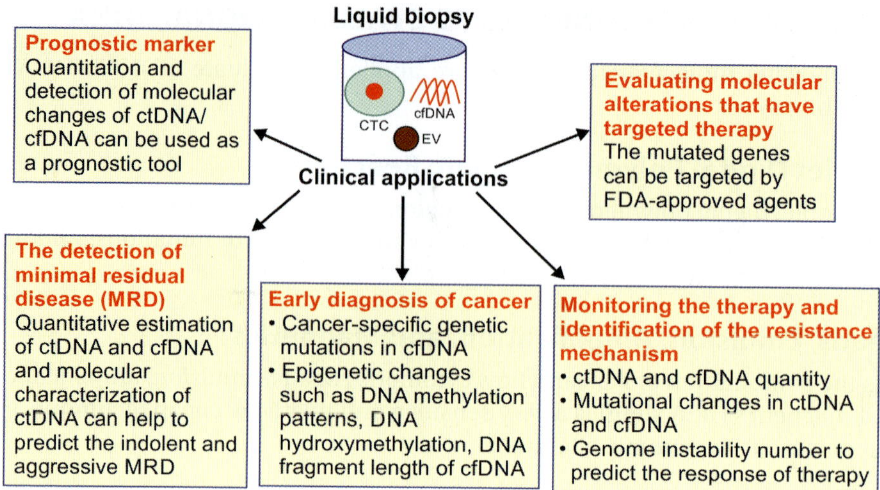

FIG. 4: Clinical applications of liquid biopsy.

Early Diagnosis of Cancer

Early diagnosis of cancer before any symptoms, imaging, or biochemical markers have drawn immense interest. There is a high expectation that liquid biopsy may play a significant role in this area. However, it is challenging to use liquid biopsy in cancer screening or early diagnosis due to extremely low levels of ctDNA in the blood and low incidence of cancer in the general population. The various approaches were based on cancer-specific genetic and epigenetic mutations in cfDNA.[29,30]

In addition, DNA methylation patterns may also play an important role. Distinct DNA-methylation patterns have been described in different cancer types.[31]

The various other epigenetic changes can also be assessed from cfDNA, such as DNA hydroxymethylation, DNA fragment length, etc.

In a prospective study,[32] 10,006 women without any prior history of cancer were studied by CancerSeek platform. Out of these, 26 women were detected as cancer by CancerSeek platform. These women had cancer of early to late stage. In this study, 70 out of 96 cancers were detected by standard screening tests. The result raises the clinical utility of liquid biopsy. In another study,[33] cfDNA was used to evaluate several groups of nonmetastatic clinically established cancers with no known screening test. The sensitivity of liquid biopsy was 70–98%, and specificity was 99%. So, liquid biopsy can be used for screening of cancer.

The major challenges in cancer screening by liquid biopsy are (1) Limited shedding of ctDNA by early-stage cancer that decreases the sensitivity of the test; (2) Only a few mutations are pathognomonic for any specific type of cancer; (3) Recent studies have shown that aging individuals may show mutation of cancer driver genes.[34,35]

This has been seen largely in leukocytes and is known as clonal hematopoiesis of indeterminate potential (CHIP). The elimination of CHIP is necessary from the total cfDNA mutation to increase the sensitivity of liquid biopsy.

Monitoring the Therapy and Identification of the Resistance Mechanism

The serum biomarkers or/and imaging are usually used for monitoring of treatment response of a tumor. Imaging exposes the patient to radiation and serum tumor biomarker may not represent the therapy response. Many researchers have attempted to monitor treatment response by CTC. These studies have shown that a fall of CTC count is associated with a good therapeutic response.[36,37]

The optimal time of measurement and threshold for the CTC burden needs to be validated.

Immune check point inhibitors are currently used in cancer therapy to activate the immune system of the body. ctDNA and cfDNA can be used to assess the immune checkpoint response. In nonsmall cell carcinoma of lung, ctDNA was used to predict the response of immunotherapy based treatment. Decreased ctDNA level was associated with better response and longer median survival.[38] Zhang et al.[39] analyzed pretreatment and on-treatment ctDNA in patients with advanced cancer on immunotherapy. They noted that both pretreatment and on-treatment variant allele frequencies measured in ctDNA are related to overall prognosis. Higher pretreatment variant allele frequencies are associated with reduced survival, whereas, on-treatment lower variant alleles are related to longer survival.

Jensen et al.[40] calculated genome instability number (GIN) from the quantity and magnitude of copy-number alterations across the genome in cfDNA. They noted that GIN can be used to predict the response to immunotherapy. Continuously decreasing GIN levels indicates the response to immunotherapy. GIN level can be used to discriminate progression, peudoprogression, and hyperprogression of the disease. The liquid biopsy is also helpful to identify the resistant mechanism during chemotherapy.[41-44]

In a subset of colorectal cancer, EGFR blockage by monoclonal antibody is effective. However, the development of resistance to therapy limits the treatment. The emergence of resistance to therapy is often associated with RAS mutations. The molecular profile of cfDNA in liquid biopsy is helpful to detect the resistance of the therapy.[41] Siravegna et al.[42] studied the molecular profile of ctDNA in the liquid biopsy samples in patients with colorectal cancer who were in therapies with the anti-EGFR antibodies and developed drug resistance. They detected mutations in *KRAS, NRAS, MET, ERBB2, FLT3, EGFR,* and MAPK2K1 in ctDNA of the patients. The mutated clone of the *RAS* gene decreases on withdrawal of the EGFR blocking antibodies. It indicates the clonal evolution of the mutated *RAS* gene.

In the breast cancer case with treatment by *PI3K*-α inhibitor therapy, it was noted that the loss of function *PTEN* mutations and *ESPR1*-activating mutations are associated with drug resistance.[44]

In brief, acquired resistance to drug therapy emerges by clonal evolution of mutated genes, and serial evaluation of ctDNA can give early prediction of resistance to targeted therapy.

Evaluating Molecular Alterations that have Targeted Therapy

The identification of actionable mutation of the solid tumor is important for the targeted therapy. Traditionally, it is done from the tumor tissue by biopsy. However, currently, all the information of molecular patterns can be assessed from ctDNA, cfDNA, and CTC in liquid biopsy. The food and drug administration (FDA) has approved several diagnostic tests on ctDNA such as Cobas EGFR mutation test V2 in nonsmall cell lung cancer, therascreen PIK3CA RGQ PCR kit to detect PIK3CA mutation in carcinoma of the breast, and Guardant 360 for the detection of molecular profiling.

It is a challenge to decide on chemotherapy protocols in the carcinoma of unknown primary (CUP) and many times empirical chemotherapy regimens are given.

Kato et al.[45] studied ctDNA alteration of the CUP by NGS. They noted that 66% of patients had pathogenic alterations and almost all the patients had actionable alterations.

Okamura et al. detected alterations in ctDNA in advanced esophageal and gastric adenocarcinomas by NGS. They noted that 76% of patients had >1 genomic alteration and 69% of patients had characteristic genetic alteration. *TP53, PIK3CA, ERBB2,* and *KRAS* genes were commonly affected. The mutated genes can be targeted by FDA-approved agents. Interestingly, patients with at least one characterized alteration were different than other patients indicating personalized therapy.[46]

Charo et al.[47] studied the molecular profile of several gynecological cancers and noted at least one characterized alteration in ctDNA in 75% of patients. Therapy matched to ctDNA alteration in 31% of patients showed better overall survival.

Pathogenic mutation of ctDNA in advanced breast cancer was noted in >68% of patients.[48]

Schwaederle et al.[49] noted that >82% of nonsmall cell lung carcinoma showed ≥1 alteration that is potentially actionable by the targeted therapy approved by FDA.

All this evidence suggests that ctDNA/cfDNA may provide useful information on the alteration of genes that are actionable by the targeted therapy or may guide in therapeutic decisions.

Detection of Minimal Residual Disease

The CTC and cfDNA can help in real time monitoring of the patients with potentially curable malignancies but at higher risk of minimal residual disease. To validate the cfDNA in monitoring the minimal residual disease (MRD), it is essential to have the following criteria: (1) cfDNA should be detected with high sensitivity and specificity, (2) there should be a period of gap between the detection by cfDNA and conventional biomarkers, (3) the treatment by available therapy should help the patient in long-term survival. Various studies have shown that molecular relapse can be detected several months before detection by conventional methods such as imaging or biomarkers.[50,51] The choice of drug is crucial in this context. It is also not clear that therapy at this stage will cure the patient.

Quantitative estimation of ctDNA and cfDNA and molecular characterization of ctDNA can help to predict the indolent and aggressive MRD. In case of indolent MRD, the circulating cells are not proliferating or balanced by apoptosis. So, there is no progression of disease. However, in the case of aggressive MRD, the disseminated tumor cells proliferate significantly. This can be detected by molecular characterization of ctDNA.

Liquid Biopsy as a Prognostic Marker

The risk of poor outcomes for the patient after treatment is important to make further decisions about aggressive therapy. In this context, ctDNA/cfDNA can be used as a prognostic tool. It has been noted that ctDNA amount >5% and at least one gene alteration had a poor overall survival rate.[52] Jensen et al. did genome-wide sequencing from the cfDNA and showed that elevation of genomic instability number correlated with poor prognosis.[53]

Various studies have shown that in preoperative or postoperative malignancies the elevated ctDNA/cfDNA had a significantly shorter overall survival rate.[54,55]

CHALLENGES IN APPLICATIONS OF LIQUID BIOPSY

There are several challenges in the applications of liquid biopsy. The main difficulty is an extremely low amount of ctDNA/cfDNA in the blood, particularly those patients with low tumor burden. Due to the low amount of ctDNA/cfDNA, the sequencing may be expensive. Standardization of CTC/ctDNA in different laboratories is variable. It also requires expert skills.

The CTC is usually separated by an EpCAM-based immunological approach. However, the surface markers may not be expressed in certain tumors and this may be a major limitation of the detection of CTC.[56]

Mutations of cfDNA may not always related to the tumor and clonal hematopoiesis of indeterminate potential (CHIP) mostly in elderly individuals is the other source of mutations.

CONCLUSION

Liquid biopsy has emerged as a new field of technology with immense possibilities in the last few years. They are particularly used for evaluating the molecular profiling of the tumor with many possible clinical applications.

The tumors release ctDNA/CTC into the blood. Various sophisticated technologies such as ddPCR, BEAMing, TAM-Seq, and WGBSeq are available to isolate and evaluate ctDNA. In comparison, the isolation of CTC is difficult, and various enrichment technologies are available in the market. Specific biomarkers expressed on CTC and also different biophysical properties are used to enrich CTC.

The ctDNA/CTC are usually isolated from blood. However, other body fluids such as urine, cerebrospinal fluid (CSF), and ascites can be used for study.

The ctDNA/CTC can be applied in the detection of early cancer, disease monitoring and detection of resistance, detection of actionable mutations, cancer prognosis, and the detection of minimal residual disease. Large clinical validation studies are mandatory for the successful and reproducible clinical utility of liquid biopsy. The ctDNA/CTC can be collected serially and can provide real-time information on molecular profiles. The combination of liquid biopsy along with tissue biopsy and imaging technology can provide critical information regarding the clinical management of the patient.

The ctDNA is used to evaluate druggable mutation in cancer therapy. In comparison, CTC can provide additional information, particularly tumor heterogeneity. CTC can be used to assess transcriptional plasticity. Different organ of the body has different microenvironments and transcriptional analysis of CTC can predict the possible site of metastasis. In the future, exploration of additional analytes such as RNA, cell-free RNA, microRNA, and exosomes, will be possible from CTC.

In conclusion, liquid biopsy is a very promising technology in the personalized treatment of cancer. However, it needs standardization of the isolation of its components and clinical validation before the routine clinical application.

REFERENCES

1. McGranahan N, Swanton C. Clonal heterogeneity and tumor evolution: Past, present, and the future. Cell. 2017;168(4):613-28.
2. Eslami SZ, Cortes-Hernandez LE, Alix-Panabieres C. Epithelial cell adhesion molecule: an anchor to isolate clinically relevant circulating tumor cells. Cells. 2020;9(8):1836-52.
3. Rushton AJ, Nteliopoulos G, Shaw JA, Coombes RC. A review of circulating tumour cell enrichment technologies. Cancers (Basel). 2021;13(5):970.
4. Harb W, Fan A, Tran T, Danila DC, Keys D, Schwartz M, Ionescu-Zanetti C. Mutational analysis of circulating tumor cells using a novel microfluidic collection device and qPCR assay. Transl Oncol. 2013;6(5):528-38.
5. Ferreira MM, Ramani VC, Jeffrey SS. Circulating tumor cell technologies. Mol Oncol. 2016;10(3):374-94.
6. Miltenyi S, Müller W, Weichel W, Radbruch A. High gradient magnetic cell separation with MACS. Cytometry. 1990;11(2):231-8.
7. Talasaz AH, Powell AA, Huber DE, Berbee JG, Roh K-H, Yu W, et al. Isolating highly enriched populations of circulating epithelial cells and other rare cells from blood using a magnetic sweeper device. Proc Natl Acad Sci USA. 2009;106(10):3970-5.
8. Junttila MR, Saarinen S, Schmidt T, Kast J, Westermarck J. Single-step Strep-tag purification for the isolation and identification of protein complexes from mammalian cells. Proteomics. 2005;5(5):1199-203.
9. Xu Y, Liu B, Ding F, Zhou X, Tu P, Yu B, et al. Circulating tumor cell detection: A direct comparison between negative and unbiased enrichment in lung cancer. Oncol Lett. 2017; 13(6):4882-6.
10. Sequist LV, Nagrath S, Toner M, Haber DA, Lynch TJ. The CTC-chip: An exciting new tool to detect circulating tumor cells in lung cancer patients. J Thorac Oncol. 2009;4(3):281-3.

11. Stott SL, Hsu CH, Tsukrov DI, Yu M, Miyamoto DT, Waltman BA, et al. Isolation of circulating tumor cells using a microvortex-generating herringbone-chip. Proc Natl Acad Sci USA. 2010;107(43):18392-7.
12. Kaburagi T, Kiyoshima M, Nawa T, Ichimura H, Saito T, Hayashihara K, et al. Acquired EGFR T790M mutation after relapse following EGFR-TKI therapy: A population-based multi-institutional study. Anticancer Res. 2018;38(5):3145-50.
13. Tulley S, Zhao Q, Dong H, Pearl ML, Chen W-T. Vita-AssayTM method of enrichment and identification of circulating cancer cells/circulating tumor cells (CTCs). Methods Mol Biol. 2016;1406:107-19.
14. Loeian MS, Mehdi Aghaei S, Farhadi F, Rai V, Yang HW, Johnson MD, et al. Liquid biopsy using the nanotube-CTC-chip: Capture of invasive CTCs with high purity using preferential adherence in breast cancer patients. Lab Chip. 2019;19(11):1899-915.
15. Harouaka RA, Zhou MD, Yeh Y-T, Khan WJ, Das A, Liu X, et al. Flexible micro spring array device for high-throughput enrichment of viable circulating tumor cells. Clin Chem. 2014;60(2):323-33.
16. Desitter I, Guerrouahen BS, Benali-Furet N, Wechsler J, Jänne PA, Kuang Y, et al. A new device for rapid isolation by size and characterization of rare circulating tumor cells. Anticancer Res. 2011;31(2):427-41.
17. Hosokawa M, Hayata T, Fukuda Y, Arakaki A, Yoshino T, Tanaka T, et al. Size-Selective microcavity array for rapid and efficient detection of circulating tumor cells. Anal Chem. 2010;82(15):6629-35.
18. Hou HW, Warkiani ME, Khoo BL, Li ZR, Soo RA, Tan D.S.-W, et al. Isolation and retrieval of circulating tumor cells using centrifugal forces. Sci Rep. 2013;3:1259.
19. Miller MC, Robinson PS, Wagner C, O'Shannessy DJ. The Parsortix™ Cell Separation System-A versatile liquid biopsy platform. Cytometry A. 2018;93(12):1234-9.
20. Lemaire CA, Liu SZ, Wilkerson CL, Ramani VC, Barzanian NA, Huang K-W, et al. Fast and label-free isolation of circulating tumor cells from blood: from a research microfluidic platform to an automated fluidic instrument, VTX-1 liquid biopsy system. SLAS Technol. 2018;23(1):16-29.
21. Königsberg R, Gneist M, Jahn-Kuch D, Pfeiler G, Hager G, Hudec M, et al. Circulating tumor cells in metastatic colorectal cancer: Efficacy and feasibility of different enrichment methods. Cancer Lett. 2010;293(1):117-23.
22. Ramirez AB, U'Ren L, Campton DE, Stewart D, Nordberg JJ, Stilwell JL, et al. RareCyte® CTC Analysis Step 1: AccuCyte® Sample Preparation for the Comprehensive Recovery of Nucleated Cells from Whole Blood. Methods Mol Biol. 2017;1634:163-72.
23. Le Du F, Fujii T, Kida K, Davis DW, Park M, Liu DD, et al. EpCAM-independent isolation of circulating tumor cells with epithelial-to-mesenchymal transition and cancer stem cell phenotypes using ApoStream(R) in patients with breast cancer treated with primary systemic therapy. PLoS one. 2020;15:e0229903.
24. Fachin F, Spuhler P, Martel-Foley JM, Edd JF, Barber TA, Walsh J, et al. Monolithic chip for high-throughput blood cell depletion to sort rare circulating tumor cells. Sci Rep. 2017;7(1): 10936.
25. Lee AC, Svedlund J, Darai E, Lee Y, Lee D, Lee HB, et al. OPENchip: An on-chip in situ molecular profiling platform for gene expression analysis and oncogenic mutation detection in single circulating tumour cells. Lab Chip. 2020;20:912-22.
26. Fischer JC, Niederacher D, Topp SA, Honisch E, Schumacher S, Schmitz N, et al. Diagnostic leukapheresis enables reliable detection of circulating tumor cells of nonmetastatic cancer patients. Proc Natl Acad Sci. 2013;110(41):16580-5.
27. Zhang BO, Xu CW, Shao Y, Wang HT, Wu YF, Song YY, et al. Comparison of droplet digital PCR and conventional quantitative PCR for measuring EGFR gene mutation. Exp Ther Med. 2015;9(4):1383-8.
28. Imperial R, Nazer M, Ahmed Z, Kam AE, Pluard TJ, Bahaj W, et al. Matched Whole-Genome Sequencing (WGS) and Whole-Exome Sequencing (WES) of Tumor Tissue with Circulating

Tumor DNA (ctDNA) Analysis: Complementary Modalities in Clinical Practice. Cancers (Basel). 2019;11(9):1399.

29. Bettegowda C, Sausen M, Leary RJ, Kinde I, Wang Y, Agrawal N, et al. Detection of circulating tumor DNA in early- and late-stage human malignancies. Sci Transl Med. 2014;6(224): 224ra24.
30. Phallen J, Sausen M, Adleff V, Leal A, Hruban C, White J et al. Direct detection of early-stage cancers using circulating tumor. Sci Transl Med. 2017;9(403):eaan2415.
31. Hoadley KA, Yau C, Hinoue T, Wolf DM, Lazar AJ, Drill E, et al. Cell-of-origin patterns dominate the molecular classification of 10,000 tumors from 33 types of cancer. Cell. 2018;173(2): 291-304.e6.
32. Lennon AM, Buchanan AH, Kinde I, Warren A, Honushefsky A, Cohain AT, et al. Feasibility of blood testing combined with PET-CT to screen for cancer and guide intervention. Science. 2020;369(6499):eabb9601.
33. Cohen JD, Li L, Wang Y, Thoburn C, Afsari B, Danilova L, et al. Detection and localization of surgically resectable cancers with a multi-analyte blood test. Science. 2018;359(6378): 926 30.
34. Genovese G, Kahler AK, Handsaker RE, Lindberg J, Rose SA, Bakhoum SF, et al. Clonal hematopoiesis and blood-cancer risk inferred from blood DNA sequence. N Engl J Med. 2014;371(26):2477-87.
35. Chan H-T, Nagayama S, Chin Y-M, Otaki M, Hayashi R, Kiyotani K, et al. Clinical significance of clonal hematopoiesis in the interpretation of blood liquid biopsy. Mol Oncol. 2020; 14(8):1719-30.
36. Economos C, Morrissey C, Vessella RL. Circulating tumor cells as a marker of response: implications for determining treatment efficacy and evaluating new agents. Curr Opin Urol. 2012;22(3):190-6.
37. Li Y, Wu S, Bai F. Molecular characterization of circulating tumor cells-from bench to bedside. Semin Cell Dev Biol. 2018;75:88-97.
38. Ricciuti B, Jones G, Severgnini M, Alessi JV, Recondo G, Lawrence M, et al. Early plasma circulating tumor DNA (ctDNA) changes predict response to first-line pembrolizumab-based therapy in non-small cell lung cancer (NSCLC). J Immunother Cancer. 2021;9(3): e001504.
39. Zhang Q, Luo J, Wu S, Si H, Gao C, Xu W, et al. Prognostic and predictive impact of circulating tumor DNA in patients with advanced cancers treated with immune checkpoint blockade. Cancer Discov. 2020;10(12):1842-53.
40. Jensen TJ, Goodman AM, Kato S, Ellison CK, Daniels GA, Kim L, et al. Genome-wide sequencing of cell-free DNA identifies copy-number alterations that can be used for monitoring response to immunotherapy in cancer patients. Mol Cancer Ther. 2019;18(2):448-58.
41. Van Emburgh BO, Arena S, Siravegna G, Lazzari L, Crisafulli G, Corti G, et al. Acquired RAS or EGFR mutations and duration of response to EGFR blockade in colorectal cancer. Nat Commun. 2016;7:13665.
42. Siravegna G, Mussolin B, Buscarino M, Corti G, Cassingena A, Crisafulli G, et al. Clonal evolution and resistance to EGFR blockade in the blood of colorectal cancer patients. Nat Med. 2015;21(7):827.
43. Cao H, Liu X, Chen Y, Yang P, Huang T, Song L, et al. Circulating tumor DNA Is capable of monitoring the therapeutic response and resistance in advanced colorectal cancer patients undergoing combined target and chemotherapy. Front Oncol. 2020;10:466.
44. Razavi P, Dickler MN, Shah PD, Toy W, Brown DN, Won HH, et al. Alterations in PTEN and ESR1 promote clinical resistance to alpelisib plus aromatase inhibitors. Nat Cancer. 2020;1: 382-93.
45. Kato S, Weipert C, Gumas S, Okamura R, Lee S, Sicklick JK, et al. Therapeutic actionability of circulating cell-free DNA alterations in carcinoma of unknown primary. JCO precision oncology. 2021;5:1687-98.

46. Kato S, Okamura R, Baumgartner JM, Patel H, Leichman L, Kelly K, et al. Analysis of circulating tumor DNA and clinical correlates in patients with esophageal, gastroesophageal junction, and gastric adenocarcinoma. Clin Cancer Res. 2018;24(24):6248-56.
47. Charo LM, Eskander RN, Okamura R, Patel SP, Nikanjam M, Lanman RB, et al. Clinical implications of plasma circulating tumor DNA in gynecologic cancer patients. Mol Oncol. 2021;15:67-79.
48. Shatsky R, Parker BA, Bui NQ, Helsten T, Schwab RB, Boles SG, et al. Next-generation sequencing of tissue and circulating tumor DNA: the UC San Diego Moores center for personalized cancer therapy experience with breast malignancies. Mol Cancer Ther. 2019;18(5):1001-11.
49. Schwaederle MC, Patel SP, Husain H, Ikeda M, Lanman RB, Banks KC, et al. Utility of genomic assessment of blood-derived circulating tumor DNA (ctDNA) in patients with advanced lung adenocarcinoma. Clin Cancer Res. 2017;23(17):5101-11.
50. Chaudhuri AA, Chabon JJ, Lovejoy AF, Newman AM, Stehr H, Azad TD, et al. Early detection of molecular residual disease in localized lung cancer by circulating tumor DNA profiling. Cancer Discov. 2017;7(12):1394-403.
51. Haselmann V, Gebhardt C, Brechtel I, Duda A, Czerwinski C, Sucker A, et al. Liquid profiling of circulating tumor DNA in plasma of melanoma patients for companion diagnostics and monitoring of BRAF inhibitor therapy. Clin Chem. 2018;64(5):830-42.
52. Schwaederle M, Husain H, Fanta PT, Piccioni DE, Kesari S, Schwab RB, et al. Use of liquid biopsies in clinical oncology: pilot experience in 168 patients. Clin Cancer Res. 2016;22(22): 5497-505.
53. Jensen TJ, Goodman AM, Ellison CK, Holden KA, Kato S, Kim L, et al. Genome-wide sequencing of cell-free dna enables detection of copy-number alterations in patients with cancer where tissue biopsy is not feasible. Mol Cancer Ther. 2021;20(11):2274-9.
54. Cabel L, Jeannot E, Bieche I, Vacher S, Callens C, Bazire L, et al. Prognostic impact of residual HPV ctDNA detection after chemoradiotherapy for anal squamous cell carcinoma. Clin Cancer Res. 2018;24(22):5767-71.
55. Cristofanilli M, Budd GT, Ellis MJ, Stopeck A, Matera J, Miller MC, et al. Circulating tumor cells, disease progression, and survival in metastatic breast cancer. N Engl J Med. 2004;351(8): 781-91.
56. Su DW, Nieva J. Biophysical technologies for understanding circulating tumor cell biology and metastasis. Transl Lung Cancer Res. 2017;6(4):473-85.

8

CHAPTER

Updates in Neuroendocrine Tumors

Prasenjit Das, Arghya Bandyopadhyay

INTRODUCTION

Neuroendocrine neoplasms (NENs) are heterogeneous tumors with common phenotypes but differ greatly in origin and biology. NENs occur in almost every organ system or region of the body. "Neuroendocrine" (NE) terminology is applied to widely dispersed cells with neuro and endocrine properties.[1] The "neuro" property is based on the identification of dense core granules (DCG), a similar substance present in serotonergic neurons that store monoamines (unlike neurons, NE cells do not contain synapses). The "endocrine" property refers to the synthesis and secretion of these monoamines. Several components of peptide hormones and amines act as NE markers, they include: (a) Transcription factors of NE differentiation (e.g., INSM1), (b) peptide hormones in dense core vesicles (e.g., chromogranin), (c) small chemical mediators stored in small synaptic-like vesicles (e.g., synaptophysin), (d) receptors involved in NE cell control [e.g., somatostatin receptor, or somatostatin receptor (SSTR)], (e) location-specific transcription factors (e.g., TTF1 and SATB2), and (f) hormones and enzymes required for hormone processing.[2]

The NE cell system can be divided into: (a) Cell aggregates that constitute glands (e.g., pituitary, parathyroid, paraganglia, and adrenal medulla) and (b) diffusely distributed dispersed cells that constitute a disseminated system [diffuse neuroendocrine system (DNES)] that consists of approximately 17 different cell types. These cells, either individually or in aggregates, are present in the skin, thyroid, lung, thymus, gastroenteropancreatic (GEP) tract, and urogenital tract. They are the largest group of hormone-producing cells in the body.[3]

NEUROENDOCRINE TUMORS AND CARCINOMAS: COMMON SITES

Given the varied distribution of the NE cells in the human body, NENs can occur in almost every organ system but are the most common in the gastrointestinal tract (GIT), pancreas, and lungs **(Table 1)**. They account for approximately 0.5% of all newly diagnosed malignancies.[4]

TABLE 1: Organ-specific distribution of neuroendocrine neoplasms.

Organ system	Proportion (%)
Gastroenteropancreatic NEN	70
Respiratory NEN	25
NEN of other sites	5

(NEN: neuroendocrine neoplasm)

Most patients are in the sixth to eighth decade with a female preponderance of around 2.5:1. The incidence of NEN is on the rise possibly due to improved awareness and a better detection system.[5] A web-based registry data on GEP-neuroendocrine tumor (NET) in India was published in 2017 with a reporting span between 2001 and 2006 including 6 tertiary care centers identifying 407 GEP-NET cases. Primary sites were the pancreas (42.9%), small intestine (22.1%), colorectum (9%), and the appendix (2.7%). Most commonly well-differentiated NETs were identified, while grade 3 and poorly differentiated NE carcinomas (NEC) were reported in 8.8% of cases. At diagnosis, metastasis was present in approximately 45% of these cases.[6]

Before we discuss the current World Health Organization (WHO) classification, diagnostic methods, and prognostic parameters of NEN, we will present the historical perspective and concept behind the evolution of the current (5th edition) uniform classification framework by WHO.

EVOLUTION OF TERMINOLOGIES USED, CLASSIFICATION, CONTROVERSIES, AND UPDATES

How has the Terminology Changed and Why?

The evolution of our concepts of DNES and its tumors started in 1897 with the Russian scientist Nikolai Kultschisky detecting enterochromaffin cells at the base of the normal Lieberkühn intestine crypts.[7] In 1907, Siegfried Oberndorfer described a small tumor in the appendix and coined the term "carcinoid" which means "carcinoma-like" lesion.[8] In 1914, Pierre Masson described a novel silver-stain technique to classify endocrine cells and in collaboration with Antonin Gosset, he postulated the origin of intestinal carcinoid and brilliantly suggested the relation between neural and endocrine lesions in the appendix, laying the basis of the concept behind NETs. The existence of DNES in humans was first proposed by Friedrich Feyrter in 1938.[9] In his influential paper, the author proposed that the endocrine system comprises not only compact epithelial organs that release hormones into the lymph and blood but also dispersed clear endocrine cells. These cells can be found individually or in groups throughout the system. He also proposed that DNES is developed by chemotactic migration of nervous tissue to a specific body site.[10] In 1966, AGE Pearse provided a classification system that unified the variety of diffusely scattered endocrine cells by introducing the term "APUD". This acronym (amine precursor uptake and decarboxylation) recognized the common biochemical characteristics of all these cells.[11] He also boldly suggested that their origin is the neural crest, a

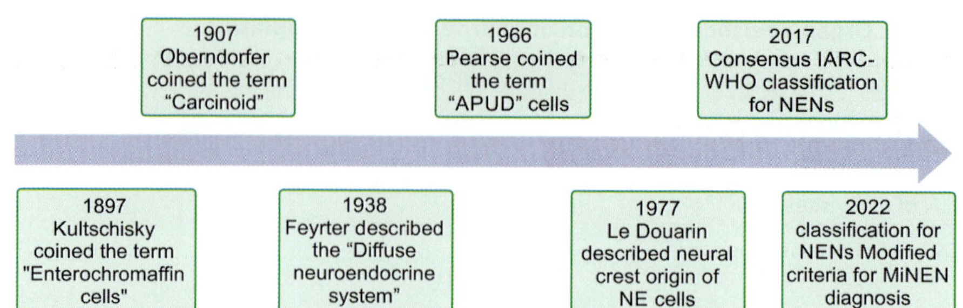

FIG. 1: Evolution of neuroendocrine neoplasm, terminologies, and classification.

(APUD: amine precursor uptake and decarboxylation; IARC: International Agency for Research on Cancer; MiNeN: mixed neuroendocrine-non-neuroendocrine neoplasms; NE: neuroendocrine; NEN: neuroendocrine neoplasms; WHO: World Health Organization)

transient neural structure already known to be the progenitor of the autonomic ganglia, paraganglia, and melanocytes. Later, Le Douarin et al. were able to confirm that ganglion cells of submucosa and myenteric plexus of the GIT, cells of paraganglia, melanocytes, and thyroid C cells were indeed of neural crest origin by their famous quail-chick chimeric model.[12] However, the cells of the gastrointestinal diffuse endocrine system lacked the markers of neural crest origin indirectly favoring their local origin from endodermal origin cells **(Fig. 1)**.[13]

There has been prolonged controversy regarding the origin of the gut NE system. Recent studies indicate that NE cells in the stomach, intestines, and pancreas are believed to come from a shared stem cell precursor. This precursor is located at the base of intestinal crypts or the neck of gastric glands in the stomach, while in the pancreas it is thought to reside within the ductal epithelium, giving rise to pancreatic islet cells. Transcription factors such as protein atonal homolog 1 (PATCH 1), neurogenin 3 (NGN3), and neuro D possibly are responsible for lineage transformation.[3]

Thus, currently, NE cells are divided into two subfamilies: Epithelial NE cells derived mainly from the embryonic endoderm, and nonepithelial NE cells (paraganglia, also called paraneurons) derived from embryonic neuroectoderm. The epithelial NE cells include pituitary adenohypophysial cells, parafollicular C cells, parathyroid cells, Merkel cells of the skin, and islet cells of the pancreas, and diffuse NE cells populate the mucosa of the gastrointestinal, respiratory, and genitourinary system.[14]

Paraganglia, derived from the sympathetic and parasympathetic autonomic nervous system, is present in soft tissue from the base of the skull to the bottom of the vertebral column. They include bilateral adrenal medulla, para-aortic paraganglia, the carotid body, the jugulotympanic paraganglia (glomus jugulare), the organ of Zuckerkandl, and paraganglia of the lung and porta hepatis. All NE cells express several proteins including neuron-specific enolase (NSE), chromogranin, synaptophysin, PGP 9.5, CD56, and INSM1. Chromogranin and INSM1 are specific biomarkers for NE differentiation, while others are nonspecific.[15] Moreover, most epithelial NE cells express keratin, which distinguishes them from nonepithelial paraganglia cells. These NE cells also exhibit specific transcription factors and hormones, allowing their

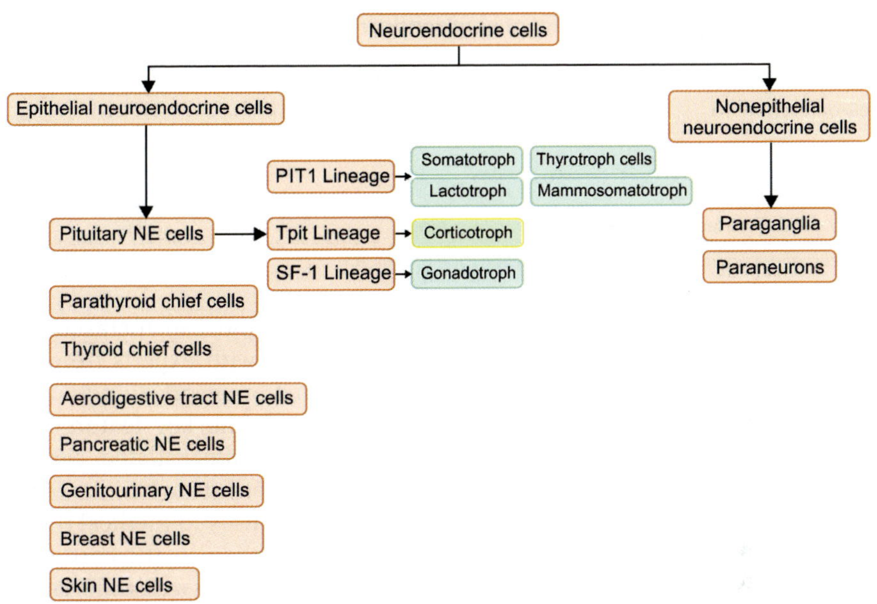

FLOWCHART 1: Families of neuroendocrine cells.

(NE: neuroendocrine)

identification and classification according to cell type. The paraganglia expresses the transcription factor GATA3 and tyrosine hydroxylase, an enzyme critical in catecholamine synthesis[16] **(Flowchart 1)**.

Epithelial NENs have been described under the terms of carcinoid tumor, argentaffinoma, APUDoma, small cell carcinoma, islet cell tumor, medullary thyroid carcinoma, Merkel cell tumor, NET, and NEC. Neoplasms with non-neuroendocrine origin include paraganglioma, pheochromocytoma, neuroblastoma, and olfactory neuroblastomas.[17] In the WHO classification of NENs in 2022, NENs have been broadly classified into NENs of endocrine organ origin and NENs of nonendocrine organ origin. NENs that arise in the GIT, lungs, upper airways, urogenital system, breast, and skin have been classified into the latter category.[18]

In the following section, we will discuss the evolution of the current 5th edition WHO classification of NEN following the consensus conference of the International Agency for Research on Cancer (IARC) and the World Health Organization (WHO) in 2017.

Common Classification Framework for Neuroendocrine Neoplasms

The evolution of the NEN classification system began with the "Munich Classification 1995", which served as a basis for subsequent WHO classifications in 2000 and 2014.[19,20] It also provides insight into the staging and grading system of NEN proposed by the European Neuroendocrine Tumor Society (ENETS) in 2006 and 2007.[17] From the year 2000 onwards the term "carcinoid"

TABLE 2: Common grading system of neuroendocrine tumors (NETs).

Differentiation	Mitosis/2 mm^2	Ki-67 labeling index	Nomenclature
Well-differentiated	<2	<3%	NET G1
	2–20	3–20%	NET G2
	>20	>20%	NET G3
Poorly differentiated	>20	>20%	NEC

(NEC: neuroendocrine carcinoma; NET: neuroendocrine tumor)

was abolished as all NENs are potentially malignant and can metastasize. In 2017, a consensus meeting was held in Lyon, France, with experts from IARC and WHO who proposed a common classification framework to standardize concepts between NEN of different anatomic sites.[21] The key feature of the common classification is a distinction between well-differentiated NET and poorly differentiated NEC, both sharing common expressions of NE markers but varying in biological aggressiveness and different responses to medical therapy. Morphology on hematoxylin and eosin (H&E) stained slides is the cornerstone of the differential diagnosis between NET and NEC. The well-differentiated NET is subdivided into NETs of G1, G2, and G3 corresponding to NETs of low, intermediate, and high grade based on mitotic count and Ki-67 labeling index (LI) **(Table 2)**. The poorly differentiated NEC does not have the typical histological characteristics of NETs, shows usually necrosis, and is aggressive. Based on morphological features, NECs are further divided into small-cell neuroendocrine carcinoma (SCNEC) and large-cell neuroendocrine cell carcinoma (LCNEC), the latter often mimicking any other epithelial malignancy. It was proposed that the mitotic count be expressed in numbers per mm^2 area, ideally counted to 10 mm^2 to assure accuracy (except in the breast where "hot spots" are counted). Ki-67 LI should be performed using a validated antibody (i.e., MIB antibody) in regions of most intense labeling (hotspots of at least 0.4 mm^2). The presence or absence of necrosis should be mentioned as focal (punctate) or diffuse (geographical) **(Figs. 2A to I)**.

Site-specific Characteristics and Classification System of Neuroendocrine Neoplasms

This section will examine the classification of NENs based on their specific anatomical sites within both endocrine and nonendocrine systems. We will stress the minor differences in organ-specific NEN classification of the 5th edition WHO.[18]

Pancreatic and Gastrointestinal Neuroendocrine Neoplasms

For most of the GIT NETs, the common 2017 grading system for NET is applicable as detailed earlier. In the past, GIT NETs were classified as per their embryological origin as foregut, midgut, and hindgut NETs and their functional characteristics. However, from 2010 onwards uniform classification has been used based on their proliferation index and mitotic counting, which was eventually revised in 2017.[22] Well-differentiated NENs (G1–G3) show characteristic

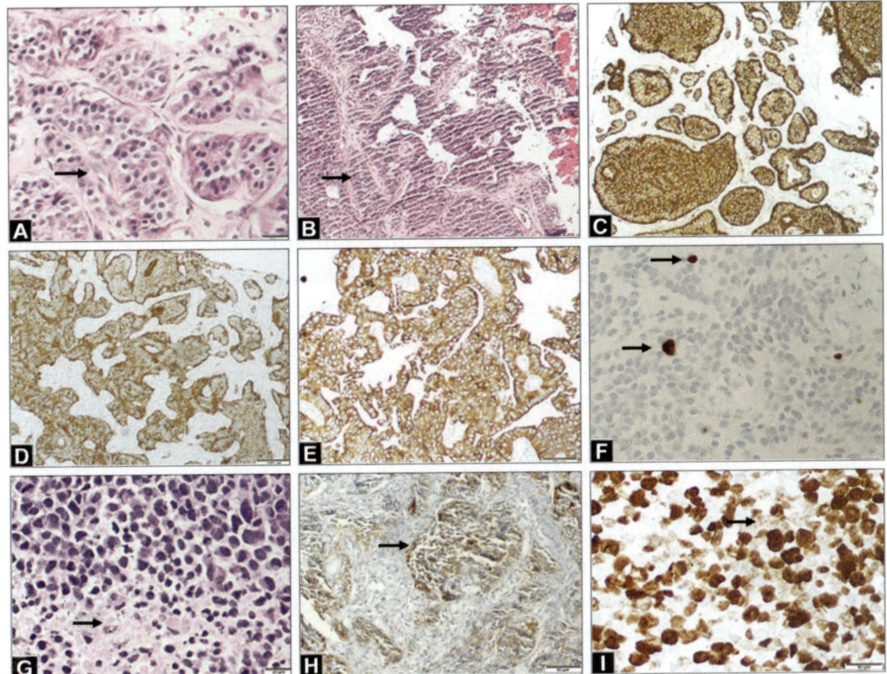

FIGS. 2A TO I: (A to F) The differences in well-differentiated neuroendocrine tumor (NET) and (G to I) a neuroendocrine carcinoma (NEC).

A well-differentiated NET shows characteristic monomorphic tumor cells and salt-and-pepper chromatin, with abundant eosinophilic granular cytoplasm and typical nested (arrow), (**Fig. 2A:** ×200) or ribbon-like arrangements (arrow) (**Fig. 2B:** ×100). A well-differentiated NET usually shows strong positivity for chromogranin (CG) (**Fig 2C:** ×200), synaptophysin (Syn) (**Fig. 2D:** ×100), Keratin (**Fig. 2E:** ×100), and low Ki-67 LI (arrows, positive nuclei) (**Fig. 2F:** ×400). A poorly differentiated NEC shows a sheet-like arrangement of pleomorphic tumor cells with necrosis (arrow) and molding (in the case of small cell-NEC, **Fig. 2G:** ×400). In NEC, CG stain is usually absent/focal/faint (arrow) (**Fig. 2H:** ×100). Ki-67 LI is very high (>20%). During a Ki-67 stain interpretation, counting should be performed in a hot spot and darkly and lightly stained nuclei (arrow) should be taken into account (**Fig. 2I:** ×400).

NET findings such as organoid architecture, monomorphic nuclear characteristics, and stippled or "salt-and-pepper"chromatin.[23] Also, commonly the cells can be arranged in nests, cords, ribbons, trabecula, and acinar patterns. Necrosis is not seen. Whereas in NECs organoid architecture is not seen, but it is rather characterized by sheet-like cell arrangements, nuclear atypia, frequent mitoses, apoptosis, and necrosis. Among NECs, SCNEC cells show scant cytoplasm and hyperchromatic nuclei with nuclear molding, and LCNEC cells mimic other carcinomas and have moderate-to-abundant cytoplasm, pleomorphic nuclei with prominent nucleoli, and necrosis. Whereas in the GIT, the SCNEC is common in the esophagus and anorectal region, the LCNEC occurs frequently in the stomach and intestine.[24,25] Also, GIT NECs can develop secondarily in patients receiving radiation therapy and such tumors are common in the esophagus, colon, and rectum. Ironically, these secondary NECs show a better outcome than usual NECs.[26] Mixed neuroendocrine-non-neuroendocrine neoplasms (MiNeN) show unquestionable non-neuroendocrine and NEN components, and both components should be identifiable morphologically and immunohistochemically. Compared to previous criteria of the NE area of at least 30% of the tumor area, the WHO 2022 classification of NENs has revised the definition to unquestionable identification of two areas regardless of their amounts.[27] The earlier nomenclature of mixed adeno-neuroendocrine carcinoma (MANEC) is no longer in use as in MiNeN the non-NE component can show squamous differentiation.[28] The NE differentiation should have morphological characteristics of NENs on H&E-stained sections, and such areas should show at least Syn and INSM1 positivity. CG is mostly negative or very focal/faint. Recently, MiNeNs have been classified prognostically as "high-grade malignant"—comprising mixed adenocarcinoma, or squamous cell carcinoma and NEC components; "intermediate-grade malignant"—mixed adenocarcinoma and NET; and "low-grade" comprising mixed adenoma and NET (MANET)[18] **(Figs. 3A to C)**. However, the 2019 WHO classification does not recognize MANET as a MiNeN. Further subgrading of MiNeN is important as in high-grade MiNeN, the prognosis is dependent on the NEC component, while in intermediate-grade MiNeN, prognosis depends on the nonepithelial component.[18] MiNeNs can be seen at the gastroesophageal (GE) junction, the pancreatobiliary region, and the rectum.[22] Regarding the diagnostic criteria of MiNeN, note that the previous cutoff point of 30% tumor area has been still provisionally maintained for GIT MiNeNs, and even when focal NEN differentia-

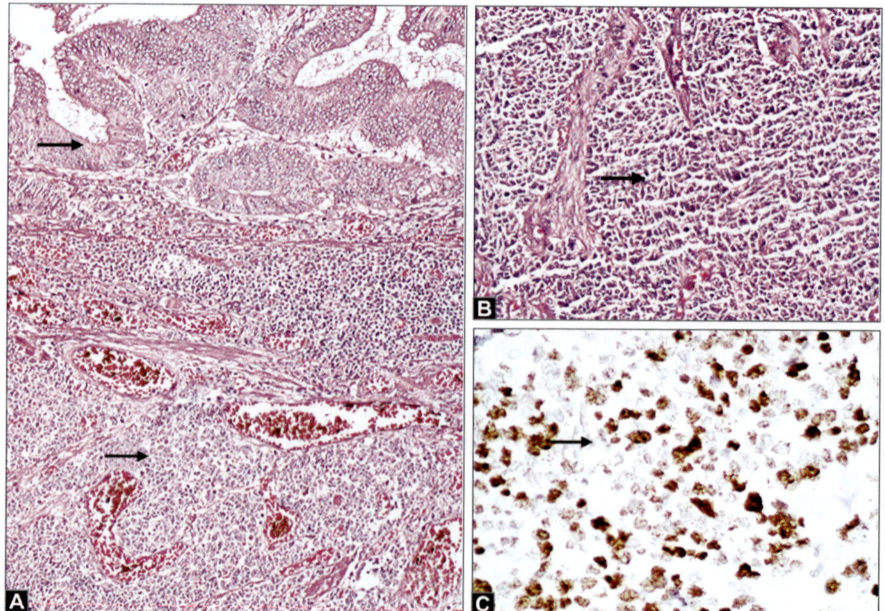

FIGS. 3A TO C: (A: ×40 and B: ×100) Sections of an intestinal MiNeN show features of adenoma with high-grade dysplasia at the top (upper arrow) and below features of a poorly differentiated NEC (lower arrow). (C: ×400) The NEC component shows a high Ki-67 labeling index (arrow).

(MiNeN: Mixed neuroendocrine-non-neuroendocrine neoplasms; NEC: neuroendocrine carcinoma)

tion is observed in an epithelial tumor, the same should be documented and the area of such differentiation should be mentioned.[18]

Also, based on genetic studies, it seems logical to use the unitary grading system for both GIT and pancreatic NENs. TP53 and RB1 mutations are identified in both GIT NEC and pancreatic NET. However, in NETs, these mutations are not identified. *MEN1*, *DAXX*, and *ATRX* mutations on the other hand are common in well-differentiated NETs.[29,30] The GIT and pancreatic NENs on the other hand commonly express SSTR2 and SSTR5, neuropeptide receptors responsible for mitogen-activated protein kinase (MAPK) pathway, and calcium-channel activators.[18] Multiple NENs in the GIT (especially in the duodenum) and pancreas or NENs in association with multiple gastrointestinal stromal tumors are usually associated with inherited syndromes such as autosomal dominant Von Hippel–Lindau (VHL) syndrome, MEN1, NF1, or tuberous sclerosis. In such cases, specific hormonal stains should be performed to identify the somatostatinomas (NF1 associated), gastrinomas (MEN1 associated), or insulinomas (TS associated) along with genetic studies.[31]

In addition, it should be remembered that, though the unified NET grading system can be used throughout the GIT, a close examination of the background changes in gastric NETs can give vital clues regarding etiopathogenesis. Based on the etiological association, gastric NENs are classified into three types: Type 1 NEN, which is the most common type, arises in a background of atrophic gastritis **(Figs. 4A and B)**; type 2 NEN, which are rarest of the three types, are associated with MEN1 and Zollinger–Ellison syndromes; while type 3 NENs are sporadic. Therefore, when experiencing autoimmune or *Helicobacter pylori*-induced atrophic gastritis, enterochromaffin-like (ECL) cell hyperplasia or dysplastic NE nodules should always be screened for at least CG stain. While the type I and 2 gastric NENs are usually of WHO grade 1 type, type 3 NENs show higher grades and commonly show metastasis.[32,33] In the appendix, as stated earlier, NENs are common. However, unlike the GE junction or rectum,

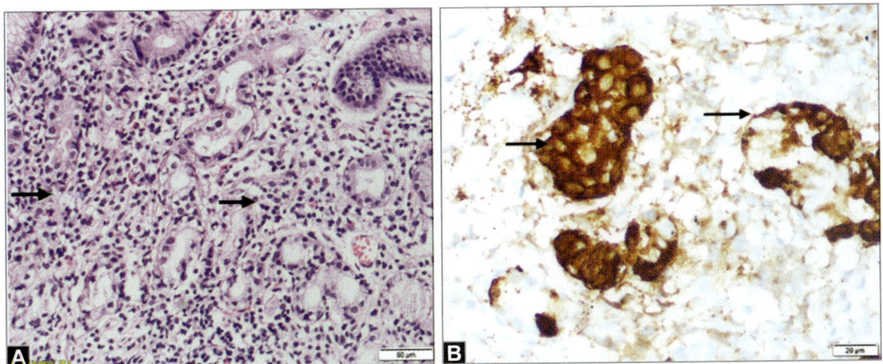

FIGS. 4A AND B: Biopsy from the gastric body shows complete antralization (atrophy), i.e., replacement of the oxyntic glands by pyloric glands with dense intraepithelial lymphocytic infiltrate (arrows) (A: ×100), and/ or replacement of glands by fibrosis. In atrophic gastritis, always a chromogranin (CG) stain must be performed to rule out the possibility of neuroendocrine (NE) cell hyperplasia/adenoma. In this example, both micronodular NE cell hyperplasia and linear hyperplasia are noted (arrows) (B: ×400).

in the appendix, G3-NET or NEC are rare.[18] However, high-grade MiNeNs or goblet cell carcinomas can be seen in the appendix; the latter, though they show NE differentiation, are not considered NEC per se. However, the WHO 2022 classification of NENs reserved the term "amphicrine carcinomas", for which single tumor cells show epithelial and NE differentiation. Goblet cell carcinoma possibly fits best to this group of distinct tumors.[18,34] On the basis of the cell type, NENs in the appendix are also classified as enterochromaffin cell (EC) type (serotonin producing), L-cell type (which produces glucagon-like peptide), and PP/YY producing type. However, these subtypes do not have any prognostic or therapeutic implications.[35]

Neuroendocrine Neoplasms in Lungs

The classification of lung NEN is composed of low-grade typical carcinoid (TC), intermediate-grade atypical carcinoid (AC), high-grade small cell lung carcinoma (SCLC), and LCNEC.[36] Therefore, the terminology and diagnostic criteria used in the fifth edition for lung NENs remained unchanged since the 1999 WHO classification **(Table 3)**. When lung NEC has other components such as squamous cell carcinoma or adenocarcinoma, tumors are classified as combined SCLC or LCNEC. The criteria to distinguish between TCs and ACs were initially established based on lung resection samples rather than samples obtained from metastatic sites or small biopsies/cytology samples.

As in small biopsy and cytological samples, a distinction between typical carcinoid and atypical carcinoid may not be possible, in such a scenario the term "carcinoid tumor, not otherwise specified (NOS)" should be used and the mitotic count, the presence/absence of necrosis, and Ki-67 LI should be documented. The term "carcinoid tumor, NOS" is also recommended for use in cases of metastatic carcinoids and during the slide review of resected lung carcinoids, especially when the complete set of tumor slides is not available for examination. There are some controversies about the usefulness of the Ki-67 index in lung NENs, but it can be especially useful in small biopsies with crush artifacts, where carcinoids may be misdiagnosed as SCLC.[37]

Neuroendocrine tumor of the lung with elevated mitotic count and/or Ki-67 proliferation index: Recent reports document lung NETs with carcinoid tumor's morphological characteristics but with mitotic count >10/2 mm^2 and/or Ki-67

TABLE 3: Diagnostic criteria for lung NENs.

	Typical carcinoid	Atypical carcinoid	SCLC	LCNEC
Mitosis per 2 mm^2	<2	2–10	>10 (median 80)	>10 (median 70)
Necrosis	No	Focal, if any	Yes	Yes
Neuroendocrine morphology	Yes	Yes	Unlike typical carcinoid	No
Ki-67 index	Up to 5%	Up to 30%	30–100%	30–100%

(SCLC: small cell lung carcinoma; LCNEC: large cell neuroendocrine carcinomas; NEN: neuroendocrine neoplasms)

LI higher than expected (>30%). These tumors generally correspond to those classified as grade 3 NETs in the pancreas (PanNET). However, due to insufficient data regarding their prognosis, this subset of tumors is classified as LCNEC according to the current WHO classification scheme. Limited genomic analysis data for these tumors show a relationship with carcinoid rather than SCLC or LCNEC based on the *RC1* or *TP53* mutation.[38]

Neuroendocrine Neoplasms in Breast

According to the current fifth edition WHO classification for breast tumors, NENs of the breast are classified into: (a) Well-differentiated NETs; these are low-to-intermediate-grade tumors with peripheral myoepithelial layer. They are also classified as either in-situ or invasive disease; (b) Poorly differentiated NECs, histologically classified into SCNECs and LCNECs.[21] The grading system of NEN of other organs in the body (like PanNET) does not apply to NETs of the breast, they are graded according to the Nottingham grading system, and most NETs are G1 or G2.[39] Invasive carcinoma-no special type (NST) with NE differentiation should not be diagnosed as NEN until the NE histological characteristics and marker expression are distinct and uniform enough. Similarly, solid papillary carcinoma and the hypercellular subtype of mucinous carcinoma could express NE markers but should not be classified as NET or NEN.[40] Most NETs in the breast represent mixed NENs and most SCNECs in the breast show components of conventional mammary carcinoma. Cancers with a >90% NEN pattern should be classified as NET or NEC. It should be remembered, that outside the context of rare SCNEC, NE differentiation in other breast carcinomas has no therapeutic significance.

Skin Neuroendocrine Neoplasms

The primary cutaneous NEN is called Merkel cell carcinoma (MCC). It is a high-grade poorly differentiated neoplasm categorized as NEC in the current WHO classification framework. However, neither proliferation parameters nor necrosis are needed to designate it as a high-grade carcinoma. There are two subtypes: Merkel cell polyoma virus-positive MCC and virus-negative MCC.[41] Most MCCs develop de novo; however, some primary cutaneous NE carcinoma can arise from dysplastic squamous epithelium.[42] Primary cutaneous well-differentiated NET is exceedingly rare, few reported cases of low-grade NEN in the skin are either metastatic deposits or low-grade sweat gland carcinoma showing NE differentiation.[43,44]

Head and Neck Neuroendocrine Neoplasms

The current fifth edition of WHO classification for head and neck tumors reflects the common WHO/IARC classification framework. The upper aerodigestive tract and salivary NENs are dichotomously classified into well-differentiated NET (assigned to three grades G1, G2, and G3) and poorly differentiated NEC (including small cell and large cell carcinoma). However, the G3 category remains provisional. Grade 1 NET has <2 mitosis/2 mm^2 and lacks necrosis; Grade 2 NET exhibits necrosis (often punctate or coagulative) and/or 2–10 mitosis/2 mm^2. Grade 3 NET have mitosis >10/2 mm^2. The Ki-67 LI is <20%.[45]

The optimal Ki-67 index has not yet been defined to classify between the G1 and G2 NETs in the head and neck region.[46] In this region, the larynx is the most common site for NEN. In the nasal cavity, the WHO classification includes only NEC.[47] However, MiNEN has been well documented.[48]

The *middle ear neuroendocrine tumor* (MeNET), previously known as middle ear adenoma is a neoplasm arising from the middle ear mucosa showing epithelial and neuroendocrine differentiation. The grading system of MeNET is still under investigation, however, they have a very low Ki-67 LI (<2%).[21]

Female Genital Organ Neuroendocrine Neoplasms

Neuroendocrine neoplasms are rare in the female genital tract (FGT). In the current WHO 5th edition, the classification of NEN in the FGT is like other body parts and divided into NET and NECs. The only exception is the ovary, where the "ovarian carcinoid" is still in use. They are the most common type of NEN in the FGT and are considered monodermal teratomas arising from NE cells within the intestinal epithelium of mature cystic teratoma.[49] The SCNEC and LCNEC of the FGT are morphologically similar to all other body parts, most commonly occurring in the cervix followed by the endometrium. In the cervix, they are associated with high-risk human papillomavirus (HPV) (HPV 16 and 18) and show diffuse block positivity for p16.[50] It should be remembered that hypercalcemia-type ovarian SCNEC genetically does not show common NEN-related genes, and commonly shows the *SMARCA4* gene mutation.[51]

Pituitary Neuroendocrine Neoplasms

In the fifth edition of the WHO classification of endocrine tumors and NET, the nomenclature of NET has been changed. Pituitary neuroendocrine tumor (PitNET) is now the preferred terminology for pituitary NEN, formerly known as pituitary adenoma.[52] When metastatic, the term metastatic PitNET is preferred instead of pituitary carcinoma.[53]

Unlike NENs of other body parts, no formal grading (based on mitosis and Ki-67 LI) or staging system is applied to PitNET. Such tumors show prognosis based on their cytodifferentiation. That means, the differentiation of cells in a tumor denotes their aggressiveness, risk of recurrence, and therapeutic response.[53] PitNETs are classified according to their origin from three major families of adenohypophysial cells [driven by pituitary-specific positive transcription factor 1 (PIT1), PIT1 and T box transcription factor (TPIT), steroidogenic factor 1 (SF1), and six terminally differentiated cell types (i.e., corticotroph, lactotroph, somatotroph, mammosomatotroph, thyrotroph, and gonadotroph)]. Immunohistochemistry (IHC) for pituitary transcription factors (PIT1, TPIT, and SF1), adenohypophysial hormones, and keratins (especially CAM 5.2) are now essential for the classification of PitNET. The term PitNET-NOS can be used when ancillary tools for subtyping are not available. Although SSTR IHC is not required for routine PitNET reporting, immunoreactivity of SSTR2 and SSTR5 has been shown to predict the response to somatostatin analog.[54] **Flowchart 2** shows the detailed classification schema for PitNET based on transcription factors, cell types, and low molecular weight keratin (LMWK) expression pattern.

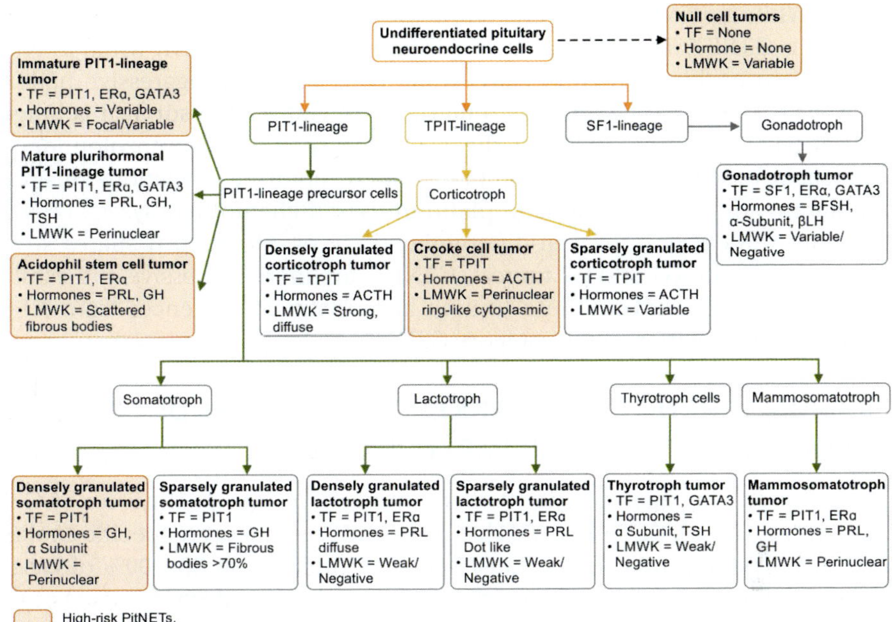

FLOWCHART 2: A detailed schema of classifying the PitNETs. The high-risk subtypes have been highlighted.

(ACTH: adrenocorticotropic hormone; BFSH: bovine follicle-stimulating hormone; GH: growth hormone; LMWK: low molecular weight keratin; PRL: prolactin; TF: transcription factor; TSH: thyroid-stimulating hormone)

Why was there a Need to Classify G3-Neuroendocrine Tumor and Neuroendocrine Carcinoma?

The WHO tumor classification was published in 2018, and a category was created—G3-NET—for a group of well-differentiated NETs that showed a poorer prognosis than G1 and G2 NETs. Although G3-NET clinically shows syndromes due to hormone production, NEC presents aggressive clinical features with disseminated disease.[18] Histologically, these NENs show similarities with well-differentiated NETs and lack the characteristics of NEC and necrosis. However, compared to G1 and G2 NETs, G3 NET shows vesicular nuclei, membrane irregularities, atypia, and a reduced tumor-to-stroma ratio. Most commonly, G3 NET is detected in the pancreas, whereas NECs are common in luminal GIT.[18] CG stain is mostly diffusely expressed in G3-NET, while in NECs, CG is expressed focally/faintly or with dot-like positivity. Clinically, while the G3 NET shows high avidity for somatostatin receptor scintigraphy, the NEC shows low avidity. However, fludeoxyglucose-18 positron emission tomography (FDG-PET) uptake is seen in NEC, but that is unlikely in G3 NET. While the Ki-67 LI is between 20 and 35% in G5NET, in NEC the range is nearly 20–90%, with a median cut-off of 55%.[18] Due to proven mutations of RB1 and SMAD4 in NEC, these markers lack expression, while in G3NET, these markers are retained. TP53 expression also shows a mutant pattern in NEC (in 95%), not in G3NET. The expression of ATRX and DAXX is lost in G3NET, while its expression is retained in NEC. While up to 60% of NECs show the KRAS mutation, the same is not detected in G3NET. The expression of SSTR2A is seen in G3NET, while in NEC it is not seen or faint. Prognostically, while NEC shows an aggressive pattern (survival 11–17 months) with early metastasis, in G3NET the survival is longer (survival 54–99 months).[18] While the G3NET responds to temozolomide or streptozocin-based therapies and somatostatin receptor-based peptide receptor radiotherapy, the NEC responds to platinum-based chemotherapy.[24,55] G3NET falls under the category of well-differentiated NENs. Although it shares some characteristics with G1 and G2 tumors, G3NETs are more aggressive and exhibit a high proliferation index. These tumors have distinct differences from NEC, which led to the creation of the category G3NET.

IMMUNOPHENOTYPIC MARKERS OF NEUROENDOCRINE NEOPLASMS AND THEIR IMPLICATIONS

Among the cell lineage-specific markers, most NENs are positive for (CG-A, synaptophysin (Syn), CD56 (NCAM1), CD57 (Leu7), and neuron-specific enolase (NSE).[23,31] Synaptophysin is the most sensitive (positive in 95–100% of cases) and CG A is the most specific NE marker.[56] Although CG and Syn are used as the first-line routine NE markers; in higher-grade NE tumors, CG staining can be focal or lost. In addition, CG stain can vary depending on the site of origin of the NEN; for example, while most GIT foregut NENs are CG positive, only about 40–60% of colorectal NENs are CG positive and appendicular L-cell NETs are negative.[18] Hence, in a morphologically suspected case, adding additional markers is needed if only one of the CG and Syn markers is positive. Syn positivity in other epithelial tumors has been reported.[57] CD56, CD57, and NSE lack specificity,[1] however, CD56 can be used in poorly differentiated NECs as CG might not help. Insulinoma-associated protein 1 (INSM1) is considered the first-line NE marker in NET of the thoracic, head, and neck and has high sensitivity comparable to Syn. All primary and nearly 90% of the metastatic pancreatic NENs show INSM1 positivity. In the luminal GIT, INSM1 can be of value mainly in ileal NETs, while it may not always be reliable in other sites.[5] In summary, it must be remembered that at least two lineage-specific NE markers should be positive before calling any tumor NET. In addition to lineage-specific markers, several transcription factors, such as CDX2, SATB2, CDH17, ISL-1, and PAX-8, can be positive in NET; however, their expression varies depending on the tumor origin site. For example, while CDX2 is expressed in most NETs arising from luminal GIT and pancreas, in the lung its expression is uncommon.[4] On hindgut other hand, while the NENs are positive for SATB2, foregut and midgut NENs are rarely positive.[4] CDH17 is expressed in the majority of small intestinal, appendiceal, and rectal NETs, and in a small proportion of pancreatic and pulmonary NETs.[4] ISL-1 and PAX-8 are commonly expressed in the lung, pancreatic, duodenal, and rectal NETs, and at low frequency in other GI NETs.[4,6] Lung NENs and medullary thyroid carcinomas can express TTF1, but the expression is antibody clone dependent, and SPT24 is the most reliable for this purpose.[58] Based on their cell of origin and functionality, tumor cells can also stain for insulin, glucagon, somatostatin, or pancreatic polypeptide (PP).

However, routine application of these hormonal markers is not necessary, although nonfunctional NENs are supposed to be less aggressive.[6] In addition to these, in a few organs, a classification and characterization of specific markers of NENs is needed. For example, for pituitary NET, the PIT1, TPIT, and SF1 transcription factors, adenohypophysial hormonal markers, and keratin (especially CAM 5.2) staining are now essential for classification. CG positivity can be seen in appendicular goblet cell carcinoma; however, the same should not be classified as a NEN as detailed earlier **(Figs. 5A to D)**.[18] Also, to differentiate between epithelial and nonepithelial NEN, pan-keratin staining (AE1/AE3) is a must in all NENs along with other markers. Keratin will be positive in all epithelial NENs, while negative in nonepithelial NENs, such as in paraganglioma or pheochromocytoma. In this regard, CAM 5.2 is most reliable. The latter mostly on the other hand show positivity for GATA3. Hence, a keratin stain may be of value in case of metastatic NEN of unknown origin.[59] Another second-generation NE marker, secretagogin (SECG) is positive in most epithelial-origin NENs including, lung, pancreas, and GIT, and can be of help if first-line NE markers are noncontributory.[18] A combination of PDX1 and CDX2 can help identify NEN of higher GIT origin, while islet hormone markers such as insulin, glucagon, somatostatin, and gastrin can help identify pancreatic and duodenal NENs in the case of metastasis of unknown origin (MUO).[18] Although most NENs are dual negative for CK7/CK20, metastatic Merkle cell carcinomas can show paranuclear dot positivity with CK20 and are also positive for SATB2, CM2B4, and tdT.[60]

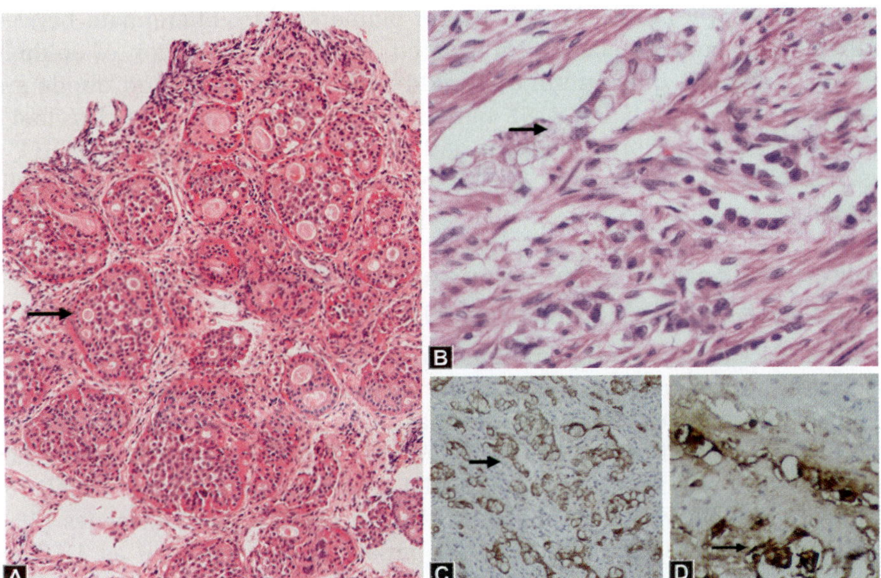

FIGS. 5A TO D: (A: ×100) Nested morphology is a frequent feature of ileal neuroendocrine tumor (NET) (arrow); (B: ×400) An appendicular goblet cell carcinoma showing unilayered tubules with goblet cells (arrow); (C: ×100) A goblet cell carcinoma showing positivity for Keratin (arrow); and (D: ×200) chromogranin (CG) (arrow).

Some markers have been identified to give prognostic information and guide therapy. PanNETs are negative for O^6-methylguanine-DNA methyltransferase (MGMT) (expression in 10% tumor cells) and show a better response to alkylating agents (temozolomide, dacarbazine, and streptozotocin)-based therapy and progressive free survival is better in this group than in cases positive for MGMT.[61] MGMT deficiency is observed in about half of PanNETs.[62] However, a major limitation is the heterogeneity of the detection method and criteria used for methylation detection, especially using the polymerase chain reaction (PCR)-based methylation test. However, succinate dehydrogenase complex iron sulfur subunit B (SDHB) stain loss or SDHB mutation in pheochromocytoma, head and neck paraganglioma, thoracic–abdominal–pelvic paragangliomas are found to indicate germline mutation and malignant potential in such NENs.[63] More recently *SDH* gene mutations have been identified in pituitary adenomas and PanNENs also, making it essential to screen for SDHB loss for identifying a pathogenic mutant.[64] Though not routinely indicated, SSRTA 1–5 expression (in 70–80% in PanNETs and rarely in lung NENs) indicates better disease-free and overall survival in NENs.[18] The loss of e-cadherin and expression of β-catenin have also been associated with poor outcomes. CK19, CD117, p18, and p21 stain expressions are also associated with a poor prognosis. Microsatellite instability or mismatch repair (MMR) protein deficiency may be detected in 10–12% of NEN. MMR-deficient NECs show a relatively better prognosis and may be identified shortly as another prognostic subgroup.[65] PD-L1 expression has been identified in about half of the poorly differentiated NECs and G3 NETs and is also a marker of poor prognosis. However, NENs expressing high PD-L1 may be candidates for targeted therapy[66] **(Table 4)**. The use of biomarkers to differentiate between epithelial and nonepithelial NENs resulted in the reclassification of epithelial NETs in the spine, duodenum, and middle ear. In the spine and duodenum, composite neuronal/glial and NE tumors are observed, currently classified as "composite gangliocytoma/neuroma and neuroendocrine tumor (CoGNET)" in the 2022 WHO classification of NENs, instead of earlier terminology of gangliocytic paraganglioma.[18]

Molecular Changes in Neuroendocrine Neoplasms and Implications of Molecular Analysis

About 90–95% of NENs are sporadic, while 5% are hereditary. Genetic alterations associated with hereditary NENs have already been discussed earlier. But in recent years, considerable overlap has been noted between sporadic and hereditary NEN and *alterations in the MEN1, VHL, NF1, or TSC* genes have been observed in both. In sporadic PanNET, somatic mutations of *MEN1* (37–44%),[67,68] mutually exclusive mutations in the *DAXX* and *ATRX* genes (45%), 37 *CDKN1B* (1%), VHL (1%) and DNA repair machinery, such as *MUTYH1* (MuT Y homolog), *BRCA2*, and *CHEK2* (checkpoint kinase 2) genes have been observed.[18] *DAXX/ATRX* inactivation also causes chromosomal instability and alternative lengthening of telomeres (ALT), especially in the NETs.[69] The loss of *ATRX*, *DAXX*, and Menin is common in PanNETs. Other rare genetic alterations

TABLE 4: Common markers used for NENs.

Lineage-specific markers	First-line NE markers	Chromogranin A, synaptophysin, and INSM1
	Second-line NE markers	CD56, CD57, and NSE
Transcription factors expressed in NENs	Site-specific	CDX2, SATB2, CDH17, ISL1, PAX8, PDX1, SECG, PIT1, TPIT, and SF1
Peptide hormones	Pancreatic and duodenal NETs	Insulin, glucagon, somatostatin, gastric, or pancreatic polypeptide (PP)
Epithelial markers	Pankeratin	All epithelial NENs
	CK20	Dot-like positivity in Merkle cell carcinoma
	CK7/CK20	Most NENs are dual negative
Prognostic markers	Marker of better prognosis	SSRTA1–5+, MGMT-loss, and MSI/MMRd
	Markers of poor prognosis	E-cadherin loss, β-catenin+, CK19+, CD117+, p18+, p21+, SDHB loss/mutant, and PD-L1 expression
Therapeutic indicator		MGMT-negative Pan-NETs show better response to alkylating agents (temozolomide, dacarbazine, and streptozotocin); SSTR expressing NETs can be treated with SSA and PRRT

(INSM1: insulinoma-associated protein 1; MSI: microsatellite instability; MGMT: O6-methylguanine-DNA methyltransferase; MMRd: mismatch repair deficiency; NE: neoendocrine; NEN: neuroendocrine neoplasms; PanNET: pancreas neuroendocrine tumor; PRRT: peptide receptor radiotherapy; SSA: somatostatin analogs; SSTR: somatostatin receptor)

observed are in the set-domain-containing 2 (*SETD2*), *MLL3* (myeloid/lymphoid or mixed lineage leukemia protein 3), *ARID2* (AT-rich interaction domain 2), and *SMARCA4* (SWI/SNF-related, matrix-associated, actin-dependent regulator of chromatin, subfamily a, member 4) genes, mammalian target of rapamycin (mTOR) pathway (10–15%), with loss of function mutations of *PTEN*, *TSC1*, or *TSC2*, and *DEPDC5*, and activating mutations of the *PI2KCA* kinase domain.[70] In the poorly differentiated NECs, *RB*, *TP*53, *KRAS*, *APC*, and *ARID1A* mutations have been commonly identified.[30] Unlike PanNETs, in small intestinal NETs, *CDKN1B* (5–8%), *APC* (7.7%), *BRAF* (3.8%), *CDKN2C* (7.7%), *KRAS* (3.8%), *PIK3C* (3.8%), and *TP53* (3.8%) mutations and copy number variations (CNVs), especially loss of heterozygosity (LOH) of chromosome 18 has been detected. Upregulation of IGF has been identified in half of the small-intestinal (SI) NETs. *RB* mutation is relatively uncommon in SI-NETs.[18] In lung NECs, inactivation of *TP53* and *RB*, overexpression of Bcl-2 and *MYC*, and activation of the *PI3K*/*AKT*/mTOR pathway have been identified.[18] CNV involving chromosome 3p has been identified in up to 90% of SCNECs of the lung. On the other hand, in lung carcinoids, the *MEN1* mutation is common. In the WHO classification of NENs in 2022, LCNECs have been subdivided into three additional molecular subtypes: (1) LCNEC with pulmonary SCNEC-like characteristics—these tumors show T*P53* and *RB* mutations, along with *MYC* amplification and *PTEN* mutations; (2) LCNEC with NSCLC-like characteristics—characterized by *KRAS* and *PIK3CA* mutations and without *TP53* and *RB* mutations; and (3) LCNEC with characteristics similar to NET (carcinoid)—LCNECs with MEN1 alterations, low mutation burden, and without *TP53* and *RB* mutations.[18]

Molecular analysis of MiNeNs indicates the origin of both endocrine and nonendocrine components from a single precursor. *APC, KRAS,* and *SMAD4* mutations and microsatellite instability frequently noted in colorectal adenocarcinomas have also been documented in colorectal MiNeNs.[71]

Epigenetic alterations, such as CpG island methylator phenotype, have been described in around 80% of the PanNETs.[72,73] The role of MGMT expression and methylation profiling has already been highlighted earlier. The role of the *DAXX/ATRX* complex in DNA methylation has been observed and *DAXX/ATRX* mutated tumors show a different methylation profile.[74] Based on epigenetic changes, the WHO 2022 classification has further divided nonfunctional PanNETs into three subtypes: A cell-like, A cell-like > B cell-like, and B cell-like/other.[18] Shortly, analyses of genetic alterations, epigenetic changes, and CNV studies may become routine in comprehensive subtyping of NENs.

CHALLENGES IN PATHOLOGICAL EVALUATION AND GRADING, SOLUTIONS, AND APPROACH

Histological Considerations

The primary necessity for pathologists is understanding that the classification of "well-differentiated" and "poorly differentiated" NENs depends on simple histological evaluation and not on the Ki-67 LI. We have described earlier the classical histological pattern in NENs. Depending on nuclear monomorphism, granular eosinophilic cytoplasm in tumor cells, and nested (or type A), trabecular, pseudo glandular, and diffuse pattern, a NET is suspected. The nested morphology is the most common and frequent in NETs of the ileal and jejunum[75] **(Figs. 5A to D)**. In PitNETs, the cytoplasm can be basophilic, eosinophilic, or chromophobic. The small bowel EC NETs show basophilic cell nests and stromal fibrosis, because of the abundant serotonin produced by them.[18] While the central lung NENs show typical morphology, peripheral lung NENs can show spindling. Amyloid-like material can be seen in duodenal-pancreatic NEN. Somatostatinomas show abundant hepatoid cytoplasm and prominent psammoma bodies.[18] L-cell tumors in the rectum and appendix can show prominent ribbons.[18] It should be remembered that architectural patterns can overlap between different sites. Some of the NENs also can have prominent fibrous stroma, though overall NENs are stroma-poor.[18] Not all NETs show monomorphic nuclei, nuclear pleomorphism, and membrane irregularities, and vesicular nuclei can be seen in G3 NET. G3-NET can also show a reduced tumor-to-stroma ratio. In NEC, typically a solid high-grade tumor with necrosis, frequent apoptotic bodies, and high Ki-67 LI (>55%) are seen. However, this cut-off point is arbitrary, though mostly applicable. As mentioned, in addition to SCNEC and LCNEC, Merkle cell carcinoma of the skin is considered a site-specific type of NEC **(Flowchart 3)**.[18]

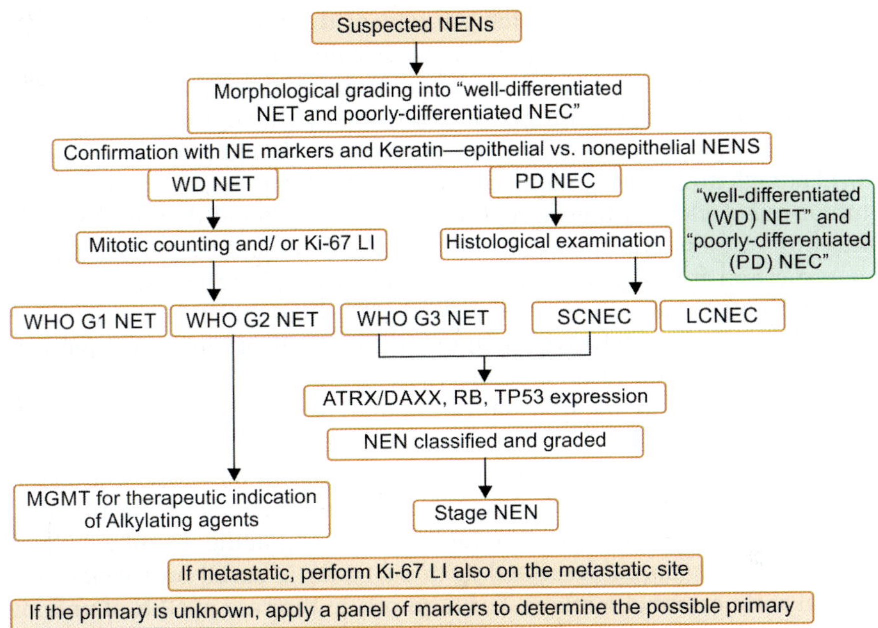

FLOWCHART 3: A schema to approach the diagnosis and histological grading of NENs.

(LI: labeling index; LCNEC: large-cell neuroendocrine cell carcinoma; MGMT: O^6-methylguanine-DNA methyltransferase; NEC: neuroendocrine carcinoma; NENs: neuroendocrine neoplasms; NET; neuroendocrine tumor; SCNEC: small-cell neuroendocrine carcinoma; WHO: World Health Organization)

Minimum Marker Criteria

The second issue is that pathologists must adhere to a minimum requirement of at least two positive NE markers before diagnosing an NEN. Also, a keratin stain must be performed to differentiate between an epithelial NEN and a non-epithelial NEN.

Issues with Histological Classification of Neuroendocrine Neoplasms

Then comes the issue of histological grading in NEN. For grading, both the mitotic index and Ki-67 LI can be performed. However, it must be remembered that in small-core biopsies, in samples where the exact fixation protocol was not followed and in thick sections, the mitotic count may not be reliable and Ki-67 LI is needed. However, pathologists must follow the protocol for these assessments. The mitotic index is expressed per 2 mm^2, which equals 10 high-power fields at 40× magnification when using an ocular field diameter of 0.5 mm giving an area per field of 0.2 mm^2. Fifty such fields are to be counted. The Ki-67 LI is determined by counting at least 500 cells in hotspots identified at the scanner power. Where both parameters can be assessed, but there is a discrepancy between the grades assigned by either parameter, the higher grade is taken, which is usually by the Ki-67 LI.[76] The eyeballing method for calculating the Ki-67 LI is discouraged. Automated image analysis is preferred; however, falsely high indices may be recorded as it does not differentiate between labeled tumor cells and lymphocytes and, this method is time-consuming. The most accurate method is to take a color printout of the hotspots with the highest Ki-67 labeling and calculate the percentage of stained cells by manual counting. Both strongly and faintly stained nuclei are to be counted as positive.[77] When printing or automated counting is not possible, pathologists should identify the hotspot. Without moving the field further, they should manually count the Ki-67 LI at high power by carefully tallying the number of positive nuclei against all tumor cell nuclei. Furthermore, it must be remembered that, in the case of multicentric tumors and metastatic sites, Ki-67 LI should be performed in all primary foci and at least in one of the metastatic foci, to determine whether any of these tumor foci shows a higher histological grade than the other. In such a case, the overall prognosis will be based on the higher grade of tumor. As mentioned earlier, for lung NENs, Ki-67 labeling is not mandatory. Phosphohistone H3 (pHH3) staining for the identification of mitotic figures is less well recognized but can be helpful.

Pathologists should also remember that along with diagnosis and classification, proper staging of NEN along with the performance of the prognostic panel of markers are necessary. Though histological grading is unified, classification in some organs as described in this chapter is based on specific transcriptional and hormonal markers. Furthermore, in the case of NEN of unknown primary origin, applying a site-specific panel of markers to identify the possible site of origin will help in clinical decision-making. SDHB staining may help to determine hereditary tumors, and MGMT methylation status may help to decide on the outcome of alkylating agents in NETs **(Figs. 3A to C)**.

Newer Considerations for the Diagnosis of Mixed Neuroendocrine-Non-neuroendocrine Neoplasms

Another issue for pathologists is the diagnosis of mixed endocrine and non-endocrine neoplasms, as in the 2022 WHO classification the previous area cut-off of 30% has been abolished. However, as stated above, to diagnose MiNeN, both these differentiations must be identified in the H&E sections, supported by the Syn and INSM1 copositivity. In the absence of histological differentiation, immunohistochemical differentiation only does not qualify for a diagnosis of MiNeN, however, such a differentiation must be reported, and percentage of the area of IHC differentiation must be mentioned.[18] When a diagnosis of MiNeN is made, further subgrading should be done following the **Flowchart 3**.

Another issue that must be remembered is that NEN in most organs has a distinct staging system. However, MiNeNs should be staged in a site-specific manner using the current non-neuroendocrine cancer-related American Joint Committee on Cancer (AJCC)/Union for International Cancer Control (UICC) TNM classification.[78]

CONCLUSION

The classification of NENs in various organs is evolving. Though the 2017 WHO classification of NENs applies to most organs, site-specific differences must be remembered especially in the lung, pituitary, middle ear, appendix, etc. The WHO 2022 classification retains the criteria of the unified histological NEN grading system. Appropriate protocol for mitotic counting and Ki-67 labeling studies must be followed to increase interobserver agreements. A pathologist should follow a systematic approach to identify NEN, confirm with applicable marker studies, differentiate between epithelial and nonepithelial NEN, and perform WHO grading and staging. For the diagnosis of MiNeN, the 2022 WHO classification has abolished the 30% area criteria for NE differentiation in a nonendocrine neoplasm. However, both differentiations must be identifiable histologically, undisputed, and supported with synaptophysin and INSM1 staining. Further prognostic subgrading is necessary in MiNeN. Although NENs are categorized according to the AJCC/UICC staging system for NENs, the site-specific AJCC/UICC staging system for non-neuroendocrine tumors for MiNeNs should be followed. Differentiation of G3-NET and NEC is important and histological analysis, marker studies, and molecular analyses help. Both prognostic and therapeutic markers and molecular analysis can help to individualize NEN therapy.

REFERENCES

1. Oronsky B, Ma PC, Morgensztern D, Carter CA. Nothing but NET: A review of neuroendocrine tumors and carcinomas. Neoplasia. 2017;19(12):991-1002.
2. Rindi G, Wiedenmann B. Neuroendocrine neoplasms of the gut and pancreas: New insights. Nat Rev Endocrinol. 2011;8(1):54-64.
3. Schimmack S, Svejda B, Lawrence B, Kidd M, Modlin IM. The diversity and commonalities of gastroenteropancreatic neuroendocrine tumors. Langenbecks Arch Surg. 2011;396(3): 273-98.
4. Taal BG and Visser O. Epidemiology of neuroendocrine tumours. Neuroendocrinology. 2004;80(Suppl 1);3-7.
5. Das S, Dasari A. Epidemiology, incidence, and prevalence of neuroendocrine neoplasms: Are there global differences? Curr Oncol Rep. 2021;23(4):43.
6. Palepu J, Shrikhande SV, Bhaduri D, Shah RC, Sirohi B, Chhabra V, et al. Trends in diagnosis of gastroenteropancreatic neuroendocrine tumors (GEP-NETs) in India: A report of multicenter data from a web-based registry. Indian J Gastroenterol. 2017;36(6):445-51.
7. Kultschitzky N. Zur Frage über den Bau des Darmkanals. Arch Mikrosk Anat. 1897;49:7-35.
8. Oberndorfer S. Karzinoide Tumoren des Dónndarms. Frankf Z Pathol. 1907;1:426-32.
9. Gosset A, Masson P. Tumeurs endocrines de l'appendice. Presse Med. 1914;22:237.
10. Feyrter F. Über die peripheren endokrinen (parakrinen) Drüsen des Menschen. Germany: Verlag, Wien-Dusseldorf; 1953.
11. Pearse AGE. The APUD cell concept and its implications in pathology. Pathol Annu 1974;9: 27-41.
12. Fontaine J, Le Douarin NM. Analysis of endoderm formation in the avian blastoderm by the use of quail-chick chimaeras. The problem of the neuroectodermal origin of the cells of the APUD series. J Embryol Exp Morphol. 1977;41:209-22.
13. Rosai J. An evolutionary view of neuroendocrine cells and their tumors. Int J Surg Pathol. 2001;9(2):87-92.
14. Asa SL, Mete O, Cusimano MD, McCutcheon IE, Perry A, Yamada S, et al; Attendees of the 15th Meeting of the International Pituitary Pathology Club, Istanbul October 2019. Pituitary neuroendocrine tumors: A model for neuroendocrine tumor classification. Mod Pathol. 2021;34(9):1634-50.
15. Rosenbaum JN, Guo Z, Baus RM, Werner H, Rehrauer WM, Lloyd RV. INSM1: A novel immunohistochemical and molecular marker for neuroendocrine and neuroepithelial neoplasms. Am J Clin Pathol. 2015;144(4):579-91.

16. Asa SL, Ezzat S, Mete O. The diagnosis and clinical significance of paragangliomas in unusual locations. J Clin Med. 2018;7(9):280.
17. Klöppel G. Neuroendocrine Neoplasms: Dichotomy, origin and classifications. Visc Med. 2017;33(5):324-30.
18. Rindi G, Mete O, Uccella S, Basturk O, La Rosa S, Brosens LAA, et al. Overview of the 2022 WHO classification of neuroendocrine neoplasms. Endocr Pathol. 2022;33(1):115-54.
19. Bosman FT, Carneiro F, Hruban RH, Theise ND (Eds): WHO Classification of Tumours of the Digestive System Volume 3, 4th edition. Lyon: IARC Press; 2010. p. 417.
20. Lloyd RV, Osamura RY, Klöppel G, Rosai J: WHO Classification of Tumours of Endocrine Organs, 4th edition. Lyon: IARC Press' 2017.
21. Rindi G, Klimstra DS, Abedi-Ardekani B, Asa SL, Bosman FT, Brambilla E, et al. A common classification framework for neuroendocrine neoplasms: An International Agency for Research on Cancer (IARC) and World Health Organization (WHO) expert consensus proposal. Mod Pathol. 2018;31(12):1770-86.
22. Sharma N, Sharma D. An overview of pancreatic neuroendocrine tumors. Challenges in Pancreatic Cancer. 2021:79.
23. Kyriakopoulos G, Mavroeidi V, Chatzellis E, Kaltsas GA, Alexandraki KI. Histopathological, immunohistochemical, genetic and molecular markers of neuroendocrine neoplasms. Ann Transl Med. 2018;6(12):252.
24. Sorbye H, Welin S, Langer SW, Vestermark LW, Holt N, Osterlund P, et al. Predictive and prognostic factors for treatment and survival in 305 patients with advanced gastrointestinal neuroendocrine carcinoma (WHO G3): The NORDIC NEC study. Ann Oncol. 2013;24: 152-60.
25. Huang Q, Wu H, Nie L, Shi J, Lebenthal A, Chen J, et al. Primary high-grade neuroendocrine carcinoma of the esophagus: A clinicopathologic and immunohistochemical study of 42 resection cases. Am J Surg Pathol. 2013;37(4):467-83.
26. Hadoux J, Blanchard P, Scoazec JY, Burtin P, Planchard D, Malka D, et al. Post-radiation grade 3 neuroendocrine carcinoma: A new entity? Neuroendocrinology. 2021;111(1-2):139-45.
27. La Rosa S, Sessa F, Uccella S. Mixed neuroendocrine-nonneuroendocrine neoplasms (MiNENs): Unifying the concept of a heterogeneous group of neoplasms. Endocr Pathol. 2016;27(4):284-311.
28. Uccella S, La Rosa S. Looking into digestive mixed neuroendocrine-nonneuroendocrine neoplasms: Subtypes, prognosis, and predictive factors. Histopathology. 2020;77(5):700-17.
29. Popa O, Taban SM, Pantea S, Plopeanu AD, Barna RA, Cornianu M, et al. The new WHO classification of gastrointestinal neuroendocrine tumors and immunohistochemical expression of somatostatin receptor 2 and 5. Exp Ther Med. 2021;22(4):1179.
30. Puccini A, Poorman K, Salem ME, Soldato D, Seeber A, Goldberg RM, et al. Comprehensive genomic profiling of gastroenteropancreatic neuroendocrine neoplasms (GEP-NENs). Clin Cancer Res. 2020;26(22):5943-51.
31. Kim JY, Hong SM. Recent updates on neuroendocrine tumors from the gastrointestinal and pancreatobiliary tracts. Arch Pathol Lab Med. 2016;140(5):437-48.
32. O'Toole D, Delle Fave G, Jensen RT. Gastric and duodenal neuroendocrine tumours. Best Pract Res Clin Gastroenterol. 2012;26(6):719-35.
33. Li TT, Qiu F, Qian ZR, Wan J, Qi XK, Wu BY. Classification, clinicopathologic features and treatment of gastric neuroendocrine tumors. World J Gastroenterol. 2014;20(1):118-25.
34. Hrabe J. Neuroendocrine tumors of the appendix, colon, and rectum. Surg Oncol Clin N Am. 2020;29(2):267-79.
35. Misdraji J, Carr NJ, Pai RK. Appendiceal goblet cell adenocarcinoma. In: WHO Classification of Tumours Editorial Board (Eds). WHO Classification of Tumours of Digestive system, 5th edition. Lyon; IARC Press. pp. 149-51.
36. WHO Classification of Tumours Editorial Board. Thoracic tumours. WHO classification of tumours series Volume 5, 5th edition. Lyon, France: International Agency for Research on Cancer; 2021.

37. Pelosi G, Rindi G, Travis WD, Papotti M. Ki-67 antigen in lung neuroendocrine tumors: Unraveling a role in clinical practice. J Thorac Oncol. 2014;9(3):273-84.
38. Rekhtman N, Desmeules P, Litvak AM, Pietanza MC, Santos-Zabala ML, Ni A, et al. Stage IV lung carcinoids: Spectrum and evolution of proliferation rate, focusing on variants with elevated proliferation indices. Mod Pathol. 2019;32(8):1106-22.
39. WHO Classification of Tumours Editorial Board. Breast tumours. WHO classification of tumours series, Volume 2, 5th edition. Lyon, France: International Agency for Research on Cancer; 2019.
40. Lakhani SREI, Schnitt SJ, Tan PY, van de Vijver MJ. WHO classification of tumours of the breast, 4th edition. Lyon: International Agency for Research on Cancer; 2012. p. 240.
41. Duncavage EJ, Le BM, Wang D, Pfeifer JD. Merkel cell polyomavirus: A specific marker for Merkel cell carcinoma in histologically similar tumors. Am J Surg Pathol. 2009;33(12): 1771-7.
42. Paik JY, Hall G, Clarkson A, Lee L, Toon C, Colebatch A, et al. Immunohistochemistry for Merkel cell polyomavirus is highly specific but not sensitive for the diagnosis of Merkel cell carcinoma in the Australian population. Hum Pathol. 2011;42(10):1385-90.
43. Jedrych J, Busam K, Klimstra DS, Pulitzer M. Cutaneous metastases as an initial manifestation of visceral well-differentiated neuroendocrine tumor: A report of four cases and a review of literature. J Cutan Pathol. 2013;41:113-22.
44. Goto K, Anan T, Nakatsuka T, Kaku Y, Sakurai T, Fukumoto T, et al. Low-grade neuroendocrine carcinoma of the skin (primary cutaneous carcinoid tumor) as a distinctive entity of cutaneous neuroendocrine tumors: A clinicopathologic study of 3 cases with literature review. Am J Dermatopathol. 2017;39(4):250-8.
45. WHO Classification of Tumours Editorial Board. Head and neck tumours. WHO classification of tumours series, Volume 9, 5th edition. Lyon (France): International Agency for Research on Cancer; 2023.
46. Bal M, Sharma A, Rane SU, Mittal N, Chaukar D, Prabhash K, et al. Neuroendocrine neoplasms of the larynx: A clinicopathologic analysis of 27 neuroendocrine tumors and neuroendocrine carcinomas. Head Neck Pathol. 2022;16(2):375-87.
47. La Rosa S, Uccella S. Classification of neuroendocrine neoplasms: Lights and shadows. Rev Endocr Metab Disord. 2021;22(3):527-38.
48. Uccella S, Ottini G, Facco C, Maragliano R, Asioli S, Sessa F, et al. Neuroendocrine neoplasms of the head and neck and olfactory neuroblastoma. Diagnosis and classification. Pathologica. 2017;109(1):14-30.
49. Robboy SJ, Scully RE. Strumal carcinoid of the ovary: An analysis of 50 cases of a distinctive tumor composed of thyroid tissue and carcinoid. Cancer. 1980;46(9):2019-34.
50. Castle PE, Pierz A, Stoler MH. A systematic review and meta-analysis on the attribution of human papillomavirus (HPV) in neuroendocrine cancers of the cervix. Gynecol Oncol. 2018;148(2):422-9.
51. Patibandla JR, Fehniger JE, Levine DA, Jelinic P. Small cell cancers of the female genital tract: Molecular and clinical aspects. Gynecol Oncol. 2018;149(2):420-7.
52. WHO Classification of Tumours Editorial Board. Endocrine and neuroendocrine tumours. WHO classification of tumours series, Volume 10, 5th edition. Lyon (France): International Agency for Research on Cancer; 2022.
53. Asa SL. Challenges in the Diagnosis of Pituitary Neuroendocrine Tumors. Endocr Pathol. 2021;32(2):222-7.
54. Asa SL, Mete O, Perry A, Osamura RY. Overview of the 2022 WHO Classification of Pituitary Tumors. Endocr Pathol. 2022;33(1):6-26.
55. Rinke A, Gress TM. Neuroendocrine Cancer, Therapeutic Strategies in G3 Cancers. Digestion. 2017;95(2):109-14.
56. Wang HL, Kim CJ, Koo J, Zhou W, Choi EK, Arcega R, et al. Practical immunohistochemistry in neoplastic pathology of the gastrointestinal tract, liver, biliary tract, and pancreas. Arch Pathol Lab Med. 2017;141(9):1155-80.

57. Mukhopadhyay S, Dermawan JK, Lanigan CP, Farver CF. Insulinoma-associated protein 1 (INSM1) is a sensitive and highly specific marker of neuroendocrine differentiation in primary lung neoplasms: An immunohistochemical study of 345 cases, including 292 whole-tissue sections. Mod Pathol. 2019;32(1):100-9.
58. Baloch Z, Mete O, Asa SL. Immunohistochemical biomarkers in thyroid pathology. Endocr Pathol. 2018;29(2):91-112.
59. Mete O, Asa SL, Gill AJ, Kimura N, de Krijger RR, Tischler A. Overview of the 2022 WHO classification of paragangliomas and pheochromocytomas. Endocr Pathol. 2022;33(1): 90-114.
60. Juhlin CC, Zedenius J, Höög A. Metastatic neuroendocrine neoplasms of unknown primary: Clues from pathology workup. Cancers (Basel). 2022;14(9):2210.
61. Yagi K, Ono H, Kudo A, Kinowaki Y, Asano D, Watanabe S, et al. MGMT is frequently inactivated in pancreatic NET-G2 and is associated with the therapeutic activity of STZ-based regimens. Scientific Reports. 2023;13(1):7535.
62. de Mestier L, Couvelard A, Blazevic A, Hentic O, de Herder WW, Rebours V, et al. Critical appraisal of MGMT in digestive NET treated with alkylating agents. Endocrine-related cancer. 2020;27(10):R391-405.
63. Gul AE, Keser SH, Barisik NO, Gurbuz YS, Sensu S, Erdogan N. Succinate dehydrogenase complex iron sulfur subunit B (SDHB) immunohistochemistry in pheochromocytoma, head and neck paraganglioma, thoraco-abdomino-pelvic paragangliomas: is it a good idea to use in routine work? Asian Pac J Cancer Prev. 2021;22(6):1721-9.
64. Niemeijer ND, Papathomas TG, Korpershoek E, De Krijger RR, Oudijk L, Morreau H, et al. Succinate dehydrogenase (SDH)-deficient pancreatic neuroendocrine tumor expands the SDH-related tumor spectrum. J Clin Endocrinol Metab. 2015;100(10):E1386-93.
65. Sahnane N, Furlan D, Monti M, Romualdi C, Vanoli A, Vicari E, et al. Microsatellite unstable gastrointestinal neuroendocrine carcinomas: A new clinicopathologic entity. Endocr Relat Cancer. 2015;22(1):35-45.
66. Cavalcanti E, Armentano R, Valentini AM, Chieppa M, Caruso ML. Role of PD-L1 expression as a biomarker for GEP neuroendocrine neoplasm grading. Cell Death Dis. 2017;8(8):e3004.
67. Jiao Y, Shi C, Edil BH, de Wilde RF, Klimstra DS, et al. DAXX/ATRX, MEN1, and mTOR pathway genes are frequently altered in pancreatic neuroendocrine tumors. Science. 2011;331(6021):1199-203.
68. Scarpa A, Chang DK, Nones K, Corbo V, Patch AM, Bailey P, et al.; Australian Pancreatic Cancer Genome Initiative Whole-genome landscape of pancreatic neuroendocrine tumours. Nature. 2017;543(7643):65-71.
69. Lovejoy CA, Li W, Reisenweber S, Thongthip S, Bruno J, de Lange T, et al. Loss of ATRX, genome instability, and an altered DNA damage response are hallmarks of the alternative lengthening of telomeres pathway. PLoS Genet. 2012;8(7):e1002772.
70. Raj NP, Soumerai T, Valentino E, Hechtman JF, Berger MF, Reidy DL. Next-generation sequencing (NGS) in advanced well differentiated pancreatic neuroendocrine tumors (WD pNETs): A study using MSK-IMPACT. J Clin Oncol. 2016;34:246.
71. Jesinghaus M, Konukiewitz B, Keller G, Kloor M, Steiger K, Reiche M, et al. Colorectal mixed adenoneuroendocrine carcinomas and neuroendocrine carcinomas are genetically closely related to colorectal adenocarcinomas. Mod. Pathol. 2017;30:610-9.
72. House MG, Herman JG, Guo MZ, Hooker CM, Schulick RD, Lillemoe KD, et al. Aberrant hypermethylation of tumor suppressor genes in pancreatic endocrine neoplasms. Ann. Surg. 2003;238(3):423-32.
73. Stefanoli M, La Rosa S, Sahnane N, Romualdi C, Pastorino R, Marando A, et al. Prognostic relevance of aberrant DNA methylation in G1 and G2 pancreatic neuroendocrine tumors. Neuroendocrinology. 2014;100:26-34.
74. Pipinikas CP, Dibra H, Karpathakis A, Feber A, Novelli M, Oukrif D, et al. Epigenetic dysregulation and poorer prognosis in DAXX-deficient pancreatic neuroendocrine tumours. Endocr Relat Cancer. 2015;22:L13-8.

75. Manneh Kopp R, Espinosa-Olarte P, Alonso-Gordoa T. Diagnosis in neuroendocrine neoplasms: From molecular biology to molecular imaging. Cancers. 2022;14(10):2514.
76. McCall CM, Shi C, Cornish TC, Klimstra DS, Tang LH, Basturk O, et al. Grading of well-differentiated pancreatic neuroendocrine tumors is improved by the inclusion of both Ki67 proliferative index and mitotic rate. Am J Surg Pathol. 2013;37:1671-7.
77. Reid MD, Bagci P, Ohike N, Saka B, Erbarut Seven I, Dursun N, et al. Calculation of the Ki67 index in pancreatic neuroendocrine tumors: a comparative analysis of four counting methodologies. Mod Pathol. 2015;28:686-94.
78. Brierley JD, Gospodarowicz MK, Wittekind C. (Eds). TNM classification of malignant tumours, 8th edition. Oxford: Wiley Blackwell; 2017.

9

CHAPTER

Recent Advances and Changing Landscape of Endometrial Carcinoma

Divya Midha

INTRODUCTION

In 1983, Bokhman described a dualistic classification of endometrial carcinoma (EC) based on clinical, endocrine, metabolic, and histopathological features **(Table 1)**. Type 1 EC are low-grade endometrioid carcinomas which are estrogen-dependent and often clinically indolent, while type 2 EC are nonendometrioid, clinically aggressive carcinomas that are unrelated to estrogen stimulation and include serous and clear cell carcinomas.[1] This traditional classification did not reflect the full heterogeneity of EC and the accurate histotyping of EC was inconsistent, limited by suboptimal reproducibility, did not yield prognostic and predictive information which consequently adversely affected the clinical

TABLE 1: Traditional dualistic model of classification of endometrial carcinoma.

	Type 1 EC	Type 2 EC
Histotype	Endometrioid carcinoma	• Nonendometrioid carcinoma • Serous or clear cell carcinoma
Tumor grade	Low	High
Precursor lesion	Hyperplasia	Atrophy
Distribution	70–80%	20–30%
Body habitus	Obese	Not obese
Hormonal status	Estrogen dependent	Estrogen independent
Age	Perimenopausal	Postmenopausal
Risk factors	Nulliparity, diabetes, late menopause	None
Mutations	• *PTEN* inactivation • *KRAS* mutation • Microsatellite instability	• p53 mutation • p16 mutation • HER2 overexpression
Prognosis	Favorable	Poor

(EC: endometrioid carcinoma)

management of patients with EC.[2] In recent years, there has been tremendous improvement and progress in our understanding of pathogenic mechanisms underlying EC. Genomic data from The Cancer Genome Atlas Research Network (TGCA) published 30 years later in 2013 supported classification of EC into four prognostically significant nonoverlapping subgroups: POLE-mutated/ultramutated, MSI-high (MSI-H)/hypermutated, copy number low and copy number high.[3] The 2020 World Health Organization (WHO) classification of EC acknowledges the molecular subgroups of EC but continues to use histomorphology as essential criteria aided by immunohistochemistry (IHC) as desirable criteria for classification into EC histotypes.[4] With the emergence of the molecular classification of EC, the new International Federation of Gynecology and Obstetrics (FIGO) staging system of EC published in 2023 metamorphosed from an anatomical staging system (FIGO 2009) to a staging system which encompasses histological typing, lymphovascular space invasion (LVSI), size of nodal metastasis and integrates molecular classification into its domain while distinguishing between synchronous and metastatic endometrioid endometrial and ovarian cancers.[5]

ENDOMETRIAL CARCINOMA: HISTOTYPING

The 2020 WHO classification of EC with key histologic findings and immunoprofiles is summarized in **Table 2**.

This new WHO classification includes novel tumor types, such as mesonephric-like adenocarcinoma and gastric-type mucinous carcinoma. Endometrial mucinous carcinoma is now regarded as a pattern of endometrioid carcinoma, and not a distinct tumor type.[4]

The low grade EC or nonaggressive histological types comprise low-grade (grade 1 and 2) endometrial endometrioid carcinomas (EECs). The high grade EC or aggressive histological types comprise high-grade (grade 3) EECs, serous, clear cell, undifferentiated, mixed, mesonephric-like, gastrointestinal mucinous type carcinomas, and carcinosarcomas **(Figs. 1 to 7)**.[4,5]

The histotype diagnosis in EC shows high interobserver variation especially in high grade EC and histotype diagnosis does not consistently predict clinical outcome. Prognostic separation by tumor histotyping is therefore often found to be unreliable and inaccurate especially in high-grade tumors.[2]

ENDOMETRIAL CARCINOMA: TUMOR GRADE

The EECs are graded on the basis on proportion of solid nonsquamous areas: Low grade = grade 1 (≤5% solid nonsquamous areas) and grade 2 (6–50% solid nonsquamous areas); and high grade = grade 3 EEC (>50% solid nonsquamous areas) **(Fig. 1)**. Nuclear atypia excessive for the grade raises the grade of a grade 1 or 2 tumor by one. The presence of unusual nuclear atypia in an architecturally low-grade tumor should prompt the consideration of serous carcinoma.[4,6-8]

Since the clinical management of FIGO grades 1 and 2 endometrioid adenocarcinomas is similar, a "binary FIGO" grading system has been proposed and accepted by WHO 2020 classification of EC, which endorses combining

TABLE 2: The 2020 WHO classification of endometrial carcinoma with key histologic findings and immunoprofiles.

Histotype	Histological features	PAX8	ER PR	p16	p53	Napsin-A HNF-1B AMACR	MMR	Nuclear β-catenin	Pan-CK	Others
Endometrioid carcinoma, low grade **(Figs. 1A and B)**	• ≤50% solid growth • Oval or round glands with smooth outlines lined by columnar to cuboidal cells • Pseudostratified low-grade oval to round nuclei • Squamous or mucinous metaplasia • Background atypical hyperplasia	+	+	–	Wild	Napsin-A– HNF-1B +/– AMACR –	Loss (40–60%)	+/–	+	Loss of PTEN/ ARID1A
Endometrioid carcinoma, high grade **(Fig. 1C)**	• >50% solid growth • Gland formation is seen at least focally • The cells in the solid component resemble those lining the glandular spaces • Nuclei usually have moderate (grade 2) atypia • Squamous or mucinous metaplasia • Background atypical hyperplasia	+	+	–	Abn 25%	Napsin-A– HNF-1B ± AMACR –	Loss (40–60%)	+/–	+	Loss of PTEN/ ARID1A

Continued

Continued

Histotype	Histological features	PAX8	ER PR	p16	p53	Napsin-A HNF-1B AMACR	MMR	Nuclear β-catenin	Pan-CK	Others
Serous carcinoma **(Fig. 2)**	• Develops in a background of atrophic endometrium/polyp • Focal areas of papillary growth • Budding and exfoliation of tumor cells • Irregular glands, often with slit-like spaces • Psammoma bodies (one-third of cases) • Hyperchromatic nuclei with macronucleoli (grade 3 nuclei) • Pleomorphic/bizarre forms • Numerous mitotic figures	+	+/–	+	Abn	Napsin-A ± HNF-1B– AMACR–	Intact	–	+	HER2 IHC as one-third show HER2 amplification
Clear cell carcinoma **(Fig. 3)**	• Tubulocystic, papillary, or solid growth • Cuboidal-polygonal cells • Variable nuclear pleomorphism (not marked) • Low mitotic rate • Nuclear hob-nailing • Cytoplasmic clearing • Hyalinized stromal cores, hyaline droplets	+	–	–	Abn 30%	Napsin-A ++ HNF-1B ++ AMACR ++	Loss/Intact	–	+	

Continued

Continued

Histotype	Histological features	PAX8	ER PR	p16	p53	Napsin-A HNF-1B AMACR	MMR	Nuclear β-catenin	Pan-CK	Others
Un/De-differentiated carcinoma **(Fig. 5)**	• Undifferentiated carcinoma is a solid-pattern tumor lacking overt morphologic evidence of epithelial differentiation showing diffuse sheets of monomorphic small to intermediate-sized discohesive cells • Dedifferentiated carcinoma is an undifferentiated carcinoma found in combination with an endometrioid carcinoma that is typically low-grade • Focal rhabdoid/ plasmacytoid morphology • Focal marked nuclear pleomorphism, multinucleation, spindling, and "abrupt" keratinization	–	–	–	Wild	Napsin-A– HNF-1B– AMACR–	Loss (50–60%)	–	+/–	• Loss of E-cadherin in un/de-differentiated component • Loss of IN1/ BRG1 in 30% • NE marker expression in <10% tumour cells

Continued

Continued

Histotype	Histological features	PAX8	ER PR	p16	p53	Napsin-A HNF-1B AMACR	MMR	Nuclear β-catenin	Pan-CK	Others
Mesonephric-like carcinoma **(Fig. 6)**	• Small tubules with dense eosinophilic colloid-like material • Diverse array of morphologies including papillary, ductal, retiform, solid, and spindled architecture	±	–	±	Wild	Napsin-A– HNF-1B– AMACR–	Intact	–	+	• GATA3 and TTF1 + (inverse pattern of staining) • Calretinin + CD10 + (luminal)
Gastrointestinal-type carcinoma **(Fig. 7)**	• Presence of gastric-type morphology and/or goblet cells with no evidence of any other primary site • Absence of typical endometrioid component • Absence of cervical glandular or stromal involvement (with complete sampling of the cervix)	±	±	±	Abn/ Wild	Napsin-A– HNF-1B– AMACR–	Limited studies	–	+	• At least focal IHC expression of one or more gastrointestinal markers (e.g., MUC6, CK20, and CDX2) • Absent or minimal (< 5%) expression of ER • CK7 +/–
Carcinosarcoma **(Fig. 4)**	• Biphasic endometrial carcinoma composed of a component of high-grade sarcoma (with or without heterologous elements) juxtaposed with a component of high-grade carcinoma	+/–	+/–	+	Abn	Napsin-A– HNF-1B– AMAC–	Loss/Intact	–	+/–	• Desmin, Myogenin and MyoD1 in heterologous RMS component

Continued

Continued

Histotype	Histological features	PAX8	ER PR	p16	p53	Napsin-A HNF-1B AMACR	MMR	Nuclear β-catenin	Pan-CK	Others
	• The sarcomatous component should measure at least 1 mm in one dimension as per ISGyP guidelines									• HER2 IHC as 15–20% show HER2 amplification
Mixed carcinoma	• Endometrial carcinoma with two distinct histological types, in which at least one component is either serous or clear cell carcinoma • Exclude de-differentiated carcinoma and carcinosarcoma • *Desirable*: Immunohistochemical demonstration of the two distinct carcinoma types	+	±	±	Abn/ Wild	Napsin-A ± HNF-1B ± AMACR ±	Loss/Intact	+/–	+	• No minimum amount of serous carcinoma/clear cell carcinoma component is needed (as long it is recognized confidently) • IHC depends on the components of mixed carcinoma

Note:
- ± denotes variable staining.
- For p16 staining + denotes diffuse, block-like expression;—denotes negative, focal, or patchy staining.

(Abn: abnormal; ER/PR: estrogen and progesterone receptors; ISGyP: International Society of Gynecological Pathologists; MMR: mismatch repair; Pan-CK: pan-cytokeratin; NE: neuroendocrine; RMS: rhabdomyosarcoma)

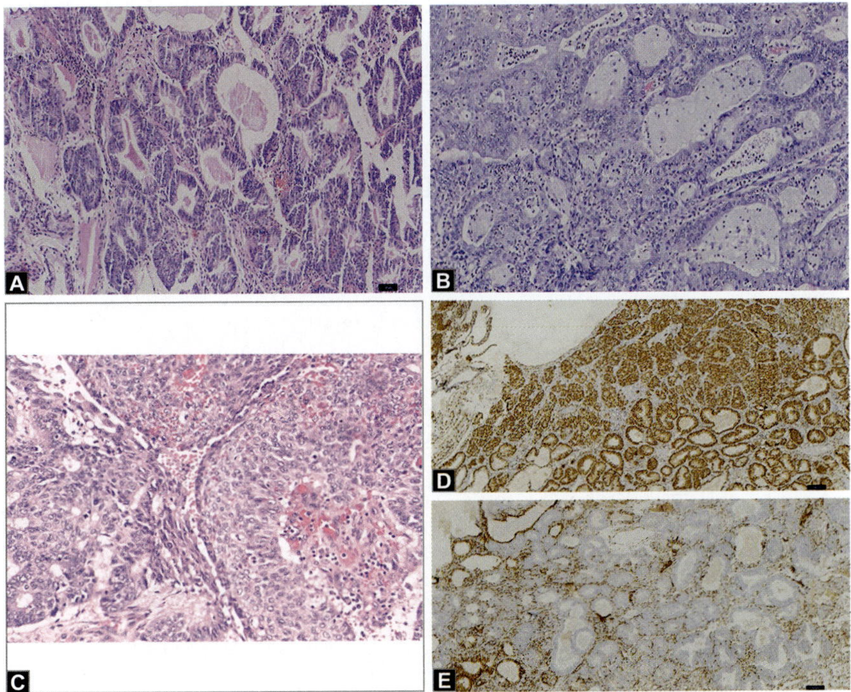

FIGS. 1A TO E: (A) International Federation of Gynecology and Obstetrics FIGO Grade 1 endometrial carcinoma (EEC); (B) FIGO Grade 2 EEC; (C) FIGO Grade 3 EEC; (D) ER in low-grade EEC; (E) Lack of block positivity for p16 in low-grade EEC.

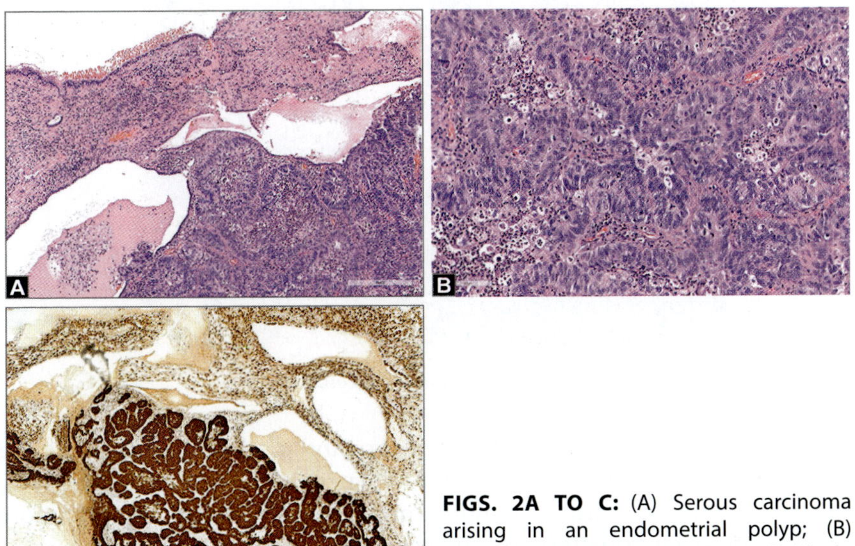

FIGS. 2A TO C: (A) Serous carcinoma arising in an endometrial polyp; (B) Endometrial serous carcinoma; (C) Block-like p16 in endometrial serous carcinoma.

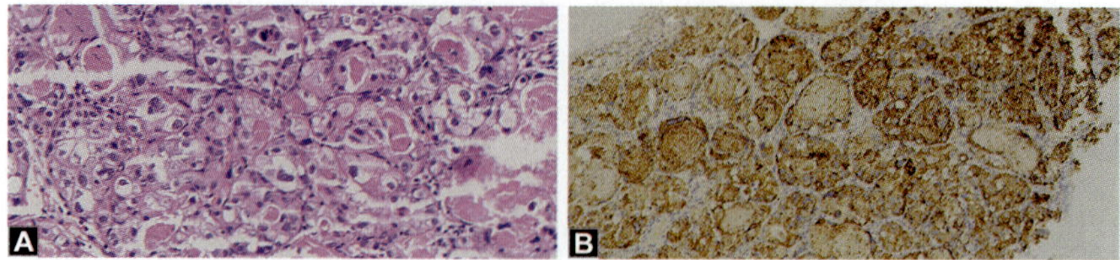

FIGS. 3A AND B: (A) Endometrial clear cell carcinoma; (B) Strong and diffuse Napsin-A expression in endometrial clear cell carcinoma.

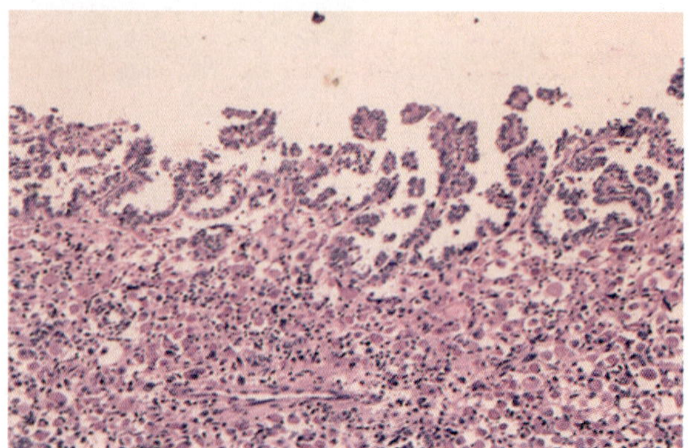

FIG. 4: Endometrial carcinosarcoma.

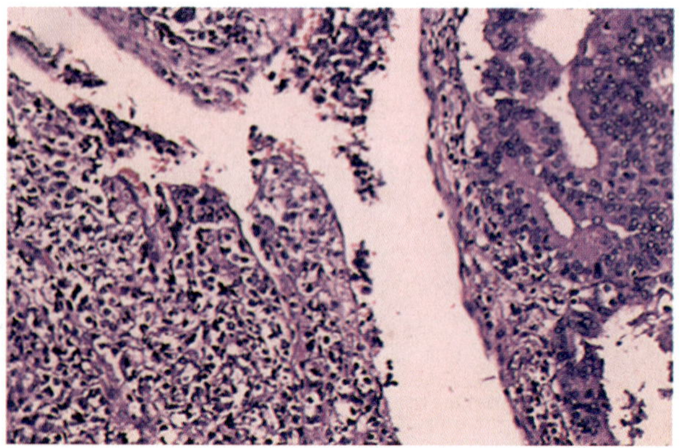

FIG. 5: De-differentiated endometrial carcinoma.

FIGO grades 1 and 2 into a low-grade category and grade 3 tumors into a high-grade category.[9,10] International Society of Gynecological Pathologists (ISGyP) as part of ISGyP endometrial carcinoma project endorses the interpretation of a confluent microacinar pattern as solid growth.[7]

Binary FIGO grading system is considered appropriate in hysterectomy specimens or when comprehensive surgical staging is planned. Distinguishing between FIGO grades 1 and 2 would still be necessary for patients desiring fertility preservation because grade 1 tumors are often treated with hormonal

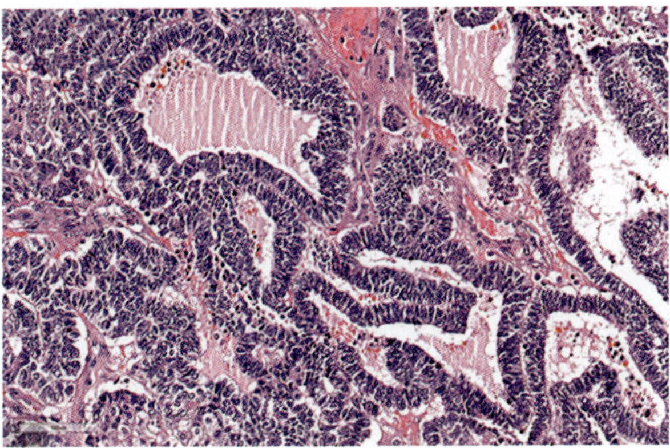

FIG. 6: Endometrial mesonephric-like carcinoma.

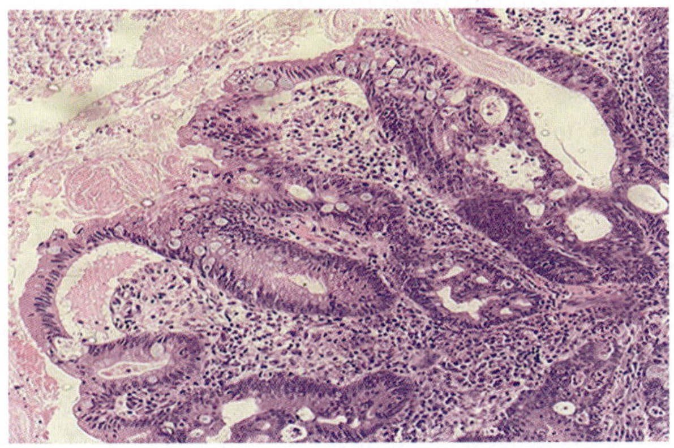

FIG. 7: Gastrointestinal-type endometrial carcinoma.

therapy. It would be acceptable to report both the binary FIGO grade and the FIGO grade, e.g., low-grade EEC (FIGO grade 2).[4,7]

Adenocarcinomas with squamous differentiation are graded according to the microscopic features of the glandular component.[4,6]

Serous adenocarcinomas, clear cell adenocarcinomas, mesonephric-like carcinomas, gastrointestinal-type mucinous EC, undifferentiated carcinomas, and carcinosarcomas are considered high-grade by definition **(Figs. 2 to 7)**.[4,8]

ENDOMETRIAL CARCINOMA: GROSS AND MACROSCOPIC EVALUATION

Since recommendations for adjuvant treatment for EC by the National Comprehensive Cancer Network (NNCN)[11] and the European Society of Gynecological Oncology (ESGO), the European Society for Radiotherapy and Oncology (ESTRO), and the European Society of Pathology (ESP)[12] are based almost entirely on pathologic findings, great care must be taken during gross and macroscopic evaluation of the tumor. **Table 3** highlights the guidelines for gross reporting of EC as proposed by ISGyP.[13]

TABLE 3: Recommendations for gross/macroscopic examination in a case of endometrial carcinoma.

Recommendation	Description	Significance
Specimen orientation	• *Use anatomical landmarks:* ○ Peritoneal reflection is higher anteriorly, lower posteriorly • *The sequence of structures in the adnexal region*: ○ Ovary, fallopian tube, and round ligament (posterior to anterior)	
Opening uterus	• Open immediately upon receipt • Open along the lateral walls (3 o' clock and 9 o' clock) • Do not amputate the cervix	• Allows better visualization and measurement of the tumor • Prevents autolysis which may affect accurate histotyping and grading • Avoids preanalytical issues for ancillary tests
Inking	• Inking of peritoneal and/or nonperitoneal surfaces • Inking paracervical/parametrial resection margins and ectocervical/vaginal cuff margin	• For orientation purposes • To confirm tumor at the serosal surface • Inking paracervical/parametrial resection margins and ectocervical/vaginal cuff margin aids in accurate assessment of the depth of cervical stromal invasion and margin status
Sectioning of the uterus	• Use horizontal/transverse sectioning from the lower uterine segment to the fundus • Vertical sectioning of lower uterine segment in conjunction with upper cervix	Accurate sampling for microscopic assessment
Grossly visible tumor	• 1 section per cm of the largest tumor dimension or at least 4 blocks • Submit ≤3 cm tumors entirely • At least 1 full thickness section of the uterine wall (including uterine serosa) representing the deepest myoinvasion	• Adequate tumor sampling minimizes the risk of missing a high-grade carcinoma component • Full-thickness sections of endomyometrium and cervix are required for accurate assessment of the depth of myoinvasion and depth of cervical stromal invasion, respectively

Continued

Continued

Recommendation	Description	Significance
	• Sample the tumor/nontumor interface • Take 1–2 full-thickness sections of non-neoplastic endomyometrium • Sample any other grossly visible endometrial lesions • Take at least two longitudinal sections (1 anterior, 1 posterior) from the lower uterine segment • Take at least two full-thickness sections (1 anterior, 1 posterior) of cervix, whether grossly unremarkable or involved by tumor • Include the ectocervical or vaginal cuff margin especially if involved by tumor	• Submitting the entire endometrium increases the probability of identifying microscopic tumors • Sampling the tumor/nontumor interface aids in the assessment of deepest myometrial invasion and identification of precursor lesions, such as atypical hyperplasia, atrophy, and polyp • Assessment of the depth of cervical stromal invasion is used for adjuvant radiotherapy planning
Parametrium	Submit parametrium entirely in sequential slices, if present, before opening the uterus	Parametrial sampling before opening the uterus minimizes the chance of carryover
Ovaries	• Section ovaries perpendicularly to long axis 2–3 mm apart • Submit at least 2 sections of each ovary	Identification of microscopic involvement of ovaries
Fallopian tubes	• If fallopian tube is uninvolved, submit entirely as per SEE-FIM protocol, or • Sample at least the fimbriae entirely as per SEE-FIM protocol and representative sections of the rest of the fallopian tube	Identification of microscopic involvement of fallopian tubes
Omentum	• Submit 1–2 representative sections of the omentum if grossly positive • Submit 1 section per 2–3 cm of maximal dimension or at least 4 blocks if grossly negative	• Important for staging • Involvement implies stage IVB
Atypical hyperplasia or no grossly visible tumor	• Submit the entire endometrium and adjacent inner myometrium • Submit cornual blocks in cases of biopsy-proven carcinoma	Identification of residual atypical hyperplasia or carcinoma

Continued

Continued

Recommendation	Description	Significance
Lynch syndrome	• Submit the entire endometrium if no gross lesions, including the endomyometrial interface and lower uterine segment with upper endocervix • Submit all grossly visible lesions • Submit the adnexa entirely	Identification of microscopic atypical hyperplasia or carcinoma and microscopic involvement of the adnexa
Lymph nodes	• Submit grossly positive lymph nodes representatively • Submit grossly uninvolved lymph nodes entirely • Section sentinel nodes at 2.0–3.0 mm intervals perpendicular to the long axis • Ultrastaging methods for sentinel nodes Memorial Sloan Kettering Cancer Center Protocol • If the initial H&E-stained slide is positive for carcinoma, no further workup is required • *If the initial H&E-stained slide is negative for carcinoma, cut 2 additional levels 50 μm apart including 2 slides at each level:* 1 for H&E and 1 for Pan-CK IHC MD Anderson Cancer Center Protocol • If the initial H&E-stained slide is positive for carcinoma, no further workup is required • If the initial H&E-stained slide is negative for carcinoma, cut 3 serial sections 250 μm apart, including 1 for H&E and 2 unstained slides • If additional H&E slide is negative, use 1 of the 2 unstained slides for Pan-CK IHC	• Identification of isolated tumor cells (≤0.2 mm or <200 cells) • Identification of micrometastases (>0.2 to ≤2 mm) • Identification of macrometastases (>2 mm)

(IHC: immunohistochemistry; SEE-FIM: sectioning and extensively examining the fimbria; Pan-CK: pan-cytokeratin)

ENDOMETRIAL CARCINOMA: PROGNOSTIC FACTORS, OTHER THAN HISTOTYPE AND TUMOR GRADE

The molecular classification of EC that has emerged from the TCGA study provides superior prognostic information to tumor histotyping and grading. This molecular classification, however, cannot replace the clinicopathologic risk assessment based on parameters other than histotype and grade.[14] The

TABLE 4: Pathological parameters that need to be recorded in every case of endometrial carcinoma.

Pathological parameters	Significance
Tumor size	May predict nodal involvement and recurrence
Tumor histotype	• In biopsy—extent of surgical staging • In hysterectomy—adjuvant treatment
Tumor grade	• In biopsy—extent of surgical staging • In hysterectomy—adjuvant treatment
Depth of myometrial invasion	pT1a versus pT1b
Cervical stromal invasion	pT2
Adnexal involvement	pT3a
Uterine serosal involvement	pT3a
Parametrial and vaginal involvement	pT3b
Regional lymph node involvement with size of metastasis	pN
Omentum	pM1

molecular and clinicopathologic prognostic risk grouping systems when applied together is likely to risk stratify the patients more accurately and this concept also forms the basis of FIGO 2023 staging of EC.[5,11,12]

The staging parameters that need to be recorded in every case of EC has been tabulated **(Table 4)** and has been described below along with the challenges in its interpretation.[5,14-16]

Myometrial Invasion

- The absence or presence of myometrial invasion is required for staging (pT1a, no or <50% myoinvasion; pT1b, ≥50% myoinvasion). If myometrial invasion is present, percentage of invasion, and/or measurements of depth of myoinvasion and total myometrial thickness at point of maximum invasion should be reported **(Fig. 8)**.
- The depth of myometrial invasion should always be measured from the endomyometrial junction if possible. This includes tumors involving polyps and tumors involving the lower uterine segment (LUS).
- In case of an exophytic tumor, the depth of myometrial invasion and not tumor thickness should be measured by identifying the adjacent endomyometrial junction and by correlating with the macroscopic appearance.
- Invasion into polyp stroma should not be considered invasion and should not be used for staging in the absence of myoinvasion.
- In EC invading a leiomyoma, the leiomyoma should be included when measuring the thickness of the myometrial wall.
- Sections from the uterine cornual should not be used for determining myoinvasion unless the tumor is limited only to the cornual region or involves the uterine serosa in the cornual region.

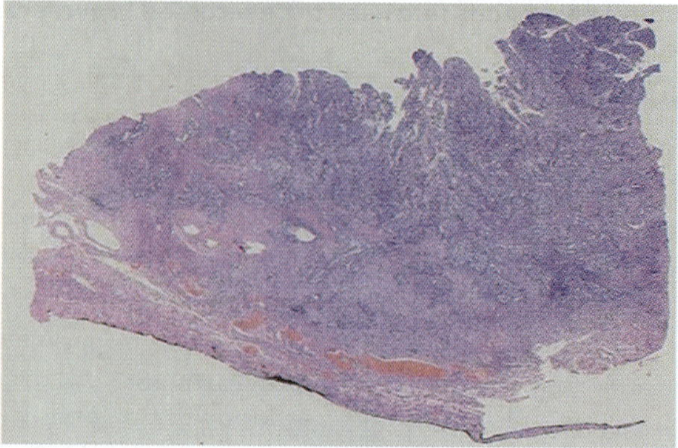

FIG. 8: Endomyometrial junction not identifiable on the slide showing deepest myoinvasion: Invasion into deep myometrial vascular arcuate plexus is considered as >50% myoinvasion.

- If myometrial invasion occurs from carcinoma within adenomyosis, the deepest myoinvasive point should be reported according to where this is located in the myometrium, and regardless of whether or not it arises from adenomyosis.
- The most easily recognized pattern of myoinvasion is diffusely infiltrating glands (single gland pattern) in the myometrium with or without desmoplastic reaction.

Challenges Faced While Assessing Myometrial Invasion

- *Carcinoma involving adenomyosis:* Depth of myoinvasion can be assessed either from the endomyometrial junction or from the edge of adenomyotic focus. ISGyP guidelines recommend reporting the deepest point of myoinvasion from the endomyometrial junction, irrespective of the nearest focus of adenomyosis.
- *Myoinvasive cancer with an irregular or nonidentifiable endomyometrial junction or pushing type of invasion:* When the endomyometrial junction cannot be easily identified because of its obliteration by tumor or when there is no identifiable endomyometrial junction on the slide showing deepest myoinvasion, invasion into deep myometrial vascular arcuate plexus is considered as >50% myoinvasion.
- *Microcystic, elongated, and fragmented (MELF) pattern* **(Fig. 9)**: MELF pattern of invasion is seen in 16% cases of EC and is associated with endometrioid morphology, mismatch repair deficiency (MMRd), LVSI, and involved lymph nodes. The glands are microcystic, slit-like; tumor cells appear squamoid, eosinophilic or deceptively bland and histiocytoid; surrounded by focal myxoid change and lymphocytes. This pattern of invasion is subtle, may be missed at low power examination, thus underestimating depth of invasion. MELF pattern of invasion may be mistaken as LVSI and may need deeper levels and immunohistochemistry (IHC) confirmation with cytokeratin and D2-40 immunostains.

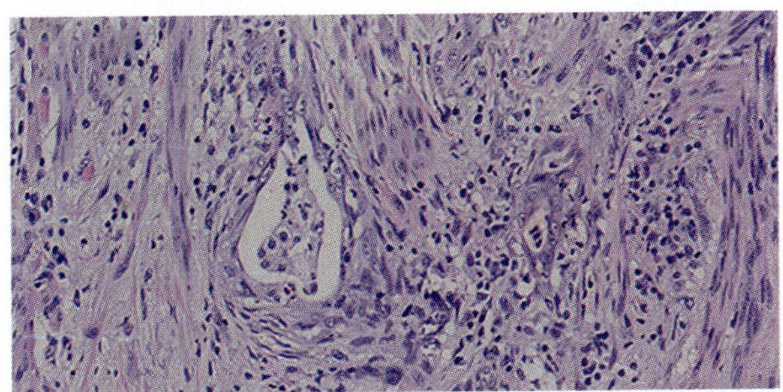

FIG. 9: Microcystic, elongated, and fragmented (MELF) pattern: Microcystic, slit-like glands; tumor cells appear deceptively bland and histiocytoid, surrounded by focal myxoid change and lymphocytes.

- *Adenoma malignum type of myoinvasion:* These are widely spaced, irregular glands haphazardly infiltrating the myometrium without significant cytologic atypia and stromal desmoplasia. Careful microscopic examination shows at least focal cytologic atypia, pseudo-stratification of glands, focal stromal edema, inflammatory infiltrate in and around the atypical glands, and LVSI.

Lymphovascular Space Invasion

- LVSI is defined as the presence of smooth bordered and cohesive clusters of tumor cells in an endothelial-lined space within the myometrium beyond the invasive front of the tumor, conforming to the shape of the vascular space.
- Proximity to larger vessels, more eosinophilic cytoplasm in the tumor emboli, and the presence of a perivascular lymphocytic infiltrate composed of >20 lymphocytes are other supportive criteria for LVSI.
- LVSI should be unequivocal when reported.
- LVSI is reported as no LVSI, focal LVSI, and extensive/substantial LVSI. The determination of the precise number of involved vessels to discriminate between focal and extensive/substantial LVSI requires additional scientific evidence, however, for staging purposes the recommendation by WHO 2020 (≥5 vessels) is adopted.
- LVSI should not be included in assessment of depth of myometrial invasion.
- Presence of LVSI alone on the uterine serosa, parametrium, adnexal, or periadnexal tissues does not constitute true involvement and should not be used for staging.

Challenges While Assessing Lymphovascular Space Invasion

- *True versus pseudoinvasion:* Pseudoinvasion includes disaggregated tumor fragments intermixed with inflammation and/or stroma floating within large vessels and retraction artifacts (tumor fragments within smooth, rounded contours without endothelial lining).
- *MELF pattern of myoinvasion:* MELF pattern of invasion may be mistaken as LVSI **(Fig. 9)** and may need deeper levels and IHC confirmation with cytokeratin and D2-40 immunostains as mentioned earlier.

- *WHO 2020 and FIGO 2023 definition of extensive/substantial LVSI:* Most resources do not clarify whether the extent of LVSI is based on the maximum involvement in a single tissue section or on the cumulative extent across all tissue sections. This will have an impact on the reproducibility of LVSI quantification which may lead to potential difficulties in comparability between practices and regions.

Cervical Stromal Involvement

- The presence of cervical stromal invasion upstages EC to pT2.
- Absence or presence of cervical stromal invasion should be reported.
- For the purposes of standard reporting, the uppermost endocervical mucinous gland identified in the section should be taken as the upper limit of the endocervix.
- In tumors with cervical stromal invasion, depth of cervical wall invasion (from the surface in relation to the cervical wall thickness or the proportion of the cervical wall thickness) and status of radial and distal margins (with minimum distance to tumor) should also be included.

Challenges in Assessing Cervical Stromal Invasion

- *Cervical stromal invasion versus cervical mucosal involvement*: Mere colonization of cervical mucosal glands by tumor does not amount to cervical stromal invasion. Absence of lobular architecture of benign endocervical glands within the neoplastic glands, confluent glandular growth, presence of neoplastic glands admixed with benign endocervical glands, and surrounding stromal desmoplastic/inflammatory reaction are supportive criteria of cervical stromal invasion **(Figs. 10A and B)**.
- *Cervical stromal invasion versus LUS involvement:* LUS and upper endocervix are not clearly demarcated, often showing alternating mucinous and ciliated LUS glands microscopically. The uppermost endocervical gland (with mucin-containing cells) should be considered the upper limit of the endocervix. Additional sampling may be useful in equivocal cases.
- *Polypoid uterine cancer prolapsing into endocervical canal:* This does not upstage the tumor to pT2 in absence of cervical stromal invasion.
- Stage II endometrial cancer versus stage I endocervical cancer **(Table 5) (Figs. 11A to D)**.

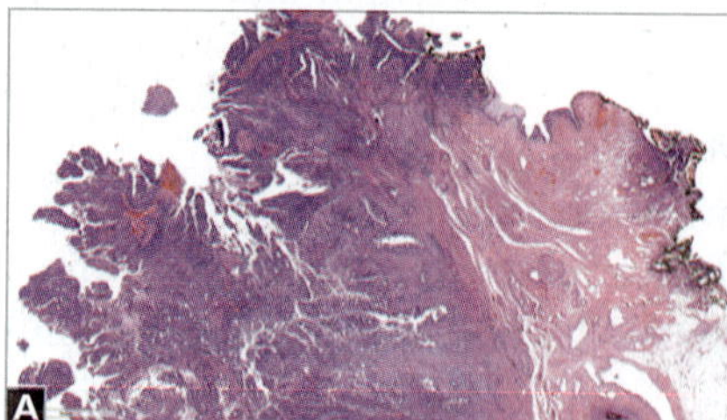

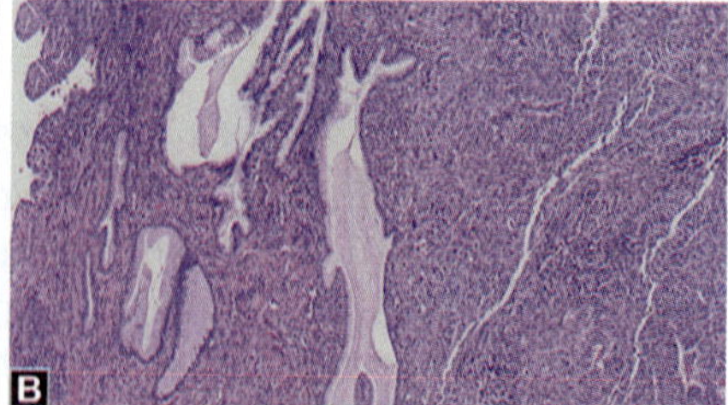

FIGS. 10A AND B: Cervical stromal invasion. (A) Absence of lobular architecture of benign endocervical glands within the neoplastic glands and confluent glandular growth. (B) Presence of neoplastic glands admixed with benign endocervical glands and surrounding stromal desmoplastic/inflammatory reaction.

TABLE 5: Endometrial endometrioid carcinoma versus endocervical adenocarcinoma.

	Endometrial endometrioid carcinoma	Endocervical adenocarcinoma
Gross and clinical features	Bulk of tumor in endometrium/LUS	Bulk of tumor in cervix; barrel-shaped cervix
Microscopy	• *Precursor:* Atypical hyperplasia • Squamous morules • Tall columnar cells with stromal foamy histiocytes	• *Precursor:* Adenocarcinoma in situ • Intracytoplasmic mucin, goblet cells • Floating mitoses • Basal apoptosis
IHC	• ER, PR + • p16– • Vimentin + • CEA– • PAX8 + • MMR loss/intact	• ER, PR– • p16 +/HPV-ISH +ve • Vimentin– • CEA– • PAX8 ± • MMR intact

Note:
- ± denotes variable staining.
- For p16 staining + denotes diffuse, block-like expression;—denotes negative, focal, or patchy staining.
- HPV-ISH, HPV DNA in-situ hybridization.

(CEA: carcinoembryonic antigen; ER: estrogen receptor; MMR: mismatch repair; IHC: immunohistochemistry; HPV-ISH: hybridization for human papillomavirus; LUS: lower uterine segment)

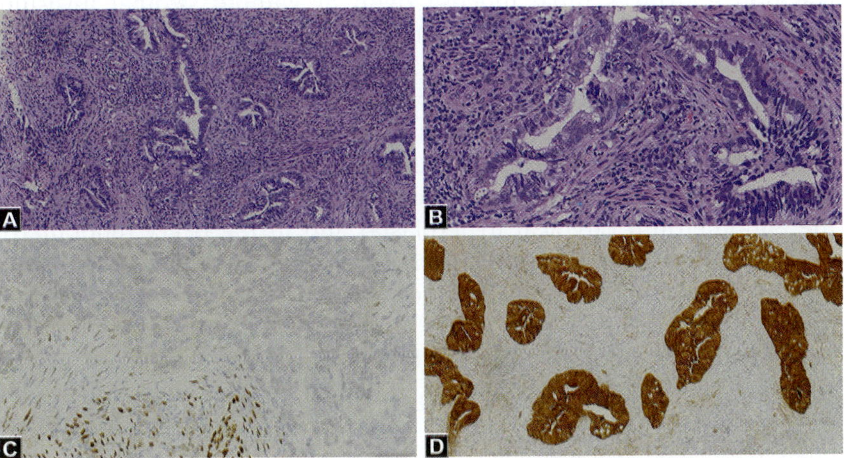

FIGS. 11A TO D: Endocervical adenocarcinoma, human papillomavirus (HPV) associated. (A) Endometrioid morphology on low power. (B) Floating mitoses and basal apoptosis on high power. (C) Estrogen receptor (ER) and progesterone receptors (PR) negative (PR not in figure, internal control-stromal cells are positive); (D) Block positive staining for p16; surrogate marker of HPV etiology.

Adnexal Involvement

- It is important to distinguish ovarian involvement in EC as metastatic or synchronous.

- The 2023 FIGO staging for EC endorses the view of WHO 2020 classification and ESGO/ESTRO/ESP guidelines for EC and establishes the category of stage IA3 when the following criteria are met in a low-grade EEC:
  - No more than superficial myometrial invasion is present (<50%).
  - The absence of extensive/substantial LVSI.
  - The absence of additional metastases; and
  - The ovarian tumor is unilateral, limited to the ovary without capsule invasion/breach (equivalent to pT1a).

  The cases not fulfilling these criteria should be interpreted as extensive spread of EC to the ovary (stage IIIA1).
- Tumor involvement of the fallopian tube should also be recorded and staged as IIIA1.
- In cases of serous EC with coexisting tubal intraepithelial (mucosal) carcinoma, with or without stromal invasion, WT1 immunostaining should be undertaken to help define whether the fallopian lesion is an independent synchronous or metastatic. Diffuse, strong WT1 staining is seen in primary adnexal high-grade serous carcinoma versus negative to focal staining in primary endometrial serous carcinoma.

Challenges in Assessing Adnexal Involvement

- *Presence of intraluminal tubal floating tumor fragments:* This is a controversial issue, particularly in serous carcinoma, but is not considered for staging purposes. Fallopian tube involvement should be diagnosed when carcinoma involves tubal mucosa (with or without stromal invasion) or wall/serosa (except for endometrioid or clear cell carcinoma arising in endometriosis).
- *Different resources state different criteria for synchronous versus metastatic involvement:* Bilateral ovarian involvement by tumor is a criterion of unfavorable outcome in the 2023 FIGO and ISGyP recommendations but not in the 2020 WHO classification. Precursors to endometrioid carcinoma in the endometrium (atypical hyperplasia) and in the ovary (endometriosis, adenofibroma) are among the criteria for classification of favorable outcome by ISGyP recommendations, but not by WHO 2020 or 2023 FIGO staging system.
- *Equivocal cases:* There will be borderline cases, e.g., low-grade EEC cases with 60% myometrial invasion and unilateral ovarian involvement without extrauterine or extraovarian spread. Discussion in a multidisciplinary tumor board may help in such equivocal cases.

Serosal Involvement

- Serosal involvement upstages EC to pT3a.
- Serosal involvement denotes full-thickness involvement of the myometrium with the tumor reaching the mesothelial layer or submesothelial fibro connective tissue, even when tumor is not present on the surface or when no desmoplastic reaction is seen as per ISGyP guidelines.
- Inking the serosa during grossing is a useful exercise.

Challenges in Assessing Serosal Involvement

Concept of "uterine subserosa": FIGO 2023 has introduced stage IIIA2 defined as involvement of uterine subserosa or spread through uterine serosa. Uterine subserosa is not defined in a way that can be reproducibly evaluated by pathologists. ISGyP recommendations already include the submesothelial fibro connective tissue as part of the definition of serosal involvement and can be used to define subserosal involvement.

Vaginal and Parametrial Involvement

- Vaginal and parametrial invasion upstages EC to pT3b.
- Vaginal involvement may take the form of direct extension or so-called drop-metastasis, in which there is no connection between the vaginal tumor and the dominant mass.
- Parametrial invasion denotes stromal infiltration by carcinoma as a result of direct extension or discrete metastases due to discontinuous spread **(Fig. 12)**.

Challenges in Assessing Vaginal and Parametrial Invasion

- Free floating tumor fragments should be not be considered as true involvement.
- Presence of LVSI at these sites should be not be used for staging purposes.

Lymph Node Status

- Lymph node status including sentinel lymph node status reports the total number of lymph nodes found and the number of positive lymph nodes and the presence of extranodal extension **(Figs. 13A and B)**.
- Micrometastasis (>0.2 mm and up to 2 mm) are reported as pN1(mi).
- Isolated tumor cells (ITCs) no greater than 0.2 mm in regional lymph nodes should be reported as pN0(i+).
- The FIGO 2023 staging system distinguishes between micrometastasis and macrometastasis, classifying them separately as IIIC1i and IIIC1ii for pelvic lymph node involvement and IIIC2i and IIIC2ii for para-aortic lymph node involvement.

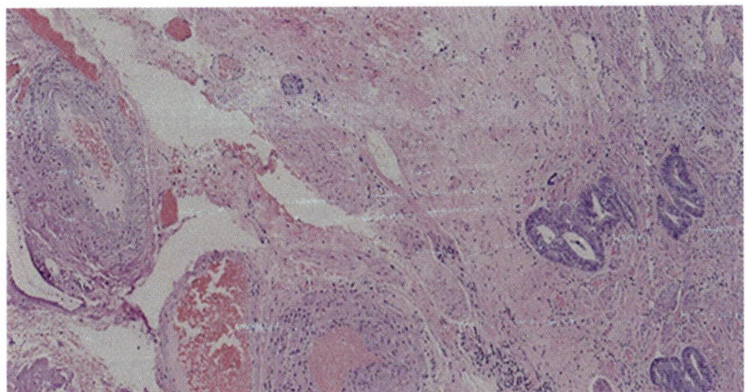

FIG. 12: Parametrial invasion by endometrial carcinoma (EC).

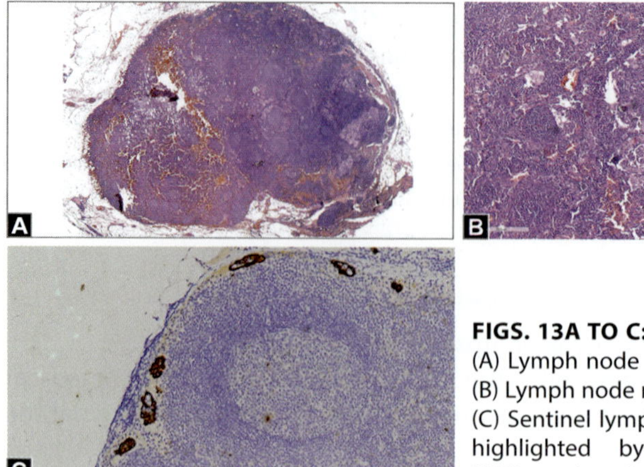
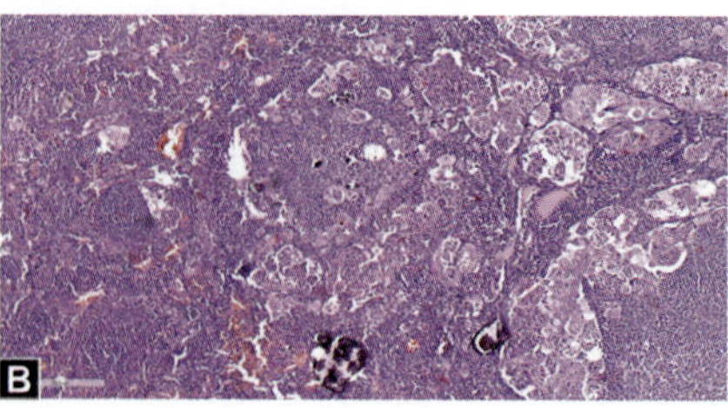

FIGS. 13A TO C: Lymph node metastasis. (A) Lymph node metastasis on low-power. (B) Lymph node metastasis on high-power. (C) Sentinel lymph node ultrastaging: ITCs highlighted by immunohistochemistry (IHC)-cytokeratin (AE1/AE3).

- A finding of ITCs alone does not upstage a carcinoma **(Fig. 13C)**.
- Lymph node ultra staging is recommended for the analysis of sentinel lymph nodes (see **Table 3**) **(Fig. 13)**.[13]

Peritoneal Cytology

- Positive peritoneal cytology is no longer included in staging of EC but is recommended as part of the surgical procedure by NNCN guidelines.[11]
- There is lack of consensus in literature with regard to its prognostic significance in the absence of other evidence of extrauterine spread.
- If peritoneal washings are positive for malignant cells, this should be recorded as this is taken to be an adverse risk factor when considering adjuvant therapy.[11]

Omentum

Omental involvement by EC is considered abdominal peritoneal metastasis (Stage IVB).[5]

ENDOMETRIAL CARCINOMA: MOLECULAR CLASSIFICATION

An integrated genomic characterization of endometrial cancer by the TCGA Research Network identified 4 prognostically different genomic types, including POLE-mutated/ultramutated, microsatellite instability (MSI)-high (MSI-H)/hypermutated, copy number low, and copy number high **(Table 6)**.[3]

High-grade EEC (grade 3) which is a prognostically, clinically, and molecularly heterogeneous disease benefits most from applying molecular classification. Molecular profiling of grade 3 endometrioid carcinoma is able to discriminate an excellent prognosis group (*POLEmut* in early-stage disease) from a bad prognosis group [p53 abnormal (p53abn)].[17,18] Recent data have demonstrated that high-grade EECs falling into the nonspecific molecular profile (NSMP) group, especially when estrogen receptor (ER)-negative, also have a bad prognosis.[19]

TABLE 6: Molecular classification of endometrial carcinoma.

	POLEmut	MMRd	NSMP	p53abn
Molecular features	*Ultramutated:* • >100 mutations/ megabase (Mb) • Very low CNA • Microsatellite stable (MSS)	*Hypermutated:* • 10–100 mutations/Mb • Low CNA • Microsatellite instability (MSI)	*Variants common in PTEN, CTNNB1, PIK3CA, KRAS, ARID1A:* • < 10 mutations/Mb • Low CNA • MSS	*TP53 variants*: • < 10 mutations/Mb • Very high CNA • MSS
Key histological features	• High grade • Ambiguous morphology • Tumor giant cells • Prominent tumor-infiltrating lymphocytes (TILs) **(Fig. 21)**	• High grade • Endometrioid • Mucinous differentiation • MELF pattern of invasion • LVSI • Prominent TILs **(Fig. 15)**	• Low grade • Squamous differentiation/ morules • TILs not prominent **(Figs. 1A and 1B)**	• High grade • Diffuse cytological atypia • Typically serous carcinoma **(Fig. 2)**
Diagnostic tests	*Pole mutational analysis*: • NGS/Sanger sequencing/ hotspot analysis • 11 pathogenic variants • No IHC surrogate	• *MMR IHC*: MLH1, MSH2, MSH6, PMS2— ○ 4 IHC or 2 IHC approach • MSI assay • NGS	• MMR-proficient • p53-wildtype • Pathogenic POLE variant absent • Further stratification by using ER,PR • CTNNB1 • L1-CAM	• p53 mutational analysis • p53 IHC

Continued

Continued

	POLEmut	**MMRd**	**NSMP**	**p53abn**
Clinical features	Younger age	Association with Lynch syndrome	Higher body mass index	Advanced stage at presentation
Treatment	De-escalation for stage I, II	• Highly responsive to immunotherapy • Adjuvant radiation • ? No benefit from chemotherapy	• Highly favorable de-escalation, vault brachytherapy, endocrine therapy • Unfavorable chemotherapy + Radiotherapy	• Chemotherapy • PARP inhibitor • Anti-HER2 treatment
Prognosis	Excellent	Intermediate	Intermediate to excellent	Poor
Adjuvant clinical trials	• PORTEC 4a (de-escalation) • RAINBO Blue (de-escalation) • TAPER (de-escalation)	• NRG GY 020 (+ICB, Pembrolizumab) • RAINBO Green (+ICB, Durvalumab) • ADELE (+ICB, Tislelizumab)	• RAINBO Orange (+ endocrine therapy) • TAPER (de-escalation)	• RAINBO Red (+PARPi, Olaparib) • CAN STAMP (+PARPi, Niraparib) • NRG GY 026 (+HER2, Trastuzumab/ Pertuzumab)

(CNA: copy number alterations; ICB: Immune checkpoint blockade therapy; LVSI: lympho-vascular space invasion; MELF: microcystic, elongated and fragmented; MMRd: mismatch repair deficiency; MSI: microsatellite instability; MSS: microsatellite stable; NGS: next generation sequencing; NSMP: No specific molecular profile; p53abn: p53 abnormal; PARPi: PARP inhibitor; *POLE*mut: POLE utramutated; TILs: tumor infiltrating lymphocytes)

The TCGA molecular classification system required very costly analysis of unfixed tumor samples. However, in order to make diagnosis of EC more reproducible, accurate, and clinically actionable, it has become very clear that the way forward is to incorporate strategies in routine practice that reflect molecular subtype of EC. This therefore translates to the use of surrogate markers of the TCGA molecular groups that are inexpensive, applicable to formalin-fixed paraffin-embedded tissue, and can be applied in routine practice.

Both the PORTEC group and the Proactive Molecular Risk Classifier for Endometrial Cancer (PRoMisE) study group have classified the molecular subgroups by using surrogate markers in paraffin embedded tissues. Sequencing for mutations in the *POLE* exonuclease domain (EDM) is a surrogate for the *POLE* ultramutated (*POLEmut)* group. IHC for mismatch repair (MMR) proteins is a surrogate for MSI-high (MSI-H)/hypermutated group. TP53 mutational analysis or abnormal p53 immunostaining can serve as surrogate markers for the presence of high somatic copy-number abnormalities, with the latter being less expensive and used more readily in practice.[20,21]

Thus, the TCGA molecular categories of EC can be replicated in practice using surrogate markers: MMR and p53 IHC and sequencing for *POLE* EDM (PRoMisE classifier).

These must be interpreted using a particular algorithm as the two categories characterized by high mutational rates, *POLE*mut and MMRd EC, can show multiple mutations and adherence to the algorithm ensures correct interpretation of MMR and p53 IHC **(Fig. 14)**.

Whenever resources permit, complete molecular classification (*POLEmut*, MMRd, NSMP, and p53abn) is encouraged in all cases of EC for prognostic risk-group stratification as these influence adjuvant or systemic treatment decisions. ESGO/ESTRO/ESP guidelines for EC define the prognostic risk groups both when molecular classification is known and unknown.[12]

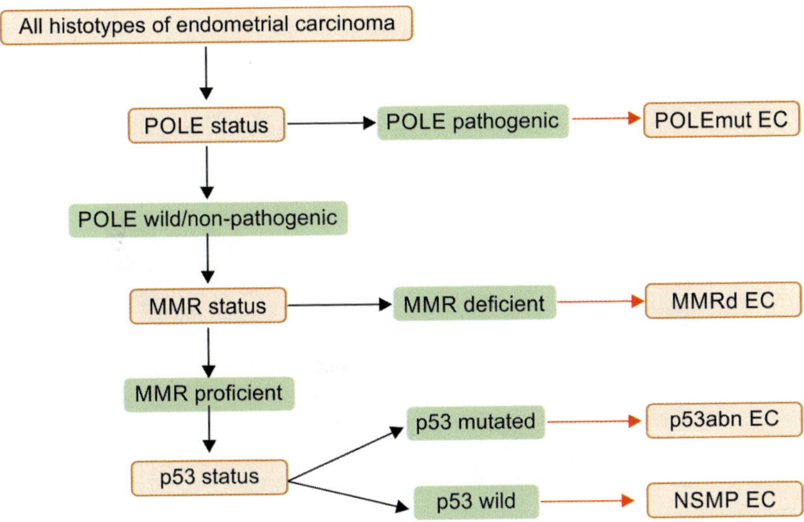

FIG. 14: Algorithmic approach to POLE testing, mismatch repair (MMR) immunohistochemistry (IHC), and p53 IHC for molecular classification of endometrial carcinoma (EC).

Molecular subtype assignment can be conducted on a biopsy specimen, in which appropriate handling and control of fixation conditions may allow for a better performance of immunohistochemical and molecular techniques than on the final hysterectomy specimen.[22]

ANCILLARY TESTING IN ENDOMETRIAL CARCINOMA

Ancillary Testing in Endometrial Carcinoma in Performed in Following Scenarios

- Diagnostic IHC which is used to subclassify EC into different histotypes **(Table 2)** and to differentiate endometrial primary from endocervical primary in small biopsy specimens **(Table 5) (Fig. 11)**.
- Biomarker testing in EC includes IHC for MMR proteins, HER2, and p53 IHC.[22,23]
- *POLE* testing in EC.[22]

Mismatch Repair Testing in Endometrial Carcinoma

- *Lack of MMR expression (MMR deficiency) has been described in approximately 20–30% of EC*: Majority occurs sporadically as a result of methylation of the *MLH1* promoter region and resultant epigenetic silencing of *MLH1*. 5–6% are associated with Lynch syndrome.
- *MMR testing is essential for the following reasons:*
    - Lynch syndrome screening
    - Aids in histotyping—MMRd/MSI is considered a marker for endometrioid-type EC **(Fig. 15)**.
    - Aids in genotyping—MMR/MSI testing of all cases for identification of the hypermutated MMRd/MSI category of EC.
    - Prognostic—MMRd EC have an intermediate prognosis.
    - Predictive—MMRd tumors of all sites are eligible for targeted treatment with immune checkpoint inhibitors.

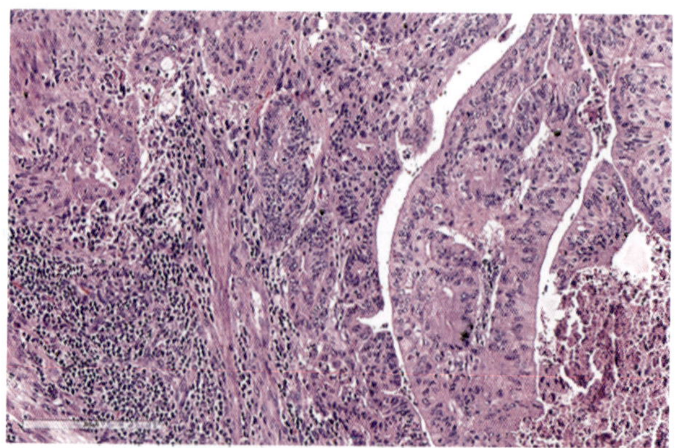

FIG. 15: Mismatch repair-deficient endometrial carcinoma (MMRd EC) with prominent tumor-infiltrating lymphocytes (TILs).

- *Testing for a mismatch repair defects*: Detection of MMRd can be carried out through IHC for MMR proteins (*MLH1, PMS2, MSH2,* and *MSH6*) or through MSI analysis by polymerase chain reaction (PCR). The two methods have comparable sensitivity and show approximately 96% concordance.

The MMR IHC simply detects the presence or absence of the four MMR proteins within cancer cells. MMR IHC is straightforward to interpret in most cases based on the fact that MMR proteins function in dimers: loss of MLH1 nuclear expression is usually accompanied by PMS2 loss, whereas MSH2 loss is accompanied by MSH6 loss in the context of satisfactory internal positive control (lymphocytes, endometrial stromal cells). MMR IHC has the advantages of being cheaper, easily accessible to pathologists, amenable to IHC external quality assurance schemes, allowing correlation with morphology, and enabling identification of the defective protein, thereby guiding downstream testing.

The MSI testing detects differences in the lengths of a selection of microsatellites, resulting from indel errors, between normal cells and tumor cells. Several approved commercial platforms are available for MSI testing by PCR; this test is currently more expensive than IHC. MSI testing is carried out on DNA extracted from tumor tissue and its interpretation requires a high level of expertise as the changes seen in EC are reported to be more subtle than those in colonic cancer. In addition, detection of MSI would require IHC to identify the gene that may have a mutation, and PCR may miss *MSH6*-deficient tumors.

- MMR protein expression in normal tissues is seen as nuclear staining, generally uniform but may be of variable intensity. More rapidly proliferating cells show more intense staining. In cancer cells, the staining intensity is strong and higher than stroma, normal glands, or inflammatory cells.
- *Testing approach:* The most cost-effective screening approach involves two IHC approach for *MSH6* and *PMS2,* with subsequent *MSH2* IHC (if *MSH6* loss) and/or MLH1 IHC (if *PMS2* loss). Alternatively, all four MMR proteins (*MLH1, PMS2, MSH2,* and *MSH6*) are tested.
- *Normal result in tumor (mismatch repair proficient tumors):* All four MMR proteins (*MLH1, PMS2, MSH2,* and *MSH6*) are tested or only *PMS2* and *MSH6* tested. If there is intact nuclear staining, there is no immunohistochemical evidence of aMMRd.
- *Abnormal result 1 in tumors:*
    - Loss of nuclear staining of *MLH1* and *PMS2* **(Figs. 16A and B)**: This MMRd is likely to be sporadic and rarely Lynch syndrome. Testing for *MLH1 Promoter* hypermethylation is recommended (by methylation-specific PCR or by methylation specific, multiplex, and ligation-dependent probe amplification) **(Fig. 17)**.
- *Abnormal result 2 in tumors:*
    - Loss of nuclear staining of *MSH2* and *MSH6.*
    - Loss of nuclear staining of *MSH6.*
    - Loss of nuclear staining of *PMS2.*
    - Loss of nuclear staining of *MLH1* and *PMS2* without *MLH1* promoter methylation. These MMRd patterns are associated with Lynch syndrome and germline testing is indicated.

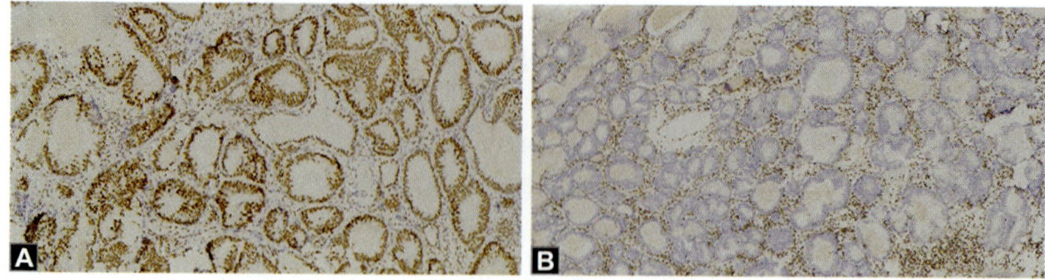

FIGS. 16A AND B: (A) Retained *MSH2* and *MSH6* (figure shows only *MSH2*); (B) Loss of *MLH1* and *PMS2* (figure shows only PMS2).

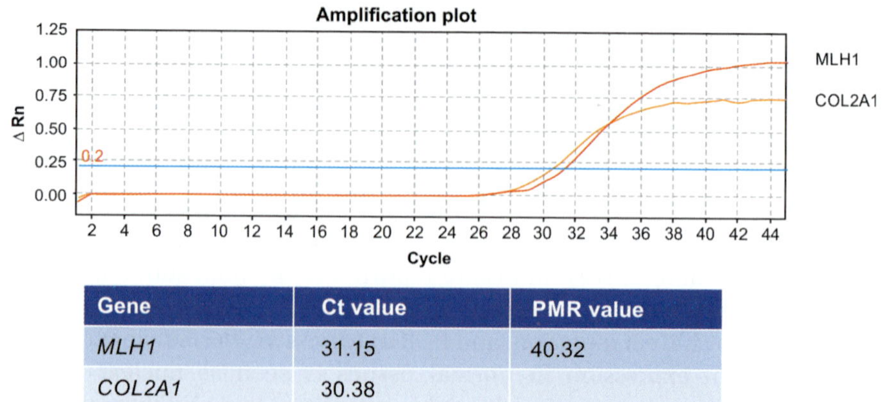

Gene	Ct value	PMR value
MLH1	31.15	40.32
COL2A1	30.38	

PMR value >4 indicates MLH1 promoter methylation

FIG. 17: MLH1 hypermethylation—reverse transcription-polymerase chain reaction (RT-PCR) assay.

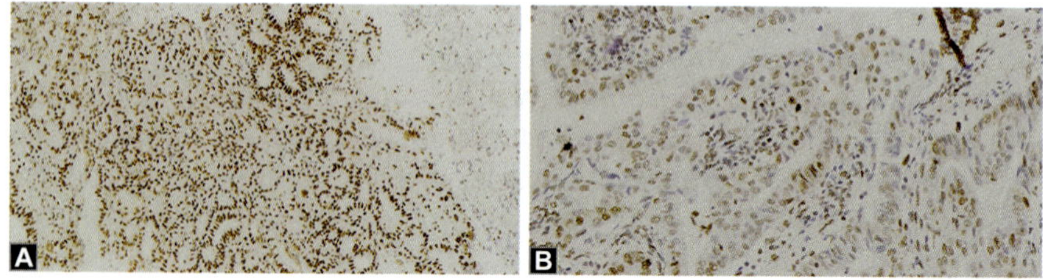

FIGS. 18A AND B: (A) *MSH6* in endometrial biopsy (intact nuclear staining). (B) *MSH6* in same case in hysterectomy specimen; Note weak staining/loss of staining due to poor fixation.

- *Pitfalls during MMR testing:*
  - Pitfall due to poor fixation—fixation affects IHC detection and can show loss of nuclear staining in tumor cells in areas of poor fixation (false positive) **(Figs. 18A and B)**. This is why biopsy is preferred over hysterectomy because of better fixation and antigenicity in biopsy specimens as compared to hysterectomy specimens **(Figs. 18A and B)**. Staining protocol should be standardized with appropriate quality assurance. Presence of internal control (stromal cells, lymphocytes, and normal glands) should be noted in areas showing loss of nuclear staining.

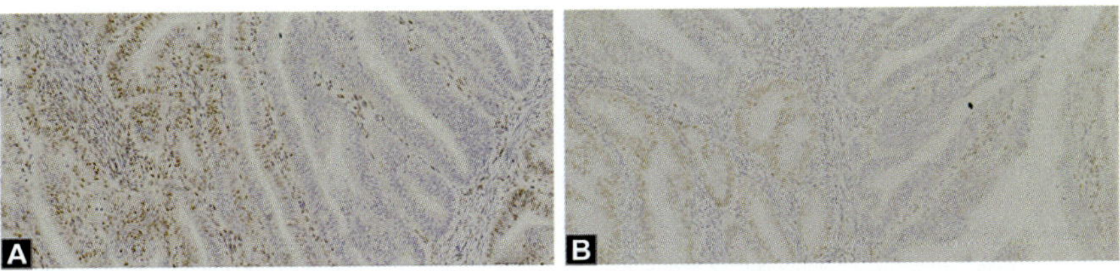

FIGS. 19A AND B: (A) Subclonal loss of MLH1; note intact internal control in area of subclonal loss. (B) Subclonal loss of PMS2 in same case; note intact internal control in area of subclonal loss.

  - Very focal expression in MMRd—some missense mutations can result in weak/focal expression. Very weak staining/very focal expression (in comparison to internal control) is best regarded as "loss".
  - Subclonal expression—Subclonal expression is defined as abrupt and complete regional loss of staining in tumor cell nuclei in the presence of positive internal controls (i.e., stromal cells, lymphocytes) **(Figs. 19A and B)**. Subclonal expression has to be distinguished from variable expression due to fixation artefact. Normal staining must be seen in the internal control in the area showing loss of expression in tumor cells. An arbitrary cutoff of 10% is suggested to avoid reporting this pattern in cases where it is extremely focal and of unlikely clinical significance.[24]
  - Cytoplasmic/Membranous staining—cytoplasmic/membranous staining does not constitute normal expression and should be reported as abnormal.
  - False negative result—nonfunctional protein with retained antigenicity (most commonly *MLH1*).

p53 Immunohistochemistry in Endometrial Carcinoma

- p53 IHC is interpreted as abnormal and wild-type staining patterns.
- Normal (wild-type) expression is characterized by a heterogeneous staining pattern in which there are variable number of positive cells with variable staining intensity admixed with negative cells.
- Three abnormal or mutation-type IHC patterns of p53 expression have been described which predict underlying *TP53* gene mutations with 96% sensitivity and 100% specificity **(Figs. 20A to D)**.[25]
  - Overexpression type (nuclear overexpression in 80–100% of cells) associated with nonsynonymous missense mutations seen in ~70% cases.
  - Complete absence (null pattern) associated with loss-of-function mutations seen in ~25% cases.
  - Cytoplasmic expression (associated with loss-of-function mutation disrupting nuclear localization domain) seen in <5% cases.
  - Rarely (<5%), truncating or splice site mutations can result in wild-type expression (because of a nonfunctional p53 protein).
- Subclonal abnormal p53 expression has been identified in 5% of ECs in biopsy specimens, predominantly associated with *POLE* mutations or MMR deficiency. Subclonal abnormal p53 expression is defined as ≥10% tumor cells showing abrupt change from wild-type to mutant-pattern

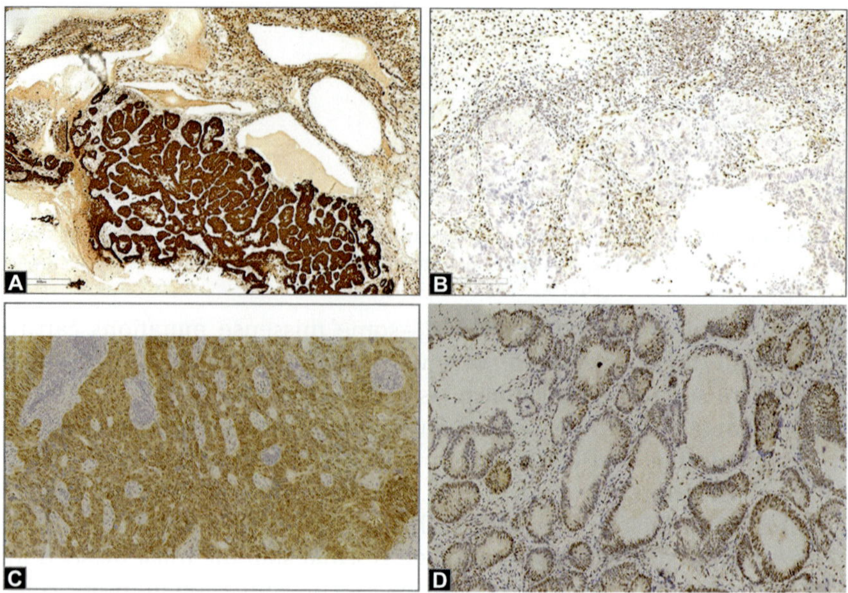

FIGS. 20A TO D: (A) Overexpression pattern of abnormal (mutated) p53 expression; (B) Null pattern of abnormal (mutated) p53 expression; (C) Cytoplasmic pattern of abnormal (mutated) p53 expression; (D) Wild-type p53 expression.

staining and is reported as p53 abnormal noting the presence and extent of subclonal staining. POLE-mutated or MMR deficient tumors are assigned to these subtypes if found associated regardless of their p53 status, because the behavior of these tumors seems to be driven by *POLE* mutation status or MMR deficiency rather than their p53 status. The significance of abnormal subclonal p53 expression in tumors lacking *POLE* mutations or MMR deficiency is unknown.[26]

Human Epidermal Growth Factor Receptor 2 Immunohistochemistry in Endometrial Carcinoma

Endometrial serous carcinoma and carcinosarcoma have aggressive metastatic potential with low effectivity of traditional platinum-based chemotherapy and high rates of resistance and recurrence. HER2 overexpression is seen in ~30–35% of serous carcinoma and in ~15–20% of carcinosarcoma and is a potential target for anti-HER2 therapy.[27]

College of American Pathologists (CAP) suggests using a reporting format as that used for reporting the results of HER2 testing for breast cancer, with modifications **(Tables 7 and 8)**.[23]

POLE Testing in Endometrial Carcinoma

- Mutational analysis for *POLE* is recommended by the WHO wherever resources permit. *POLE* mutated EC represent 5–10% of all endometrial cancers. Patients are typically younger than patients with non-*POLE*

TABLE 7: Reporting results of HER2 testing by immunohistochemistry for endometrial serous carcinoma as per CAP guidelines.

Result	Criteria
Negative (score 0)	No staining observed
Negative (score 1+)	Incomplete membrane staining that is faint/barely perceptible in any proportion of cells or weak complete staining in <10% of tumor cells*
Equivocal (score 2+)†	Intense complete or *basolateral/lateral membrane* staining in ≤30% tumor cells* or weak-to-moderate staining in ≥10% of tumor cells*
Positive (score 3+)	Intense complete or *basolateral/lateral membrane* staining in >30% of tumor cells*

*Readily appreciated using a low-power objective and observed within a homogeneous and contiguous population of invasive tumor cells.

†Must order reflex test (same specimen using ISH) or order a new test (new specimen if available, using IHC or ISH).

TABLE 8: Reporting results of HER2 testing by fluorescent in situ hybridization (dual-probe assay) as per CAP guidelines.

Result	Criteria
Negative	FISH HER2/CEP17 ratio <2.0 and average HER2 copy number <6 per nucleus
Positive	• FISH HER2/CEP17 ratio ≥2.0, or • FISH HER2/CEP17 ratio <2.0 with average HER2 copy number ≥6 per nucleus

(FISH: fluorescence in situ hybridization)

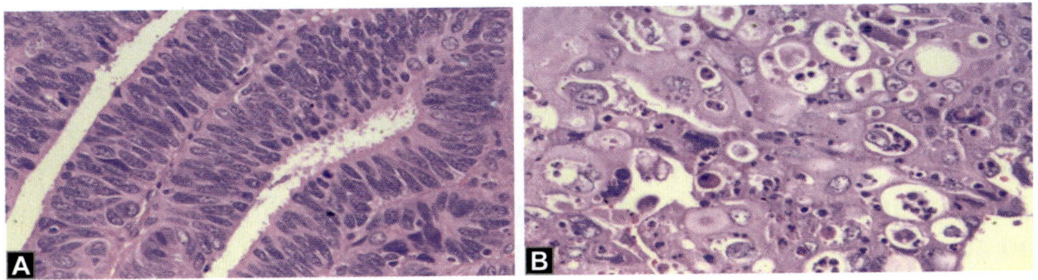

FIGS. 21A AND B: Ambiguous histology of *POLE*mut endometrial cancer (EC).

mutated EC and generally present at a low stage. *POLE* mutated carcinomas have been shown to be associated with abundant tumor infiltrating and peritumoral lymphocytes, tumor giant cells, intratumoral heterogeneity, and serous-like/ambiguous morphology **(Figs. 21A and B)**.[28]

- Methods for *POLE* testing include next generation sequencing, sanger sequencing, hotspot single nucleotide SNaPshot assay, droplet digital PCR test **(Fig. 22)**. There is no IHC surrogate for *POLE* testing.[29]
- Detected *POLE* mutation should be pathogenic, involving the exonuclease domain (EDM) and correlated with ultramutated phenotype. Interpretation of *POLE* results should be based on published data. 11 mutations have been established as being pathogenic. Majority of pathogenic mutations are within exons 9, 11, 13, and 14.[29]

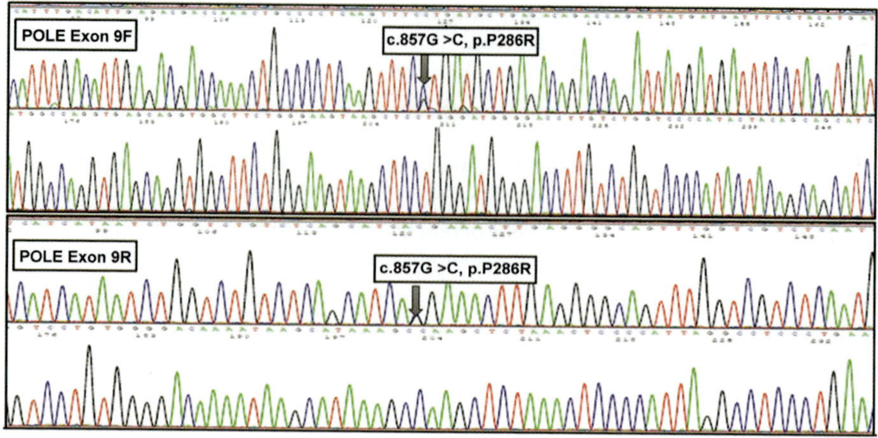

FIG. 22: Sanger sequencing for *POLE exonuclease domain* (EDM), positive for heterozygous missense variant at exon 9 (P286R).

BOX 1 Molecular classification of endometrial carcinoma in presence of multiple classifiers.

- Pathogenic *POLE* exonuclease domain mutation, p53 abnormal tumors → classified as *POLE*mut
- MMR deficient, p53 abnormal tumors → classified as MMRd
- Pathogenic *POLE* exonuclease domain mutation, MMR deficient (subclonal) tumors → classified as *POLE*mut
- Nonpathogenic *POLE* mutation, MMR deficient tumor → classified as MMRd

(MMR: mismatch repair; MMRd: mismatch repair deficiency)

- 3–5% of EC harbor >1 molecular classifying alteration and are referred to as multiple classifier **(Box 1)**. p53 alterations in the presence of *POLE* pathogenic mutation or MMR deficiency are likely secondary events acquired in tumor progression (passenger mutations) and are typically subclonal. In the presence of mutant p53 or MMRd staining patterns, performing a *POLE* mutation analysis is advisable to avoid misclassification into the p53*abn* and MMRd groups.
- A recently developed test is QPOLE, which is a POLE hotspot test that is both quick (taking approximately 2 hours) and cost-effective. The test uses a quantitative polymerase chain reaction (qPCR) assay and promises to be an efficient and accurate testing procedure for POLE in endometrial biopsy and hysterectomy specimens.[30]

STAGING OF ENDOMETRIAL CARCINOMA

The updated FIGO staging system for EC was published in 2023 and represents a paradigm change from the traditional 2009 FIGO staging of EC which was a purely anatomic staging system agnostic of parameters such as tumor type, tumor grade, LVSI, and molecular subtype. The updated system incorporates all of these "nonanatomical" parameters in an attempt to make staging more personalized and relevant to patient prognostication and management, and to align with ESGO/ESTRO/ESP risk stratification of EC.[5,12]

The main highlights of FIGO 2023 staging system of EC is as follows:

- Incorporates tumor type and tumor grade as staging parameters by distinguishing EC into two principal categories based on their degree of aggressiveness: Aggressive and nonaggressive histologic types.
- Incorporates LVSI as a staging parameter.
- Incorporates size of lymph node metastasis as a staging parameter.
- Introduces stage IA3 for synchronous low grade endometrial and ovarian endometrioid carcinomas.
- Integrates molecular classification of EC into staging of EC.

The application and acceptability of FIGO 2023 staging system of EC comes with its challenges as the new staging has its strengths and weaknesses.[16]

- Advantages of FIGO 2023 staging system of EC include adoption of parameters important for management and prognostication, inclusion of size of lymph node metastasis and separation of tumors with synchronous involvement of the uterine corpus, and ovary to avoid overtreatment of either category.
- Disadvantages of FIGO 2023 staging system of EC include complexity of the new system when compared to the prior version which will hinder its easy adoption and applicability. It has incorporated pathological variables for which definitions are still evolving, as well as variables that are subject to considerable interobserver variability in their assessment (e.g., requirement to distinguish between a superficially myoinvasive low grade EEC, stage 1A2 and one confined to the endometrium, and stage 1A1). FIGO 2023 has introduced the concept of "uterine subserosa" to define stage IIIA2; however uterine subserosa is not defined in a way that can be reproducibly evaluated by pathologists. With regard to the definition of extensive/substantial LVSI, FIGO 2023 does not clarify whether the extent of LVSI is based on the maximum involvement in a single tissue section or on the cumulative extent across all tissue sections. This will have an impact on the reproducibility of LVSI quantification which may lead to potential difficulties in application of this staging system. Lastly, in under-resourced settings where ancillary testing is limited, it will be difficult to routinely apply FIGO 2023 staging.

CLINICAL IMPLICATIONS AND FUTURE DIRECTIONS IN ENDOMETRIAL CARCINOMA

The molecular subgroups of EC provide the basis for a more robust classification with prognostic significance. Molecular classification besides being prognostic, has also been shown to predict response to chemotherapy and to be associated with specific molecular targets against which targeted drugs are available. Studies using immune checkpoint inhibitors for patients with MMRd EC have shown high rates of response. PARP inhibitors targeting homologous recombination deficiency and antibodies targeting HER2 overexpression within the p53abn group, have shown promising results.[31,32] Thus, better selection of adjuvant treatment can be achieved when treatment is based on molecular group **(Table 6)**.

With regard to trials, the comprehensive RAINBO trials program for patients with high-risk and advanced-stage EC is selecting and comparing adjuvant treatments based on the molecular group. For patients with *POLE*mut EC, de-escalation of adjuvant treatment will be studied in a registry; for those with MMRd EC, radiation will be compared with radiation plus checkpoint inhibition; for patients with p53abn EC, chemoradiation will be compared with chemoradiation followed by PARP inhibition; and for those with no specific molecular profile (NSMP) cancers, adjuvant chemoradiation will be compared with approaches including hormonal treatment. Many studies on novel targeted agents and combination treatments as adjuvant treatment or treatment of recurrent or metastatic disease are ongoing. Results of these trials are likely to have profound impact on treatment guidelines in the coming years **(Table 6)**.[31,32]

Despite recommendations for integrating molecular classification of EC into routine pathology reporting and clinical management, uptake is inconsistent. To assign ProMisE subtype, all molecular components must be available (*POLE* mutation status, MMR, and p53 IHC) and these often these are assessed at different stages of care and/or at different centers resulting in delays in treatment. Recently a single-test DNA-based targeted next generation sequencing (NGS) molecular classifier (ProMisE NGS) has been developed which demonstrates excellent concordance with the original ProMisE classifier and maintains prognostic value. Reliable molecular subtyping can be obtained at diagnosis using a single-test NGS targeted gene assay, providing an alternative means to obtain molecular classification for patients with EC.[33]

CONCLUSION

The new WHO classification emphasizes the importance of histology supported by adjunct IHC. This is particularly important for accurate distinction of endometrioid from nonendometrioid EC. Recent years have shown that histotyping of EC alone does not reflect the true biology of EC and is not highly reproducible especially in high grade tumors. The landscape of EC diagnosis has changed from a histotype based classification system to a biomarker based classification. The staging system for EC has also metamorphosed from an anatomical staging system to one which integrates molecular classification into its domain and is more aligned to risk stratification models. Thus, molecular classification of EC has proven that genomic data can be made to be practical, accessible, interpretable, informative, and actionable. This chapter gives an overview on changing landscape of EC, highlights guidelines for specimen handling and reporting, morphologic assessment, ancillary testing, and genomic subtyping with a brief insight into the future directions.

ACKNOWLEDGMENTS

We would like to thank Dr Geetashree Mukherjee, Dr Deepak Kumar Mishra, Dr Mayur Parihar, Dr Lateef Zameer, Dr Sushant Vinarkar, Dr Anand Bardia, Dr Bhagat Singh Lali, Dr Shivani Sarkar, Disease Management Group, Gynecological Oncology, Tata Medical Center, Kolkata for their contribution.

REFERENCES

1. Bokhman JV. Two pathogenetic types of endometrial carcinoma. Gynecol Oncol. 1983;15(1):10-7.
2. Gilks CB, Oliva E, Soslow RA. Poor interobserver reproducibility in the diagnosis of high-grade endometrial carcinoma. Am J Surg Pathol. 2013;37(6):874-81.
3. Cancer Genome Atlas Research Network, Kandoth C, Schultz N, Cherniack AD, Akbani R, Liu Y, Robertson GA, et al. Integrated genomic characterization of endometrial carcinoma. Nature. 2013;497(7447):67-73.
4. Publication of the WHO Classification of Tumours, 5th Edition, Volume 4: Female Genital Tumours – IARC. [online] Available from https://www.iarc.who.int/news-events/publication-of-the-who-classification-of-tumours-5th-edition-volume-4-female-genital-tumours/ [Last accessed November, 2024].
5. Berek JS, Matias-Guiu X, Creutzberg C, Fotopoulou C, Gaffney D, Kehoe S, et al. FIGO staging of endometrial cancer: 2023. J Gynaecol Oncol. 2023;34(5):e85.
6. Rabban JT, Gilks CB, Malpica A, Matias-Guiu X, Mittal K, Mutter GL, et al. Issues in the differential diagnosis of uterine low-grade endometrioid carcinoma, including mixed endometrial carcinomas: Recommendations from the International Society of Gynecological Pathologists. Int J Gynecol Pathol. 2019;38(Iss 1 Suppl 1):S25-39.
7. Soslow RA, Tornos C, Park KJ, Malpica A, Matias-Guiu X, Oliva E, et al. Endometrial carcinoma diagnosis: Use of FIGO grading and genomic subcategories in clinical practice: Recommendations of the International Society of Gynecological Pathologists. Int J Gynecol Pathol. 2019;38(Iss 1 Suppl 1):S64-74.
8. Murali R, Davidson B, Fadare O, Carlson JA, Crum CP, Gilks CB, et al. High-grade endometrial carcinomas: Morphologic and immunohistochemical features, diagnostic challenges and recommendations. Int J Gynecol Pathol. 2019;38(Iss 1 Suppl 1):S40-63.
9. Alkushi A, Abdul-Rahman ZH, Lim P, Schulzer M, Coldman A, Kalloger SE, et al. Description of a novel system for grading of endometrial carcinoma and comparison with existing grading systems. Am J Surg Pathol. 2005;29(3):295-304.
10. Conlon N, Leitao MM, Abu-Rustum NR, Soslow RA. Grading uterine endometrioid carcinoma: a proposal that binary is best. Am J Surg Pathol. 2014;38(12):1583-7.
11. Abu-Rustum N, Yashar C, Arend R, Barber E, Bradley K, Brooks R, et al. Uterine Neoplasms, Version 1.2023, NCCN Clinical Practice Guidelines in Oncology. J Natl Compr Cancer Netw JNCCN. 2023;21(2):181-209.
12. Concin N, Creutzberg CL, Vergote I, Cibula D, Mirza MR, Marnitz S, et al. ESGO/ESTRO/ESP guidelines for the management of patients with endometrial carcinoma. Virchows Arch Int J Pathol. 2021;478(2):153-90.
13. Malpica A, Euscher ED, Hecht JL, Ali-Fehmi R, Quick CM, Singh N, et al. Endometrial carcinoma, grossing and processing issues: Recommendations of the International Society of Gynecologic Pathologists. Int J Gynecol Pathol. 2019;38(Iss 1 Suppl 1):S9-24.
14. Singh N, Hirschowitz L, Zaino R, Alvarado-Cabrero I, Duggan MA, Ali-Fehmi R, et al. Pathologic prognostic factors in endometrial carcinoma (other than tumor type and grade). Int J Gynecol Pathol. 2019;38(Iss 1 Suppl 1):S93-113.
15. Turashvili G, Hanley K. Practical Updates and Diagnostic Challenges in Endometrial Carcinoma. Arch Pathol Lab Med. 2024;148(1):78-98.
16. McCluggage WG, Bosse T, Gilks CB, Howitt BE, McAlpine JN, Nucci MR, et al. FIGO 2023 endometrial cancer staging: too much, too soon? Int J Gynecol Cancer. 2023;34(1):138-43.
17. Bosse T, Nout RA, McAlpine JN, McConechy MK, Britton H, Hussein YR, et al. Molecular classification of Grade 3 endometrioid endometrial cancers identifies distinct prognostic subgroups. Am J Surg Pathol. 2018;42(5):561-8.
18. Zheng W. Molecular Classification of endometrial cancer and the 2023 FIGO staging: Exploring the challenges and opportunities for pathologists. Cancers. 2023;15(16):4101.
19. Vermij L, Jobsen JJ, León-Castillo A, Brinkhuis M, Roothaan S, Powell ME, et al. Prognostic refinement of NSMP high-risk endometrial cancers using oestrogen receptor immunohistochemistry. Br J Cancer. 2023;128(7):1360-8.

20. León-Castillo A, de Boer SM, Powell ME, Mileshkin LR, Mackay HJ, Leary A, et al. Molecular classification of the PORTEC-3 trial for high-risk endometrial cancer: Impact on prognosis and benefit From adjuvant therapy. J Clin Oncol. 2020;38(29):3388-97.
21. Talhouk A, McConechy MK, Leung S, Li-Chang HH, Kwon JS, Melnyk N, et al. A clinically applicable molecular-based classification for endometrial cancers. Br J Cancer. 2015; 113(2):299-310.
22. Casey L, Singh N. POLE, MMR, and MSI testing in endometrial cancer: Proceedings of the ISGyP companion society session at the USCAP 2020 annual meeting. Int J Gynecol Pathol. 2021;40(1):5-16.
23. Hagemann IS, Bridge JA, Tafe LJ, Hameed MR, Moncur JT, Bellizzi AM, et al. Current laboratory testing practices for assessment of ERBB2/HER2 in endometrial serous carcinoma and colorectal carcinoma. Arch Pathol Lab Med. 2023;147(10):1148-57.
24. Mendoza RP, Wang P, Schulte JJ, Tjota MY, Jani I, Martinez AC, et al. Endometrial carcinomas with subclonal loss of mismatch repair proteins: A clinicopathologic and genomic study. Am J Surg Pathol. 2023;47(5):589-98.
25. Köbel M, Ronnett BM, Singh N, Soslow RA, Gilks CB, McCluggage WG. Interpretation of P53 Immunohistochemistry in Endometrial Carcinomas: Toward Increased Reproducibility. Int J Gynecol Pathol. 2019;38 (Iss 1 Suppl 1):S123-31.
26. Huvila J, Thompson EF, Vanden Broek J, Lum A, Senz J, Leung S, et al. Subclonal p53 immunostaining in the diagnosis of endometrial carcinoma molecular subtype. Histopathology. 2023;83(6):880-90.
27. McNamara B, Mutlu L, Greenman M, Harold J, Santin A. HER2 oncogene as molecular target in uterine serous carcinoma and uterine carcinosarcoma. Cancers. 2023;15(16):4085.
28. Hoang LN, McConechy MK, Köbel M, Han G, Rouzbahman M, Davidson B, et al. Histotype-genotype correlation in 36 high-grade endometrial carcinomas. Am J Surg Pathol. 2013;37(9):1421-32.
29. León-Castillo A, Britton H, McConechy MK, McAlpine JN, Nout R, Kommoss S, et al. Interpretation of somatic POLE mutations in endometrial carcinoma. J Pathol. 2020; 250(3):323-35.
30. Van den Heerik ASVM, Ter Haar NT, Vermij L, Jobsen JJ, Brinkhuis M, Roothaan SM, et al. QPOLE: A quick, simple, and cheap alternative for POLE sequencing in endometrial cancer by multiplex genotyping quantitative polymerase chain reaction. JCO Glob Oncol. 2023;9:e2200384.
31. Jamieson A, Barroilhet LM, McAlpine JN. Molecular classification in endometrial cancer: Opportunities for precision oncology in a changing landscape. Cancer. 2022;128(15):2853-7.
32. van den Heerik ASVM, Horeweg N, de Boer SM, Bosse T, Creutzberg CL. Adjuvant therapy for endometrial cancer in the era of molecular classification: radiotherapy, chemoradiation and novel targets for therapy. Int J Gynecol Cancer. 2021;31(4):594-604.
33. Jamieson A, McConechy MK, Lum A, Leung S, Thompson EF, Senz J, et al. Harmonized molecular classification; assessment of a single-test ProMisE NGS tool. Gynecol Oncol. 2023;175:45-52.

10

CHAPTER

Computational Pathology: An Emerging Discipline with Vast Potential

Pranab Dey

INTRODUCTION

Since the introduction of the light microscope, histopathology has been the basis of understanding the pathology. The tissue diagnosis and classification of the disease are mainly based on the microscopic images. The first revolution occurred around the year 1980 when immunohistochemistry (IHC) was introduced with the application of monoclonal antibodies. Later on, the second revolution happened after the introduction of molecular pathology in laboratory service. Molecular pathology is a developing branch with a significant impact on pathology bypassing the microscopic study. With the introduction of whole-slide imaging (WSI), digital pathology is now playing a crucial role in pathology. Instead of glass slides digital slides are increasingly used for reporting. In the meantime, artificial intelligence (AI) has been growing as a newer and promising branch with great impact and is considered the third revolution in pathology.[1,2] The rapid development of digital imaging, bioinformatics, increased computational power, molecular genetics, and AI has urged to creation of a new discipline in pathology, known as computational pathology (CPath) **(Fig. 1)**. The following main factors are responsible for the emergence of CPath: (1) Digital imaging system, (2) powerful and flexible laboratory information system, and (3) the structural database of clinical information to integrate with the pathology findings. CPath incorporates the raw data from multiple sources and provides relevant clinical information. It helps to make the mathematical model at the molecular, individual, and population levels for better diagnosis and also disease prediction. In this new discipline of CPath, the role of pathologists will be to provide multidimensional interpretations of digital imaging by applying molecular pathology and clinical raw data. In addition, the discipline of CPath will also provide valuable information to physicians, patients, and healthcare providers. The simple definition of CPath is given as *"using computation for the interpretation of multiparameter data to improve health care"*.[3] In fact, CPath combines the digital image data and metadata of the patient to extract patterns, and it analyzes features using an

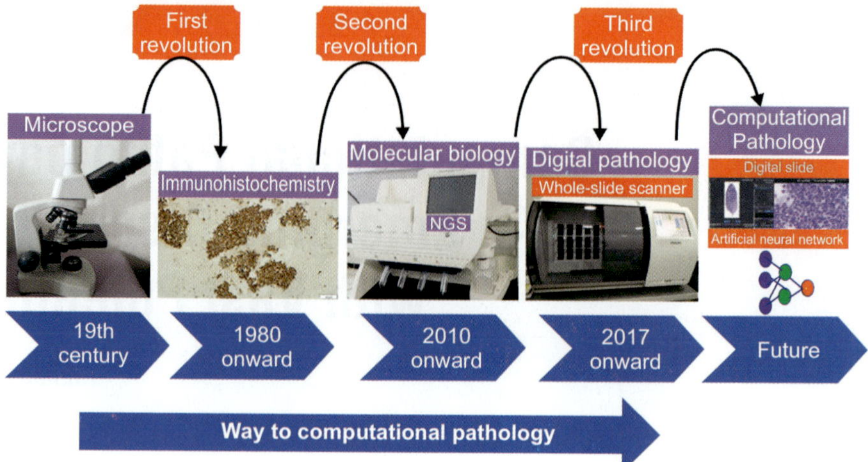

FIG. 1: Historical background of computational pathology.

artificial neural network (ANN). Till now, there are very few CPath models validated by pathologists indicating the barriers in the applications of CPath in clinical practice.

CONSTITUENTS OF COMPUTATIONAL PATHOLOGY

The major components of CPath include the following **(Fig. 2)**:

- *Clinical data*: The patients' chief complaints, past medical history, and other relevant information are recorded in natural language.
- *Hospital data*: It includes the duration of the patient's stay, expenditure, etc.
- *Digital imaging*: The introduction of WSI is the major advancement of digital pathology.[4] The whole glass slide is captured in digital format. Each image is composed of small units known as pixels. Each pixel has three color components: Red, green, and blue. Depending on the optical density, the color component of the pixel is recorded in digital format on the computer. At the time of viewing, the computer generates the complete image from the digital format. WSI simulates a microscopic view of the slide and any part of the digital slide can be viewed with any magnification. Most of the WSI system enables to scan the image in the Z-axis with high-resolution facilities. So, WSI provides the total information of the glass slide. The IHC and other special stains can also be acquired and restored with the help of WSI. The main advantages of digital slides are easy storage of the slide, rapid sharing of the slide, and rapid access to the same type of lesions. In addition, quantitative assessment of different immune markers, including cell phenotype, is possible by digital slides. Moreover, digitized slides are ideal for applying deep neural networks (DNNs) for various purposes. The workflow of digitized images is highlighted in **Figure 3**.
- *Molecular and other metadata*: The details of molecular genetics and other laboratory investigations are also recorded. Currently next-generation sequence (NGS) data may be available with all the molecular changes. Many

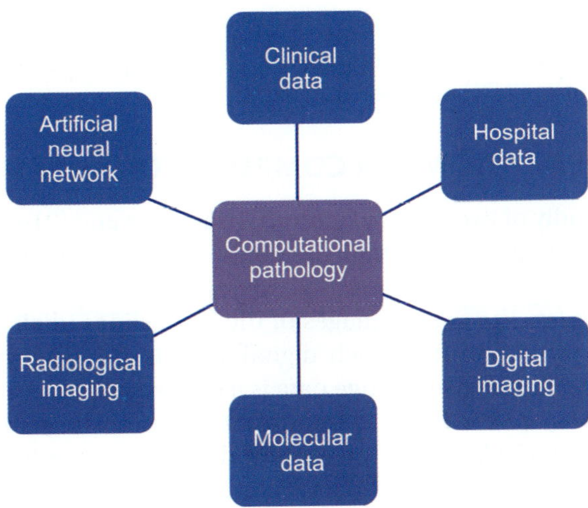

FIG. 2: The components of computational pathology.

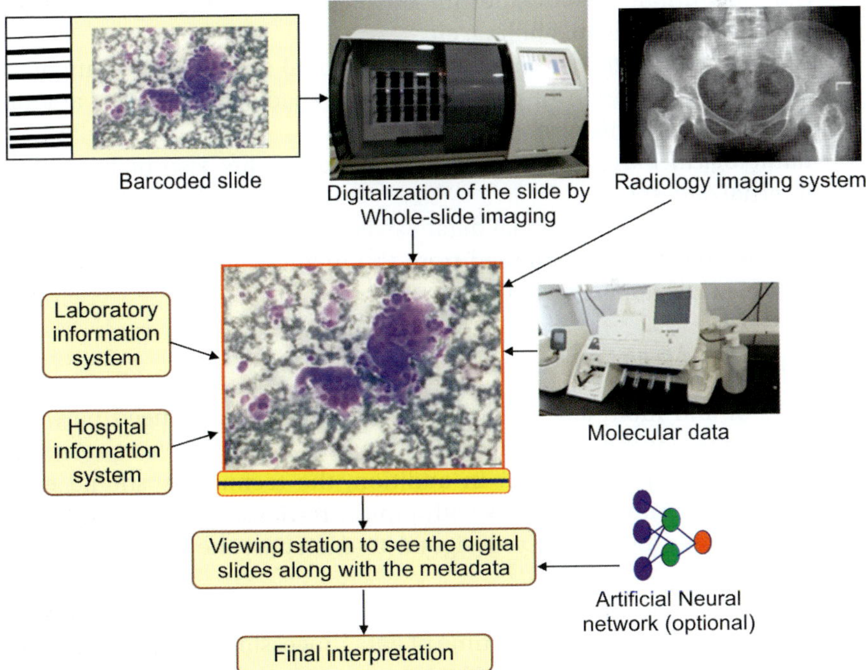

FIG. 3: Workflow of digital pathology.

of the molecular changes are now actionable and are treatable by small drug inhibitors. So, the prediction of personalized treatment will be possible.

- *Imaging*: Radiological imaging such as ultrasound, computerized tomography scans, etc. are also important databases.

- *ANN*: It is a rapidly growing branch with vast impact in diagnosis, management, and prediction of prognosis. DNN and particularly convolutional neural network (CNN) are used in CPath.[5]

DATA PREPARATION FOR COMPUTATIONAL PATHOLOGY

The data are broadly of two types: (1) Internal database and (2) external database.

- *Internal database*: The internal database is generated in the individual laboratories.
  - *Digital slides*: The digital images of the glass slides (digital slides) are the primary source of data. Each digital slide is 1–3 gigabytes in size and, therefore, handling such huge data is a challenge.
  - *Molecular genetics*: The next important internal data set is the molecular data that includes both genetic and epigenetic information. Tumor heterogeneity and genetic data from different tissue samples may be a potential challenge.
  - *Laboratory investigations*: These include various laboratory investigations such as biochemical, hematological, and tumor markers.
  - *Administration*: This includes the hospital stay of the patient, number of outdoor visits, hospital billing, etc.
  - *Clinical information*: It includes the personal details of the patient such as age, sex, duration of complaints, past medical history, or any other relevant clinical history.
  - *Radiological imaging*: The radiological images are also included in the internal data set.
- *External database*: The external database is not directly linked to the patient. It provides information obtained from the medical literature, clinical trials, and molecular databases from other patients.

DATA PREPARATION

The storage of and rapid access to a huge dataset need advanced networking technologies. The advanced technologies should handle huge compressed data and it should be object-oriented. In addition, the technology should encode different types of complex data sets with rapidly retrieval of the data. Moreover, the network should be properly designed to transport the data to the CPath system.

The pathology and radiology reports are mainly descriptive and written in natural language as text data. At the time of data processing, it is essential to make the structured data in a more meaningful way from these raw data. The more challenging is the data processing of the huge molecular data obtained from NGS. The various mutational changes should be identified and incorporated into the network.

Bioinformatics applies the computational pipeline software where the multiple data sets are modified serially. The multiple data processing elements are connected in a series and the output of an earlier algorithm functions as input of the next algorithm. Once the data passes through all the steps, the data processing is then complete. The resultant data is then transferred to a new destination. The destination stores the data. The data storage in the destination may be obtained from the multiple pipelines working parallel. Even the same data can be split into multiple pipelines to get the resultant data. The pipeline can handle the volume, variety, and velocity of the big data and is essential for doing complex analysis. The successful application of pipelines in CPath needs proper designing and supporting infrastructure.

MODELING IN COMPUTATIONAL PATHOLOGY

Designing the ANN model: At first, the pathologists should identify the problem area and based on the specific problem, the model is built up. The model may solve the diagnostic problem or classification or management of the case. It may also show the hospital expenditure or usage of different drugs or any other hospital-related problems. The model in CPath may be individual patient-specific, molecular, or population-level. The patient-specific model helps in the interpretation of clinical information in the context of tissue diagnosis, and it is essential for precision medicine. The molecular-level model helps to understand the disease process. The population-level model helps in the effective allocation of resources in the laboratory and health care system. The deep neural network is useful for making the model from the WSI images.[5] Each neural network model consists of input nodes, hidden nodes, and output nodes **(Flowchart 1)**.[1,6] To have a successful robust neural network model, a large number of cases are needed and the data is used to make the input nodes. The hidden layer with hidden nodes should be well-designed. The neural network model should be trained by repeated iterations. Each neural network model should be evaluated to assess its success. Usually, the receiver operating curve (ROC) and confusion matrix with true-positive, false-positive, true-negative, and false-negative estimation are used for evaluating the computational model. So after deciding the aims, the model can be prepared. The model preparation has three steps: (1) Dataset preparation by collection of data and formatting for ANN; (2) ANN model to make; and (3) Deployment of the model. The model should be verified in real life. If needed, the model should be modified accordingly **(Flowchart 1)**.

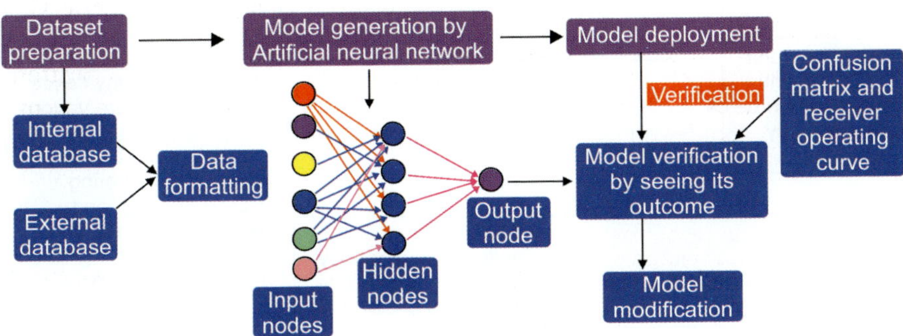

FLOWCHART 1: Model development in computational pathology.

APPLICATIONS OF COMPUTATIONAL PATHOLOGY

There are various potential applications of CPath in clinical laboratories **(Flowchart 2)**.

Diagnosis, Subtyping, Grading, and Scoring of Different Markers on Digital Slides

The CPath-based CNN model can help in the diagnosis and grading of histopathology cases. It also provides expert-level opinion with consistency and minimum interobserver variability. Chen et al.[7] classified the lung carcinomas accurately by applying CNN from the WSI slides.[7,8] Kanavati et al.[8] used the CNN model with transfer learning and weakly supervised learning to identify and accurately classification of lung carcinomas from non-neoplastic lesions. They noted highly promising results for differentiating between lung carcinoma and non-neoplastic lesions. In the case of prostatic carcinoma, better diagnosis and Gleason's grading were obtained by DNN done on WSI images. The neural network reduces interobserver variability and provides consistent results.[9-11]

Deep learning neural networks identified and quantified various histological features particularly tumor budding in colorectal carcinoma.[12] Tumor microenvironment particularly immature desmoplastic stroma, inflammatory stroma, and epithelial tumor-infiltrating lymphocytes (TIL) in colorectal carcinoma were successfully evaluated by DNN in colorectal carcinoma.[12] The DNN picked up the characteristic morphological features that have prognostic importance.

Computational pathology with the application of CNN can score various diagnostic and prognostic markers such as mitotic index, Ki-67 scoring, PD-L1 scoring, and human epidermal growth factor receptor 2 (HER-2) scoring. Overall automated scoring is superior to digital scoring regarding high precision, consistency, and speed. Saha et al.[13] successfully scored Ki-67 in the hotspot region of breast carcinoma by using deep convolutional network.

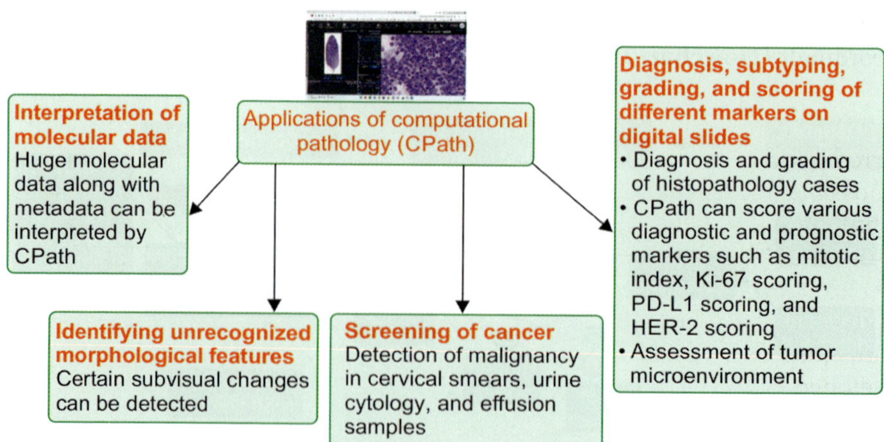

FLOWCHART 2: Clinical application of computational pathology.

Choschzick et al.[14] standardized Ki-67 scoring detection by DNN in vulval carcinoma cases with an accuracy of 96%. In another study, Ki-67 scoring was compared between manual and digital image analysis. The digital image analysis was considered as superior than manual counting.[15] Automated PD-L1 scoring was done with the help of convolutional neural network (CCN) in WSI image of metastatic head and neck squamous cell carcinoma. The study showed a good correlation between automated scoring and human scoring.[16] In another study, deep learning-based detection of PDL1 scoring was done on WSI images of small cell carcinoma of lung. The study showed good agreement between AI and pathologists.[17]

Screening of Cancer

Deep neural networks can bypass the extraction of details about morphological features on WSI images. DNN in WSI is widely used in the detection of malignancy in cervical smears, urine cytology, and effusion samples.[18-20]

Cheng et al.[21] made a recurrent neural network based model to classify cells in WSI images of cervical smears. They had 93.5% *specificity* and 95.1% *sensitivity*. Wang et al.[22] developed a complete automated system on WSIs of conventional Pap smear samples. They concluded that the automated analysis on WSI by DNN is fast and reliable. Zhang et al.[19] applied machine learning algorithms to identify abnormal urothelial cells. Ou et al.[23] successfully classified urothelial cell on urine according to Paris system with the help of AI-assisted WSI of urine.

Deep CNN was also used in the identification of malignant cells on pleural effusion. Most of the network model showed high sensitivity and specificity.[20,24]

Identifying Unrecognized Morphological Features

The pathologist usually studies selected morphological features to assess the prognosis of a case. However, there may be subvisual changes in WSI, which may be related with the patient's outcome.[25] Beck et al.[25] studied comprehensive analysis of automatically quantitated morphological features of breast carcinoma cases. They noted that certain stromal features of breast carcinoma cases are strongly associated with the overall survival of the patient's prognosis.

Molecular Study

Currently large amount of molecular data is available by NGS. It is quite impossible to interpret these data successfully. Zhao et al.[26] developed a novel technique of NGS data analysis. The entire process consists of four steps: (1) Retrieval of NGS data, (2) preprocessing the data, (3) topic modeling with the help of machine learning, which can interpret large data set from the text, and (4) data mining. Simple data extraction may not be enough as CPath needs to integrate the NGS data with WSI and clinical information. Dander et al.[27] developed a bioinformatics platform that can integrate all relevant clinical data, NGS data, and WSI images of the tissue. This bioinformatics platform is web-based and it is scalable, flexible, and expandable. The application is open-sourced and can be downloaded to use. A late fusion technology has been developed by integrating RNA sequencing data and WSI images of the histopathology of the tumor to accurately classify the non-small cell lung carcinomas.[28] So, this fusion methodology may be useful for the classification of different tumor.

CHALLENGES IN THE IMPLEMENTATION OF COMPUTATIONAL PATHOLOGY

There are several hurdles in the implementation of CPath. These are described in the following text.

Adequate Infrastructure

The proper infrastructure is required for the successful implementation of CPath. At first, there should be proper organization of the whole system such as collection of digitalized images, clinical data, data formatting, and building the AI model. So each laboratory needs a data operator to procure WSI images and clinical data. The bioinformatics person and computer software engineers are also needed for making the AI model. Implementation of CPath needs a huge amount of financial investment. WSI is costly and many laboratories cannot afford it. Moreover, the cost of trained manpower should also be considered.

Data Source and Storage

To build any successful AI model, a large amount of data is needed. This is not feasible for a single institution. Active collaboration from multiple institutes is needed for the data collection. Moreover, the text data should be formatted properly for use in the AI model. The other major problem is the storage of data. WSI takes up huge data space. So the storage of data is the major challenge in CPath.

Performance of the Computer

The data processing of the computer should be fast to deal with WSI images. The computer should have a powerful graphic processing unit. The speed of processing is very important as CNN may take a longer time to implement. To date, most of the laboratories have the standard computer that cannot handle huge data. Cloud-based image processing may be a solution to this problem.

Data Security

In cloud-based data use, cyber security is one of the major challenges of CPath. The patient's medical history is personal and each patient deserves the protection of his or her data. As the data is available on the internet and accessible by different laboratories, there is a high chance of misuse of the data.

Ethics

Medical ethics is another important aspect of CPath. There is a high chance of commercial use of the patient's data. This should be properly controlled. Hence, a proper guideline is required about the part of the data that can be used for CPath.

CONCLUSION

There is rapid development in the areas of digital images, molecular data, proteomics, and bioinformatics. It is high time to integrate these data by CPath. The CPath will be applicable for various areas of clinical oncology, particularly to detect the subvisual changes in tissue sections. In real life, there is no such established discipline like CPath. Many laboratories have only part of it. For the successful implementation of CPath, we need proper vision, good funding, human resources, and well collaborations among different laboratories. In addition, the intention of the pathologists to accept the newer technology is very important. Overall, most of us try to resist any newer technologies at the beginning. There are many hurdles to implementing the CPath particularly infrastructure, computer power, data collection, and medical ethics. It is expected that we will overcome these problems in the future and will implement CPath in the clinical laboratories.

REFERENCES

1. Dey P. Artificial neural network in diagnostic cytology. Cytojournal. 2022;19:27.
2. Dey P. The emerging role of deep learning in cytology. Cytopathology. 2021;32(2):154-60.
3. Louis DN, Feldman M, Carter AB, Dighe AS, Pfeifer JD, Bry L, et al. Computational Pathology: A Path Ahead. Arch Pathol Lab Med. 2016;140(1):41-50.
4. Saini T, Bansal B, Dey P. Digital cytology: Current status and future prospects. Diagn Cytopathol. 2023;51(3):211-8.
5. Dey P, Bansal B, Saini T. An emerging era of computational cytology. Diagn Cytopathol. 2023;51(4):270-5.
6. Dey P, Dey R. Artificial neural network--mechanism and application in pathology. Indian J Pathol Microbiol. 2002;45(3):371-4.
7. Chen CL, Chen CC, Yu WH, Chen SH, Chang YC, Hsu TI, et al. An annotation-free whole-slide training approach to pathological classification of lung cancer types using deep learning. Nat Commun. 2021;12(1):1193.
8. Kanavati F, Toyokawa G, Momosaki S, Rambeau M, Kozuma Y, Shoji F, et al. Weakly-supervised learning for lung carcinoma classification using deep learning. Sci Rep. 2020; 10(1):9297.
9. Singhal N, Soni S, Bonthu S, Chattopadhyay N, Samanta P, Joshi U, et al. A deep learning system for prostate cancer diagnosis and grading in whole slide images of core needle biopsies. Sci Rep. 2022;12(1):3383.
10. Bulten W, Pinckaers H, van Boven H, Vink R, de Bel T, van Ginneken B, et al. Automated deep-learning system for Gleason grading of prostate cancer using biopsies: a diagnostic study. Lancet Oncol. 2020;21(2):233-41.
11. Pantanowitz L, Quiroga-Garza GM, Bien L, Heled R, Laifenfeld D, Linhart C, et al. An artificial intelligence algorithm for prostate cancer diagnosis in whole slide images of core needle biopsies: a blinded clinical validation and deployment study. Lancet Digit Health. 2020;2(8):e407-e416.
12. Pai RK, Hartman D, Schaeffer DF, Rosty C, Shivji S, Kirsch R, et al. Development and initial validation of a deep learning algorithm to quantify histological features in colorectal carcinoma including tumour budding/poorly differentiated clusters. Histopathology. 2021;79(3):391-405.

13. Saha M, Chakraborty C, Arun I, Ahmed R, Chatterjee S. An Advanced Deep Learning Approach for Ki-67 Stained Hotspot Detection and Proliferation Rate Scoring for Prognostic Evaluation of Breast Cancer. Sci Rep. 2017;7(1):3213.
14. Choschzick M, Alyahiaoui M, Ciritsis A, Rossi C, Gut A, Hejduk P, et al. Deep learning for the standardized classification of Ki-67 in vulva carcinoma: A feasibility study. Heliyon. 2021;7(7):e07577.
15. Stålhammar G, Robertson S, Wedlund L, Lippert M, Rantalainen M, Bergh J, et al. Digital image analysis of Ki67 in hot spots is superior to both manual Ki67 and mitotic counts in breast cancer. Histopathology. 2018;72(6):974-89.
16. Puladi B, Ooms M, Kintsler S, Houschyar KS, Steib F, Modabber A, et al. Automated PD-L1 Scoring Using Artificial Intelligence in Head and Neck Squamous Cell Carcinoma. Cancers (Basel). 2021;13(17):4409.
17. van Eekelen L, Spronck J, Looijen-Salamon M, Vos S, Munari E, Girolami I, et al. Comparing deep learning and pathologist quantification of cell-level PD-L1 expression in non-small cell lung cancer whole-slide images. Sci Rep. 2024;14(1):7136.
18. Liang Y, Pan C, Sun W, Liu Q, Du Y. Global context-aware cervical cell detection with soft scale anchor matching. Comput Methods Programs Biomed. 2021;204:106061.
19. Zhang Z, Fu X, Liu J, Huang Z, Liu N, Fang F, et al. Developing a Machine Learning Algorithm for Identifying Abnormal Urothelial Cells: A Feasibility Study. Acta Cytol. 2021;65(4):335-41.
20. Xie X, Fu CC, Lv L, Ye Q, Yu Y, Fang Q, et al. Deep convolutional neural network-based classification of cancer cells on cytological pleural effusion images. Mod Pathol. 2022;35(5): 609-14.
21. Cheng S, Liu S, Yu J, Rao G, Xiao Y, Han W, et al. Robust whole slide image analysis for cervical cancer screening using deep learning. Nat Commun. 2021;12(1):5639.
22. Wang CW, Liou YA, Lin YJ, Chang CC, Chu PH, Lee YC, et al. Artificial intelligence-assisted fast screening cervical high grade squamous intraepithelial lesion and squamous cell carcinoma diagnosis and treatment planning. Sci Rep. 2021;11(1):16244.
23. Ou C, Tsao Y, Chang C, Lin S, Yang L, Hang F, et al. Evaluation of an artificial intelligence algorithm for assisting the Paris System in reporting urinary cytology: A pilot study. Cancer Cytopathol. 2022;130(11):872-80.
24. Sanyal P, Dey P. Using a deep learning neural network for the identification of malignant cells in effusion cytology material. Cytopathology. 2023;34(5):466-71.
25. Beck AH, Sangoi AR, Leung S, Marinelli RJ, Nielsen TO, van de Vijver MJ, et al. Systematic analysis of breast cancer morphology uncovers stromal features associated with survival. Sci Transl Med. 2011;3(108):108ra113.
26. Zhao W, Chen JJ, Perkins R, Wang Y, Liu Z, Hong H, Tong W, Zou W. A novel procedure on next generation sequencing data analysis using text mining algorithm. BMC Bioinformatics. 2016;17(1):213. Erratum in: BMC Bioinformatics. 2016;17:301.
27. Dander A, Baldauf M, Sperk M, Pabinger S, Hiltpolt B, Trajanoski Z. Personalized Oncology Suite: integrating next-generation sequencing data and whole-slide bioimages. BMC Bioinformatics. 2014;15(1):306.
28. Carrillo-Perez F, Morales JC, Castillo-Secilla D, Molina-Castro Y, Guillén A, Rojas I, et al. Non-small-cell lung cancer classification via RNA-Seq and histology imaging probability fusion. BMC Bioinformatics. 2021;22(1):454.

11

CHAPTER

Impact of Molecular Testing in Recent WHO Classification of Thyroid Lesions

Shruti Gupta, Niraj Kumari

INTRODUCTION

Thyroid lesions are a common occurrence in clinical practice with increased frequency of lesions occurring in women and adult population. Thyroid cancers (TCAs) are the most common endocrine malignancy in the world. More than 70% of these lesions are benign; however, the initial diagnosis is based on radiological and cytological evidence that affect the management of these lesions. Histomorphological features are also often overlapping and have significant interobserver variation in diagnosis. In everyday practice, thyroid malignancies pose a diagnostic challenge. To overcome these issues, tools such as immunohistochemistry, digital image analysis, and artificial neural networks have been explored with variable results.[1] Over the past two decades, with rapidly increasing knowledge of molecular mechanisms of thyroid cancers, interobserver variation in cytomorphologic evaluation of indeterminate lesions, and variable outcome, molecular methods have emerged as diagnostic, prognostic, and predictive markers of therapeutic significance.

The World Health Organization (WHO) classification of tumors essentially is an amalgamation of existing knowledge and emerging concepts for establishing a standard guideline for classification, accurate diagnosis, and uniform treatment of diseases. Over the last decade, the pathogenesis and multistage carcinogenesis of TCAs have been extensively studied. More than 90% of TCAs harbor driver mutations, gene fusions, and copy-number alterations. The WHO classification released in 2022 has been instrumental in emphasizing the role of molecular testing for classification and stratifying risk of thyroid lesions. The increased database of molecular mechanisms of thyroid dictates the inclusion of rare variants based on molecular features in the WHO classification. The latest WHO classification categorizes follicular cell derived lesions by strategic risk stratification based on the molecular pathways of tumorigenesis and with the basic understanding that driver genes implicated in well-differentiated thyroid cancers are mutually exclusive.[2]

MUTATIONAL LANDSCAPE OF THYROID LESIONS

Most TCAs arise from the multiple genetic alterations in thyroid follicular epithelial cells. The two major signaling pathways involved in development and progression of thyroid malignancies include the mitogen-activated protein kinase (MAPK) pathway and the PI3K/AKT pathway. The dysregulation in these two pathways contributes to development of most follicular cell derived malignancies of thyroid. For the instigation of papillary thyroid carcinomas (PTCs), MAPK activation is critical and for the instigation of follicular thyroid carcinomas, the activation of PI3K/AKT is crucial and key to the progression and development. PI3K/AKT pathway is also related with the downregulation of the iodide-handling machinery in thyroid cells. **Figure 1** illustrates the mechanisms and pathways for development and progression of thyroid malignancies. The NF-κB pathway has also been implicated to control antiapoptotic signaling pathway in cancer cells and upregulating the oncoproteins in the MAP kinase pathway.[3]

Kalarani et al. have discussed multiple candidate genes for thyroid carcinogenesis including *BAX* (BCL-2 associated X), *XRCC1* (X-ray repair cross-complementing group 1), *XRCC3* (X-ray repair cross-complementing group 3), *XP05* (exportin 5), *IL-10, BRAF, RET,* and *K-RAS.*[4]

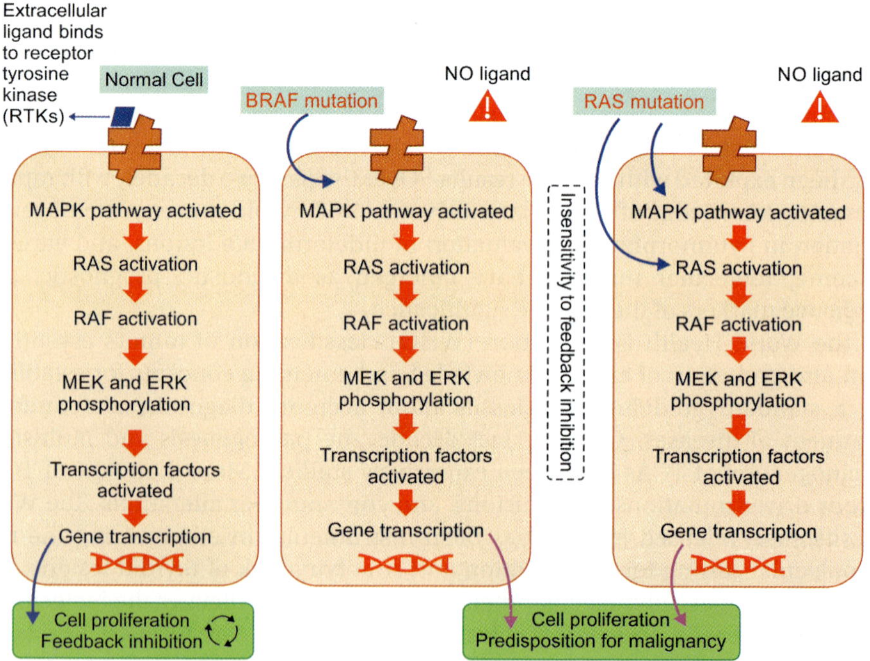

FIG. 1: Mechanisms and pathways for development and progression of thyroid malignancies. The MAPK pathway is activated in the absence of any ligand owing to BRAF and RAS mutations.

(BRAF: v-Raf murine sarcoma viral oncogene homolog B1; ERG: erythroblast transformation-specific-related gene; MAPK: mitogen-activated protein kinase; MEK: mitogen-activated protein kinase; RAS: rat sarcoma)

BRAF

The B-Raf proto-oncogene (*BRAF*) encodes for a cytoplasmic serine/threonine kinase and has a crucial role in regulating the MAP kinase pathway. BRAF mutations are noted in various malignancies including malignant melanoma, PTCs, pediatric low-grade gliomas, and colorectal and ovarian cancers. The most common BRAF mutation is the V600E caused due to thymidine to adenosine transversion at exon 15 nucleotide 1799 of the *BRAF* gene located on chromosome 7.[5] The prevalence of BRAFV600E mutation is noted in 35–60% in PTCs with higher prevalence among Asians, ranging from 45% to 76%. Among Asians, East Asians reported highest rates of BRAFV600E mutations (76.4%).[6] In patients with the classical PTCs, BRAFV600E mutation has been reported to have significant association with increased age, nodal and distant metastases, and recurrences, thus considered as a poor prognostic factor.[7] Other BRAF mutations are also known, of which the most common is the BRAFK601E mutation.

The cases harboring K601E follow the course of RAS-driven tumors and are often follicular patterned on histology.[8] Approximately 6% of FV-PTCs (follicular variant of PTC) harbor BRAFV601E mutations.[9]

RAS

The *RAS* gene family consists of primarily three small proteins KRAS, NRAS, and H-RAS that regulate signaling pathways for transduction. RAS mutations are the second most common mutations in thyroid tumors. They selectively activate the PI3K/AKT pathway in development of follicular cell derived tumors and cause constitutive RAS signaling.[8] Missense mutations in NRAS occur at codons 12, 13, 61, 141, and 146 in decreasing order of frequency. NRAS mutation at codon 61 has more oncogenic potential in follicular patterned lesions.[10] It is noteworthy that both benign and malignant thyroid lesions can harbor gain of function RAS mutations. Approximately 20–40% follicular adenomas (FA), 30–60% non-invasive follicular thyroid neoplasm with papillary-like nuclear features (NIFTP), 14–20% thyroid tumors with uncertain malignant potential, 15–43% FV-PTC, 30–50% follicular thyroid carcinoma (FTC) and 18–50% poorly differentiated thyroid carcinoma (PDTC) harbor RAS mutations.[11] A meta-analysis published by Riccio et al. discussing indeterminate thyroid nodules (ITNs) and RAS mutations has demonstrated that thyroid nodules with RAS-like mutations are less likely to have extrathyroidal extension and lymph node metastases. They have shown that RAS subtype can be utilized for its prognostic value as nodules with NRAS and KRAS mutations are associated with less aggressive disease compared to the HRAS counterpart.[12]

RET

RET proto-oncogene presents on paracentric region in the long arm of chromosome 10 and encodes a transmembrane tyrosine kinase receptor. Normally, receptor tyrosine kinases are not expressed in thyroid follicular cells and are restricted to parafollicular cells only. RET molecular alterations are linked with almost 95–98% of multiple endocrine neoplasias MEN2A and MEN2B, familial medullary thyroid carcinomas (MTCs), and 50% of sporadic MTCs.[13]

Germline RET point mutations are found in exon 10, 11, 16, 13, 14, and 15 in patients and family members of MTCs; however, RET-PTC rearrangements are detected in 35% of sporadic and 60% of radiation-induced PTC.[14]

RET point mutations act as an independent prognostic marker in risk stratification of MTC, where prophylactic thyroidectomies are recommended in relatives of MTC patients harboring high-risk RET mutations. The codons 883, 918, and 922 at exon 16 are at the highest risk of developing MTCs, followed by codons 611, 618, 620, and 634 located at exon 10 and 11. The codons 609, 768, 790, 804, and 891 are at lowest risk for development of MTCs.[13] Somatic RET mutations are associated with nodal metastases and worse prognosis.[15] PTC classically shows RET rearrangements of which most frequent is RET/PTC1 and RET/PTC3 in 90% of cases. Till date, more than 10 genotypes of RET/PTC rearrangements are reported in malignant thyroid lesions. RET/PTC3 rearrangements are associated with history of radiation exposure, younger age, and higher stage at presentation.[16]

PAX8/PPARG

PAX8 (Paired box-8) is a transcription factor responsible for normal development of thyroid, renal apparatus, and genital tracts. Peroxisome proliferator-activated receptor (PPAR) is a nuclear receptor, necessary for adipocyte and thyrocyte differentiation along with cell development. PAX8/PPARG rearrangements result in a fusion protein (PPFP), due to a chromosomal translocation between regions 2q13 and 3p25. This fusion protein stimulates oncogenesis through various mechanisms including transcriptional activation, proteasomal degradation, and novel transcriptional activity.[17]

Approximately 10–35% of FTCs harbor PAX8/PPARG rearrangement and PPFP fusion protein. Such lesions are more prone to have vascular and capsular invasion. Although few follicular adenomas (FAs) and PTCs also have the PAX8/PPARG rearrangement, the presence of PPFP fusion protein can be an important factor in making management decision and necessitating the need for surgical intervention in indeterminate thyroid cytology.[18] Detection of the fusion protein in thyroid lesions has therapeutic relevance as PPARG agonists can be used in clinical practice. PPARG agonist pioglitazone has been found to show treatment response in transgenic mice.[19]

TERT

TERT known as the telomerase reverse transcriptase protein is a critical protein for apoptosis and cell ageing. A gain of mutation in the TERT activates telomerase and promotes tumorigenesis. The hot-spot TERT mutations are cytidine to thymidine transition at 228 and 250 position, of which C228T is more frequent. In 2013, Liu et al. reported these hot-spot TERT promoter mutations in TCAs and noted that these are prevalent in aggressive thyroid cancers and BRAFV600E positive PTCs. They noticed the C228T mutation was noted in 37.5% of PDTC, 42.6% ATCs, and 11.7% PTCs. The frequency of TERT mutations was higher in

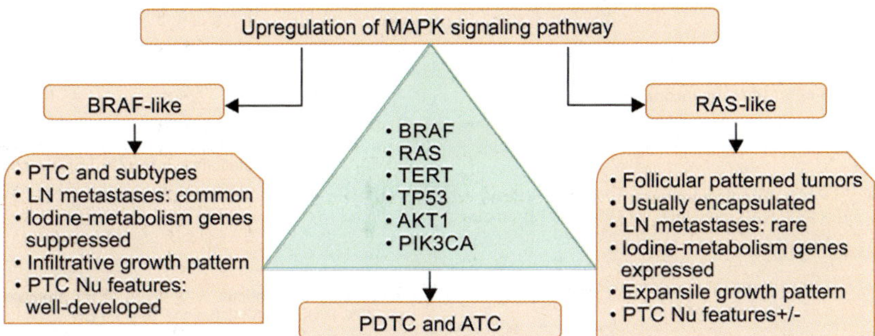

FLOWCHART 1: The frequency of molecular alterations in the various thyroid malignancies.
(LN: lymph node; MAPK: mitogen-activated protein kinase; PTC: papillary thyroid carcinoma; RAS: rat sarcoma; TERT: telomerase reverse transcriptase)

aggressive morphological PTC variants.[20] Recent studies have postulated that approximately 73% of anaplastic carcinoma and 40% poorly differentiated TCAs harbor TERT promoter mutation.[16] A large number of studies have shown that PTCs and FTCs with TERT promoter mutations show increased tendency of extrathyroidal extension, nodal, and distant metastases. A higher rate of TERT mutations was seen in BRAFV600E-mutated PTCs. A study of 182 PTCs by Muzza et al. has shown that higher rates of recurrence are noted in PTCs with TERT promoter mutations.[21]

Thus, the detection of TERT promoter mutations is of diagnostic relevance in preoperative fine needle aspirate and of predictive relevance for post-thyroidectomy patients with thyroid tumors for prognostic and aggressive management.

Flowchart 1 illustrates a plot portraying the frequency of molecular alterations in different types of TCAs.

THE CANCER GENOME ATLAS[22]

The Cancer Genome Atlas (TCGA) project gathered multidimensional genomic findings by comprehensive analysis of 496 cases of PTC using multiple techniques by combining the analysis of multiple genomic variations, gene expressions, methylation, and microRNA alterations. The collaborative efforts have not only clarified the mutational landscape of PTC but also establish the relationship between tumor histology, differentiation, and genotype.

The TCGA reemphasizes the fact that PTCs are driven by the MAP kinase pathway, and BRAF and RAS mutations are mutually exclusive to each other. TCGA has classified PTCs into RAS-like and BRAF-like tumors, which have prominent signaling differences, leading to different genomic and morphological characteristics. **Figure 2** depicts the key features of RAS-like and BRAF-like tumors. A BRAFV600E-RAS gene expression score (BRS) has been developed during the TCGA analysis, which delineates the two classifiers. The BRAF-like tumors have classical PTC-like morphology, exhibit higher MAP kinase activity, harbor lower iodine metabolic capacity, and lower hormone differentiation.

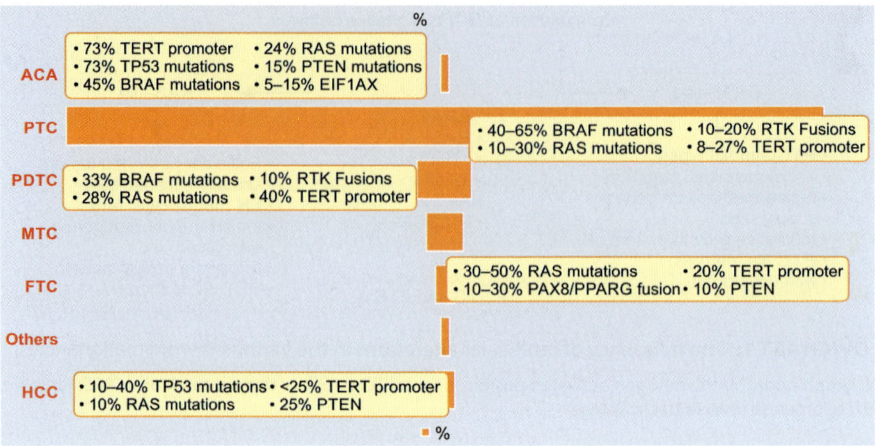

FIG. 2: The key features of RAS-like and BRAF-like tumors are illustrated along with key molecular alterations in poorly differentiated and anaplastic thyroid carcinomas.

(ACA: anaplastic thyroid carcinoma; FTC: follicular thyroid carcinoma; HCC: hepatocellular carcinoma; MTC: medullary thyroid cancer; PTC: papillary thyroid carcinoma; PTDC: poorly differentiated thyroid carcinoma; PTEN: phosphatase and tensin homolog; RAS: rat sarcoma; TERT: telomerase reverse transcriptase)

The RAS-like tumors retain the expression of thyroid differentiation factors and signaling occurs through both MAP kinase and PI3K. A thyroid differentiation score (TDS) was devised using 16 thyroid metabolism and function genes.[22]

The reclassification of PTCs in the fifth edition has been done owing to the characteristic molecular profiles as IEFVPTC which has RAS-like profile while infiltrative follicular variant of PTC which has BRAF-like profile.

In addition, TCGA has identified mutations in other genes such as *EIF1AX, RET,* and *ALK* in PTC and also classifies BRAF-PTC into molecular subtypes.

BRAF-mutant tumors can be categorized based on the "tumor differentiation score" into BRAF-TDS-hi and BRAF-TDS-lo. The TDS-hi group has preserved expression of iodine metabolism genes and correlates with smaller sized tumors and less nodal involvement. The TDS-lo group has larger sized tumors, increased tendency for nodal and distant metastases.[23]

The TCGA has identified markers for prognostication of PTC using expression of miR-21 and TERT promoter mutations as an indicator of aggressive behavior. The TCGA associates TERT promoter mutation with higher patient age and increased rate of recurrence.

The multiplatform TCGA analysis had a huge impact on the management of ITNs. The discoveries have encouraged researchers for the reclassification of follicular-derived neoplasms in the latest classification.

Lim et al. have utilized the TCGA database information and analyzed the RNA sequencing data of 503 PTCs and have demonstrated that the tumor microenvironment plays a crucial role in tumor progression in BRAF-like PTCs.[24]

MOLECULAR TESTS

Based on the extensive molecular profiling, different molecular tests have been introduced and validated across various institutions. The role of molecular

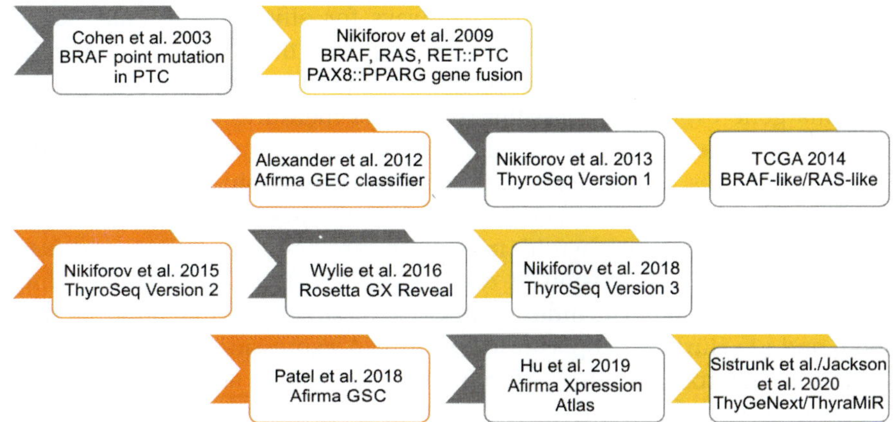

FIG. 3: Timeline of development of laboratory assays for molecular testing in thyroid lesions.
(GEC: gene expression classifier; GSC: gene sequence classifier; PTC: papillary thyroid carcinoma; RAS: rat sarcoma)

testing and its correlation with the TBSRTC ITNs have become the mainstay of preoperative thyroid nodule assessment mainly for diagnostic purposes.[25] Postoperative molecular tests are being increasingly used for risk stratification and targeted therapy in advanced thyroid cancers.

The history of molecular testing has been discussed by Bayan et al. in detail. The testing dates back four decades back when Fusco et al. tested five cases of PTC and found TRK and RET rearrangements. Later, Lemoine et al. noted N and H RAS mutations in various stages of thyroid tumorigenesis which was followed by Namba et al. Further, the identification of steps in tumorigenesis, and laboratory assays came into the picture in the early 2000s.[26] The timeline of development of laboratory assays is depicted in **Fig. 3**. Cohen et al. successfully identified the BRAFV600E mutation in PTCs and correlated with the histological diagnosis creating a breakthrough for development of laboratory assays for detection of PTC in ITNs.[27]

Since then, molecular tests are increasingly used for risk stratification in ITNs. The detection of specific somatic mutations, gene rearrangements, and microRNA expression profiles can have high specificity and high positive predictive values (PPV) for TCAs.[28] It is noteworthy that molecular testing is not essential but may be parallelly carried in indeterminate thyroid cytology in subjects with nodule size more than 4 cm and/or any compressive symptoms.[29]

The goal of molecular testing is to effectively "rule in" or "rule out" a malignant thyroid lesion. To predict malignancy, a test should have "high" PPV and to predict benignity, a test should have a "high" negative predictive value (NPV).[30] However, the testing is not straight forward and the larger challenge is that the NPV and PPV depend on the prevalence of thyroid malignancies in the given population. Validation studies for different populations need to be done for different populations before any definite guidelines could be set.[31]

A combination of cancer mutations and gene expression profiling, identification of new mutations and miRNA expression profiles, and next-generation sequencing (NGS) analysis are the pathways for efficient molecular testing. **Flowchart 2** depicts an algorithmic approach for the various commercially available laboratory developed assays available in the market.

Afirma gene expression classifier (GEC) test measures the transcription of 142 gene expression panel for thyroid lesions and 25 gene expression panel to rule out metastases, medullary carcinoma, and parathyroid lesions. The Afirma gene sequence classifier (GSC) comprises of a sequence of classifiers that detect mRNA expression for parathyroid, medullary carcinoma and BRAF, and fusion transcripts for RET/PTC fusion. It also includes: (1) Follicular content index (mRNA expression), (2) HC index (mRNA expression and mitochondrial transcripts), and (3) Hürthle neoplasm index (mRNA expression and chromosomal level loss of heterozygosity).[6,29] Afirma GSC has definite advantages over GEC including improved specificity and PPV and improved performance with oncocytic neoplasms. The high sensitivity and NPV attained with GEC are maintained in GSC. The study by Vuong et al. concluded that Afirma GSC can classify a larger percentage of nodules with indeterminate thyroid cytology as benign.[32]

Next-generation sequencing forms the mainstay of many available molecular tests. The major benefit of NGS is that meagre quantity of cellular material can be exploited to detect multiple genetic alterations in a single test. ThyroSeq v.2 is a test that uses NGS technology for the analysis of 14 genes, 42 gene fusions, and expression levels of 16 genes. BRAF, *RAS* genes, PIK3CA, TP53, RET, promoter of TERT, and others are screened for point mutations at DNA level. The gene fusions are detected by mRNA expression. ThyroSeq v3 is another test using DNA- and RNA-based NGS assay that analyses 112 genes for point mutations, insertions/deletions, gene fusions, copy-number variations, and abnormal gene expression. This approach utilizes a genomic classifier to separate malignant lesions from benign lesions. ThyroSeq v3 has an added advantage over ThyroSeq v2 by including benign and malignant oncocytic lesions.[33]

ThyGenX is a commercially available 7-gene panel using NGS to detect genetic alterations. ThyraMIR is a microRNA expression-based classifier which evaluates 10 microRNA. It can enhance specificity and sensitivity with ThyGenX. RosettaGX Reveal is a microRNA expression-based classifier which evaluates 24 microRNA. It has an added advantage that it can be performed on pre-existing FNA smears. Of these, the Afirma-GEC and Rosetta GX Reveal are considered as rule-out tests. ThyroSeq v2 and ThyGenX clubbed with ThyraMIR are considered as both, "rule-in" and "rule-out" tests.[34,35]

Molecular risk groups have been created based on the various tests comprising: Low-risk—lesions having a single RAS mutation or a RAS-like variant; Intermediate-risk: lesions having BRAFV600E mutation, BRAF-like variants and copy-number alterations, and High-risk: lesions with TERT, TP53, AKT1, and PIK3CA alterations.[35]

A new classifier based on real-time polymerase chain reaction (real-time PCR) and a neural network program named as ThyroidPrint has been developed recently. This is a multiplexed quantitative PCR test based on 10-gene signature has been reported to have a sensitivity of 91%, a PPV of 95%, and NPV of 78% in validation studies.[36]

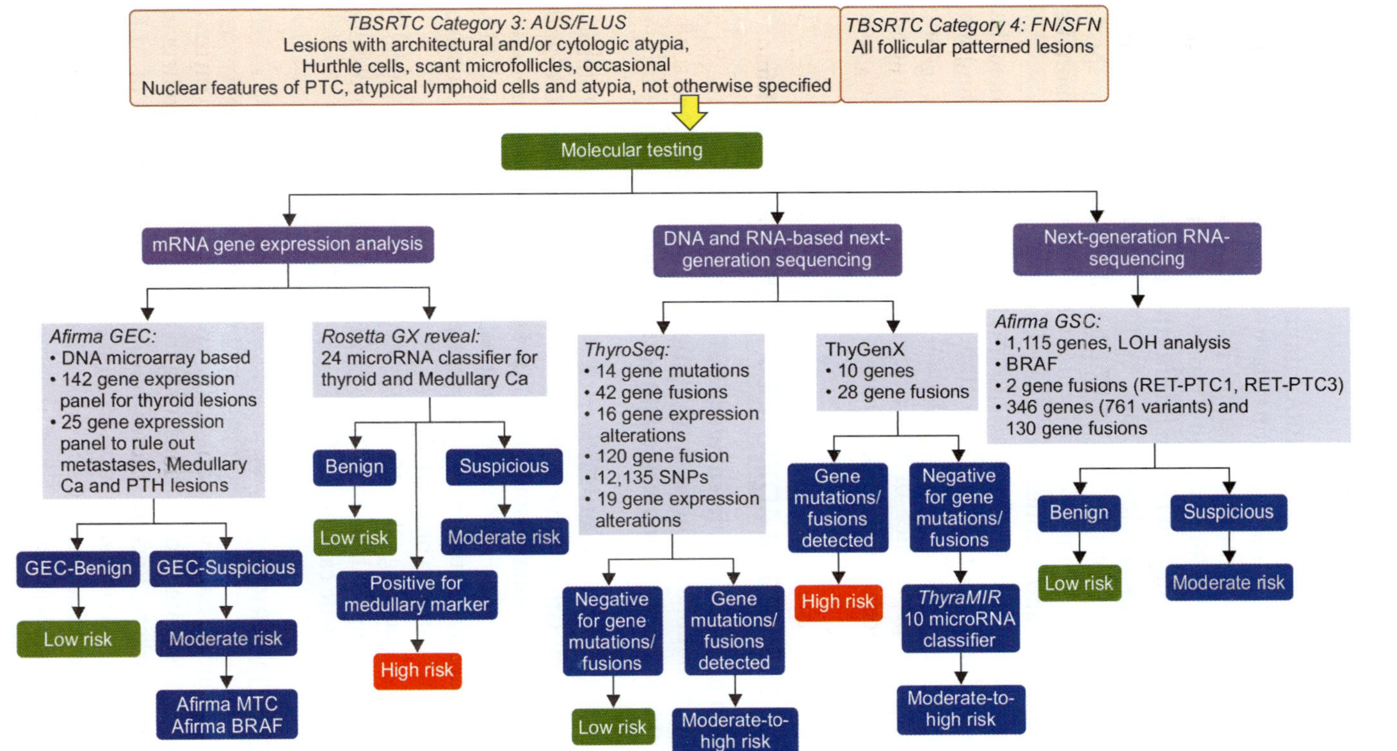

FLOWCHART 2: An algorithmic approach for the various commercially available laboratory developed assays.

(GEC: gene expression classifier; GSC: gene sequence classifier; PTC: papillary thyroid carcinoma)

Another mi-RNA-based classifier is the mir-THYpe, which is being utilized for TBSRTC III and IV and evaluates 11 mi-RNA expression profiles. A multicenter study by Santos et al. has reported sensitivity of 89%, PPV of 66%, and NPV of 95%.[36]

Owing to the increased prevalence of BRAF mutations in Asians, molecular testing for BRAFV600E and RAS mutations have been tried in the Indian perspectives using thyroid fine needle aspirates by using standardized kits for real-time PCR technology.[37,38] **Figures 4A to F** represent a picture panel portraying the utility of molecular testing in ITN on fine needle aspiration.

A wide range of cytology specimens such as FNA smears (cyto-scrapes), aspirate in nucleic acid preservative, cell blocks, liquid-based cytology specimens, and supernatants can be used for molecular testing, depending upon the availability of the platform and routine standardized protocols.

It is significant to understand that the interpretation of these molecular testing must be done with the correlation of clinical and radiological findings owing to substantial heterogeneity in the individual tumors as well as the testing platforms available and prevalence of TCa across the continents. A prudent management decision needs a multidisciplinary approach of the pathologists and the surgeons.

MOLECULAR TESTING IN ADVANCED THYROID CANCERS

Molecular testing in high grade, differentiated, and advanced thyroid cancers is targeted to identify mutations for therapeutic purposes. Advanced TCAs usually have multiple mutations, copy-number alterations, and fusions which contribute to the aggressive behavior.

American Head and Neck Society Endocrine Surgery Section and International Thyroid Oncology Group have extensively reviewed the literature and issued guidelines for mutational testing in TCAs. For advanced, differentiated TCAs, multistep testing for BRAFV600E, RET fusions, NTRK1/2 fusions, and ALK fusions is recommended for initiation of appropriate therapy. A comprehensive tissue-based NGS panel can also be used.[39]

A tissue-based NGS covering all SNVs, indels, copy-number alterations, and gene rearrangements along with a simultaneous BRAFV600E mutation testing is recommended in anaplastic carcinoma.[39]

EMERGING BIOMARKERS[40]

Whole-genome sequencing has revolutionized the oncology practice, and thyroid lesions are being investigated for various diagnostic, prognostic, predictive, and therapeutic biomarkers. Recent studies have implicated the role of ALK translocations with a range of fusion partners in a small subset of PTC, PDTC, and anaplastic thyroid carcinomas (ACAs). ALK alterations are more frequently noted in female PTC patients who have undergone radiation therapy. The availability of crizotinib mandates ALK testing, which can be performed by ALK immunohistochemistry.

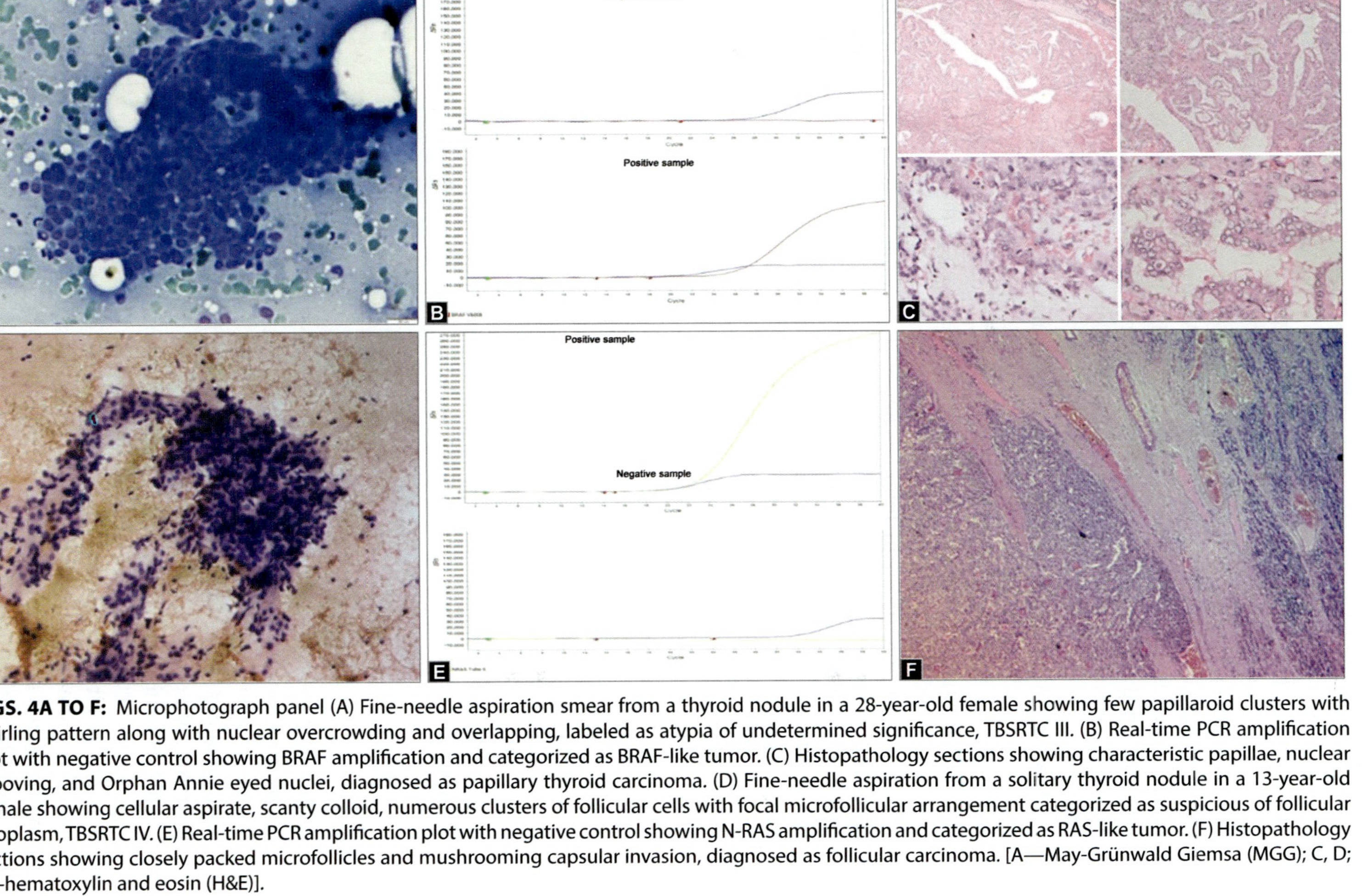

FIGS. 4A TO F: Microphotograph panel (A) Fine-needle aspiration smear from a thyroid nodule in a 28-year-old female showing few papillaroid clusters with swirling pattern along with nuclear overcrowding and overlapping, labeled as atypia of undetermined significance, TBSRTC III. (B) Real-time PCR amplification plot with negative control showing BRAF amplification and categorized as BRAF-like tumor. (C) Histopathology sections showing characteristic papillae, nuclear grooving, and Orphan Annie eyed nuclei, diagnosed as papillary thyroid carcinoma. (D) Fine-needle aspiration from a solitary thyroid nodule in a 13-year-old female showing cellular aspirate, scanty colloid, numerous clusters of follicular cells with focal microfollicular arrangement categorized as suspicious of follicular neoplasm, TBSRTC IV. (E) Real-time PCR amplification plot with negative control showing N-RAS amplification and categorized as RAS-like tumor. (F) Histopathology sections showing closely packed microfollicles and mushrooming capsular invasion, diagnosed as follicular carcinoma. [A—May-Grünwald Giemsa (MGG); C, D; F—hematoxylin and eosin (H&E)].

Basic tests such as immunohistochemistry can be used as surrogate markers to detect molecular alterations. Antibodies for BRAFV600E, RAS, PTEN, ALK mutations, and NTRK fusions are being used for TCA management.

NTRK rearrangements have been noted in PTCs presenting as multinodular lesions with infiltrative growth pattern and follicular patterned lesions with papillae and solid areas. NTRK-rearranged TCAs are associated with lymphovascular invasion, nodal metastases, and extrathyroidal extension. NTRK fusion proteins, on the other hand, encode for transmembrane proteins TrkA, TrkB, and TrkC which respectively activate the MAP kinase, RAS-ERK, and PI3/AKT pathway.

Apart from the embryonal thyroid neoplasms, DICER1 mutations are also noted in 75% females and 17% males clinically presenting with multinodular goiter (MNG). Individuals with germline DICER1 mutations are predisposed to thyroid follicular hyperplasia. It is recommended that pediatric MNG patients be tested for DICER1 mutations.

The role of microRNA in thyroid cancers forms the basis of various commercially available miRNA classifiers. miR-21, miR-127, miR-136, miR-146b, miR-221, miR-222, and miR-181b have been shown to be upregulated in PTCs, while miR-146b, miR-221, and miR-222 are upregulated in ACAs. Among MTCs, upregulation of miR-21, miR-183, and miR-375 has been related to poor prognosis.[40]

Currently, the role of liquid biopsy in diagnosis and monitoring of TCa is also being investigated. Newer technologies are enabling ease of detection of cell free DNA, circulating tumor cells and microRNA in the blood. Attempts for detection of BRAFV600E mutations and NTRK fusions in PTC can be instrumental in the patient management. RET mutation detection is now widely practiced liquid biopsy in family members of MTC patients.[41]

Anaplastic thyroid carcinoma has shown higher expression of programmed death-ligand 1 (PD-L1), and multiple clinical trials are exploring the role of immunotherapy for TCa. PD-L1 can be detected immunohistochemically easily using specific clones.[42]

2022 WHO CLASSIFICATION OF THYROID TUMORS

The WHO classification 2022 encompasses novel concepts in thyroid pathology including the relevant changes in nomenclature and grading of thyroid lesions based on histomorphology and molecular features.[2] The present edition has taken into account the cell of origin and molecular profile in detail. The pathologic characteristics have been discussed in the light of molecular profile, along with the clinical outcome. The follicular cell derived neoplasms have been graded as benign, low-risk, and malignant lesions based on their clinicopathological characteristics and genetic alterations. The previous WHO classification has dealt with molecular-genetic characterization of well-differentiated follicular-patterned thyroid tumors with limited success.[43] The new classification lays emphasis on classification based on cell of origin and tumor differentiation. Immunohistochemical markers and gene expression analysis can be used as effective tools for the classification.[44] **Figure 5** illustrates the latest WHO

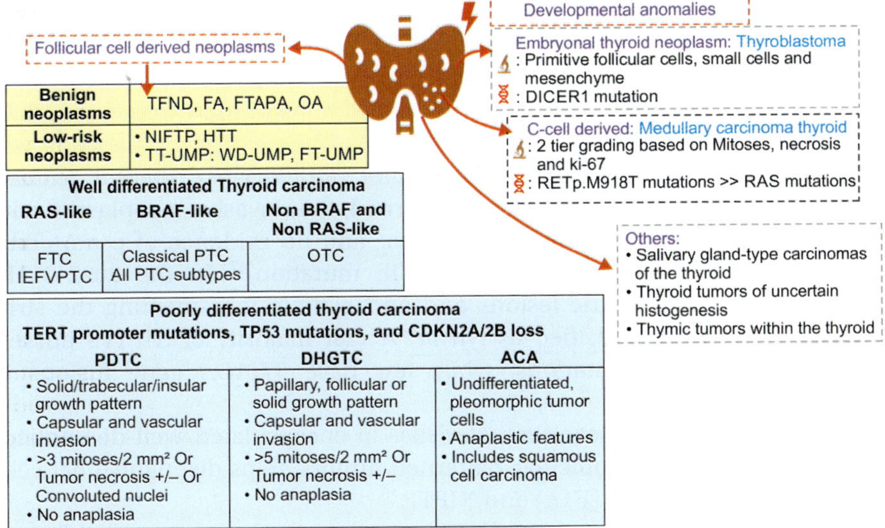

FIG. 5: 2022 WHO classification of thyroid neoplasms and its correlation with the molecular features.

(ACA: anaplastic thyroid carcinoma; FA: follicular adenoma; FTAPA: follicular adenoma with papillary architecture; FTC: follicular thyroid carcinoma; IEFVPTC: invasive encapsulated follicular variant of papillary thyroid carcinoma; PTC: papillary thyroid carcinoma; PDTC: poorly differentiated thyroid carcinoma; TFND: thyroid follicular nodular disease; TT-UMP: thyroid tumors of uncertain malignant potential)

classification of thyroid neoplasms and its correlation with the molecular features.[2]

FOLLICULAR CELL DERIVED NEOPLASMS

Benign Neoplasms

Owing to the molecular profiling studies, it is now clear that the spectrum of multifocal benign nodules can be clonal and thus have been christened as *"Thyroid follicular nodular disease"* (TFND) which encompasses the entities previously labeled as hyperplastic nodule, multinodular/adenomatous/colloid goiter. 70% TFNDs are known to have TSHR mutation.[44]

Follicular adenoma with papillary architecture (FTAPA) is a benign, encapsulated tumor which has intrafollicular papillary architecture but no nuclear features of PTC. FTAPA are autonomous hyperfunctioning nodules and have mutations in TSHR, GNAS, PRKAR1A, and EZH1, unlike the classical FAs which have RAS mutations. Few of these can also possess DICER1 mutations. FTAPA need careful histomorphological assessment of the nuclear features and should not be mistaken for PTC.[45]

The usage of term Hurthle cell has been discouraged and is replaced by oncocytic cells as the term "Hurthle" was originally used by German histologist Karl Hurthle to describe parafollicular C cells.[2,45] Later, another German pathologist Herwig Hamperl coined the term "oncocytic" for the polyhedral cells with abundant, oxyphilic cytoplasm, and central round nucleus.[46]

Oncocytic adenomas (OAs) are benign, encapsulated tumors consisting of >75% oncocytic cells. OAs have specific gene mutations in the mitochondrial biosynthesis system, such as ESRRA and PPARGC1A.[44]

Low-risk Neoplasms

Noninvasive follicular thyroid neoplasm with papillary-like nuclear features (NIFTPs) are described as follicular patterned, noninvasive neoplasms with PTC-like nuclear features, mitoses <3/2 mm^2 and no evidence of psammoma bodies, tumor necrosis, and BRAF p.V600E mutation.[47] In the 2022 WHO classification, subcentimetric lesions and oncocytic lesions meeting the strict diagnostic criteria are classified as NIFTP. A vast majority of NIFTPs possess RAS and BRAFV601E mutations, while few have *THADA* gene fusions or PAX8::PPARG.[45]

The assessment of nuclear characteristics in encapsulated/well-demarcated noninvasive RAS-mutant follicular-patterned tumors helps distinguish between follicular thyroid adenoma (FTA) and NIFTP.[48]

Hyalinizing trabecular tumors (HTT) are described as tumors with pure trabecular architecture, extracellular hyaline matrix, and PTC-like nuclear features. GLIS3 regulates thyroid gland development and hormone synthesis.[40] HTTs have specific PAX8::GLIS fusions which can be used as a diagnostic marker. Few authors have utilized surrogate immunohistochemical marker using an antibody to C-terminus region of GLIS3.[49] Ki-67 cell membrane reactivity (with MIB1 Mab) is another unique feature of HTT.[45,47]

The term "Thyroid tumors of uncertain malignant potential (TT-UMP)" is reserved for those thyroid neoplasms where extensive examination of capsule shows questionable capsular/vascular invasion. TT-UMPs with PTC-like nuclear features are termed as WDT-UMP and those without the nuclear features are called FT-UMP. These tumors carry various driver mutations including RAS, EIF1AX, TSHR, and PAX8::PPARG rearrangements.[44] Vigorous guidelines for assessment of capsular/vascular invasion need to be identified.

Table 1 tabulates the key identification features of benign and low-risk thyroid neoplasms.

Malignant Neoplasms

Follicular thyroid carcinomas (FTCs) are tumors with predominant follicular growth pattern, classically divided based on capsular/vascular invasion as minimally invasive, encapsulated angioinvasive, and widely invasive. This stratification shows direct correlation with patient prognosis and survival and it is important to look closely for these features. Morphologically, FTCs show no features of PTC-like nuclear atypia. The 5th edition maintains the categorization and emphasizes on the RAS-like character of these neoplasms.[2,45]

Assessment of the tumor interface and examination of entire capsule at multiple levels is of paramount importance. NRASQ61R-specific immunohistochemistry can be used for identifying invasion.[48]

Invasive encapsulated follicular variant of papillary thyroid carcinoma (IEFVPTC) are distinct entities with fibrous capsule but can show angioinvasion

TABLE 1: The key identification features of benign and low-risk thyroid neoplasms as per WHO 2022 classification.

Follicular cell derived neoplasms			Key identification features	Capsular/ vascular invasion	Characteristics genetic alterations
Benign		TFND	• Multinodular • Encapsulated	No	• TSHR6 mutation (70%) • Others: GNAS, EZH1, ZNF148, and SPOP
		FA	• Solitary nodule/ encapsulated	No	• RAS-like mutations
		FTAPA	• Solitary nodule/ encapsulated • Intrafollicular papillary architecture	No	• Increased frequency of ESRRA and PPARGC1A
		OA	• Solitary nodule/ encapsulated • >75% oncocytic tumor cells	No	• RAS mutations • PAX8::PPARG translocations
Low-risk	TT-UMP	NIFTP	• Encapsulated • Follicular growth pattern • PTC-like nuclear features	No	• BRAFV600E • RET rearrangements • TERT promoter mutations
		FT-UMP	• Follicular growth pattern • Non-PTC-like nuclear features	Questionable	• RAS-like mutations • Mutations in EIF1AX and TSHR • PAX8::PPARG rearrangements
		WD-UMP	• Follicular growth pattern • PTC-like nuclear features	Questionable	
		HTT	• PTC-like nuclear atypia • Trabecular growth pattern • Extracellular hyaline matrix • Ki-67 membranous staining	No	• PAX8::GLIS1 and PAX8::GLIS3 fusions

(FA: follicular adenoma; FTAPA: follicular adenoma with papillary architecture; FT-UMP: follicular tumor of uncertain malignant potential; HTT: hyalinizing trabecular tumor; NIFTP: noninvasive follicular thyroid neoplasm with papillary-like nuclear features; PTC: papillary thyroid carcinoma; RAS: rat sarcoma; TERT: telomerase reverse transcriptase; TFND: thyroid follicular nodular disease; TT-UMP: thyroid tumors of uncertain malignant potential) and can metastasize. IEFVPTC is included under the RAS-driven tumors, and this distinction from PTC has been done owing to the different molecular profiles of PTC and IEFVPTC. The RNA expression profiling of IEFVPTC is similar to FA, FTC, and not PTC.[50] Thus, these tumors have better prognosis than the invasive follicular variant of PTCs.

PTC and subtypes: The TCGA project has extensively studied the molecular landscape of PTCs and its correlation with histological subtypes. The WHO 2022 classification emphasizes the importance of histological subtyping of PTC along with detection of the BRAF-like and RAS-like characteristics. The term variant is replaced by the term subtypes and various subtypes including *classic, encapsulated classic, infiltrative follicular, diffuse sclerosing, solid/trabecular, tall cell, columnar cell, hobnail, clear cell, spindle cell, Warthin-like, oncocytic, and PTC with fibromatosis/fasciitis-like/desmoid-type stroma* are described.[50]

The *classical PTCs* have true papillae with a fibrovascular core, nuclear features of papillary carcinoma and are essentially BRAFV600E driven tumors.

The *infiltrative follicular PTCs (IF-PTCs)* have follicular architecture with a infiltrative growth pattern and a BRAF-like phenotype. IF-PTCs show atypical nuclear features, psammoma bodies, stromal fibrosis, and increased risk of lymphatic invasion.[51]

The more aggressive subtypes of PTC include the tall cell, columnar cell, and hobnail morphology. The 2022 WHO defines the tall cell variant with the tall cells ≥3 times tall than wide. The diagnosis of hobnail subtype is based on the cut-off of 30% hobnail cells. However, the aggressive clinical presentation and increased nuclear atypia along with mixed papillary and micropapillary pattern with 10–30% hobnail cells should prompt a diagnosis of Hobnail PTCs. However, the aggressive clinical presentation and increased nuclear atypia along with mixed papillary and micropapillary pattern with hobnail cells should prompt a diagnosis of Hobnail PTCs.[51] These subtypes are associated with increased risk of nodal metastasis, recurrences, distant metastases, and worse outcomes.[2,45]

The entity papillary thyroid microcarcinoma based on tumor size has been disregarded and histological subtyping of the subcentimetric PTCs is recommended as it is for the conventional PTCs. Similarly, the solid PTC subtype should show >50% of solid/trabecular tumor growth pattern. In the 4th edition, the cribriform morular tumor was classified as PTC variant, but molecular profiling has defied the follicular cell derivation of these tumors, and they have been included under the tumors of uncertain histogenesis in the 2022 update.[43,45]

Oncocytic carcinomas (OCAs) are described as invasive lesions with >75% oncocytic cells, <5 mitoses/mm^2, and absence of tumor necrosis. OCAs are differentiated from oncocytic adenomas on the account of capsular and vascular invasion. Based on the invasion, three subtypes minimally invasive, encapsulated angioinvasive, and invasive neoplasms are described. Approximately 81% OCAs harbor copy-number alterations.[51] OCAs are uncommon lesions and should not be mistaken for oxyphilic PTCs which harbor BRAFV600E mutations.

OCAs can harbor *RAS, TSHR, EIF1AX, TP53, PTEN, BRAF, PAX8-PPAR*γ, and *MEN1* mutations.[46]

It is important to note that the 2022 WHO classification emphasized on the reporting of well differentiated TCa after excluding high-grade features such as tumor necrosis and/or ≥5 mitoses per 2 mm^2.[51] All differentiated TCAs (PTCs/FTCs/OTCs) with these high-grade features, the term *"differentiated high-grade thyroid carcinoma" (DHGTC)* is specified. This encourages the histopathologists to actively look for mitoses and tumor necrosis in cases designated as PTCs/FTCs/OTCs and thus better prognostication at histological level.

The term poorly differentiated TCa (PDTC) is explained by two consensus protocols: The Turin consensus and the Memorial Sloan Kettering Cancer Center (MSKCC). The WHO 2022 has espoused the Turin consensus and defines PDTCs as poorly differentiated carcinomas with solid/trabecular/insular growth pattern and at least one of the following characteristics: convoluted nuclei, ≥3 mitosis per 2 mm^2, and tumor necrosis.[51]

Both PDTCs and DHGTCs harbor BRAF and RAS mutations along with poor prognostic genetic alterations such as: TP53, CDKN2A, PIK3CA, AKT1, and TERT promoter mutations. It is postulated that DHGTCs are mostly derived from BRAF-driven PTCs, while PDTCs often exhibit aberrant RAS signaling.[45]

A combination of BRAF p.V600E and TERT promoter mutations referred to as "genetic duet".[44] The occurrence of this genetic duet is associated with poor prognosis and poor curative effect of radioiodine therapy in PTC.[52]

The major changes in the 5th edition *anaplastic thyroid carcinoma (ACA)* is the inclusion of squamous cell carcinoma (SCC) as a subtype based on the molecular profile. It was noted that most SCC express TTF-1 and PAX-8 and also have BRAFV600E mutations and poor outcome such as the ACAs. The indicators of outcome in ACAs include gross residual disease, size of the tumor, encapsulation, margin status, and TERT promoter mutations.[53]

The 2022 WHO classification recommends the use of BRAF p.V600E mutation-specific VE1 immunohistochemistry in all patients with ACAs for targeted therapy against BRAF and MEK inhibitor.[45]

C-cell Derived Neoplasms

Medullary carcinoma of thyroid, derived from parafollicular C cells, is characterized by RET mutations. Most hereditary cases have RET mutation while sporadic cases harbor RET mutations followed by RAS mutations.[44] The 2022 WHO classification recommends two-tier grading of MTCs based on presence and absence of necrosis, proliferation index, Ki-67 ≥5%, and mitoses ≥5 cells/2 mm^2. This grading system is an innovative scheme for risk stratification and survival analysis of MTCs. Based on this grading, majority of MTCs are found to be low grade. However, for adequate prognostication, adequate sampling and thorough clinical assessment are pertinent.[2]

Others[2]

There are four other categories described on the basis of cell of origin: Embryonal thyroid neoplasms, Salivary gland type carcinomas, thyroid tumors of uncertain histogenesis, and thymic tumors. Thyroblastoma is a rare embryonal tumor of thyroid with primitive differentiation, showing DICER1 mutation and

SALL4 immunopositivity. Salivary gland carcinomas of the thyroid include mucoepidermoid carcinomas (MECs) and secretory carcinoma (SeC). Thyroid MECs are histologically similar to MECs arising in the salivary gland and few cases show CRTC1::MAML2 fusion. Thyroid SeCs are also histologically similar to SeC arising in the salivary gland and always show ETV6::NTRK3 fusions.[2] Among the intrathyroidal thymic tumors, the term "thyroid carcinoma showing thymic-like differentiation" is replaced by "intrathyroid thymic carcinoma".

Thyroid tumors of uncertain histogenesis are a newer entity in the 2022 classification and has been introduced based on the fact that these tumors do not express thyroglobulin or PAX-8 and show focal TTF-1 expression. The cell of origin and differentiation of lesions under this category (Sclerosing mucoepidermoid carcinoma with eosinophilia and Cribriform morular thyroid carcinoma) is a matter of debate.[2,45]

TARGETED THERAPY IN THYROID CANCERS[42]

The role of molecular profiling lies in understanding the pathogenesis, and thus affecting the treatment protocols. The benign and low-risk are easily managed by surgical resection and adequate follow-up, while advanced thyroid cancers with systemic involvement are increasing tested for molecular alterations and instigation of targeted treatment.

For BRAFV600E mutant locally advanced, unresectable, or metastatic solid tumors, a combination of dabrafenib (BRAF inhibitor) and trametinib (MEK inhibitor) is approved by US-FDA. For locally advanced, unresectable, or metastatic solid tumors with NTRK fusions selective TRK inhibitors as larotrectinib and multikinase inhibitors as entrectinib are recommended.

A vast majority of MTC patients are treated by surgical resection; however, residual disease and recurrence pose a treatment challenge for oncologists. The FDA has approved selpercatinib (selective RET kinase inhibitor) and pralsetinib (tyrosine kinase inhibitor) for RET-mutant positive MTCs.[42]

CONCLUSION

With the advancing knowledge and inclusion of molecular tests for thyroid cancers, new insights regarding tumorigenesis of thyroid lesions have come into light. This chapter discusses the molecular alterations in thyroid cancers along with various commercially available assays. The chapter also discusses the key updates of the 2022 WHO classification. The latest WHO classification has integrated molecular testing for a better understanding of the origin and differentiation of thyroid tumors. The integration of molecular testing has a huge impact on management and targeted treatment of thyroid cancers.

REFERENCES

1. Gupta S, Savala R, Gupta N, Dey P. Fractal dimension and chromatin textural analysis to differentiate follicular carcinoma and adenoma on fine needle aspiration cytology. Cytopathology. 2020;31(5):491-3.

2. Christofer Juhlin C, Mete O, Baloch ZW. The 2022 WHO classification of thyroid tumors: novel concepts in nomenclature and grading. Endocr Relat Cancer. 2022;30(2):e220293.
3. Xing M. Molecular pathogenesis and mechanisms of thyroid cancer. Nat Rev Cancer. 2013;13(3):184-99.
4. Kalarani IB, Sivamani G, Veerabathiran R. Identification of crucial genes involved in thyroid cancer development. J Egypt Natl Canc Inst. 2023;35(1):15.
5. Tang KT, Lee CH. BRAF mutation in papillary thyroid carcinoma: pathogenic role and clinical implications. J Chin Med Assoc. 2010;73(3):113-28.
6. Rashid FA, Munkhdelger J, Fukuoka J, Bychkov A. Prevalence of *BRAFV600E* mutation in Asian series of papillary thyroid carcinoma-a contemporary systematic review. Gland Surg. 2020;9(5):1878-900.
7. Jasmine F, Aschebrook-Kilfoy B, Rahman MM, Zaagman G, Grogan RH, Kamal M, et al. Association of DNA Promoter Methylation and *BRAF* Mutation in Thyroid Cancer. Curr Oncol. 2023;30(3):2978-96.
8. Giordano TJ. Genomic Hallmarks of Thyroid Neoplasia. Annu Rev Pathol. 2018;13:141-62.
9. Matrone A, Citro F, Gambale C, Prete A, Minaldi E, Ciampi R, et al. BRAF K601E Mutation in Oncocytic Carcinoma of the Thyroid: A Case Report and Literature Review. J Clin Med. 2023;12(22):6970.
10. Marotta V, Bifulco M, Vitale M. Significance of RAS Mutations in Thyroid Benign Nodules and Non-Medullary Thyroid Cancer. Cancers (Basel). 2021;13(15):3785.
11. Kakudo K. Different Threshold of Malignancy for *RAS*-like Thyroid Tumors Causes Significant Differences in Thyroid Nodule Practice. Cancers (Basel). 2022;14(3):812.
12. Riccio IR, LaForteza AC, Hussein MH, Linhuber JP, Issa PP, Staav J, et al. Diagnostic utility of *RAS* mutation testing for refining cytologically indeterminate thyroid nodules. EXCLI J. 2024;23:283-99.
13. Accardo G, Conzo G, Esposito D, Gambardella C, Mazzella M, Castaldo F, et al. Genetics of medullary thyroid cancer: An overview. Int J Surg. 2017;41 (Suppl 1):S2-S6.
14. Bunone G, Uggeri M, Mondellini P, Pierotti MA, Bongarzone I. RET Receptor Expression in Thyroid Follicular Epithelial Cell-derived Tumors. Cancer Res. 2000;60 (11):2845-9.
15. Luzón-Toro B, Fernández RM, Villalba-Benito L, Torroglosa A, Antiñolo G, Borrego S. Influencers on Thyroid Cancer Onset: Molecular Genetic Basis. Genes (Basel). 2019;10(11): 913.
16. Niciporuka R, Nazarovs J, Ozolins A, Narbuts Z, Miklasevics E, Gardovskis J. Can We Predict Differentiated Thyroid Cancer Behavior? Role of Genetic and Molecular Markers. Medicina (Kaunas). 2021;57(10):1131.
17. Reddi HV, McIver B, Grebe SK, Eberhardt NL. The paired box-8/peroxisome proliferator-activated receptor-gamma oncogene in thyroid tumorigenesis. Endocrinology. 2007; 148(3):932-5.
18. Hu J, Yuan IJ, Mirshahidi S, Simental A, Lee SC, Yuan X. Thyroid Carcinoma: Phenotypic Features, Underlying Biology and Potential Relevance for Targeting Therapy. Int J Mol Sci. 2021;22(4):1950.
19. Raman P, Koenig RJ. Pax-8-PPAR-γ fusion protein in thyroid carcinoma. Nat Rev Endocrinol. 2014;10(10):616-23.
20. Liu X, Bishop J, Shan Y, Pai S, Liu D, Murugan AK, et al. Highly prevalent TERT promoter mutations in aggressive thyroid cancers. Endocr Relat Cancer. 2013;20(4):603-10.
21. Muzza M, Colombo C, Rossi S, Tosi D, Cirello V, Perrino M, et al. Telomerase in differentiated thyroid cancer: promoter mutations, expression and localization. Mol Cell Endocrinol. 2015;399:288-95.
22. Cancer Genome Atlas Research Network. Integrated genomic characterization of papillary thyroid carcinoma. Cell. 2014;159(3):676-90.
23. Boucai L, Seshan V, Williams M, Knauf JA, Saqcena M, Ghossein RA, et al. Characterization of Subtypes of BRAF-Mutant Papillary Thyroid Cancer Defined by Their Thyroid Differentiation Score. J Clin Endocrinol Metab. 2022;107(4):1030-9.

24. Lim J, Lee HS, Park J, Kim KS, Kim SK, Cho YW, et al. Different Molecular Phenotypes of Progression in BRAF- and RAS-Like Papillary Thyroid Carcinoma. Endocrinol Metab (Seoul). 2023;38(4):445-54.
25. Baloch Z, LiVolsi VA. The Bethesda System for Reporting Thyroid Cytology (TBSRTC): From look-backs to look-ahead. Diagn Cytopathol. 2020;48(10):862-6.
26. Alzumaili B, Sadow PM. Update on Molecular Diagnostics in Thyroid Pathology: A Review. Genes (Basel). 2023;14(7):1314.
27. Cohen Y, Xing M, Mambo E, Guo Z, Wu G, Trink B, et al. BRAF mutation in papillary thyroid carcinoma. J Natl Cancer Inst. 2003;95(8):625-7.
28. Rossi ED, Pantanowitz L, Faquin WC. The Role of Molecular Testing for the Indeterminate Thyroid FNA. Genes (Basel). 2019;10(10):736.
29. Sahli ZT, Smith PW, Umbricht CB, Zeiger MA. Preoperative Molecular Markers in Thyroid Nodules. Front Endocrinol (Lausanne). 2018;9:179.
30. Danilovic DLS, Marui S. Critical analysis of molecular tests in indeterminate thyroid nodules. Arch Endocrinol Metab. 2018;62(6):572-5.
31. Kannan S. Molecular Markers in the Diagnosis of Thyroid Cancer in Indeterminate Thyroid Nodules. Indian J Surg Oncol. 2022;13(1):11-6.
32. Vuong HG, Nguyen TPX, Hassell LA, Jung CK. Diagnostic performances of the Afirma Gene Sequencing Classifier in comparison with the Gene Expression Classifier: A meta-analysis. Cancer Cytopathol. 2021;129(3):182-9.
33. Borowczyk M, Szczepanek-Parulska E, Olejarz M, Więckowska B, Verburg FA, Dębicki S, et al. Evaluation of 167 Gene Expression Classifier (GEC) and ThyroSeq v2 Diagnostic Accuracy in the Preoperative Assessment of Indeterminate Thyroid Nodules: Bivariate/HROC Meta-analysis. Endocr Pathol. 2019;30(1):8-15.
34. Ferraz C. Can current molecular tests help in the diagnosis of indeterminate thyroid nodule FNAB? Arch Endocrinol Metab. 2018;62(6):576-84.
35. Rajab M, Payne RJ, Forest VI, Pusztaszeri M. Molecular Testing for Thyroid Nodules: The Experience at McGill University Teaching Hospitals in Canada. Cancers (Basel). 2022;14(17): 4140.
36. Santos MT, Rodrigues BM, Shizukuda S, Oliveira AF, Oliveira M, Figueiredo DLA, et al. Clinical decision support analysis of a microRNA-based thyroid molecular classifier: A real-world, prospective and multicentre validation study. EBioMedicine. 2022;82:104137.
37. Gupta O, Gautam U, Chandrasekhar M, Rajwanshi A, Radotra BD, Verma R, et al. Molecular Testing for BRAFV600E and RAS Mutations from Cytoscrapes of Thyroid Fine Needle Aspirates: A Single-Center Pilot Study. J Cytol. 2020;37(4):174-81.
38. Chirayath SR, Pavithran PV, Abraham N, Nair V, Bhavani N, Kumar H, et al. Prospective Study of Bethesda Categories III and IV Thyroid Nodules: Outcomes and Predictive Value of BRAFV600E Mutation. Indian J Endocrinol Metab. 2019;23(3):278-81.
39. Shonka DC Jr, Ho A, Chintakuntlawar AV, Geiger JL, Park JC, Seetharamu N, et al. American Head and Neck Society Endocrine Surgery Section and International Thyroid Oncology Group consensus statement on mutational testing in thyroid cancer: Defining advanced thyroid cancer and its targeted treatment. Head Neck. 2022;44(6):1277-300.
40. Agarwal S, Bychkov A, Jung CK. Emerging Biomarkers in Thyroid Practice and Research. Cancers (Basel). 2021;14(1):204.
41. Romano C, Martorana F, Pennisi MS, Stella S, Massimino M, Tirrò E, et al. Opportunities and Challenges of Liquid Biopsy in Thyroid Cancer. Int J Mol Sci. 2021;22(14):7707.
42. Garcia-Alvarez A, Hernando J, Carmona-Alonso A, Capdevila J. What is the status of immunotherapy in thyroid neoplasms? Front Endocrinol (Lausanne). 2022;13:929091.
43. Patel N, Bavikar R, Lad YP, Singh M, Dharwadkar A, Viswanathan V. A comparison of the WHO 2004 and WHO 2017 thyroid tumor classifications. J Cancer Res Ther. 2024;20(1): 311-4.
44. Chiba T. Molecular Pathology of Thyroid Tumors: Essential Points to Comprehend Regarding the Latest WHO Classification. Biomedicines. 2024;12(4):712.

45. Rossi ED, Baloch Z. The Impact of the 2022 WHO Classification of Thyroid Neoplasms on Everyday Practice of Cytopathology. Endocr Pathol. 2023;34(1):23-33.
46. McFadden DG, Sadow PM. Genetics, Diagnosis, and Management of Hürthle Cell Thyroid Neoplasms. Front Endocrinol (Lausanne). 2021;12:696386.
47. Lebrun L, Salmon I. Pathology and new insights in thyroid neoplasms in the 2022 WHO classification. Curr Opin Oncol. 2024;36(1):13-21.
48. Hernandez-Prera JC, Wenig BM. RAS-Mutant Follicular Thyroid Tumors: A Continuous Challenge for Pathologists. Endocr Pathol. 2024;18:1-8.
49. Nikiforova MN, Nikitski AV, Panebianco F, Kaya C, Yip L, Williams M, et al. GLIS Rearrangement is a Genomic Hallmark of Hyalinizing Trabecular Tumor of the Thyroid Gland. Thyroid. 2019;29(2):161-73.
50. Jung CK, Bychkov A, Kakudo K. Update from the 2022 World Health Organization Classification of Thyroid Tumors: A Standardized Diagnostic Approach. Endocrinol Metab (Seoul). 2022;37(5):703-18.
51. Basolo F, Macerola E, Poma AM, Torregrossa L. The 5th edition of WHO classification of tumors of endocrine organs: changes in the diagnosis of follicular-derived thyroid carcinoma. Endocrine. 2023;80(3):470-6.
52. Cao J, Zhu X, Sun Y, Li X, Yun C, Zhang W. The genetic duet of BRAF V600E and TERT promoter mutations predicts the poor curative effect of radioiodine therapy in papillary thyroid cancer. Eur J Nucl Med Mol Imaging. 2022;49(10):3470-81.
53. Xu B, Fuchs T, Dogan S, Landa I, Katabi N, Fagin JA, et al. Dissecting Anaplastic Thyroid Carcinoma: A Comprehensive Clinical, Histologic, Immunophenotypic, and Molecular Study of 360 Cases. Thyroid. 2020;30(10):1505-17.

12

CHAPTER

Cancer Stem Cells and Their Implications

Soundarya Ravi, Debasis Gochhait

INTRODUCTION TO STEM CELLS

Stem cells are a unique type of undifferentiated or partially differentiated cells characterized by their self-renewal capacity and the ability to differentiate into a variety of cell types.[1] Stem cells are found in embryo as well as adults. The primary role of embryonic stem cells (ESCs) is the formation of multiple organ systems, as they possess the ability to differentiate into any mature cell types of the trilaminar germ lines. In adults, these stem cells possess the potential to regenerate and repair certain damaged tissues.

CLASSIFICATION OF STEM CELLS

Based on the differentiation potential, the stem cells are classified into the following subtypes:

- *Totipotent stem cells (TSCs)*: These stem cells have the greatest ability to differentiate and can form both the embryo and the extra-embryonic tissues. The best example of TSC is a zygote, which is formed by the fertilization of an oocyte by a sperm.[2]
- *Pluripotent stem cells (PSCs)*: These stem cells have the ability to differentiate into the cells of the three germ layers but cannot form extra-embryonic tissues like the placenta. The inner cell mass of the blastocyst stage forms the ESCs, which are a classic example of PSCs.[3] Additionally, PSCs can be artificially created by genetic reprogramming of mature somatic cells, known as induced pluripotent stem cells (iPSCs).[4]
- *Multipotent stem cells (MSCs)*: These stem cells have limited differentiation potential compared to PSCs. They can form a variety of cells within a specific cell lineage. Adult stem cells (ASCs), also known as tissue-specific stem cells (TSSCs), fall under this category. For example, hematopoietic stem cells (HSCs) are a type of ASC that can develop into different types of terminally differentiated myeloid and lymphoid cells.[5]

- *Unipotent stem cells (USCs)*: These stem cells can differentiate into only a particular cell type and also have self-renewal properties. A few examples are muscle stem cells, type 2 pneumocytes, epidermal stem cells, etc.

STEM CELL NICHES

The stem cells reside in a microenvironment at particular anatomic locations known as the stem cell niche, which helps to control the rate of proliferation and differentiation of stem cells through signals.[6] This "stem cell niche" hypothesis was postulated by Raymond Schofield in the year 1978, in which he stated that the behavior of the stem cells was determined by the cells associated with it.[7] Niches are composed of an extracellular matrix (ECM), which acts as a scaffold for the stem cells, stromal support cells, blood vessels, and neuronal connections. The various ASCs and the locations of their niches are outlined below:

- HSCs are located close to the blood vessels (vascular niche) and along the endosteal surface of the trabecular bone (endosteal niche).[8,9]
- The epidermal stem cells of the skin are located in the bulge of the hair follicles.[10] Similarly, the stem cells of the cornea are located in the limbus.[11]
- In the gastrointestinal tract, the intestinal stem cells are located at the base of the crypts among the Paneth cells.[12] The hepatic stem cells, also known as the oval cells, are located in the canal of Hering.[13]

CANCER STEM CELLS: HISTORY, ORIGIN, AND DEVELOPMENT

Cancer stem cells (CSCs) also known as tumor-initiating cells (TICs) are a small group of cells among the malignant cells, which possess the ability for self-renewal and differentiation and are responsible for cancer initiation and propagation. They exhibit properties similar to those of normal PSCs. However, CSCs show high genetic instability due to the accumulation of multiple molecular alterations.[14]

History of Cancer Stem Cells

The field of CSC research has made significant strides over the past 20 years. In the early 1970s, Barry G Pierce introduced the concept of cancer initiation from CSCs.[15] He found that when embryonal carcinoma cells from teratocarcinoma were transplanted into mice, they were able to differentiate into various cell types of different lineages. Following this, many experiments conducted by John Dick, Bonnet, and Lapidot et al. validated the existence of CSCs by inducing acute myeloid leukemia (AML) in severely immunocompromised mouse models.[16-18] Lapidot et al. specifically isolated a subpopulation of cells expressing high CD34 and low CD38, which were able to initiate AML in immunodeficient mice upon transplantation and identified them as leukemia-initiating cells (LICs).

This concept of CSCs has since been implicated in a variety of solid organ malignancies like brain, breast, gastrointestinal tract, liver, lung, oral cavity, prostate, etc.[19-21] In 2003, Al-Hajj et al. isolated TICs expressing high CD44 and low CD24 cell-surface markers from breast cancer patients. Similarly, CD44 and CD133 markers have been utilized to isolate CSCs from brain and prostate malignancies.[19,22] Additionally, various cell-surface markers and transcription factors expressed by CSCs have been identified, aiding in the isolation and distinction of this subset from the remaining tumor cell population. Researches have shown that differentiated cancer cells can acquire stem cell properties by activating genes responsible for epithelial-mesenchymal transition (EMT).[23] Despite the vast developments and improvements in CSC research, uncertainty prevails regarding the origin and development of CSCs. However, future research on cancer and its stemness is expected to further refine our understanding of CSCs in the coming years.

Origin of Cancer Stem Cells

Even after extensive research on CSCs, their origin remains unclear. However, cancer researchers have proposed two potential pathways for the generation of CSCs, which are as follows **(Figs. 1A and B)**.

Conversion of Normal Stem Cells to Cancer Stem Cells

Due to certain genetic mutations, normal stem cells transform into premalignant stem cells. With the accumulation of additional genetic and epigenetic

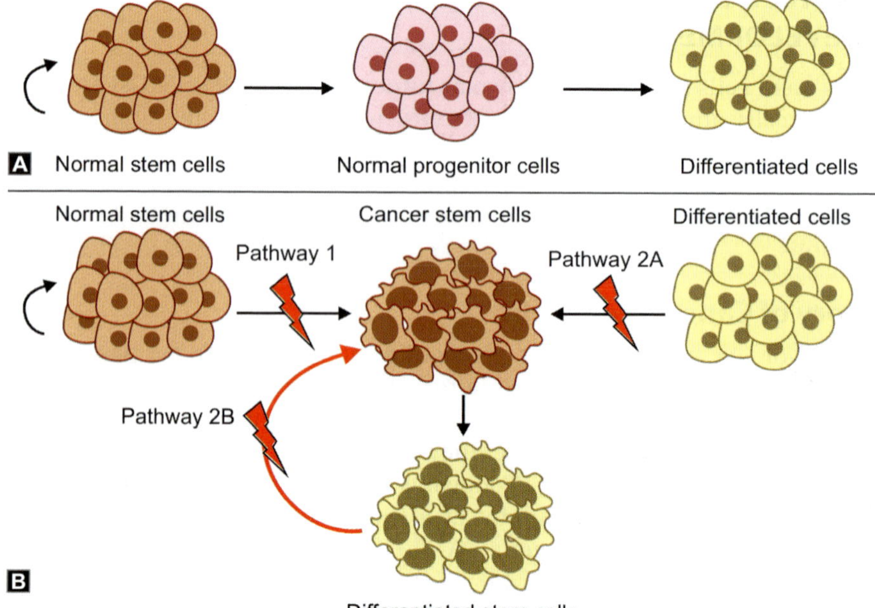

FIGS. 1A AND B: (A) The normal physiological proliferation and self-renewal of stem cells and differentiation into a mature cell; (B) the pathways hypothesized in the origin of cancer stem cells (CSCs); pathway 1 shows the conversion of normal stem cells CSCs. Pathway 2 shows formation of CSCs from dedifferentiation of mature cells.

Note: Red lightning bolt symbol represents acquisition of multiple genetic and epigenetic mutations.

alterations, these premalignant stem cells further develop into CSCs.[24-27] Since normal stem cells already possess self-renewal capacity and proliferation potential, their conversion into CSCs results in uncontrolled proliferation and the spread of cancer. This is the most accepted hypothesis among scientists.

The "Moolgavkar–Venzon–Knudson two-stage model" best explains the development of cancer from CSCs.[28,29] In this model, cancer progression occurs through two phases: *Initiation* and *promotion* phases. In the *initiation* phase, normal stem cells undergo significant genetic damage to form premalignant stem cells. Due to their self-renewal capacity, these mutated stem cells proliferate and maintain this genetic mutation. During the *promotion* phase, these mutated stem cells undergo malignant transformation to form cancer by acquiring further genetic mutations.

Reprogramming and Dedifferentiation of Mature Differentiated Cells to Form Cancer Stem Cells

Repetitive insults to differentiated cells, such as infections, chronic inflammation, toxin or radiation exposure, and tissue repair, can induce mutations that result in de-differentiation and reprogramming, causing these cells to acquire stem cell characteristics.[27,30] This concept was studied by Takahashi et al., who demonstrated that mouse embryonic cells and adult fibroblasts could be induced to form PSCs (iPSCs) by increasing the expression of four factors, known as Yamanaka factors: OCT3/4, Sox2, c-Myc, and Klf4. These iPSCs led to the development of malignancies in mice upon transplantation.[4]

In certain instances, after the development of cancer, some of the differentiated cancer cells or cancer progenitor cells undergo dedifferentiation and acquire stem cell properties through EMT. These dedifferentiated, stem cell-like cancer cells are usually responsible for invasion and distant metastasis.[23,31]

Mechanisms of Development of Cancer Stem Cells

Many theories have been put forth in literature, which explain the mechanisms of development of CSCs. Some of the important theories are listed below:

- Symmetric and asymmetric division model of development of CSCs
- Signaling pathways involved in the development of CSCs
- Microenvironment model of development of CSCs
- Embryonic model of development of CSCs

Symmetric and Asymmetric Division Model of Development of Cancer Stem Cells

Stem cells proliferate and undergo two types of cell division, i.e., symmetric and asymmetric division.[32]

1. *Symmetric division*: In symmetric division, the parent stem cell undergoes mitosis to form two identical daughter cells that possess the same genotype and phenotypic characteristics. The purpose of symmetric division is to expand the stem cell population through proliferation. It is observed in ESCs during fetal development and in ASCs during wound healing and regeneration.

2. *Asymmetric division*: In asymmetric division, the parent stem cell divides into two daughter cells: One retains the stem cell characteristics, while the other differentiates to acquire a different phenotype. Therefore, the purpose of asymmetric division is to increase the number of differentiated cells without depleting the stem cell population. Both symmetric and asymmetric division processes are tightly regulated by intrinsic and extrinsic mechanisms.

In malignancies, a balanced tumor heterogeneity is maintained by the asymmetric division of CSCs, which produces both differentiated cancer cells as well as maintains the CSC population. However, when there is a disruption in asymmetric division, an imbalance develops, leading to an excessive production of undifferentiated CSCs, resulting in aggressive tumor behavior.[33] This link between carcinogenesis and imbalanced asymmetric division was initially identified in *Drosophila melanogaster* and was later found in humans as well.[34-36] Some tumor suppressor genes like adenomatosis polyposis coli (*APC*), human variant of lethal giant larvae (*HUGL-1* and *HUGL-2*), *p63*, brain tumor (*BRAT*), etc., play an active role in mitotic spindle apparatus regulation.[37-39] Alterations in these tumor suppressor genes lead to dysregulation of asymmetric cell division and are observed in malignancies such as colorectal cancers, melanoma, etc.

Signaling Pathways Involved in the Development of Cancer Stem Cells

Many signaling pathways play a major role in regulating stem cell behavior and characteristics, such as cell survival, proliferation, and self-renewal.[40] These signaling pathways are either excessively activated or suppressed leading to the development of CSCs. Some of the important signaling pathways, such as JAK/STAT (Janus kinase/signal transducers and activators of transcription), Wnt (wingless-related integration site), NOTCH, and Hedgehog are outlined below.

- *JAK/STAT signaling pathway*: The JAK/STAT signaling pathway is stimulated by cytokines or growth factors that act on the corresponding tyrosine kinase receptors on the cell surface.[41] Upon phosphorylation, this pathway is stimulated, which is then involved in cell proliferation, differentiation and apoptosis. Activation of the JAK/STAT pathway is observed in myeloproliferative neoplasms such as polycythemia vera, essential thrombocythemia, and primary myelofibrosis.[42,43] The STAT pathway is also implicated in breast cancer, head and neck cancer, endometrial cancer, diffuse large B-cell lymphoma, colorectal cancer, hepatocellular carcinoma, and glioma.[44-47]

In breast carcinoma, the survival and maintenance of CSCs are due to the persistent activation of STAT3.[48,49] Interleukin-6 (IL-6) activates the JAK/STAT pathway by stimulating the downstream *Oct4* gene, leading to the production of CSCs in breast cancer and endometrial cancer.[44,50] Similarly, IL-10 induces stemness and invasive properties in nonsmall-cell lung carcinoma via the JAK/STAT pathway.[51]

- *Wnt signaling pathway*: The abnormal activation of the "wingless-related integration site" pathway, also known as the Wnt signaling pathway, is involved in the dedifferentiation of CSCs and CSC-mediated metastasis. This pathway can be activated through a canonical process, which involves the de-repression and release of beta-catenin from the Axin complex, or through a noncanonical process, by activating calcium signaling cascades.[52,53]

Certain proteins of the ECM like periostin, tenascin C, and inhibitors of bone morphogenetic protein (BMP) increase Wnt signals and promote CSC development.[54,55] Increased CD44 expression in pancreatic, colon, and lung cancers causes activation of Wnt signaling through beta-catenin and promotes CSCs mediated metastasis.[56-58]

- *NOTCH signaling pathway*: Under physiological conditions, the Delta/Serrate/lag-2 (*DSL*), also known as the NOTCH ligand, acts on the NOTCH receptor, causing proteolytic cleavage of the intracellular domain (ICD) of NOTCH. This ICD translocates to the nucleus, where it attaches to the transcription factor to form a transcriptional activation complex, which then activates the target genes of the NOTCH pathway.[59] The NOTCH signaling pathway plays an important role in mammary stem cells for cell proliferation and self-renewal. Aberrant expression of the *NOTCH4* gene in mammary stem cells induces matrix invasion properties, highlighting the carcinogenic potential of this pathway.[60,61] Likewise, abnormal *NOTCH3* signaling is closely associated with CSC stemness and its therapy resistance by upregulating genes such as programmed death ligand 1 (*PD-L1*), aldehyde dehydrogenase (*ALDH*), sirtuin 1 (*SIRT1*), and mammalian target of rapamycin (*mTOR*).[62]
- *Hedgehog signaling pathway*: The Hedgehog pathway is composed of extracellular ligands, receptors, namely patched homolog 1 (PTCH) and smoothened receptor (SMO), and various downstream signaling proteins, including glioma-associated oncogene homolog (GLI).[63] This pathway is vital for the organogenesis of the nervous system, heart, and limb development during embryonic life.[64] Germline loss of the *PTCH1* gene results in Gorlin syndrome (basal cell nevus syndrome), which is associated with multiple basal cell carcinomas and various tumors.[65] Increased signaling through hedgehog pathway promotes the proliferation of CSCs in lung adenocarcinoma.[66] Similarly, SMO and GLI1 aid in the proliferation and self-renewal of CD133+ glioma stem cells.[67]

Microenvironment Model of Development of Cancer Stem Cells

Like stem cells, CSCs seem to inhabit specialized microenvironments known as niches. The interaction of CSCs with their surrounding microenvironment is essential for their survival, proliferation, and differentiation. The tumor microenvironment (TME) is composed of stromal cells such as fibroblasts and adipocytes, immune system cells such as lymphocytes and macrophages, microvessels composed of endothelial cells, and various components of the ECM.[68] The TME provides CSCs with the suitable conditions for survival and regulates their properties through the secretion of cytokines and factors, as well as through cell-to-cell contact.[69] The TME also induces angiogenesis and promotes immune evasion, invasion, and metastasis. The role of each component of the TME in the development of CSCs is highlighted below.

- *Mesenchymal stem cells*: Mesenchymal stem cells, also known as mesenchymal stromal cells, are a type of MSCs that can differentiate into various mesenchymal cell types such as osteoblasts, chondrocytes, myocytes, and adipocytes.[70] They secrete a variety of cytokines that act on CSCs in an autocrine or paracrine manner and promote cancer stemness. These cells enhance stemness in CSCs by secreting IL-6, IL-8, and C-X-C motif chemokine ligand 12 (CXCL12), which act via the nuclear factor kappa B (NF-κB) pathway.[71-73] To maintain CSCs in an undifferentiated state, mesenchymal stem cells also produce Gremlin-1, an antagonist to BMP.[74] Furthermore, mesenchymal stem cells can differentiate into cancer-associated fibroblasts (CAFs), which interact with CSCs to promote metastasis.[75]

- *CAFs*: These are specialized stromal cells in the TME that regulate CSC functions and are involved in tumor metastasis. CAFs are derived from a variety of fibroblastic and nonfibroblastic cellular sources such as normal fibroblasts, resident stellate cells, bone marrow-derived mesenchymal stem cells, epithelial and endothelial cells as well as from CSCs.[76-78] CAFs play a major role in cell-to-cell signaling interactions and matrix remodeling by secreting cytokines and factors like CXCL12, tumor necrosis factor alpha (TNF-α), transforming growth factor beta (TGF-β), epidermal growth factor (EGF), fibroblast growth factor 2 (FGF-2), platelet-derived growth factor (PDGF), vascular endothelial growth factor (VEGF), and hepatocyte growth factor (HGF).[79,80] CAFs induce a stemness phenotype in CSCs and promote their proliferation by activating the Wnt and NOTCH signaling pathways.[81,82] Moreover, they remodel the ECM surrounding the CSCs, which favor tumor progression and metastasis.[83]
- *Inflammatory cells*: The TME is maintained in a state of chronic inflammation to enhance cancer progression and survival. The CSC niche suppresses the activity of natural killer (NK) cells and cytotoxic T-cells (CTLs) and evades the host's immune surveillance mechanisms for the survival and maintenance of CSCs.[84,85] The cancer cells produce a variety of immunosuppressive cytokines and chemokines, which recruit different inflammatory cells such as tumor-associated macrophages (TAMs), tumor-associated neutrophils (TANs), myeloid-derived suppressor cells (MDSCs), and regulatory T-cells (T-regs). These cells act synergistically to protect the CSCs from immune attack, thereby granting them immune privilege.[86-89] In response to hypoxia and cytokines IL-10 and IL-13, macrophages are polarized toward a tumor-promoting phenotype (M2 macrophages), which, in turn, produce IL-6 and TGF-β that cause the breakdown of ECM components, stimulate angiogenesis, and promote the expansion of CSCs via the JAK1-STAT3 signal transduction pathway.[50,51,86,90] MDSCs are pathologically activated immature cells of the myeloid lineage that migrate to the site of malignancy to exhibit immunosuppressive activity. They are divided into two subtypes: Monocytic and polymorphonuclear/granulocytic MDSCs.[91] MDSCs modulate the survival of CSCs through the production of prostaglandins, microRNAs, and factors that activate the STAT3 and NOTCH pathways.[87,88,92] T-regs are CD4+CD25+ T-cell subsets expressing transcription factor forkhead box P3 (FOXP3), which are known to hamper cancer immune surveillance by suppressing antitumor immune responses.[93]

- *ECM components*: The ECM forms the noncellular part of the TME, acting as a physical barrier to protect CSCs from therapeutic drugs.[69] Matrix metalloproteinases (MMPs) produced by CAFs cause degradation and remodeling of ECM components, facilitating the EMT phenotype in CSCs and enhancing tumor invasion and metastasis.[71,94] Cell-to-cell and cell-to-matrix contacts are maintained by transmembrane cell adhesion proteins known as integrins. CSCs utilize niche-integrin interactions to potentiate their stemness and other properties. Nearly eight integrins have been identified that highlight CSCs in various solid organ malignancies such as breast, colon, and prostate.[95,96]

Embryonic Model of Development of Cancer Stem Cells

The "embryonic model" of CSC development explains the development of pediatric malignancies. According to this model, pediatric malignancies tend to develop from residual ESC rests that have remained quiescent for a period of time and are later reactivated.[97,98] Teratocarcinoma is one example of a tumor developing in adult gonads, hypothesized to arise from germinal stem cells that have lost their differentiation potential due to dysregulation in their microenvironment. Ratajczak et al. also stated that some tumors attained ESC characteristics by aberrant signaling of embryonic signaling pathways such as NOTCH, Wnt, and Hedgehog.[99,100]

PLASTICITY OF CANCER STEM CELLS

There are two schools of thought that explain tumor progression and heterogeneity: The *hierarchical* model and the *stochastic* model **(Fig. 2)**. According to the *hierarchical* model, CSCs are a unique subset of cells within the cancer cell population that exhibit self-renewing properties and have the ability to produce differentiated cancer cells.[16,101] This model best explains the concept of tumor relapse stemming from CSCs that survive therapy. However, the hierarchical model does not explain how a single cancer cell can switch between a differentiated state and an undifferentiated stem cell-like phenotype.[102] On the other hand, the *stochastic* model states that each and every cell within a cancer has the potential to initiate and propagate the tumor. The behavior of different cancer cells depends on acquisition of sequential genetic mutations and their interactions with their TME.[103-105]

Plasticity is a property of cancer cells characterized by their ability to switch from a differentiated non-CSC phenotype to a CSC phenotype and vice versa **(Fig. 3)**.[105,106] Based on certain genetic mutations, epigenetic changes and cellular interactions with the TME, some differentiated cancer cells may acquire transient stemness and enter the CSC pool. This property of plasticity unites both the hierarchical and stochastic models of tumorigenesis. The diverse plasticity of CSCs also explains their phenotypic and functional heterogeneity.[107] Tumor cells adopt this strategy to convert to a CSC phenotype as a defense mechanism to become resistant to chemotherapeutic agents.[108]

Many factors regulate the dynamics of CSC plasticity, including epigenetic alterations, signals from the TME, changes in the ECM, and the metabolic state

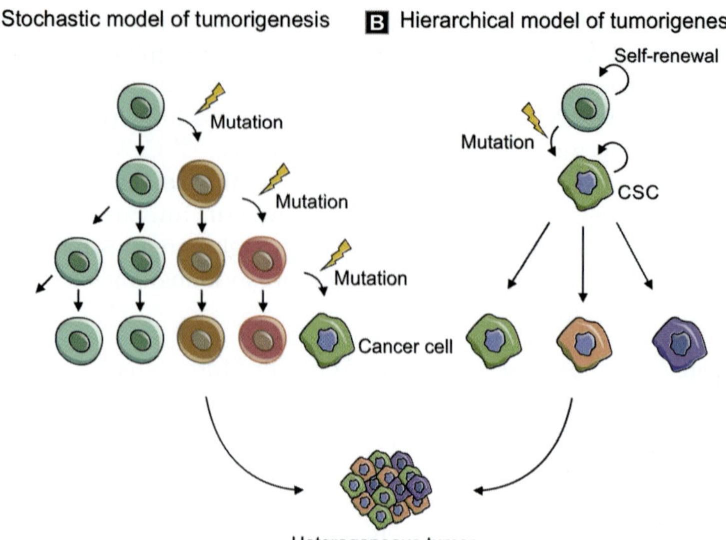

FIGS. 2A AND B: Diagrammatic illustration of the stochastic and hierarchical models of carcinogenesis. (A) In the stochastic model, each cancer cell has an equal potential to initiate tumors. The evolution of tumors from these cells is solely influenced by random factors. (B) The hierarchical model proposes that only cancer stem cells (CSCs) occupy the top of the system and possess the capability to initiate and propagate new tumors.

Source: Adapted from Carvalho LS, Gonçalves N, Fonseca NA, Moreira JN. Cancer Stem Cells and Nucleolin as Drivers of Carcinogenesis. Pharmaceuticals (Basel). 2021;14(1):60.

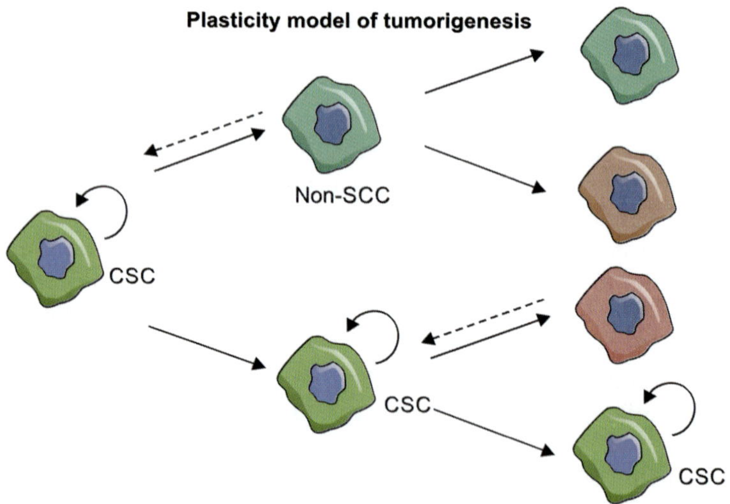

FIG. 3: Diagrammatic illustration of the plasticity model of tumorigenesis. Cancer stem cells (CSCs) have the ability to differentiate into any type of cell within a tumor. Likewise, nonstem cancer cells (non-SCCs) can also transition to a stem-like state in response to specific physiological stimuli.

Source: Adapted from Carvalho LS, Gonçalves N, Fonseca NA, Moreira JN. Cancer Stem Cells and Nucleolin as Drivers of Carcinogenesis. Pharmaceuticals (Basel). 2021;14(1):60.

of CSCs.[106,109-111] CSC plasticity is driven by engaging EMT pathways, such as the TGF-β, Wnt, and NOTCH pathways, and EMT-transcription factors like Snail, zinc finger E-box-binding homeobox (ZEB), and Twist families, which induce stemness and allow cancer cells to remain in an undifferentiated state.[112-114] Dysregulation in epigenetic modifications, such as methylation and acetylation, causes aberrant chromatin remodeling by the switch/sucrose nonfermenting (SWI/SNF) complex, resulting in CSC phenotype switching in tumor cells.[111,115,116]

Cancer stem cells have the capacity to alter mesenchymal stem cells and other neighboring cells to occupy the normal stem cell niche. Following colonization of the niche, the CSCs recruit immune cells through various signaling pathways to promote the plasticity of cancer cells.[69] The immune cells in the TME produce pro-inflammatory cytokines like TNF-α and IL-6, which upregulate the mesenchymal gene signature to induce CSC plasticity in breast carcinoma, melanoma, and lung cancer.[117,118] Hypoxic states in the TME can also trigger the plasticity of CSCs by elaboration of factors such as hypoxia-inducible factors (HIFs), TGF-β, and the proangiogenic factor VEGF.[119,120] Hypoxia also promotes cancer cells to upregulate glycolytic enzymes and switch their metabolism from oxidative phosphorylation (OXPHOS) to glycolysis. This metabolic shift to glycolysis increases the longevity of CSCs and stimulates their plasticity.[121,122]

METABOLISM OF CANCER STEM CELLS

In 1925, Otto Warburg identified that cancer cells adopt "aerobic glycolysis" as their pathway for metabolism, in which the cancer cells utilize large amounts of glucose and convert it to lactate even in the presence of ample oxygen.[123] The intermediates in the glycolytic pathway are utilized by the cancer cells for the biosynthesis of nucleic acids, proteins, and lipids, to sustain the high proliferation rates. Since then, many researchers have studied the intricacies of cancer metabolism and its role in tumor growth, spread, and therapy resistance.

The CSCs, which are a derivative of cancer cells, also exhibit alterations in their metabolic pathways, which play a crucial role in determining their plasticity.[124] Recent studies have shown that the CSCs exhibit alterations in glucose and lipid metabolism to remain in undifferentiated state and maintain its stemness. Unlike cancer cells, CSCs exhibit metabolic plasticity, allowing them to shift their metabolism between OXPHOS and glycolysis depending on their needs.[125] The metabolic program of the tumor varies across its different compartments. The actively dividing areas of the tumor with ample oxygen supply adopt a combination of both OXPHOS and glycolytic pathways, whereas in hypoxic areas, there is an upregulation of glycolytic enzymes by HIFs.[126,127] In nutrient-deprived states, CSCs adopt autophagy as their energy source to remain quiescent.[128]

Studies performed on cancers of the lung, breast, colon, and ovary, as well as glioblastoma, have shown that CSCs activate the glycolytic program to maintain stemness by upregulating glycolytic enzymes.[129-132] The transcription factor STAT3 acts as a metabolic switch by downregulating mitochondrial activity to induce aerobic glycolysis in CSCs.[133] However, recent studies have shown that in some tumors, CSCs exhibit increased mitochondrial activity and oxygen consumption, reflecting a preference for OXPHOS over glycolysis for their metabolism.[134,135] CSCs that follow the OXPHOS metabolic program show expanded mitochondrial mass, higher membrane potential, and increased mitochondrial reactive oxygen species (ROS) production.[136,137] These CSCs associated with the OXPHOS metabolic pathway are often linked to drug resistance and treatment failure.[138]

Apart from glucose, CSCs also metabolize lipids via beta oxidation of fatty acids, triggered by overexpression of peroxisome proliferator-activated receptor delta (PPAR-δ) and NANOG.[139,140] CSCs tightly regulate their fatty acid metabolic pathways to preserve its self-renewal capabilities and to resist chemotherapeutic agents. Metabolic reprogramming to fatty acid oxidation has been observed in CD133+ CSCs in hepatocellular carcinoma.[141] Glutamine is also metabolized by CSCs for the production of nicotinamide adenine dinucleotide phosphate hydrogen (NADPH) and the antioxidant glutathione (GSH).[142] The reduced NADPH pool, maintained by both fatty acid oxidation and glutamine metabolism, is utilized to decompose ROS.[143]

POTENTIAL ROLES OF CANCER STEM CELLS

Cancer Metastasis

Earlier in this chapter, we discussed the various mechanisms involved in the development of CSCs and their vital role in cancer initiation and progression. In addition to their roles in cancer initiation and progression, CSCs also have a significant impact on cancer metastasis. CSCs with metastatic potential are also known as metastatic cancer stem cells (MCSCs). Similar to other metastatic cancer cells, MCSCs possess the properties required for invasion, dissemination, differentiation, and reconstruction of tumors at distant sites from the primary tumor.[144] However, what makes MCSCs distinctive is their self-renewal capacity and stemness properties. Additionally, these cells are resistant to therapy and can remain dormant for many years to escape antitumor immune surveillance.

Interactions between CSCs and their niche modulate their survival and the development of MCSCs. At the site of the primary tumor, components of the TME such as mesenchymal stem cells, CAFs, and TAMs release cytokines and factors that generate signals, causing the breakdown of the ECM.[23,69] Dysregulation of an ECM component named tenascin-C, upregulates pro-angiogenic factors and facilitates the dissemination of CSCs.[145] Exposure of CSCs to these signals activates various EMT-transcription factors, such as Snail, ZEB, and Twist, which induce plasticity. In addition, EMT transcription factors like ZEB are associated with cellular quiescence.[146,147] Subsequently, the CSCs downregulate E-cadherin expression, which is responsible for maintaining cell-to-cell adhesion.[148] This downregulation causes the CSCs to adopt a mesenchymal phenotype, thereby acquiring invasive and migratory properties.

Meanwhile, CSCs also elaborate factors that induce a favorable microenvironment in distant organs, termed pre-metastatic niches (PMN).[149,150]

Hypoxic state at the site of primary tumor also promotes the formation of PMN by secretion of HIFs.[151] PMNs have immunosuppressive characteristics that facilitate the survival of MCSCs upon arrival. PMNs are composed of pro-tumor inflammatory cells, such as TAMs, TANs, MDSCs, and T-regs, which protect the tumor from immune-mediated destruction.[152] The TME at the distant site also undergoes structural remodeling of the ECM components with the help of MMPs to support the PMN.[153]

The MCSCs disseminate via hematogenous or lymphatic routes and colonize the primed PMN to form a metastatic niche. In due course, the MCSCs grow and proliferate in this suitable microenvironment, initially forming micrometastases, which later develop into macrometastases.[152] However, it was observed that in some tumors, such as prostate and breast cancers, the MCSCs remain dormant in the metastatic niche for a long period before manifesting as overt metastasis.[128,154] This quiescent state can be reverted back to proliferative state by restoration of epithelial phenotype by undergoing mesenchymal-to-epithelial transition (MET).[155,156] The initiation of angiogenesis by factors such as VEGF and angiopoietin, secreted by TAMs in the metastatic niche, is also essential for the growth of MCSCs in the metastatic site.[154] Thus, with the support of the primary tumor niche, PMN, and metastatic niche, MCSCs are able to self-renew and successfully metastasize to distant organs.

Therapy Resistance

The key role played by CSCs in various cancers is therapy resistance, which results in the development of relapse. Various mechanisms have been proposed by which CSCs exhibit resistance to commonly used therapeutic agents, which are outlined below.

- Routine chemotherapeutic agents target rapidly proliferating cells. However, the quiescent state of CSCs makes them resistant to these agents, as observed in AML.[157,158]
- CSCs exhibit treatment resistance by overexpressing drug efflux transporter proteins, known as ATP-binding cassette (ABC) transporters, which facilitate drug efflux. Various ABC transporters, including P-glycoprotein (P-gp), breast cancer resistance protein (BCRP), and multidrug resistance-associated proteins (MRP), have been observed to be overexpressed in the CSCs of breast, lung, colorectal, and prostate cancers.[159-163]
- Many CSCs express excess ALDH enzyme, which results in detoxification of the toxic aldehyde compounds that are formed when treated using cyclophosphamide derivates.[164] Due to this detoxification by ALDH, the CSCs which overexpress ALDH gain drug resistant properties.[165]
- Constitutive activation of certain antiapoptotic signaling pathways, such as Hedgehog, Wnt, and NOTCH, is a characteristic feature of CSCs. These pathways enhance self-renewal capabilities and maintain cellular quiescence, contributing to the drug-resistant properties of CSCs.[166-168] EMT reprogramming in CSCs activates the NOTCH signaling pathways, which ultimately take part in drug resistance.[169,170]

- The CSC niche provides a protective microenvironment that supports CSC survival and shields them from therapeutic agents. Components such as CAFs, immune cells like TAMs, cytokines they produce, various ECM components, and the hypoxic conditions within the TME all work together to maintain CSC stemness and contribute to drug resistance.[171-173] The hypoxic TME contributes to chemotherapy resistance by activating specific antiapoptotic pathways.[174] During hypoxia, HIFs are produced, which also activate DNA repair enzymes that repair double-stranded breaks. This additional mechanism further enhances drug resistance against DNA-damaging agents.[163,172,175]
- Epigenetic mechanisms, such as histone modifications and DNA methylation, can silence tumor suppressor genes or upregulate drug efflux transporter proteins, contributing to drug resistance in CSCs.[176,177]

DETECTION AND ISOLATION OF CANCER STEM CELLS

Till now, we have studied the role of CSCs in tumor initiation, progression, cancer metastasis, and therapy resistance. Therefore, the proper identification and isolation of these cells are essential to developing novel therapies that specifically target CSCs to eliminate cancer. Understanding the phenotypic and functional characteristics is necessary to isolate CSCs and distinguish them from other cancer cells and normal stem cells.

Characterization of Cancer Stem Cells and Their Biomarkers

Many biomarkers have been developed in recent years for the accurate identification of CSCs in both solid organ malignancies and hematological malignancies. Nevertheless, most of these markers are not specific to CSCs, as they are also expressed by normal tissue ASCs and ESCs.[178] Therefore, a combination of several markers needs to be applied to specifically identify CSCs. The identified biomarkers can be classified based on their location of expression as follows: (1) *Cell-surface biomarkers* and (2) *intracellular biomarkers*. **Tables 1 to 3** provide an exhaustive list of cell surface and intracellular CSC biomarkers for solid tumors and hematological malignancies, along with the tumors in which they are expressed.

Methods for Detection and Isolation of Cancer Stem Cells

Different methodologies have been adopted to identify CSCs and isolate them from other cells in the niche.[281,282] The stem cells are isolated using a combination of different methods and multiple stem cell markers. Some of the important methods are listed below and discussed in detail subsequently.

- CSC specific biomarkers expression and cell sorting by flow cytometry
- Side population (SP) analysis
- Invitro tumor-sphere formation assay
- Intracellular enzyme activity analysis
- Other cell sorting techniques

TABLE 1: List of cell-surface cancer stem cell (CSC) biomarkers (CD surface markers) along with their functions and the tumors in which they are expressed.

Cell-surface biomarkers—cluster of differentiation (CD)	Expansion of abbreviation/ other name/function	Tumors in which they are expressed with references
CD24	Heat-stable antigen, cell adhesion molecule	• Breast cancer[179] • Colorectal cancer[180] • Gastric cancer[181-183] • Liver cancer[184-186] • Pancreatic cancer[187]
CD26	Dipeptidyl peptidase-4 (DPP-4), adenosine deaminase complexing protein 2	Chronic myeloid leukemia[188-190]
CD29	β1-integrin, cell adhesion molecule	• Breast cancer[179,191] • Squamous cell carcinoma (SCC)[192]
CD44 and its variants	Cell-surface receptor for hyaluronan of ECM	• Breast cancer[193-197] • Colorectal cancer[198-201] • Gastric cancer[183,202-206] • Liver cancer[207,208] • Lung cancer[58,209,210] • Pancreatic cancer[187]
CD49f	α6-integrin, cell adhesion molecule	• Breast cancer[211,212] • Ovarian cancer[213]
CD70	Cellular ligand for TNF-receptor family member CD27 present on B cells	• Acute myeloid leukemia[214] • Breast cancer[215]
CD87	Urokinase plasminogen activator surface receptor (uPAR)	Lung cancer[216]
CD90	Thy-1 cell-surface antigen, glycophosphatidylinositol-anchored cell-surface protein	• Brain cancer[217] • Breast cancer[218] • Gastric cancer[205] • Liver cancer[219-221] • Lung cancer[222]
CD123	IL-3 receptor α chain	Acute myeloid leukemia[18,223-225]
CD133	Prominin-1, penta-span membrane glycoprotein	• Breast cancer[226-228] • Colorectal cancer[167,198,200] • Endometrial cancer[229] • Gastric cancer[230-232] • Liver cancer[185,233,234] • Lung cancer[216,235-238]
CD166	Activated leukocyte cell adhesion molecule (ALCAM)	• Colorectal cancer[239] • Lung cancer[240] • Ovarian cancer[241]

(ECM: extracellular matrix; IL-3: interleukin-3; TNF: tumor necrosis factor)

TABLE 2: List of cell-surface cancer stem cell (CSC) biomarkers (not CD surface markers) along with their functions and the tumors in which they are expressed.

Cell-surface biomarkers—not CD markers	Expansion of abbreviation/other name/function	Tumors in which they are expressed with references
CLL-1	C-type lectin-like molecule-1, type II transmembrane glycoprotein	Acute myeloid leukemia[242-246]
CXCR4	C-X-C chemokine receptor type 4	• Gastric cancer[247] • Liver cancer[220] • Lung cancer[248]
EpCAM	Epithelial cellular adhesion molecule, Ca^{2+} independent epithelial cell to cell adhesion	• Breast cancer[249] • Colorectal cancer[201] • Gastric cancer[183,250] • Liver cancer[251] • Lung cancer[252,253]
LGR5	Leucine-rich repeat-containing G-protein coupled receptor 5	• Breast cancer[254] • Colorectal cancer[201,255] • Gastric cancer[256,257] • Lung cancer[258]
LINGO2	Leucine-rich repeat and Ig domain containing 2, transmembrane receptor	Gastric cancer[259]
ProC-R	Protein C receptor	• Breast cancer[260] • Nasopharyngeal carcinoma[261]
TIM3	T-cell immunoglobulin and mucin domain-containing-3	Acute myeloid leukemia[18,246,262]

Cancer Stem Cell-specific Biomarkers Expression and Cell Sorting by Flow Cytometry

In this method, CSCs are precisely separated from a heterogeneous mixture of cancer cells using an advanced flow cytometry technique known as fluorescence-activated cell sorting (FACS).[283] Tumor cells are initially isolated from biopsy specimens, washed, dissociated to form a single-cell suspension, and cultured in appropriate media. These viable cells are then exposed to fluorochrome-labeled antibodies that adhere to CSC-specific antigens. When exposed to laser light, the cell-bound fluorochrome is excited and emits light of a different wavelength. Based on the emitted fluorescence and light scatter properties, the CSCs can be accurately identified and quantified. After flow cytometric detection, the cells are electrically charged and exposed to electromagnetic field inside the cell sorter. These cells are separated from each other and sorted into collecting tubes on the basis of their electric charge.

The working principle of FACS is illustrated in the form of diagram in **Figure 4**. Many studies in the literature have used a combination of various cell-surface biomarkers, listed in **Tables 1 and 2**, for fluorescence-based cell sorting

TABLE 3: List of intracellular cancer stem cell (CSC) biomarkers along with their functions and the tumors in which they are expressed.

Intracellular biomarkers	Expansion of abbreviation/other name/ function	Tumors in which they are expressed with references
ALDH	Aldehyde dehydrogenase	• Acute myeloid leukemia[263] • Breast cancer[193,264] • Cervical cancer[265] • Colorectal cancer[266] • Endometrial cancer[44] • Gastric cancer[203,267] • Lung cancer[236,237,258] • Prostate cancer[165]
BMI-1	B cell-specific Moloney murine leukemia virus integration site 1	• Acute myeloid leukemia • Breast cancer[268] • Gastric cancer[257] • Head and neck squamous cell carcinoma (SCC)[269] • Lung cancer[237]
LETM1	Leucine zipper-EF-hand containing transmembrane protein 1	• Colorectal cancer[270] • Gastric cancer[271]
MMP	Matrix metalloproteinases	Brain cancer[272]
NANOG	Homeobox domain stem cell transcription factor	• Breast cancer[273,274] • Colorectal cancer[275] • Gastric cancer[257,276] • Liver cancer[277]
NOTCH	Neurogenic locus notch homolog protein	• Breast cancer[278] • Liver cancer[82,185,186,219] • Lung cancer[169]
OCT-3/4	Octamer-binding transcription factor-3/4, POU domain, class 5, transcription factor 1 (POU5F1)	• Breast cancer[273,274] • Gastric cancer[276] • Liver cancer[221,277] • Lung cancer[279]
SOX2	Sex determining region Y-box 2, SRY-related HMG box family	• Breast cancer[273] • Colorectal cancer[280] • Gastric cancer[276]
Wnt/ß-catenin	Wingless-related integration site, catenin beta-1	• Breast cancer[254] • Liver cancer[186] • Lung cancer[58]

of the CSCs.[16,17,19,20,22,181,187,202,222,247,281] FACS is a highly advantageous technology, capable of accurately analyzing and classifying rare cell subpopulations within a relatively short time while preserving cell viability. Its high-throughput capacity allows it to sort thousands of cells per second, producing ultra-high

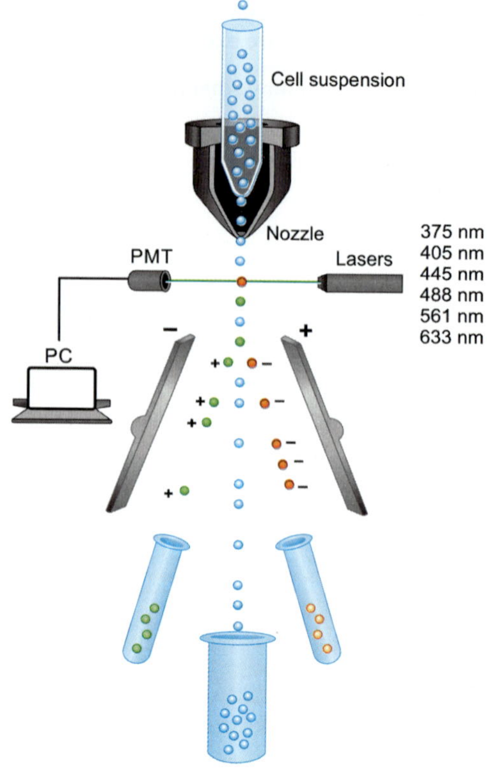

FIG. 4: Fluorescence-activated cell sorting (FACS) is a technique used to analyze and separate suspended tumor cells based on fluorescent tagging. In this process, cells are labeled with fluorochrome-tagged antibodies that target specific cell-surface markers. The cells then pass through a laser-detector system that measures their fluorescence and light scattering properties. Based on these measurements, cells are sorted in an electric field and collected into different tubes according to their characteristics. For example, in the diagram, cells labeled with green and red fluorescent proteins are isolated from those without labels, which are sorted into a separate tube.

(PMT: photomultiplier tube)

Source: Adapted from Hodne K, Weltzien FA. Single-Cell Isolation and Gene Analysis: Pitfalls and Possibilities. Int J Mol Sci. 2015;16(11):26832-49.

purity samples. However, the limitations of FACS include time-consuming sample preparation and the need for expensive instrumentation.

Side Population Analysis

In 1996, Goodell et al. identified a tiny subpopulation of cells that exhibited high efflux of the dye "Hoechst 33342" due to abundant expression of multidrug resistance (MDR) proteins like ABC family of membrane transporters.[284] These cells specifically exhibited stem cell properties such as self-renewal capacity, quiescent state, and drug resistance and were termed SP cells.[285] Due to the pumping out of the dye, the SP cells were detected as the population exhibiting low fluorescence.[286] Using the FACS technique, SP analysis detects cells in a quiescent state with the help of DNA-binding dyes such as Hoechst 33342 and

Vybrant™ DyeCycle™ Violet. This technique can be combined with biomarker-based cell sorting to enhance the enrichment of CSCs.[287] Many studies have performed SP analysis in a variety of cancers, such as breast cancer, endometrial cancer, head and neck cancer, hepatocellular carcinoma, and lung cancer, to isolate CSCs.[288-292]

In Vitro Tumor-sphere Formation Assay

The CSCs exhibit a tendency to form three-dimensional multicellular spheres when cultured in a nonadherent, serum-free medium enriched with mitogens like EGF and FGF. This colony-forming property was first studied by Reynolds et al. when they attempted to obtain neural stem cells from brain tissue.[293] Later, it was observed that these sphere-forming cells, or spheroids, exhibited stem cell properties, drug resistance and expressed CSC-specific surface biomarkers.[72,131,235,294,295] In addition, cells derived from the spheroids induced tumor formation in immunodeficient mice upon transplantation.[296] The advantage of this technique is that the serum-free medium provides a suitable environment for CSCs to propagate, as they can proliferate without any adherent layer. Despite this, the yield of CSC using this technique is low, ranging from 1 to 30%. During serial culture, the cells of the spheroid either undergo differentiation or apoptosis, thus reducing the passage numbers.[297]

Intracellular Enzyme Activity Analysis

Aldehyde dehydrogenase enzyme catalyzes the oxidation of intracellular aldehydes. The ALDH family includes three main subtypes: ALDH1, ALDH2, and ALDH3, each of which exists in various isoforms.[298] Earlier, we discussed that the CSCs exhibit increased ALDH enzyme activity, which serves as a mechanism of drug resistance.[164,165,193,203,236,258,263] Therefore, measuring intracellular ALDH activity can be a useful method for characterizing and isolating CSCs. This activity is assessed using commercially available kits such as ALDEFLUOR assay.[299] In this assay, an aminoacetaldehyde moiety tagged with the BODIPY fluorochrome, known as BODIPY-aminoacetaldehyde (BAAA), is used as a substrate for active ALDH enzyme. The cells exhibiting high ALDH activity will emit fluorescence, which are detected and sorted using the FACS technique. The test results are compared with those of a negative control, which is treated with the ALDH inhibitor "diethylaminobenzaldehyde (DEAB)".

Other Cell Sorting Techniques

Other cancer stem cell sorting techniques that warrant special mention include tumorigenicity and chemoresistance assays, cell division frequency tracking, density gradient centrifugation, immunoselection, measurement of ROS concentration, and mitochondrial membrane potential.[20,300-305] Nevertheless, a detailed discussion of these techniques is beyond the scope of this chapter.

NOVEL THERAPIES TARGETING CANCER STEM CELLS

Cancer treatment remains challenging due to the development of immune evasion properties, treatment resistance, heterogeneity, metastasis, and recurrences. These undesirable properties of tumors have led to the failure of traditional treatment strategies in certain cancers. Throughout this chapter, we have understood that CSCs play a major role in tumor progression, invasion, metastasis, and therapy resistance. Therefore, novel treatment strategies have been developed to specifically target CSCs to improve patient prognosis and enhance survival.[40,306] The different types of therapeutic agents developed against CSCs include chimeric antigen receptor (CAR) T-cells, bispecific T-cell engager molecules (BiTEs), monoclonal antibodies (mAbs), and antibody–drug conjugates (ADCs). A variety of approaches have been developed to target CSCs, some of which are discussed below.

Therapeutics Targeting the Cell-surface Biomarkers of Cancer Stem Cells

With a significant increase in the understanding of CSC surface biomarkers, new therapeutic agents have been developed to target CSC-specific cell-surface markers and eliminate them. Some of the novel CSC-directed drugs targeting these cell-surface markers and their intended uses are tabulated in **Table 4**.

Therapeutics Targeting the Signaling Pathways of Cancer Stem Cells

The signaling pathways which are responsible for stemness and survival of CSCs have become potential targets for cancer treatment. The important signaling pathways include Wnt, NOTCH, Hedgehog, TGF-β, JAK-STAT, phosphoinositide 3-kinase (PI3K), and NF-κB signaling pathways.[40] Significant advancements have been achieved in the development and clinical testing of inhibitors targeting these signaling pathways. Some of the novel CSC-directed drugs targeting the signaling pathways and their intended uses are tabulated in **Table 5**.

Therapeutics Targeting the Microenvironment of Cancer Stem Cells

The TME forms the backbone of CSC survival, nurturing and protecting them from the harmful effects of the immune system and cancer therapies. Therefore, novel therapies targeting the TME would deprive CSCs of their survival advantage. The cytokine TGF-β is one of the prime mediators of CSC-stromal crosstalk in various cancers. Many ongoing clinical trials target TGF-β and its pathway **(Table 5)** to sever the connection between CSCs and the stroma.[356-358] Newer therapies target various components of the ECM that are responsible for tumor progression. Drugs targeting MMPs, such as incyclinide (CMT-3/COL-3), have been developed to treat advanced soft-tissue sarcomas and metastatic cancers.[366,367] Angiotensin II receptor blockers such as losartan and candesartan have been shown to prolong survival in gastric cancer patients by reducing tumor-induced desmoplasia and angiogenesis.[368]

Another potential target in the TME is the tumor vasculature. A variety of Food and Drug Administration (FDA)-approved antiangiogenic agents, such as bevacizumab (a VEGF inhibitor), sorafenib, and sunitinib (both tyrosine kinase

TABLE 4: List of therapeutic agents targeting cancer stem cell (CSC)-specific cell-surface markers with their intended use.

Therapeutic target	Name of the drug	Type of drug	Intended use	References
CD24	SWA11	mAb	• Colorectal and pancreatic cancer • Lung and ovarian cancer	• Sagiv et al.[307]
	SWA11-Ricin A chain couplers	ADC	Lung cancer	Zangemeister-Wittke et al.[308]
	CD24-CAR-NK-92	CAR NK-cells	Ovarian cancer	Klapdor et al.[309]
CD33	Gemtuzumab ozogamicin	mAb	AML	Goldenson et al.[310]
	Lintuzumab-Ac225	mAb conjugated with alpha particle emitting radionuclide Ac-225	AML	Abedin et al.[311]
	Vadastuximab talirine (SGN-CD33A)	ADC	AML	Stein et al.[312]
	AMG 330	BiTE (binds to CD33 and CD3)	AML	Ravandi et al.[313]
	CD33CART	CAR-T cells	AML	Shah et al.[314]
CD36	JC63.1	mAb	Ovarian cancer	Ladanyi et al.[315]
CD44	Sulfasalazine	Suppress the effects of CD44v by inhibiting "xCT", a cystine-glutamate transporter	Gastric cancer	Shitara et al.[316]
	U36	anti-CD44v6 chimeric mAb	Head and neck SCC	Sandström et al.[317]
	RG7356	Humanized mAb	Solid tumors	Menke-van der Houven van Oordt et al.[318]

Continued

Continued

Therapeutic target	Name of the drug	Type of drug	Intended use	References
	CD44v6-targeted CAR-T cells	CAR-T cells	Head and neck SCC	Haist et al.[319]
CD47	TTI-621 (SIRPα-IgG1 Fc)	Human soluble recombinant fusion protein	• High-grade leiomyosarcoma • Sézary syndrome	• Chawla et al.[320] • Querfeld et al.[321]
	Hu5F9-G4	mAb	Malignant pediatric brain tumors	Gholamin et al.[322]
	CD47-CAR-T cells	CAR-T cells	Pancreatic cancer	Golubovskaya et al.[323]
CD96	MSH-TH111e	mAb	AML	Gramatzki et al.[324]
CD123	Talacotuzumab	mAb	AML	Montesinos et al.[325]
	IMGN632			
	Flotetuzumab	DART (bispecific for CD3ε and CD123)	AML	Uy et al.[326]
CD133	C178ABC-CD133MAb	mAb conjugated to cytolethal distending toxin (Cdt)	Head and neck SCC	Poprawa et al.[327]
	dCD133KDEL	Anti-CD133 scFv-deimmunized pseudomonas exotoxin A-KDEL fusion protein	Ovarian cancer	Skubitz et al.[328]
	MS133	BiTE (binds to CD133 and CD3)	Colorectal cancer	Zhao et al.[329]
	CD16 × 133	BiKE (binds to CD133 and CD16)	Colorectal cancer	Schmohl et al.[330]
CLL-1	CLL-1 CAR-T cells	CAR-T cells	AML	Jin et al.[331]

Continued

Continued

Therapeutic target	Name of the drug	Type of drug	Intended use	References
EpCAM	Adecatumumab	mAb	Prostate cancer	Oberneder et al.[332]
	Catumaxomab	Trifunctional mAb (binds to CD3, EpCAM and CD16 + cells)	Malignant ascites due to gynecological neoplasms	Kurbacher et al.[333]
	MT110	BiTE (binds to EpCAM and CD3)	Breast cancer	Hong et al.[334]
	chiHEA125-Ama	ADC	Pancreatic cancer	Moldenhauer et al.[335]
	EpCAM CAR T (IMC001)	CAR-T cells	Gastric cancer	Luo et al.[336]
LGR5	Petosemtamab (MCLA-158)	BiTE (binds to EGFR and LGR5)	Colorectal cancer	Herpers et al.[337]
	Anti-LGR5-MMAE	ADC	Colorectal cancer	Junttila et al.[338]
TIM-3	Sabatolimab (MBG453)	mAb	MDS	Brunner et al.[339]

(Ac-225: actinium-225; ADC: antibody drug conjugate; AML: acute myeloid leukemia; BiKE: bispecific NK-cell engager molecule; BiTE: bispecific T-cell engager molecule; CAR: chimeric antigen receptor; Cdt: cytolethal distending toxin; DART: dual affinity retargeting protein; EGFR: epidermal growth factor receptor; mAb: monoclonal antibody; MDS: myelodysplastic neoplasm; SCC: squamous cell carcinoma; scFv: single-chain fragment variable)

TABLE 5: List of therapeutic agents targeting CSC-specific signaling pathways with their intended use.

Therapeutic target	Name of the drug	Type of drug	Intended use	References
Wnt signaling pathway	Ipafricept (OMP-54F28)	Recombinant fusion protein—Frizzled family receptor 8 (Fzd8) fused to the human immunoglobulin Fc domain	Ovarian cancer	Moore et al.[340]
	Vantictumab (OMP-18R5)	mAb	Breast cancer	Diamond et al.[341]
	PRI-724	Small molecule inhibitor of β-Catenin/CBP	Hepatocellular carcinoma	Gabata et al.[342]
NOTCH signaling pathway	MK-0752	GSI	• Pancreatic cancer • Ovarian cancer	• Cook et al.[343] • Chen et al.[344]
	RO4929097	GSI	• Metastatic melanoma • Breast cancer	• Lee et al.[345] • Sardesai et al.[346]
	Nirogacestat (PF-03084014)	GSI	Desmoid tumor	Takahashi et al.[347]
	Demcizumab (OMP-21M18)	mAb directed against DLL4	Lung cancer	McKeage et al.[348]
	Enoticumab (REGN421)	mAb directed against DLL4	Solid tumors	Chiorean et al.[349]
Hedgehog signaling pathway	Vismodegib (GDC-0449)	Small-molecule inhibitor of SMO	• Metastatic solid tumors • Pancreatic cancer • Basal cell carcinoma	• LoRusso et al.[350] • Kim et al.[351] • Sekulic et al.[352]
	Sonidegib (NVP-LDE225)	Small-molecule inhibitor of SMO	Basal cell carcinoma	Pan et al.[353]
	Glasdegib	Small-molecule inhibitor of SMO	AML	Sekeres et al.[354]

Continued

Continued

Therapeutic target	Name of the drug	Type of drug	Intended use	References
TGF-β signaling pathway	Luspatercept	TGF-β ligand trap	MDS	Chan et al.[355]
	Vactosertib	Inhibitor of TGFBR1	Pancreatic cancer	Lee et al.[356]
	Galunisertib (LY2157299)	Inhibitor of TGFBR1	Hepatocellular carcinoma	Kelley et al.[357]
	Fresolimumab (GC1008)	mAb directed against TGF-β	Melanoma and renal cell carcinoma	Morris et al.[358]
JAK-STAT signaling pathway	Ruxolitinib (INCB018424)	JAK1/2 inhibitor	• Breast cancer • Colorectal cancer	• Lim et al.[359] • An et al.[360]
	Pacritinib (SB1518)	JAK2/FLT3 inhibitor	AML	Hart et al.[361]
PI3K signaling pathway	Idelalisib	PI3Kδ inhibitor	B-cell NHL	Kahl et al.[362]
	Alpelisib	PI3Kα inhibitor	Breast cancer	André et al.[363]
	Buparlisib (BKM120)	Pan-class I PI3K inhibitor	Breast cancer	Garrido-Castro et al.[364]
NF-κB signaling pathway	Selinexor	Selective inhibitor of nuclear transport	Multiple myeloma	Chari et al.[365]

(AML: acute myeloid leukemia; CBP: CREB-binding protein; DLL4: delta-like canonical notch ligand 4; GSI: gamma secretase inhibitor; JAK/STAT: Janus kinase/signal transducers and activators of transcription; mAb: monoclonal antibody; MDS: myelodysplastic neoplasm; NF-κB: nuclear factor kappa B; NHL: non-Hodgkin lymphoma; PI3K: phosphoinositide 3-kinase; SMO: smoothened receptor; TGF-β: transforming growth factor beta; TGFBR1: TGF-beta receptor type 1; Wnt: wingless-related integration site)

receptor inhibitors), are combined with standard chemotherapeutic agents for the treatment of malignancies.[369] Hypoxic state of the TME promotes CSC growth and survival. Therefore, drugs which target the hypoxic niche would cause depletion of the CSCs. Drugs that block HIF protein synthesis, such as topoisomerase inhibitors (topotecan) and mTOR inhibitors (everolimus), are employed in cancer treatment to tackle the hypoxic TME.[370,371] Currently, bioreductive drugs also termed as hypoxia-activated prodrugs (HAPs) have been developed, which specifically get activated in the hypoxic TME and target the hypoxic areas of the tumor.[372]

Many clinical trials also focus on reducing the pro-inflammatory cells of the TME, such as TAMs and MDSCs, which secrete cytokines responsible for CSC-niche crosstalk. The drugs used to target the pro-inflammatory niche in various tumors include the IL-1 receptor antagonist (anakinra), the mAbs targeting IL-1β (canakinumab), and the small-molecule inhibitor of colony-stimulating factor 1 receptor (CSF-1R) (pexidartinib).[373-375]

Immunotherapy Directed Against Cancer Stem Cells

An intact antitumor surveillance mechanism can hinder cancer progression and development. In the current era, many therapies aim to stimulate and boost the immune system to mount an effective antitumor response. Immune checkpoint inhibitors targeting cytotoxic T-lymphocyte-associated protein 4 (CTLA-4), namely ipilimumab, programmed cell death 1 (PD-1) inhibitors (nivolumab and pembrolizumab), and PDL-1 inhibitors (avelumab, durvalumab, and atezolizumab) are being tested in clinical trials in various cancers.[376-381]

The most advanced engineering techniques in immunotherapy include CAR-T-cells and CAR-NK cells. These immune cells are modified to express specific receptors directed against the antigenic proteins present on the target cell surface.[382] CAR-T-cells targeting various CSC-specific surface markers are being studied in clinical trials for CSC-directed immunotherapy **(Table 4)**.

Utility of Nanotechnology in Targeting Cancer Stem Cells

Nanotechnology is a subspeciality of science focused on the study and development of devices with dimensions ranging from 1 to 1,000 nanometers. In recent years, research in nanotechnology has led to the popularity of nanodrug delivery systems (NDDS), which utilize small-sized biodegradable particles with a high surface area, known as nanoparticles (NPs). NDDS improve the bioavailability and efficacy of drugs due to their accurate targeting mechanisms. Some of the most commonly used NPs include lipid and micelle-based NPs, polymer and nonpolymer NPs, carbon nanotubes (CNTs), graphene oxide (GO), gold nanorods (GNRs), nanobinding, nanocapsules, quantum dots (QDs), etc.[383-385] The use of NDDS can induce apoptosis, overcome drug resistance in tumors, and effectively eliminate CSCs. Several types of CSC-targeted NPs are currently being evaluated in ongoing clinical trials.[385] Despite its effective drug delivery, NDDS faces challenges such as the inability to be completely metabolized, leading to toxic accumulation and compromised biosafety.

Nanobodies (Nbs), also known as single-domain antibodies (sdAbs), are antibody fragments composed of single monomeric variable domains that target specific antigens and lack light chain domains.[386] The advantages of Nbs include their reduced immunogenicity and cost-effectiveness when produced using microbial production systems. Many Nbs have been developed to target CSC-specific biomarkers, which helps inhibit tumor growth and proliferation.[387-389] Additionally, Nbs targeting cell surface moieties can be conjugated to NDDS, enhancing their effectiveness as drug carriers.[390,391]

CONCLUSION

Cancer stem cells are a distinct subset of cancer cells characterized by their ability to self-renew, withstand challenging microenvironments in quiescent state, invade and metastasize, and develop resistance to conventional cancer treatments. These notorious properties of CSCs are primarily responsible for tumor recurrence and their lack of responsiveness to standard treatments. The survival advantage of CSCs is supported by their niche, which is specifically involved in CSC interactions and acts as a barrier against antitumor immune surveillance.

Cancer stem cells are regulated by various signaling pathways and transcription factors, as well as several factors from the TME, including cytokines, protumorigenic inflammatory cells, stromal cells, ECM components, and the hypoxic microenvironment. The plasticity of CSCs allows them to differentiate and dedifferentiate as needed for survival and to adapt their metabolic state according to the signals from the TME. Extensive research on CSCs has led to the identification of CSC-specific cell-surface and intracellular biomarkers, which can be targeted by novel therapeutic agents for more effective elimination of these cells. Notably, numerous clinical trials focusing on CSCs have been conducted, revealing promising potential for advancing cancer treatments.

Nevertheless, challenges persist in completely eliminating CSCs due to the lacunae in our understanding of their biology. The specific characteristics of CSCs and their interactions with their niche in various tumors are not yet fully understood. Many studies isolate CSCs from their niche and use immune-deficient mice for research, which does not accurately replicate the in vivo complexity of human tumors. Additionally, CSCs share signaling pathways and surface biomarkers with normal stem cells. This implies that not all regulatory factors and surface markers are suitable as specific therapeutic targets for CSCs. Factors such as epigenetics and cellular metabolism also influence CSCs and should be considered when designing novel therapies. To address these challenges, future research on CSCs and the development of promising CSC-targeted therapies must be prioritized in clinical trials to improve cancer patients' survival.

REFERENCES

1. Zakrzewski W, Dobrzyński M, Szymonowicz M, Rybak Z. Stem cells: past, present, and future. Stem Cell Res Ther. 2019;10:68.
2. Lu F, Zhang Y. Cell totipotency: molecular features, induction, and maintenance. Natl Sci Rev. 2015;2:217-25.
3. Thomson JA, Itskovitz-Eldor J, Shapiro SS, Waknitz MA, Swiergiel JJ, Marshall VS, et al. Embryonic stem cell lines derived from human blastocysts. Science. 1998;282:1145-7.

4. Takahashi K, Yamanaka S. Induction of pluripotent stem cells from mouse embryonic and adult fibroblast cultures by defined factors. Cell. 2006;126:663-76.
5. Spangrude GJ, Heimfeld S, Weissman IL. Purification and characterization of mouse hematopoietic stem cells. Science. 1988;241:58-62.
6. Ferraro F, Celso CL, Scadden D. Adult stem cells and their niches. Adv Exp Med Biol. 2010;695:155-68.
7. Schofield R. The relationship between the spleen colony-forming cell and the haemopoietic stem cell. Blood Cells. 1978;4:7-25.
8. Kiel MJ, Yilmaz OH, Iwashita T, Yilmaz OH, Terhorst C, Morrison SJ. SLAM family receptors distinguish hematopoietic stem and progenitor cells and reveal endothelial niches for stem cells. Cell. 2005;121:1109-21.
9. Calvi LM, Adams GB, Weibrecht KW, Weber JM, Olson DP, Knight MC, et al. Osteoblastic cells regulate the haematopoietic stem cell niche. Nature. 2003;425:841-6.
10. Cotsarelis G, Sun TT, Lavker RM. Label-retaining cells reside in the bulge area of pilosebaceous unit: implications for follicular stem cells, hair cycle, and skin carcinogenesis. Cell. 1990;61:1329-37.
11. Cotsarelis G, Cheng SZ, Dong G, Sun TT, Lavker RM. Existence of slow-cycling limbal epithelial basal cells that can be preferentially stimulated to proliferate: Implications on epithelial stem cells. Cell. 1989;57:201-9.
12. Barker N, van Es JH, Kuipers J, Kujala P, van den Born M, Cozijnsen M, et al. Identification of stem cells in small intestine and colon by marker gene Lgr5. Nature. 2007;449:1003-7.
13. Kuwahara R, Kofman AV, Landis CS, Swenson ES, Barendswaard E, Theise ND. The hepatic stem cell niche: identification by label-retaining cell assay. Hepatology. 2008;47:1994-2002.
14. Nowell PC. The clonal evolution of tumor cell populations. Science. 1976;194:23-8.
15. Pierce GB. Neoplasms, differentiations and mutations. Am J Pathol. 1974;77:103-18.
16. Bonnet D, Dick JE. Human acute myeloid leukemia is organized as a hierarchy that originates from a primitive hematopoietic cell. Nat Med. 1997;3:730-7.
17. Lapidot T, Sirard C, Vormoor J, Murdoch B, Hoang T, Caceres-Cortes J, et al. A cell initiating human acute myeloid leukaemia after transplantation into SCID mice. Nature. 1994;367: 645-8.
18. Sivakumar V, Ravi S, Manivannan P. Current Concepts of Leukemic Stem Cells: Origin, Characteristics, and its Clinical Implications in Acute Myeloid Leukemia. Med Res Arch. 2024;12(6).
19. Singh SK, Hawkins C, Clarke ID, Squire JA, Bayani J, Hide T, et al. Identification of human brain tumour initiating cells. Nature. 2004;432:396-401.
20. Al-Hajj M, Wicha MS, Benito-Hernandez A, Morrison SJ, Clarke MF. Prospective identification of tumorigenic breast cancer cells. Proc Natl Acad Sci U S A. 2003;100:3983-8.
21. Islam F, Gopalan V, Lam AK. Identification of Cancer Stem Cells in Esophageal Adenocarcinoma. Methods Mol Biol. 2018;1756:165-76.
22. Collins AT, Berry PA, Hyde C, Stower MJ, Maitland NJ. Prospective identification of tumorigenic prostate cancer stem cells. Cancer Res. 2005;65:10946-51.
23. Mani SA, Guo W, Liao MJ, Eaton EN, Ayyanan A, Zhou AY, et al. The epithelial-mesenchymal transition generates cells with properties of stem cells. Cell. 2008;133:704-15.
24. Reya T, Morrison SJ, Clarke MF, Weissman IL. Stem cells, cancer, and cancer stem cells. Nature. 2001;414:105-11.
25. Li L, Neaves WB. Normal stem cells and cancer stem cells: the niche matters. Cancer Res. 2006;66:4553-7.
26. Hayakawa Y, Fox JG, Wang TC. The Origins of Gastric Cancer From Gastric Stem Cells: Lessons From Mouse Models. Cell Mol Gastroenterol Hepatol. 2017;3:331-8.
27. Walcher L, Kistenmacher AK, Suo H, Kitte R, Dluczek S, Strauß A, et al. Cancer Stem Cells-Origins and Biomarkers: Perspectives for Targeted Personalized Therapies. Front Immunol. 2020;11:1280.
28. Knudson AG. Mutation and cancer: statistical study of retinoblastoma. Proc Natl Acad Sci U S A. 1971;68:820-3.

29. Moolgavkar SH, Venzon DJ. Two-event models for carcinogenesis: incidence curves for childhood and adult tumors. Math Biosci. 1979;47:55-77.
30. Basu AK. DNA Damage, Mutagenesis and Cancer. Int J Mol Sci. 2018;19:970.
31. Aktas B, Tewes M, Fehm T, Hauch S, Kimmig R, Kasimir-Bauer S. Stem cell and epithelial-mesenchymal transition markers are frequently overexpressed in circulating tumor cells of metastatic breast cancer patients. Breast Cancer Res. 2009;11:R46.
32. Morrison SJ, Kimble J. Asymmetric and symmetric stem-cell divisions in development and cancer. Nature. 2006;441:1068-74.
33. Lytle NK, Barber A, Reya T. Stem cell fate in cancer growth, progression and therapy resistance. Nat Rev Cancer. 2018;18:669-80.
34. Betschinger J, Mechtler K, Knoblich JA. Asymmetric segregation of the tumor suppressor brat regulates self-renewal in Drosophila neural stem cells. Cell. 2006;124:1241-53.
35. Bowman SK, Neumüller RA, Novatchkova M, Du Q, Knoblich JA. The Drosophila NuMA Homolog Mud regulates spindle orientation in asymmetric cell division. Dev Cell. 2006;10:731-42.
36. Bajaj J, Zimdahl B, Reya T. Fearful symmetry: Subversion of asymmetric division in cancer development and progression. Cancer Res. 2015;75:792-7.
37. Kaplan KB, Burds AA, Swedlow JR, Bekir SS, Sorger PK, Näthke IS. A role for the Adenomatous Polyposis Coli protein in chromosome segregation. Nat Cell Biol. 2001;3:429-32.
38. Yasumi M, Sakisaka T, Hoshino T, Kimura T, Sakamoto Y, Yamanaka T, et al. Direct Binding of Lgl2 to LGN during Mitosis and Its Requirement for Normal Cell Division. J Biol Chem. 2005;280:6761-5.
39. Lechler T, Fuchs E. Asymmetric cell divisions promote stratification and differentiation of mammalian skin. Nature. 2005;437:275-80.
40. Yang L, Shi P, Zhao G, Xu J, Peng W, Zhang J, et al. Targeting cancer stem cell pathways for cancer therapy. Signal Transduct Target Ther. 2020;5:8.
41. Levy DE, Darnell JE Jr. Stats: transcriptional control and biological impact. Nat Rev Mol Cell Biol. 2002;3:651-62.
42. Kralovics R, Passamonti F, Buser AS, Teo SS, Tiedt R, Passweg JR, et al. A gain-of-function mutation of JAK2 in myeloproliferative disorders. N Engl J Med. 2005;352:1779-90.
43. Levine RL, Wadleigh M, Cools J, Ebert BL, Wernig G, Huntly BJP, et al. Activating mutation in the tyrosine kinase JAK2 in polycythemia vera, essential thrombocythemia, and myeloid metaplasia with myelofibrosis. Cancer Cell. 2005;7:387-97.
44. van der Zee M, Sacchetti A, Cansoy M, Joosten R, Teeuwssen M, Heijmans-Antonissen C, et al. IL6/JAK1/STAT3 Signaling Blockade in Endometrial Cancer Affects the ALDHhi/CD126+ Stem-like Component and Reduces Tumor Burden. Cancer Res. 2015;75:3608-22.
45. Lam LT, Wright G, Davis RE, Lenz G, Farinha P, Dang L, et al. Cooperative signaling through the signal transducer and activator of transcription 3 and nuclear factor-{kappa}B pathways in subtypes of diffuse large B-cell lymphoma. Blood. 2008;111:3701-13.
46. Jiang C, Long J, Liu B, Xu M, Wang W, Xie X, et al. miR-500a-3p promotes cancer stem cells properties via STAT3 pathway in human hepatocellular carcinoma. J Exp Clin Cancer Res. 2017;36:99.
47. Karunanithi S, Levi L, DeVecchio J, Karagkounis G, Reizes O, Lathia JD, et al. RBP4-STRA6 Pathway Drives Cancer Stem Cell Maintenance and Mediates High-Fat Diet-Induced Colon Carcinogenesis. Stem Cell Reports. 2017;9:438-50.
48. Zhou J, Wulfkuhle J, Zhang H, Gu P, Yang Y, Deng J, et al. Activation of the PTEN/mTOR/STAT3 pathway in breast cancer stem-like cells is required for viability and maintenance. Proc Natl Acad Sci U S A. 2007;104:16158-63.
49. Marotta LLC, Almendro V, Marusyk A, Shipitsin M, Schemme J, Walker SR, et al. The JAK2/STAT3 signaling pathway is required for growth of CD44+CD24– stem cell–like breast cancer cells in human tumors. J Clin Invest. 2011;121:2723-35.
50. Kim SY, Kang JW, Song X, Kim BK, Yoo YD, Kwon YT, et al. Role of the IL-6-JAK1-STAT3-Oct-4 pathway in the conversion of non-stem cancer cells into cancer stem-like cells. Cell Signal. 2013;25:961-9.

51. Yang L, Dong Y, Li Y, Wang D, Liu S, Wang D, et al. IL-10 derived from M2 macrophage promotes cancer stemness via JAK1/STAT1/NF-κB/Notch1 pathway in non-small cell lung cancer. Int J Cancer. 2019;145:1099-110.
52. Katoh M. Canonical and non-canonical WNT signaling in cancer stem cells and their niches: Cellular heterogeneity, omics reprogramming, targeted therapy and tumor plasticity (Review). Int J Oncol. 2017;51:1357-69.
53. Kahn M. Can we safely target the WNT pathway? Nat Rev Drug Discov. 2014;13:513-32.
54. Malanchi I, Santamaria-Martínez A, Susanto E, Peng H, Lehr HA, Delaloye JF, et al. Interactions between cancer stem cells and their niche govern metastatic colonization. Nature. 2011;481:85-9.
55. O'Connell JT, Sugimoto H, Cooke VG, MacDonald BA, Mehta AI, LeBleu VS, et al. VEGF-A and Tenascin-C produced by S100A4+ stromal cells are important for metastatic colonization. Proc Natl Acad Sci U S A. 2011;108:16002-7.
56. Matzke-Ogi A, Jannasch K, Shatirishvili M, Fuchs B, Chiblak S, Morton J, et al. Inhibition of Tumor Growth and Metastasis in Pancreatic Cancer Models by Interference With CD44v6 Signaling. Gastroenterology. 2016;150:513-525.e10.
57. Todaro M, Gaggianesi M, Catalano V, Benfante A, Iovino F, Biffoni M, et al. CD44v6 is a marker of constitutive and reprogrammed cancer stem cells driving colon cancer metastasis. Cell Stem Cell. 2014;14:342-56.
58. Su J, Wu S, Wu H, Li L, Guo T. CD44 is functionally crucial for driving lung cancer stem cells metastasis through Wnt/β-catenin-FoxM1-Twist signaling. Mol Carcinog. 2016;55: 1962-73.
59. Schroeter EH, Kisslinger JA, Kopan R. Notch-1 signalling requires ligand-induced proteolytic release of intracellular domain. Nature. 1998;393:382-6.
60. Dontu G, Jackson KW, McNicholas E, Kawamura MJ, Abdallah WM, Wicha MS. Role of Notch signaling in cell-fate determination of human mammary stem/progenitor cells. Breast Cancer Res. 2004;6:R605-15.
61. Soriano JV, Uyttendaele H, Kitajewski J, Montesano R. Expression of an activated Notch4(int-3) oncoprotein disrupts morphogenesis and induces an invasive phenotype in mammary epithelial cells in vitro. Int J Cancer. 2000;86:652-9.
62. Xiu M, Wang Y, Li B, Wang X, Xiao F, Chen S, et al. The Role of Notch3 Signaling in Cancer Stemness and Chemoresistance: Molecular Mechanisms and Targeting Strategies. Front Mol Biosci. 2021;8.
63. Merchant AA, Matsui W. Targeting Hedgehog—a cancer stem cell pathway. Clin Cancer Res. 2010;16:3130-40.
64. Petrova R, Joyner AL. Roles for Hedgehog signaling in adult organ homeostasis and repair. Development. 2014;141:3445-57.
65. Hahn H, Wicking C, Zaphiropoulous PG, Gailani MR, Shanley S, Chidambaram A, et al. Mutations of the human homolog of Drosophila patched in the nevoid basal cell carcinoma syndrome. Cell. 1996;85:841-51.
66. Po A, Silvano M, Miele E, Capalbo C, Eramo A, Salvati V, et al. Noncanonical GLI1 signaling promotes stemness features and in vivo growth in lung adenocarcinoma. Oncogene. 2017;36:4641-52.
67. Clement V, Sanchez P, de Tribolet N, Radovanovic I, Ruiz i Altaba A. HEDGEHOG-GLI1 signaling regulates human glioma growth, cancer stem cell self-renewal, and tumorigenicity. Curr Biol. 2007;17:165-72.
68. Wang M, Zhao J, Zhang L, Wei F, Lian Y, Wu Y, et al. Role of tumor microenvironment in tumorigenesis. J Cancer. 2017;8:761-73.
69. Plaks V, Kong N, Werb Z. The cancer stem cell niche: how essential is the niche in regulating stemness of tumor cells? Cell Stem Cell. 2015;16:225-38.
70. Cuiffo BG, Karnoub AE. Mesenchymal stem cells in tumor development: emerging roles and concepts. Cell Adh Migr. 2012;6:220-30.
71. Cabarcas SM, Mathews LA, Farrar WL. The cancer stem cell niche—there goes the neighborhood? Int J Cancer. 2011;129:2315-27.

72. Sansone P, Storci G, Tavolari S, Guarnieri T, Giovannini C, Taffurelli M, et al. IL-6 triggers malignant features in mammospheres from human ductal breast carcinoma and normal mammary gland. J Clin Invest. 2007;117:3988-4002.
73. Leizer A, Alvero AB, Fu HH, Holmberg JC, Cheng YC, Silasi DA, et al. Regulation of inflammation by the NF-KB pathway in ovarian cancer stem cells. Am J Reprod Immunol. 2011;65:438-47.
74. Davis H, Irshad S, Bansal M, Rafferty H, Boitsova T, Bardella C, et al. Aberrant epithelial GREM1 expression initiates colonic tumorigenesis from cells outside the stem cell niche. Nat Med. 2015;21:62-70.
75. Spaeth EL, Dembinski JL, Sasser AK, Watson K, Klopp A, Hall B, et al. Mesenchymal Stem Cell Transition to Tumor-Associated Fibroblasts Contributes to Fibrovascular Network Expansion and Tumor Progression. PLoS One. 2009;4:e4992.
76. Kalluri R, Zeisberg M. Fibroblasts in cancer. Nat Rev Cancer. 2006;6:392-401.
77. Ezhilarasan D. Hepatic stellate cells in the injured liver: Perspectives beyond hepatic fibrosis. J Cell Physiol. 2022;237:436-49.
78. Barcellos-de-Souza P, Comito G, Pons-Segura C, Taddei ML, Gori V, Becherucci V, et al. Mesenchymal Stem Cells are Recruited and Activated into Carcinoma-Associated Fibroblasts by Prostate Cancer Microenvironment-Derived TGF-β1. Stem Cells. 2016;34: 2536-47.
79. Junttila MR, de Sauvage FJ. Influence of tumour micro-environment heterogeneity on therapeutic response. Nature. 2013;501:346-54.
80. Manoukian P, Bijlsma M, van Laarhoven H. The Cellular Origins of Cancer-Associated Fibroblasts and Their Opposing Contributions to Pancreatic Cancer Growth. Front Cell Dev Biol. 2021;9:743907.
81. Vermeulen L, De Sousa E Melo F, van der Heijden M, Cameron K, de Jong JH, Borovski T, et al. Wnt activity defines colon cancer stem cells and is regulated by the microenvironment. Nat Cell Biol. 2010;12:468-76.
82. Bai S, Zhao Y, Chen W, Peng W, Wang Y, Xiong S, et al. The stromal-tumor amplifying STC1-Notch1 feedforward signal promotes the stemness of hepatocellular carcinoma. J Transl Med. 2023;21:1-18.
83. Yeung TL, Leung CS, Wong KK, Samimi G, Thompson MS, Liu J, et al. TGF-β modulates ovarian cancer invasion by upregulating CAF-derived versican in the tumor microenvironment. Cancer Res. 2013;73:5016-28.
84. Kitamura T, Qian BZ, Pollard JW. Immune cell promotion of metastasis. Nat Rev Immunol. 2015;15:73-86.
85. Galassi C, Musella M, Manduca N, Maccafeo E, Sistigu A. The Immune Privilege of Cancer Stem Cells: A Key to Understanding Tumor Immune Escape and Therapy Failure. Cells. 2021;10:2361.
86. Wan S, Zhao E, Kryczek I, Vatan L, Sadovskaya A, Ludema G, et al. Tumor-associated macrophages produce interleukin 6 and signal via STAT3 to promote expansion of human hepatocellular carcinoma stem cells. Gastroenterology. 2014;147:1393-404.
87. Peng D, Tanikawa T, Li W, Zhao L, Vatan L, Szeliga W, et al. Myeloid-Derived Suppressor Cells Endow Stem-like Qualities to Breast Cancer Cells through IL6/STAT3 and NO/NOTCH Cross-talk Signaling. Cancer Res. 2016;76:3156-65.
88. Kuroda H, Mabuchi S, Yokoi E, Komura N, Kozasa K, Matsumoto Y, et al. Prostaglandin E2 produced by myeloid-derived suppressive cells induces cancer stem cells in uterine cervical cancer. Oncotarget. 2018;9:36317-30.
89. Yang S, Wang B, Guan C, Wu B, Cai C, Wang M, et al. Foxp3+IL-17+ T cells promote development of cancer-initiating cells in colorectal cancer. J Leukoc Biol. 2011;89:85-91.
90. Mantovani A, Marchesi F, Malesci A, Laghi L, Allavena P. Tumour-associated macrophages as treatment targets in oncology. Nat Rev Clin Oncol. 2017;14:399-416.
91. Kumar V, Patel S, Tcyganov E, Gabrilovich DI. The Nature of Myeloid-Derived Suppressor Cells in the Tumor Microenvironment. Trends Immunol. 2016;37:208-20.

92. Cui TX, Kryczek I, Zhao L, Zhao E, Kuick R, Roh MH, et al. Myeloid-derived suppressor cells enhance stemness of cancer cells by inducing microRNA101 and suppressing the corepressor CtBP2. Immunity. 2013;39:611-21.
93. Togashi Y, Shitara K, Nishikawa H. Regulatory T cells in cancer immunosuppression - implications for anticancer therapy. Nat Rev Clin Oncol. 2019;16:356-71.
94. Kessenbrock K, Plaks V, Werb Z. Matrix metalloproteinases: regulators of the tumor microenvironment. Cell. 2010;141:52-67.
95. Xiong J, Yan L, Zou C, Wang K, Chen M, Xu B, et al. Integrins regulate stemness in solid tumor: an emerging therapeutic target. J Hematol Oncol. 2021;14:177.
96. Cooper J, Giancotti FG. Integrin Signaling in Cancer: Mechanotransduction, Stemness, Epithelial Plasticity, and Therapeutic Resistance. Cancer Cell. 2019;35:347-67.
97. Sell S. Stem cell origin of cancer and differentiation therapy. Crit Rev Oncol Hematol. 2004;51:1-28.
98. Ratajczak MZ, Shin DM, Kucia M. Very Small Embryonic/Epiblast-Like Stem Cells. Am J Pathol. 2009;174:1985-92.
99. Ratajczak MZ, Bujko K, Mack A, Kucia M, Ratajczak J. Cancer from the perspective of stem cells and misappropriated tissue regeneration mechanisms. Leukemia. 2018;32:2519-26.
100. Oren O, Smith BD. Eliminating Cancer Stem Cells by Targeting Embryonic Signaling Pathways. Stem Cell Rev Rep. 2017;13:17-23.
101. Kreso A, Dick JE. Evolution of the cancer stem cell model. Cell Stem Cell. 2014;14:275-91.
102. Kreso A, O'Brien CA, van Galen P, Gan OI, Notta F, Brown AMK, et al. Variable clonal repopulation dynamics influence chemotherapy response in colorectal cancer. Science. 2013;339:543-8.
103. Li L, Tian T, Zhang X. Stochastic modelling of multistage carcinogenesis and progression of human lung cancer. J Theor Biol. 2019;479:81-9.
104. Tan WY, Chen CW, Wang W. Stochastic modeling of carcinogenesis by state space models: a new approach. Math Comput Model. 2001;33:1323-45.
105. Quail DF, Taylor MJ, Postovit LM. Microenvironmental regulation of cancer stem cell phenotypes. Curr Stem Cell Res Ther. 2012;7:197-216.
106. Das PK, Pillai S, Rakib MA, Khanam JA, Gopalan V, Lam AKY, et al. Plasticity of Cancer Stem Cell: Origin and Role in Disease Progression and Therapy Resistance. Stem Cell Rev Rep. 2020;16:397-412.
107. Tang DG. Understanding cancer stem cell heterogeneity and plasticity. Cell Res. 2012;22: 457-72.
108. Ahmed F, Haass NK. Microenvironment-Driven Dynamic Heterogeneity and Phenotypic Plasticity as a Mechanism of Melanoma Therapy Resistance. Front Oncol. 2018;8:173.
109. Greaves M. Evolutionary determinants of cancer. Cancer Discov. 2015;5:806-20.
110. Ahmed N, Escalona R, Leung D, Chan E, Kannourakis G. Tumour microenvironment and metabolic plasticity in cancer and cancer stem cells: Perspectives on metabolic and immune regulatory signatures in chemoresistant ovarian cancer stem cells. Semin Cancer Biol. 2018;53:265-81.
111. Wainwright EN, Scaffidi P. Epigenetics and Cancer Stem Cells: Unleashing, Hijacking, and Restricting Cellular Plasticity. Trends Cancer. 2017;3:372-86.
112. Krebs AM, Mitschke J, Lasierra Losada M, Schmalhofer O, Boerries M, Busch H, et al. The EMT-activator Zeb1 is a key factor for cell plasticity and promotes metastasis in pancreatic cancer. Nat Cell Biol. 2017;19:518-29.
113. Bhat GR, Sethi I, Sadida HQ, Rah B, Mir R, Algehainy N, et al. Cancer cell plasticity: from cellular, molecular, and genetic mechanisms to tumor heterogeneity and drug resistance. Cancer Metastasis Rev. 2024;43:197-228.
114. Latil M, Nassar D, Beck B, Boumahdi S, Wang L, Brisebarre A, et al. Cell-Type-Specific Chromatin States Differentially Prime Squamous Cell Carcinoma Tumor-Initiating Cells for Epithelial to Mesenchymal Transition. Cell Stem Cell. 2017;20:191-204.e5.
115. Easwaran H, Tsai HC, Baylin SB. Cancer epigenetics: tumor heterogeneity, plasticity of stem-like states, and drug resistance. Mol Cell. 2014;54:716-27.

116. Trisciuoglio D, Di Martile M, Del Bufalo D. Emerging Role of Histone Acetyltransferase in Stem Cells and Cancer. Stem Cells Int. 2018;2018:8908751.
117. Cabrera MC, Hollingsworth RE, Hurt EM. Cancer stem cell plasticity and tumor hierarchy. World J Stem Cells. 2015;7:27-36.
118. Hanahan D, Coussens LM. Accessories to the crime: functions of cells recruited to the tumor microenvironment. Cancer Cell. 2012;21:309-22.
119. Li Z, Bao S, Wu Q, Wang H, Eyler C, Sathornsumetee S, et al. Hypoxia-inducible factors regulate tumorigenic capacity of glioma stem cells. Cancer Cell. 2009;15:501-13.
120. Soleymani Abyaneh H, Gupta N, Alshareef A, Gopal K, Lavasanifar A, Lai R. Hypoxia Induces the Acquisition of Cancer Stem-like Phenotype Via Upregulation and Activation of Signal Transducer and Activator of Transcription-3 (STAT3) in MDA-MB-231, a Triple Negative Breast Cancer Cell Line. Cancer Microenviron. 2018;11:141-52.
121. Wu M, Neilson A, Swift AL, Moran R, Tamagnine J, Parslow D, et al. Multiparameter metabolic analysis reveals a close link between attenuated mitochondrial bioenergetic function and enhanced glycolysis dependency in human tumor cells. Am J Physiol Cell Physiol. 2007;292:C125-136.
122. De Francesco EM, Sotgia F, Lisanti MP. Cancer stem cells (CSCs): metabolic strategies for their identification and eradication. Biochem J. 2018;475:1611-34.
123. Warburg O. The Metabolism of Carcinoma Cells. J Cancer Res. 1925;9:148-63.
124. Zou ZW, Ma C, Medoro L, Chen L, Wang B, Gupta R, et al. LncRNA ANRIL is up-regulated in nasopharyngeal carcinoma and promotes the cancer progression via increasing proliferation, reprograming cell glucose metabolism and inducing side-population stem-like cancer cells. Oncotarget. 2016;7:61741-54.
125. Folmes CDL, Dzeja PP, Nelson TJ, Terzic A. Metabolic plasticity in stem cell homeostasis and differentiation. Cell Stem Cell. 2012;11:596-606.
126. Zhang D, Wang Y, Shi Z, Liu J, Sun P, Hou X, et al. Metabolic reprogramming of cancer-associated fibroblasts by IDH3α downregulation. Cell Rep. 2015;10:1335-48.
127. Keith B, Simon MC. Hypoxia-inducible factors, stem cells, and cancer. Cell. 2007;129:465-72.
128. Sosa MS, Bragado P, Aguirre-Ghiso JA. Mechanisms of disseminated cancer cell dormancy: an awakening field. Nat Rev Cancer. 2014;14:611-22.
129. Ciavardelli D, Rossi C, Barcaroli D, Volpe S, Consalvo A, Zucchelli M, et al. Breast cancer stem cells rely on fermentative glycolysis and are sensitive to 2-deoxyglucose treatment. Cell Death Dis. 2014;5:e1336.
130. Chen KY, Liu X, Bu P, Lin CS, Rakhilin N, Locasale JW, et al. A Metabolic Signature of Colon Cancer Initiating Cells. Ann Int Conf Proc IEEE Eng Med Biol Soc. 2014;2014:4759-62.
131. Liao J, Qian F, Tchabo N, Mhawech-Fauceglia P, Beck A, Qian Z, et al. Ovarian Cancer Spheroid Cells with Stem Cell-Like Properties Contribute to Tumor Generation, Metastasis and Chemotherapy Resistance through Hypoxia-Resistant Metabolism. PLoS One. 2014; 9:e84941.
132. Zhou Y, Zhou Y, Shingu T, Feng L, Chen Z, Ogasawara M, et al. Metabolic alterations in highly tumorigenic glioblastoma cells: preference for hypoxia and high dependency on glycolysis. J Biol Chem. 2011;286:32843-53.
133. Demaria M, Giorgi C, Lebiedzinska M, Esposito G, D'Angeli L, Bartoli A, et al. A STAT3-mediated metabolic switch is involved in tumour transformation and STAT3 addiction. Aging (Albany NY). 2010;2:823-42.
134. Sancho P, Burgos-Ramos E, Tavera A, Bou Kheir T, Jagust P, Schoenhals M, et al. MYC/PGC-1α Balance Determines the Metabolic Phenotype and Plasticity of Pancreatic Cancer Stem Cells. Cell Metab. 2015;22:590-605.
135. Janiszewska M, Suvà ML, Riggi N, Houtkooper RH, Auwerx J, Clément-Schatlo V, et al. Imp2 controls oxidative phosphorylation and is crucial for preserving glioblastoma cancer stem cells. Genes Dev. 2012;26:1926-44.
136. De Luca A, Fiorillo M, Peiris-Pagès M, Ozsvari B, Smith DL, Sanchez-Alvarez R, et al. Mitochondrial biogenesis is required for the anchorage-independent survival and propagation of stem-like cancer cells. Oncotarget. 2015;6:14777-95.

137. Lamb R, Bonuccelli G, Ozsvári B, Peiris-Pagès M, Fiorillo M, Smith DL, et al. Mitochondrial mass, a new metabolic biomarker for stem-like cancer cells: Understanding WNT/FGF-driven anabolic signaling. Oncotarget. 2015;6:30453-71.
138. Farnie G, Sotgia F, Lisanti MP. High mitochondrial mass identifies a sub-population of stem-like cancer cells that are chemo-resistant. Oncotarget. 2015;6:30472-86.
139. Ito K, Carracedo A, Weiss D, Arai F, Ala U, Avigan DE, et al. A PML–PPAR-δ pathway for fatty acid oxidation regulates hematopoietic stem cell maintenance. Nat Med. 2012;18:1350-8.
140. Liu H, Zhang Z, Song L, Gao J, Liu Y. Lipid metabolism of cancer stem cells. Oncol Lett. 2022;23:119.
141. Chen CL, Uthaya Kumar DB, Punj V, Xu J, Sher L, Tahara SM, et al. NANOG Metabolically Reprograms Tumor-Initiating Stem-like Cells through Tumorigenic Changes in Oxidative Phosphorylation and Fatty Acid Metabolism. Cell Metab. 2016;23:206-19.
142. Pacifico F, Leonardi A, Crescenzi E. Glutamine Metabolism in Cancer Stem Cells: A Complex Liaison in the Tumor Microenvironment. Int J Mol Sci. 2023;24:2337.
143. Fernandez-Marcos PJ, Nóbrega-Pereira S. NADPH: new oxygen for the ROS theory of aging. Oncotarget. 2016;7:50814-5.
144. Liao WT, Ye YP, Deng YJ, Bian XW, Ding YQ. Metastatic cancer stem cells: from the concept to therapeutics. Am J Stem Cells. 2014;3:46-62.
145. Rupp T, Langlois B, Koczorowska MM, Radwanska A, Sun Z, Hussenet T, et al. Tenascin-C Orchestrates Glioblastoma Angiogenesis by Modulation of Pro- and Anti-angiogenic Signaling. Cell Reports. 2016;17:2607-19.
146. Weidenfeld K, Barkan D. EMT and Stemness in Tumor Dormancy and Outgrowth: Are They Intertwined Processes? Front Oncol. 2018;8.
147. Francescangeli F, Contavalli P, De Angelis ML, Careccia S, Signore M, Haas TL, et al. A pre-existing population of ZEB2+ quiescent cells with stemness and mesenchymal features dictate chemoresistance in colorectal cancer. J Exp Clin Cancer Res. 2020;39:2.
148. Brabletz T, Jung A, Reu S, Porzner M, Hlubek F, Kunz-Schughart LA, et al. Variable beta-catenin expression in colorectal cancers indicates tumor progression driven by the tumor environment. Proc Natl Acad Sci U S A. 2001;98:10356-61.
149. Chin AR, Wang SE. Cancer Tills the Premetastatic Field: Mechanistic Basis and Clinical Implications. Clin Cancer Res. 2016;22:3725-33.
150. Kaplan RN, Riba RD, Zacharoulis S, Bramley AH, Vincent L, Costa C, et al. VEGFR1-positive haematopoietic bone marrow progenitors initiate the pre-metastatic niche. Nature. 2005;438:820-7.
151. Erler JT, Bennewith KL, Cox TR, Lang G, Bird D, Koong A, et al. Hypoxia-induced lysyl oxidase is a critical mediator of bone marrow cell recruitment to form the premetastatic niche. Cancer Cell. 2009;15:35-44.
152. Liu H, Zhang G, Gao R. Cellular and molecular characteristics of the premetastatic niches. Animal Model Exp Med. 2023;6:399-408.
153. Høye AM, Erler JT. Structural ECM components in the premetastatic and metastatic niche. Am J Physiol Cell Physiol. 2016;310:C955-967.
154. Ingangi V, Minopoli M, Ragone C, Motti ML, Carriero MV. Role of Microenvironment on the Fate of Disseminating Cancer Stem Cells. Front Oncol. 2019;9:82.
155. Ocaña OH, Córcoles R, Fabra A, Moreno-Bueno G, Acloque H, Vega S, et al. Metastatic colonization requires the repression of the epithelial-mesenchymal transition inducer Prrx1. Cancer Cell. 2012;22:709-24.
156. Takano S, Reichert M, Bakir B, Das KK, Nishida T, Miyazaki M, et al. Prrx1 isoform switching regulates pancreatic cancer invasion and metastatic colonization. Genes Dev. 2016;30: 233-47.
157. Stahl M, Kim TK, Zeidan AM. Update on acute myeloid leukemia stem cells: New discoveries and therapeutic opportunities. World J Stem Cells. 2016;8:316-31.
158. Guan Y, Gerhard B, Hogge DE. Detection, isolation, and stimulation of quiescent primitive leukemic progenitor cells from patients with acute myeloid leukemia (AML). Blood. 2003;101:3142-9.

159. Smalley M, Piggott L, Clarkson R. Breast cancer stem cells: Obstacles to therapy. Cancer Letters. 2013;338:57-62.
160. Ho MM, Ng AV, Lam S, Hung JY. Side population in human lung cancer cell lines and tumors is enriched with stem-like cancer cells. Cancer Res. 2007;67:4827-33.
161. Butler SJ, Richardson L, Farias N, Morrison J, Coomber BL. Characterization of cancer stem cell drug resistance in the human colorectal cancer cell lines HCT116 and SW480. Biochem Biophys Res Commun. 2017;490:29-35.
162. Sabnis NG, Miller A, Titus MA, Huss WJ. The Efflux Transporter ABCG2 Maintains Prostate Stem Cells. Mol Cancer Res. 2017;15:128-40.
163. Vinogradov S, Wei X. Cancer stem cells and drug resistance: the potential of nanomedicine. Nanomedicine (Lond). 2012;7:597-615.
164. Moreb JS. Aldehyde dehydrogenase as a marker for stem cells. Curr Stem Cell Res Ther. 2008;3:237-46.
165. van den Hoogen C, van der Horst G, Cheung H, Buijs JT, Lippitt JM, Guzmán-Ramírez N, et al. High aldehyde dehydrogenase activity identifies tumor-initiating and metastasis-initiating cells in human prostate cancer. Cancer Res. 2010;70:5163-73.
166. Kobune M, Takimoto R, Murase K, Iyama S, Sato T, Kikuchi S, et al. Drug resistance is dramatically restored by hedgehog inhibitors in CD34+ leukemic cells. Cancer Sci. 2009;100:948-55.
167. Deng YH, Pu XX, Huang MJ, Xiao J, Zhou JM, Lin TY, et al. 5-Fluorouracil upregulates the activity of Wnt signaling pathway in CD133-positive colon cancer stem-like cells. Chin J Cancer. 2010;29:810-5.
168. Wang Z, Li Y, Kong D, Banerjee S, Ahmad A, Azmi AS, et al. Acquisition of epithelial-mesenchymal transition phenotype of gemcitabine-resistant pancreatic cancer cells is linked with activation of the notch signaling pathway. Cancer Res. 2009;69:2400-7.
169. Xie M, Zhang L, He CS, Xu F, Liu JL, Hu ZH, et al. Activation of Notch-1 enhances epithelial-mesenchymal transition in gefitinib-acquired resistant lung cancer cells. J Cell Biochem. 2012;113:1501-13.
170. Meidhof S, Brabletz S, Lehmann W, Preca BT, Mock K, Ruh M, et al. ZEB1-associated drug resistance in cancer cells is reversed by the class I HDAC inhibitor mocetinostat. EMBO Mol Med. 2015;7:831-47.
171. Das M, Law S. Role of tumor microenvironment in cancer stem cell chemoresistance and recurrence. Int J Biochem Cell Biol. 2018;103:115-24.
172. Crowder SW, Balikov DA, Hwang YS, Sung HJ. Cancer Stem Cells under Hypoxia as a Chemoresistance Factor in Breast and Brain. Curr Pathobiol Rep. 2014;2:33-40.
173. Shree T, Olson OC, Elie BT, Kester JC, Garfall AL, Simpson K, et al. Macrophages and cathepsin proteases blunt chemotherapeutic response in breast cancer. Genes Dev. 2011;25:2465-79.
174. Piret JP, Cosse JP, Ninane N, Raes M, Michiels C. Hypoxia protects HepG2 cells against etoposide-induced apoptosis via a HIF-1-independent pathway. Exp Cell Res. 2006;312:2908-20.
175. Harada H, Kizaka-Kondoh S, Li G, Itasaka S, Shibuya K, Inoue M, et al. Significance of HIF-1-active cells in angiogenesis and radioresistance. Oncogene. 2007;26:7508-16.
176. Ougolkov AV, Bilim VN, Billadeau DD. Regulation of pancreatic tumor cell proliferation and chemoresistance by the histone methyltransferase enhancer of zeste homologue 2. Clin Cancer Res. 2008;14:6790-6.
177. Zhang B, Strauss AC, Chu S, Li M, Ho Y, Shiang KD, et al. Effective targeting of quiescent chronic myelogenous leukemia stem cells by histone deacetylase inhibitors in combination with imatinib mesylate. Cancer Cell. 2010;17:427-42.
178. Kim WT, Ryu CJ. Cancer stem cell surface markers on normal stem cells. BMB Rep. 2017;50:285-98.
179. Kouros-Mehr H, Bechis SK, Slorach EM, Littlepage LE, Egeblad M, Ewald AJ, et al. GATA-3 links tumor differentiation and dissemination in a luminal breast cancer model. Cancer Cell. 2008;13:141-52.

180. Was H, Czarnecka J, Kominek A, Barszcz K, Bernas T, Piwocka K, et al. Some chemotherapeutics-treated colon cancer cells display a specific phenotype being a combination of stem-like and senescent cell features. Cancer Biol Ther. 2018;19:63-75.
181. Zhang C, Li C, He F, Cai Y, Yang H. Identification of CD44+CD24+ gastric cancer stem cells. J Cancer Res Clin Oncol. 2011;137:1679-86.
182. Li K, Dan Z, Nie YQ. Gastric cancer stem cells in gastric carcinogenesis, progression, prevention and treatment. World J Gastroenterol. 2014;20:5420-6.
183. Gómez-Gallegos AA, Ramírez-Vidal L, Becerril-Rico J, Pérez-Islas E, Hernandez-Peralta ZJ, Toledo-Guzmán ME, et al. CD24+CD44+CD54+EpCAM+ gastric cancer stem cells predict tumor progression and metastasis: clinical and experimental evidence. Stem Cell Res Ther. 2023;14:16.
184. Tsai SC, Lin CC, Shih TC, Tseng RJ, Yu MC, Lin YJ, et al. The miR-200b-ZEB1 circuit regulates diverse stemness of human hepatocellular carcinoma. Mol Carcinog. 2017;56:2035-47.
185. Wang R, Li Y, Tsung A, Huang H, Du Q, Yang M, et al. iNOS promotes CD24+CD133+ liver cancer stem cell phenotype through a TACE/ADAM17-dependent Notch signaling pathway. Proc Natl Acad Sci U S A. 2018;115:E10127-36.
186. Wang R, Sun Q, Wang P, Liu M, Xiong S, Luo J, et al. Notch and Wnt/β-catenin signaling pathway play important roles in activating liver cancer stem cells. Oncotarget. 2015;7: 5754-68.
187. Li C, Heidt DG, Dalerba P, Burant CF, Zhang L, Adsay V, et al. Identification of pancreatic cancer stem cells. Cancer Res. 2007;67:1030-7.
188. Herrmann H, Sadovnik I, Cerny-Reiterer S, Rülicke T, Stefanzl G, Willmann M, et al. Dipeptidylpeptidase IV (CD26) defines leukemic stem cells (LSC) in chronic myeloid leukemia. Blood. 2014;123:3951-62.
189. Kana S, John S, Basu D, Kar R, Nachiappa Ganesh R, Dubashi B. Flow Cytometric Assessment of CD26-Positive Leukemic Stem Cells: A Rapid and Valuable Tool in the Diagnosis and Follow-Up of Chronic Myeloid Leukemia. Cureus. 16:e56944.
190. Bocchia M, Sicuranza A, Abruzzese E, Iurlo A, Sirianni S, Gozzini A, et al. Residual Peripheral Blood CD26+ Leukemic Stem Cells in Chronic Myeloid Leukemia Patients During TKI Therapy and During Treatment-Free Remission. Front Oncol. 2018;8:194.
191. Barnawi R, Al-Khaldi S, Colak D, Tulbah A, Al-Tweigeri T, Fallatah M, et al. β1 Integrin is essential for fascin-mediated breast cancer stem cell function and disease progression. Int J Cancer. 2019;145:830-41.
192. Geng S, Guo Y, Wang Q, Li L, Wang J. Cancer stem-like cells enriched with CD29 and CD44 markers exhibit molecular characteristics with epithelial-mesenchymal transition in squamous cell carcinoma. Arch Dermatol Res. 2013;305:35-47.
193. Louhichi T, Ziadi S, Saad H, Dhiab MB, Mestiri S, Trimeche M. Clinicopathological significance of cancer stem cell markers CD44 and ALDH1 expression in breast cancer. Breast Cancer. 2018;25:698-705.
194. Da Cruz Paula A, Leitão C, Marques O, Rosa AM, Santos AH, Rêma A, et al. Molecular characterization of CD44+/CD24-/Ck+/CD45- cells in benign and malignant breast lesions. Virchows Arch. 2017;470:311-22.
195. Zhang H, Brown RL, Wei Y, Zhao P, Liu S, Liu X, et al. CD44 splice isoform switching determines breast cancer stem cell state. Genes Dev. 2019;33:166-79.
196. Jin J, Krishnamachary B, Mironchik Y, Kobayashi H, Bhujwalla ZM. Phototheranostics of CD44-positive cell populations in triple negative breast cancer. Sci Rep. 2016;6:27871.
197. Wang Z, Sau S, Alsaab HO, Iyer AK. CD44 Directed Nanomicellar Payload Delivery Platform for Selective Anticancer Effect and Tumor Specific Imaging of Triple Negative Breast Cancer. Nanomedicine. 2018;14:1441-54.
198. Zhou JY, Chen M, Ma L, Wang X, Chen YG, Liu SL. Role of CD44(high)/CD133(high) HCT-116 cells in the tumorigenesis of colon cancer. Oncotarget. 2016;7:7657-66.
199. Ozawa M, Ichikawa Y, Zheng YW, Oshima T, Miyata H, Nakazawa K, et al. Prognostic significance of CD44 variant 2 upregulation in colorectal cancer. Br J Cancer. 2014;111: 365-74.

200. Tsunekuni K, Konno M, Haraguchi N, Koseki J, Asai A, Matsuoka K, et al. CD44/CD133-Positive Colorectal Cancer Stem Cells are Sensitive to Trifluridine Exposure. Sci Rep. 2019;9:14861.
201. Leng Z, Xia Q, Chen J, Li Y, Xu J, Zhao E, et al. Lgr5+CD44+EpCAM+ Strictly Defines Cancer Stem Cells in Human Colorectal Cancer. Cell Physiol Biochem. 2018;46:860-72.
202. Takaishi S, Okumura T, Tu S, Wang SSW, Shibata W, Vigneshwaran R, et al. Identification of gastric cancer stem cells using the cell surface marker CD44. Stem Cells. 2009;27:1006-20.
203. Senel F, Unal TDK, Karaman H, Inanç M, Aytekin A. Prognostic Value of Cancer Stem Cell Markers CD44 and ALDH1/2 in Gastric Cancer Cases. Asian Pac J Cancer Prev. 2017;18: 2527-31.
204. Lau WM, Teng E, Chong HS, Lopez KAP, Tay AYL, Salto-Tellez M, et al. CD44v8-10 is a cancer-specific marker for gastric cancer stem cells. Cancer Res. 2014;74:2630-41.
205. Shu X, Liu H, Pan Y, Sun L, Yu L, Sun L, et al. Distinct biological characterization of the CD44 and CD90 phenotypes of cancer stem cells in gastric cancer cell lines. Mol Cell Biochem. 2019;459:35-47.
206. Jang E, Kim E, Son HY, Lim EK, Lee H, Choi Y, et al. Nanovesicle-mediated systemic delivery of microRNA-34a for CD44 overexpressing gastric cancer stem cell therapy. Biomaterials. 2016;105:12-24.
207. Asai R, Tsuchiya H, Amisaki M, Makimoto K, Takenaga A, Sakabe T, et al. CD44 standard isoform is involved in maintenance of cancer stem cells of a hepatocellular carcinoma cell line. Cancer Med. 2019;8:773-82.
208. Morine Y, Imura S, Ikemoto T, Iwahashi S, Saito YU, Shimada M. CD44 Expression Is a Prognostic Factor in Patients with Intrahepatic Cholangiocarcinoma After Surgical Resection. Anticancer Res. 2017;37:5701-5.
209. Nishino M, Ozaki M, Hegab AE, Hamamoto J, Kagawa S, Arai D, et al. Variant CD44 expression is enriching for a cell population with cancer stem cell-like characteristics in human lung adenocarcinoma. J Cancer. 2017;8:1774-85.
210. Alamgeer M, Neil Watkins D, Banakh I, Kumar B, Gough DJ, Markman B, et al. A phase IIa study of HA-irinotecan, formulation of hyaluronic acid and irinotecan targeting CD44 in extensive-stage small cell lung cancer. Invest New Drugs. 2018;36:288-98.
211. Gomez-Miragaya J, González-Suárez E. Tumor-initiating CD49f cells are a hallmark of chemoresistant triple negative breast cancer. Mol Cell Oncol. 2017;4:e1338208.
212. Ye F, Qiu Y, Li L, Yang L, Cheng F, Zhang H, et al. The Presence of EpCAM(-)/CD49f(+) Cells in Breast Cancer Is Associated with a Poor Clinical Outcome. J Breast Cancer. 2015;18:242-8.
213. Wiechert A, Saygin C, Thiagarajan PS, Rao VS, Hale JS, Gupta N, et al. Cisplatin induces stemness in ovarian cancer. Oncotarget. 2016;7:30511-22.
214. Riether C, Schürch CM, Bührer ED, Hinterbrandner M, Huguenin AL, Hoepner S, et al. CD70/CD27 signaling promotes blast stemness and is a viable therapeutic target in acute myeloid leukemia. J Exp Med. 2017;214:359-80.
215. Liu L, Yin B, Yi Z, Liu X, Hu Z, Gao W, et al. Breast cancer stem cells characterized by CD70 expression preferentially metastasize to the lungs. Breast Cancer. 2018;25:706-16.
216. Kubo T, Takigawa N, Osawa M, Harada D, Ninomiya T, Ochi N, et al. Subpopulation of small-cell lung cancer cells expressing CD133 and CD87 show resistance to chemotherapy. Cancer Sci. 2013;104:78-84.
217. He J, Liu Y, Zhu T, Zhu J, DiMeco F, Vescovi AL, et al. CD90 is Identified as a Candidate Marker for Cancer Stem Cells in Primary High-Grade Gliomas Using Tissue Microarrays. Mol Cell Proteomics. 2012;11:M111.010744.
218. Wang X, Liu Y, Zhou K, Zhang G, Wang F, Ren J. Isolation and characterization of CD105+/CD90+ subpopulation in breast cancer MDA-MB-231 cell line. Int J Clin Exp Pathol. 2015;8:5105-12.
219. Luo J, Wang P, Wang R, Wang J, Liu M, Xiong S, et al. The Notch pathway promotes the cancer stem cell characteristics of CD90+ cells in hepatocellular carcinoma. Oncotarget. 2015;7:9525-37.
220. Zhu L, Zhang W, Wang J, Liu R. Evidence of CD90+CXCR4+ cells as circulating tumor stem cells in hepatocellular carcinoma. Tumour Biol. 2015;36:5353-60.

221. Zhao RC, Zhou J, Chen KF, Gong J, Liu J, He JY, et al. The prognostic value of combination of CD90 and OCT4 for hepatocellular carcinoma after curative resection. Neoplasma. 2016;63:288-98.
222. Yan X, Luo H, Zhou X, Zhu B, Wang Y, Bian X. Identification of CD90 as a marker for lung cancer stem cells in A549 and H446 cell lines. Oncol Rep. 2013;30:2733-40.
223. Al-Mawali A, Gillis D, Lewis I. Immunoprofiling of leukemic stem cells CD34+/CD38–/CD123+ delineate FLT3/ITD-positive clones. J Hematol Oncol. 2016;9:61.
224. Qiu S, Jia Y, Xing H, Yu T, Yu J, Yu P, et al. N-Cadherin and Tie2 positive $CD34^{+}CD38^{-}CD123^{+}$ leukemic stem cell populations can develop acute myeloid leukemia more effectively in NOD/SCID mice. Leuk Res. 2014;38:632-7.
225. Yabushita T, Satake H, Maruoka H, Morita M, Katoh D, Shimomura Y, et al. Expression of multiple leukemic stem cell markers is associated with poor prognosis in de novo acute myeloid leukemia. Leuk Lymphoma. 2018;59:2144-51.
226. Brugnoli F, Grassilli S, Al-Qassab Y, Capitani S, Bertagnolo V. CD133 in Breast Cancer Cells: More than a Stem Cell Marker. J Oncol. 2019;2019:7512632.
227. Zhang D, Sun B, Zhao X, Ma Y, Ji R, Gu Q, et al. Twist1 expression induced by sunitinib accelerates tumor cell vasculogenic mimicry by increasing the population of CD133+ cells in triple-negative breast cancer. Mol Cancer. 2014;13:207.
228. Joseph C, Arshad M, Kurozomi S, Althobiti M, Miligy IM, Al-Izzi S, et al. Overexpression of the cancer stem cell marker CD133 confers a poor prognosis in invasive breast cancer. Breast Cancer Res Treat. 2019;174:387-99.
229. Rutella S, Bonanno G, Procoli A, Mariotti A, Corallo M, Prisco MG, et al. Cells with characteristics of cancer stem/progenitor cells express the CD133 antigen in human endometrial tumors. Clin Cancer Res. 2009;15:4299-311.
230. Nosrati A, Naghshvar F, Khanari S. Cancer Stem Cell Markers CD44, CD133 in Primary Gastric Adenocarcinoma. Int J Mol Cell Med. 2014;3:279-86.
231. Lu L, Wu M, Sun L, Li W, Fu W, Zhang X, et al. Clinicopathological and prognostic significance of cancer stem cell markers CD44 and CD133 in patients with gastric cancer. Medicine (Baltimore). 2016;95:e5163.
232. Xia P, Song C, Liu J, Wang D, Xu X. Prognostic value of circulating CD133+ cells in patients with gastric cancer. Cell Prolif. 2015;48:311-7.
233. Yu GF, Lin X, Luo RC, Fang WY. Nuclear CD133 expression predicts poor prognosis for hepatocellular carcinoma. Int J Clin Exp Pathol. 2018;11:2092-9.
234. Liu K, Hao M, Ouyang Y, Zheng J, Chen D. CD133+ cancer stem cells promoted by VEGF accelerate the recurrence of hepatocellular carcinoma. Sci Rep. 2017;7:41499.
235. Zhao W, Luo Y, Li B, Zhang T. Tumorigenic lung tumorospheres exhibit stem-like features with significantly increased expression of CD133 and ABCG2. Mol Med Rep. 2016;14: 2598-606.
236. Miyata T, Oyama T, Yoshimatsu T, Higa H, Kawano D, Sekimura A, et al. The Clinical Significance of Cancer Stem Cell Markers ALDH1A1 and CD133 in Lung Adenocarcinoma. Anticancer Res. 2017;37:2541-7.
237. Koren A, Rijavec M, Kern I, Sodja E, Korosec P, Cufer T. BMI1, ALDH1A1, and CD133 Transcripts Connect Epithelial-Mesenchymal Transition to Cancer Stem Cells in Lung Carcinoma. Stem Cells Int. 2016;2016:9714315.
238. Sarvi S, Mackinnon AC, Avlonitis N, Bradley M, Rintoul RC, Rassl DM, et al. CD133+ cancer stem-like cells in small cell lung cancer are highly tumorigenic and chemoresistant but sensitive to a novel neuropeptide antagonist. Cancer Res. 2014;74:1554-65.
239. Manhas J, Bhattacharya A, Agrawal SK, Gupta B, Das P, Deo SVS, et al. Characterization of cancer stem cells from different grades of human colorectal cancer. Tumour Biol. 2016;37:14069-81.
240. Zhao M, Zhang Y, Zhang H, Wang S, Zhang M, Chen X, et al. Hypoxia-induced cell stemness leads to drug resistance and poor prognosis in lung adenocarcinoma. Lung Cancer. 2015;87:98-106.

241. Kim DK, Ham MH, Lee SY, Shin MJ, Kim YE, Song P, et al. CD166 promotes the cancer stem-like properties of primary epithelial ovarian cancer cells. BMB Rep. 2020;53:622-7.
242. Jiang YP, Liu BY, Zheng Q, Panuganti S, Chen R, Zhu J, et al. CLT030, a leukemic stem cell-targeting CLL1 antibody-drug conjugate for treatment of acute myeloid leukemia. Blood Adv. 2018;2:1738-49.
243. van Rhenen A, van Dongen GAMS, Kelder A, Rombouts EJ, Feller N, Moshaver B, et al. The novel AML stem cell associated antigen CLL-1 aids in discrimination between normal and leukemic stem cells. Blood. 2007;110:2659-66.
244. Darwish NHE, Sudha T, Godugu K, Elbaz O, Abdelghaffar HA, Hassan EEA, et al. Acute myeloid leukemia stem cell markers in prognosis and targeted therapy: potential impact of BMI-1, TIM-3 and CLL-1. Oncotarget. 2016;7:57811-20.
245. Lin TY, Zhu Y, Li Y, Zhang H, Ma AH, Long Q, et al. Daunorubicin-containing CLL1-targeting nanomicelles have anti-leukemia stem cell activity in acute myeloid leukemia. Nanomedicine. 2019;20:102004.
246. Zeijlemaker W, Kelder A, Oussoren-Brockhoff YJM, Scholten WJ, Snel AN, Veldhuizen D, et al. A simple one-tube assay for immunophenotypical quantification of leukemic stem cells in acute myeloid leukemia. Leukemia. 2016;30:439-46.
247. Fujita T, Chiwaki F, Takahashi RU, Aoyagi K, Yanagihara K, Nishimura T, et al. Identification and Characterization of CXCR4-Positive Gastric Cancer Stem Cells. PLoS One. 2015;10: e0130808.
248. Bertolini G, D'Amico L, Moro M, Landoni E, Perego P, Miceli R, et al. Microenvironment-Modulated Metastatic CD133+/CXCR4+/EpCAM- Lung Cancer-Initiating Cells Sustain Tumor Dissemination and Correlate with Poor Prognosis. Cancer Res. 2015;75:3636-49.
249. Brugnoli F, Grassilli S, Lanuti P, Marchisio M, Al-Qassab Y, Vezzali F, et al. Up-modulation of PLC-β2 reduces the number and malignancy of triple-negative breast tumor cells with a CD133+/EpCAM+ phenotype: a promising target for preventing progression of TNBC. BMC Cancer. 2017;17:617.
250. Dai M, Yuan F, Fu C, Shen G, Hu S, Shen G. Relationship between epithelial cell adhesion molecule (EpCAM) overexpression and gastric cancer patients: A systematic review and meta-analysis. PLoS One. 2017;12:e0175357.
251. Park DJ, Sung PS, Kim JH, Lee GW, Jang JW, Jung ES, et al. EpCAM-high liver cancer stem cells resist natural killer cell-mediated cytotoxicity by upregulating CEACAM1. J Immunother Cancer. 2020;8:e000301.
252. Chen L, Peng M, Li N, Song Q, Yao Y, Xu B, et al. Combined use of EpCAM and FRα enables the high-efficiency capture of circulating tumor cells in non-small cell lung cancer. Sci Rep. 2018;8:1188.
253. Thompson JC, Fan R, Black T, Yu GH, Savitch SL, Chien A, et al. Measurement and immunophenotyping of pleural fluid EpCAM-positive cells and clusters for the management of non-small cell lung cancer patients. Lung Cancer. 2019;127:25-33.
254. Yang L, Tang H, Kong Y, Xie X, Chen J, Song C, et al. LGR5 Promotes Breast Cancer Progression and Maintains Stem-Like Cells Through Activation of Wnt/β-Catenin Signaling. Stem Cells. 2015;33:2913-24.
255. Shimokawa M, Ohta Y, Nishikori S, Matano M, Takano A, Fujii M, et al. Visualization and targeting of LGR5+ human colon cancer stem cells. Nature. 2017;545:187-92.
256. Xi HQ, Cai AZ, Wu XS, Cui JX, Shen WS, Bian SB, et al. Leucine-rich repeat-containing G-protein-coupled receptor 5 is associated with invasion, metastasis, and could be a potential therapeutic target in human gastric cancer. Br J Cancer. 2014;110:2011-20.
257. Wang B, Chen Q, Cao Y, Ma X, Yin C, Jia Y, et al. LGR5 Is a Gastric Cancer Stem Cell Marker Associated with Stemness and the EMT Signature Genes NANOG, NANOGP8, PRRX1, TWIST1, and BMI1. PLoS One. 2016;11:e0168904.
258. Gao F, Zhou B, Xu JC, Gao X, Li SX, Zhu GC, et al. The role of LGR5 and ALDH1A1 in non-small cell lung cancer: Cancer progression and prognosis. Biochem Biophys Res Commun. 2015;462:91-8.

259. Jo JH, Park SB, Park S, Lee HS, Kim C, Jung DE, et al. Novel Gastric Cancer Stem Cell-Related Marker LINGO2 Is Associated with Cancer Cell Phenotype and Patient Outcome. Int J Mol Sci. 2019;20:555.

260. Wang D, Hu X, Liu C, Jia Y, Bai Y, Cai C, et al. Protein C receptor is a therapeutic stem cell target in a distinct group of breast cancers. Cell Res. 2019;29:832-45.

261. Zhang P, He Q, Wang Y, Zhou G, Chen Y, Tang L, et al. Protein C receptor maintains cancer stem cell properties via activating lipid synthesis in nasopharyngeal carcinoma. Signal Transduct Target Ther. 2022;7:1-11.

262. Kikushige Y, Miyamoto T. Identification of TIM-3 as a Leukemic Stem Cell Surface Molecule in Primary Acute Myeloid Leukemia. Oncology. 2015;89 Suppl 1:28-32.

263. Hoang VT, Buss EC, Wang W, Hoffmann I, Raffel S, Zepeda-Moreno A, et al. The rarity of ALDH(+) cells is the key to separation of normal versus leukemia stem cells by ALDH activity in AML patients. Int J Cancer. 2015;137:525-36.

264. Kim RJ, Park JR, Roh KJ, Choi AR, Kim SR, Kim PH, et al. High aldehyde dehydrogenase activity enhances stem cell features in breast cancer cells by activating hypoxia-inducible factor-2α. Cancer Lett. 2013;333:18-31.

265. Liu SY, Zheng PS. High aldehyde dehydrogenase activity identifies cancer stem cells in human cervical cancer. Oncotarget. 2013;4:2462-75.

266. Vishnubalaji R, Manikandan M, Fahad M, Hamam R, Alfayez M, Kassem M, et al. Molecular profiling of ALDH1+ colorectal cancer stem cells reveals preferential activation of MAPK, FAK, and oxidative stress pro-survival signalling pathways. Oncotarget. 2018;9:13551-64.

267. Wu D, Mou YP, Chen K, Cai JQ, Zhou YC, Pan Y, et al. Aldehyde dehydrogenase 3A1 is robustly upregulated in gastric cancer stem-like cells and associated with tumorigenesis. Int J Oncol. 2016;49:611-22.

268. Srinivasan M, Bharali DJ, Sudha T, Khedr M, Guest I, Sell S, et al. Downregulation of Bmi1 in breast cancer stem cells suppresses tumor growth and proliferation. Oncotarget. 2017;8:38731-42.

269. Herzog AE, Warner KA, Zhang Z, Bellile E, Bhagat MA, Castilho RM, et al. The IL-6R and Bmi-1 axis controls self-renewal and chemoresistance of head and neck cancer stem cells. Cell Death Dis. 2021;12:988.

270. Piao L, Feng Y, Yang Z, Qi W, Li H, Han H, et al. LETM1 is a potential cancer stem-like cell marker and predicts poor prognosis in colorectal adenocarcinoma. Pathol Res Pract. 2019;215:152437.

271. Li H, Piao L, Xu D, Xuan Y. LETM1 is a potential biomarker that predicts poor prognosis in gastric adenocarcinoma. Exp Mol Pathol. 2020;112:104333.

272. Inoue A, Takahashi H, Harada H, Kohno S, Ohue S, Kobayashi K, et al. Cancer stem-like cells of glioblastoma characteristically express MMP-13 and display highly invasive activity. Int J Oncol. 2010;37:1121-31.

273. Yang F, Zhang J, Yang H. OCT4, SOX2, and NANOG positive expression correlates with poor differentiation, advanced disease stages, and worse overall survival in HER2+ breast cancer patients. Onco Targets Ther. 2018;11:7873-81.

274. Wang D, Lu P, Zhang H, Luo M, Zhang X, Wei X, et al. Oct-4 and Nanog promote the epithelial-mesenchymal transition of breast cancer stem cells and are associated with poor prognosis in breast cancer patients. Oncotarget. 2014;5:10803-15.

275. Wang H, Liu B, Wang J, Li J, Gong Y, Li S, et al. Reduction of NANOG Mediates the Inhibitory Effect of Aspirin on Tumor Growth and Stemness in Colorectal Cancer. Cell Physiol Biochem. 2017;44:1051-63.

276. Basati G, Mohammadpour H, Emami Razavi A. Association of High Expression Levels of SOX2, NANOG, and OCT4 in Gastric Cancer Tumor Tissues with Progression and Poor Prognosis. J Gastrointest Cancer. 2020;51:41-7.

277. Chang TS, Wu YC, Chi CC, Su WC, Chang PJ, Lee KF, et al. Activation of IL6/IGFIR confers poor prognosis of HBV-related hepatocellular carcinoma through induction of OCT4/NANOG expression. Clin Cancer Res. 2015;21:201-10.

278. D'Angelo RC, Ouzounova M, Davis A, Choi D, Tchuenkam SM, Kim G, et al. Notch reporter activity in breast cancer cell lines identifies a subset of cells with stem cell activity. Mol Cancer Ther. 2015;14:779-87.
279. Li SJ, Huang J, Zhou XD, Zhang WB, Lai YT, Che GW. Clinicopathological and prognostic significance of Oct-4 expression in patients with non-small cell lung cancer: a systematic review and meta-analysis. J Thorac Dis. 2016;8:1587-600.
280. Takeda K, Mizushima T, Yokoyama Y, Hirose H, Wu X, Qian Y, et al. Sox2 is associated with cancer stem-like properties in colorectal cancer. Sci Rep. 2018;8:17639.
281. Tirino V, Desiderio V, Paino F, Papaccio G, De Rosa M. Methods for cancer stem cell detection and isolation. Methods Mol Biol. 2012;879:513-29.
282. Duan JJ, Qiu W, Xu SL, Wang B, Ye XZ, Ping YF, et al. Strategies for Isolating and Enriching Cancer Stem Cells: Well Begun Is Half Done. Stem Cells Dev. 2013;22:2221-39.
283. Bonner WA, Hulett HR, Sweet RG, Herzenberg LA. Fluorescence activated cell sorting. Rev Sci Instrum. 1972;43:404-9.
284. Goodell MA, Brose K, Paradis G, Conner AS, Mulligan RC. Isolation and functional properties of murine hematopoietic stem cells that are replicating in vivo. J Exp Med. 1996;183: 1797-806.
285. Van den Broeck A, Gremeaux L, Topal B, Vankelecom H. Human pancreatic adenocarcinoma contains a side population resistant to gemcitabine. BMC Cancer. 2012;12:354.
286. Baines P, Visser JW. Analysis and separation of murine bone marrow stem cells by H33342 fluorescence-activated cell sorting. Exp Hematol. 1983;11:701-8.
287. Pierre-Louis O, Clay D, Brunet de la Grange P, Blazsek I, Desterke C, Guerton B, et al. Dual SP/ALDH Functionalities Refine the Human Hematopoietic Lin–CD34+CD38–Stem/Progenitor Cell Compartment. Stem Cells. 2009;27:2552-62.
288. Britton KM, Kirby JA, Lennard TWJ, Meeson AP. Cancer stem cells and side population cells in breast cancer and metastasis. Cancers (Basel). 2011;3:2106-30.
289. Kato K, Takao T, Kuboyama A, Tanaka Y, Ohgami T, Yamaguchi S, et al. Endometrial Cancer Side-Population Cells Show Prominent Migration and Have a Potential to Differentiate into the Mesenchymal Cell Lineage. Am J Pathol. 2010;176:381-92.
290. Wan G, Zhou L, Xie M, Chen H, Tian J. Characterization of side population cells from laryngeal cancer cell lines. Head Neck. 2010;32:1302-9.
291. Chiba T, Miyagi S, Saraya A, Aoki R, Seki A, Morita Y, et al. The polycomb gene product BMI1 contributes to the maintenance of tumor-initiating side population cells in hepatocellular carcinoma. Cancer Res. 2008;68:7742-9.
292. Sung JM, Cho HJ, Yi H, Lee CH, Kim HS, Kim DK, et al. Characterization of a stem cell population in lung cancer A549 cells. Biochem Biophys Res Commun. 2008;371:163-7.
293. Reynolds BA, Weiss S. Clonal and population analyses demonstrate that an EGF-responsive mammalian embryonic CNS precursor is a stem cell. Dev Biol. 1996;175:1-13.
294. Zhang G, Ma L, Xie YK, Miao XB, Jin C. Esophageal cancer tumorspheres involve cancer stem-like populations with elevated aldehyde dehydrogenase enzymatic activity. Mol Med Rep. 2012;6:519-24.
295. Ponti D, Costa A, Zaffaroni N, Pratesi G, Petrangolini G, Coradini D, et al. Isolation and in vitro propagation of tumorigenic breast cancer cells with stem/progenitor cell properties. Cancer Res. 2005;65:5506-11.
296. Galli R, Binda E, Orfanelli U, Cipelletti B, Gritti A, De Vitis S, et al. Isolation and characterization of tumorigenic, stem-like neural precursors from human glioblastoma. Cancer Res. 2004;64:7011-21.
297. Pastrana E, Silva-Vargas V, Doetsch F. Eyes wide open: a critical review of sphere-formation as an assay for stem cells. Cell Stem Cell. 2011;8:486-98.
298. Duan JJ, Cai J, Gao L, Yu SC. ALDEFLUOR activity, ALDH isoforms, and their clinical significance in cancers. J Enzyme Inhib Med Chem. 38:2166035.
299. Opdenaker LM, Modarai SR, Boman BM. The Proportion of ALDEFLUOR-Positive Cancer Stem Cells Changes with Cell Culture Density Due to the Expression of Different ALDH Isoforms. Cancer Stud Mol Med. 2015;2:87-95.

300. Bapat SA, Mali AM, Koppikar CB, Kurrey NK. Stem and progenitor-like cells contribute to the aggressive behavior of human epithelial ovarian cancer. Cancer Res. 2005;65:3025-9.
301. Deleyrolle LP, Rohaus MR, Fortin JM, Reynolds BA, Azari H. Identification and isolation of slow-dividing cells in human glioblastoma using carboxy fluorescein succinimidyl ester (CFSE). J Vis Exp. 2012;3918.
302. Liu WH, Wang X, You N, Tao KS, Wang T, Tang LJ, et al. Efficient enrichment of hepatic cancer stem-like cells from a primary rat HCC model via a density gradient centrifugation-centered method. PLoS One. 2012;7:e35720.
303. Wolpert F, Roth P, Lamszus K, Tabatabai G, Weller M, Eisele G. HLA-E contributes to an immune-inhibitory phenotype of glioblastoma stem-like cells. J Neuroimmunol. 2012;250: 27-34.
304. Diehn M, Cho RW, Lobo NA, Kalisky T, Dorie MJ, Kulp AN, et al. Association of reactive oxygen species levels and radioresistance in cancer stem cells. Nature. 2009;458:780-3.
305. Ye XQ, Wang GH, Huang GJ, Bian XW, Qian GS, Yu SC. Heterogeneity of mitochondrial membrane potential: a novel tool to isolate and identify cancer stem cells from a tumor mass? Stem Cell Rev Rep. 2011;7:153-60.
306. Bisht S, Nigam M, Kunjwal SS, Sergey P, Mishra AP, Sharifi-Rad J. Cancer Stem Cells: From an Insight into the Basics to Recent Advances and Therapeutic Targeting. Stem Cells Int. 2022;2022:9653244.
307. Sagiv E, Starr A, Rozovski U, Khosravi R, Altevogt P, Wang T, et al. Targeting CD24 for treatment of colorectal and pancreatic cancer by monoclonal antibodies or small interfering RNA. Cancer Res. 2008;68:2803-12.
308. Zangemeister-Wittke U, Lehmann HP, Waibel R, Wawrzynczak EJ, Stahel RA. Action of a CD24-specific deglycosylated ricin-A-chain immunotoxin in conventional and novel models of small-cell-lung-cancer xenograft. Int J Cancer. 1993;53:521-8.
309. Klapdor R, Wang S, Morgan M, Dörk T, Hacker U, Hillemanns P, et al. Characterization of a Novel Third-Generation Anti-CD24-CAR against Ovarian Cancer. Int J Mol Sci. 2019;20: 660.
310. Goldenson BH, Goodman AM, Ball ED. Gemtuzumab ozogamicin for the treatment of acute myeloid leukemia in adults. Expert Opin Biol Ther. 2021;21:849-62.
311. Abedin S, Guru Murthy GS, Szabo A, Hamadani M, Michaelis LC, Carlson KS, et al. Lintuzumab-Ac225 with Combination with Intensive Chemotherapy Yields High Response Rate and MRD Negativity in R/R AML with Adverse Features. Blood. 2022;140:157-8.
312. Stein EM, Walter RB, Erba HP, Fathi AT, Advani AS, Lancet JE, et al. A phase 1 trial of vadastuximab talirine as monotherapy in patients with CD33-positive acute myeloid leukemia. Blood. 2018;131:387-96.
313. Ravandi F, Walter RB, Subklewe M, Buecklein V, Jongen-Lavrencic M, Paschka P, et al. Updated results from phase I dose-escalation study of AMG 330, a bispecific T-cell engager molecule, in patients with relapsed/refractory acute myeloid leukemia (R/R AML). J Clin Oncol. 2020;38:7508-7508.
314. Shah NN, Tasian SK, Kohler ME, Hsieh EM, Baumeister SHC, Summers C, et al. CD33 CAR T-Cells (CD33CART) for Children and Young Adults with Relapsed/Refractory AML: Dose-Escalation Results from a Phase I/II Multicenter Trial. Blood. 2023;142:771.
315. Ladanyi A, Mukherjee A, Kenny HA, Johnson A, Mitra AK, Sundaresan S, et al. Adipocyte-induced CD36 expression drives ovarian cancer progression and metastasis. Oncogene. 2018;37:2285-301.
316. Shitara K, Doi T, Nagano O, Imamura CK, Ozeki T, Ishii Y, et al. Dose-escalation study for the targeting of CD44v+ cancer stem cells by sulfasalazine in patients with advanced gastric cancer (EPOC1205). Gastric Cancer. 2017;20:341-9.
317. Sandström K, Nestor M, Ekberg T, Engström M, Anniko M, Lundqvist H. Targeting CD44v6 expressed in head and neck squamous cell carcinoma: preclinical characterization of an 111In-labeled monoclonal antibody. Tumour Biol. 2008;29:137-44.

318. Menke-van der Houven van Oordt CW, Gomez-Roca C, van Herpen C, Coveler AL, Mahalingam D, Verheul HMW, et al. First-in-human phase I clinical trial of RG7356, an anti-CD44 humanized antibody, in patients with advanced, CD44-expressing solid tumors. Oncotarget. 2016;7:80046-58.
319. Haist C, Schulte E, Bartels N, Bister A, Poschinski Z, Ibach TC, et al. CD44v6-targeted CAR T-cells specifically eliminate CD44 isoform 6 expressing head/neck squamous cell carcinoma cells. Oral Oncol. 2021;116:105259.
320. Chawla SP, Kelly CM, Gordon EM, Quon DV, Moradkhani A, Chua-Alcala VS, et al. TTI-621-03: A phase I/II study of TTI-621 in combination with doxorubicin in patients with unresectable or metastatic high-grade leiomyosarcoma (LMS). J Clin Oncol. 2022;40: TPS11593–TPS11593.
321. Querfeld C, Thompson JA, Taylor MH, DeSimone JA, Zain JM, Shustov AR, et al. Intralesional TTI-621, a novel biologic targeting the innate immune checkpoint CD47, in patients with relapsed or refractory mycosis fungoides or Sézary syndrome: a multicentre, phase 1 study. Lancet Haematol. 2021;8:e808-17.
322. Gholamin S, Mitra SS, Feroze AH, Liu J, Kahn SA, Zhang M, et al. Disrupting the CD47-SIRPα anti-phagocytic axis by a humanized anti-CD47 antibody is an efficacious treatment for malignant pediatric brain tumors. Sci Transl Med. 2017;9:eaaf2968.
323. Golubovskaya V, Berahovich R, Zhou H, Xu S, Harto H, Li L, et al. CD47-CAR-T Cells Effectively Kill Target Cancer Cells and Block Pancreatic Tumor Growth. Cancers (Basel). 2017;9:139.
324. Gramatzki M, Staudinger M, Kellner C, Bulduk M, Schub N, Humpe A, et al. CD96 Antibody TH-111 Eradicates AML-LSC from Autografts and the Fc- Engineered Variant MSH-TH111e May be Used In Vivo. Biol Blood Marrow Transplant. 2016;22:S200.
325. Montesinos P, Roboz GJ, Bulabois CE, Subklewe M, Platzbecker U, Ofran Y, et al. Safety and efficacy of talacotuzumab plus decitabine or decitabine alone in patients with acute myeloid leukemia not eligible for chemotherapy: results from a multicenter, randomized, phase 2/3 study. Leukemia. 2021;35:62-74.
326. Uy GL, Aldoss I, Foster MC, Sayre PH, Wieduwilt MJ, Advani AS, et al. Flotetuzumab as salvage immunotherapy for refractory acute myeloid leukemia. Blood. 2021;137:751-62.
327. Damek-Poprawa M, Volgina A, Korostoff J, Sollecito TP, Brose MS, O'Malley BW, et al. Targeted inhibition of CD133+ cells in oral cancer cell lines. J Dent Res. 2011;90:638-45.
328. Skubitz APN, Taras EP, Boylan KLM, Waldron NN, Oh S, Panoskaltsis-Mortari A, et al. Targeting CD133 in an in vivo ovarian cancer model reduces ovarian cancer progression. Gynecol Oncol. 2013;130:579-87.
329. Zhao L, Yang Y, Zhou P, Ma H, Zhao X, He X, et al. Targeting CD133high Colorectal Cancer Cells In Vitro and In Vivo With an Asymmetric Bispecific Antibody. J Immunother. 2015;38: 217-28.
330. Schmohl JU, Gleason MK, Dougherty PR, Miller JS, Vallera DA. Heterodimeric Bispecific Single Chain Variable Fragments (scFv) Killer Engagers (BiKEs) Enhance NK-cell Activity Against CD133+ Colorectal Cancer Cells. Target Oncol. 2016;11:353-61.
331. Jin X, Zhang M, Sun R, Lyu H, Xiao X, Zhang X, et al. First-in-human phase I study of CLL-1 CAR-T cells in adults with relapsed/refractory acute myeloid leukemia. J Hematol Oncol. 2022;15:88.
332. Oberneder R, Weckermann D, Ebner B, Quadt C, Kirchinger P, Raum T, et al. A phase I study with adecatumumab, a human antibody directed against epithelial cell adhesion molecule, in hormone refractory prostate cancer patients. Eur J Cancer. 2006;42:2530-8.
333. Kurbacher CM, Horn O, Kurbacher JA, Herz S, Kurbacher AT, Hildenbrand R, et al. Outpatient Intraperitoneal Catumaxomab Therapy for Malignant Ascites Related to Advanced Gynecologic Neoplasms. Oncologist. 2015;20:1333-41.
334. Hong R, Zhou Y, Tian X, Wang L, Wu X. Selective inhibition of IDO1, D-1-methyl-tryptophan (D-1MT), effectively increased EpCAM/CD3-bispecific BiTE antibody MT110 efficacy against IDO1hibreast cancer via enhancing immune cells activity. Int Immunopharmacol. 2018;54:118-24.

335. Moldenhauer G, Salnikov AV, Lüttgau S, Herr I, Anderl J, Faulstich H. Therapeutic potential of amanitin-conjugated anti-epithelial cell adhesion molecule monoclonal antibody against pancreatic carcinoma. J Natl Cancer Inst. 2012;104:622-34.
336. Luo T, Fang W, Lu Z, Tong C, Zhang H, Ai G, et al. EpCAM CAR T (IMC001) for the treatment of advanced GI cancers. J Clin Oncol. 2023;41:4034-4034.
337. Herpers B, Eppink B, James MI, Cortina C, Cañellas-Socias A, Boj SF, et al. Functional patient-derived organoid screenings identify MCLA-158 as a therapeutic EGFR × LGR5 bispecific antibody with efficacy in epithelial tumors. Nat Cancer. 2022;3:418-36.
338. Junttila MR, Mao W, Wang X, Wang BE, Pham T, Flygare J, et al. Targeting LGR5+ cells with an antibody-drug conjugate for the treatment of colon cancer. Sci Transl Med. 2015;7: 314ra186.
339. Brunner AM, Esteve J, Porkka K, Knapper S, Traer E, Scholl S, et al. Phase Ib study of sabatolimab (MBG453), a novel immunotherapy targeting TIM-3 antibody, in combination with decitabine or azacitidine in high- or very high-risk myelodysplastic syndromes. Am J Hematol. 2024;99:E32-6.
340. Moore KN, Gunderson C, Sabbatini P, McMeekin DS, Mantia-Smaldone G, Burger R, et al. A Phase 1b Dose Escalation Study of Ipafricept (OMP-54F28) in Combination with Paclitaxel and Carboplatin in Patients with Recurrent Platinum-Sensitive Ovarian Cancer. Gynecol Oncol. 2019;154:294-301.
341. Diamond JR, Becerra C, Richards D, Mita A, Osborne C, O'Shaughnessy J, et al. Phase Ib clinical trial of the anti-frizzled antibody vantictumab (OMP-18R5) plus paclitaxel in patients with locally advanced or metastatic HER2-negative breast cancer. Breast Cancer Res Treat. 2020;184:53-62.
342. Gabata R, Harada K, Mizutani Y, Ouchi H, Yoshimura K, Sato Y, et al. Anti-tumor Activity of the Small Molecule Inhibitor PRI-724 Against β-Catenin-activated Hepatocellular Carcinoma. Anticancer Res. 2020;40:5211-9.
343. Cook N, Basu B, Smith DM, Gopinathan A, Evans J, Steward WP, et al. A phase I trial of the γ-secretase inhibitor MK-0752 in combination with gemcitabine in patients with pancreatic ductal adenocarcinoma. Br J Cancer. 2018;118:793-801.
344. Chen X, Gong L, Ou R, Zheng Z, Chen J, Xie F, et al. Sequential combination therapy of ovarian cancer with cisplatin and γ-secretase inhibitor MK-0752. Gynecol Oncol. 2016; 140:537-44.
345. Lee SM, Moon J, Redman BG, Chidiac T, Flaherty LE, Zha Y, et al. Phase 2 study of RO4929097, a gamma-secretase inhibitor, in metastatic melanoma: SWOG 0933. Cancer. 2015;121:432-40.
346. Sardesai S, Badawi M, Mrozek E, Morgan E, Phelps M, Stephens J, et al. A phase I study of an oral selective gamma secretase (GS) inhibitor RO4929097 in combination with neoadjuvant paclitaxel and carboplatin in triple negative breast cancer. Invest New Drugs. 2020;38: 1400-10.
347. Takahashi T, Prensner JR, Robson CD, Janeway KA, Weigel BJ. Safety and efficacy of gamma-secretase inhibitor nirogacestat (PF-03084014) in desmoid tumor: Report of four pediatric/ young adult cases. Pediatr Blood Cancer. 2020;67:e28636.
348. McKeage MJ, Kotasek D, Markman B, Hidalgo M, Millward MJ, Jameson MB, et al. Phase IB Trial of the Anti-Cancer Stem Cell DLL4-Binding Agent Demcizumab with Pemetrexed and Carboplatin as First-Line Treatment of Metastatic Non-Squamous NSCLC. Target Oncol. 2018;13:89-98.
349. Chiorean EG, LoRusso P, Strother RM, Diamond JR, Younger A, Messersmith WA, et al. A Phase I First-in-Human Study of Enoticumab (REGN421), a Fully Human Delta-like Ligand 4 (Dll4) Monoclonal Antibody in Patients with Advanced Solid Tumors. Clin Cancer Res. 2015;21:2695-703.
350. LoRusso PM, Rudin CM, Reddy JC, Tibes R, Weiss GJ, Borad MJ, et al. Phase I trial of hedgehog pathway inhibitor vismodegib (GDC-0449) in patients with refractory, locally advanced or metastatic solid tumors. Clin Cancer Res. 2011;17:2502-11.

351. Kim EJ, Sahai V, Abel EV, Griffith KA, Greenson JK, Takebe N, et al. Pilot Clinical Trial of Hedgehog Pathway Inhibitor GDC-0449 (Vismodegib) in Combination with Gemcitabine in Patients with Metastatic Pancreatic Adenocarcinoma. Clinical Cancer Res. 2014;20: 5937-45.
352. Sekulic A, Migden MR, Oro AE, Dirix L, Lewis KD, Hainsworth JD, et al. Efficacy and safety of vismodegib in advanced basal-cell carcinoma. N Engl J Med. 2012;366:2171-9.
353. Pan S, Wu X, Jiang J, Gao W, Wan Y, Cheng D, et al. Discovery of NVP-LDE225, a Potent and Selective Smoothened Antagonist. ACS Med Chem Lett. 2010;1:130-4.
354. Sekeres MA, Montesinos P, Novak J, Wang J, Jeyakumar D, Tomlinson B, et al. Glasdegib plus intensive or non-intensive chemotherapy for untreated acute myeloid leukemia: results from the randomized, phase 3 BRIGHT AML 1019 trial. Leukemia. 2023;37:2017-26.
355. Chan O, Komrokji RS. Luspatercept in the treatment of lower-risk myelodysplastic syndromes. Future Oncol. 2021;17:1473-81.
356. Lee JE, Lee P, Yoon YC, Han BS, Ko S, Park MS, et al. Vactosertib, TGF-β receptor I inhibitor, augments the sensitization of the anti-cancer activity of gemcitabine in pancreatic cancer. Biomed Pharmacother. 2023;162:114716.
357. Kelley RK, Gane E, Assenat E, Siebler J, Galle PR, Merle P, et al. A Phase 2 Study of Galunisertib (TGF-β1 Receptor Type I Inhibitor) and Sorafenib in Patients With Advanced Hepatocellular Carcinoma. Clin Transl Gastroenterol. 2019;10:e00056.
358. Morris JC, Tan AR, Olencki TE, Shapiro GI, Dezube BJ, Reiss M, et al. Phase I Study of GC1008 (Fresolimumab): A Human Anti-Transforming Growth Factor-Beta (TGFβ) Monoclonal Antibody in Patients with Advanced Malignant Melanoma or Renal Cell Carcinoma. PLoS One. 2014;9:e90353.
359. Lim ST, Jeon YW, Gwak H, Kim SY, Suh YJ. Synergistic anticancer effects of ruxolitinib and calcitriol in estrogen receptor-positive, human epidermal growth factor receptor 2-positive breast cancer cells. Mol Med Rep. 2018;17:5581-8.
360. An HJ, Choi EK, Kim JS, Hong SW, Moon JH, Shin JS, et al. INCB018424 induces apoptotic cell death through the suppression of pJAK1 in human colon cancer cells. Neoplasma. 2014;61:56-62.
361. Hart S, Goh KC, Novotny-Diermayr V, Tan YC, Madan B, Amalini C, et al. Pacritinib (SB1518), a JAK2/FLT3 inhibitor for the treatment of acute myeloid leukemia. Blood Cancer J. 2011;1:e44.
362. Kahl BS, Spurgeon SE, Furman RR, Flinn IW, Coutre SE, Brown JR, et al. A phase 1 study of the PI3Kδ inhibitor idelalisib in patients with relapsed/refractory mantle cell lymphoma (MCL). Blood. 2014;123:3398-405.
363. André F, Ciruelos E, Rubovszky G, Campone M, Loibl S, Rugo HS, et al. Alpelisib for PIK3CA-Mutated, Hormone Receptor–Positive Advanced Breast Cancer. N Engl J Med. 2019;380: 1929-40.
364. Garrido-Castro AC, Saura C, Barroso-Sousa R, Guo H, Ciruelos E, Bermejo B, et al. Phase 2 study of buparlisib (BKM120), a pan-class I PI3K inhibitor, in patients with metastatic triple-negative breast cancer. Breast Cancer Res. 2020;22:120.
365. Chari A, Vogl DT, Gavriatopoulou M, Nooka AK, Yee AJ, Huff CA, et al. Oral Selinexor–Dexamethasone for Triple-Class Refractory Multiple Myeloma. N Engl J Med. 2019;381: 727-38.
366. Chu QSC, Forouzesh B, Syed S, Mita M, Schwartz G, Cooper J, et al. A phase II and pharmacological study of the matrix metalloproteinase inhibitor (MMPI) COL-3 in patients with advanced soft tissue sarcomas. Invest New Drugs. 2007;25:359-67.
367. Rudek MA, Figg WD, Dyer V, Dahut W, Turner ML, Steinberg SM, et al. Phase I clinical trial of oral COL-3, a matrix metalloproteinase inhibitor, in patients with refractory metastatic cancer. J Clin Oncol. 2001;19:584-92.
368. Busby J, McMenamin Ú, Spence A, Johnston BT, Hughes C, Cardwell CR. Angiotensin receptor blocker use and gastro-oesophageal cancer survival: a population-based cohort study. Aliment Pharmacol Ther. 2018;47:279-88.

369. Emmanouilides C, Pegram M, Robinson R, Hecht R, Kabbinavar F, Isacoff W. Anti-VEGF antibody bevacizumab (Avastin) with 5FU/LV as third line treatment for colorectal cancer. Tech Coloproctol. 2004;8 Suppl 1:s50-2.
370. Beppu K, Nakamura K, Linehan WM, Rapisarda A, Thiele CJ. Topotecan blocks hypoxia-inducible factor-1alpha and vascular endothelial growth factor expression induced by insulin-like growth factor-I in neuroblastoma cells. Cancer Res. 2005;65:4775-81.
371. Alam MM, Fermin JM, Knackstedt M, Noonan MJ, Powell T, Goodreau L, et al. Everolimus downregulates STAT3/HIF-1α/VEGF pathway to inhibit angiogenesis and lymphangiogenesis in TP53 mutant head and neck squamous cell carcinoma (HNSCC). Oncotarget. 2023;14:85-95.
372. Li Y, Zhao L, Li XF. Targeting Hypoxia: Hypoxia-Activated Prodrugs in Cancer Therapy. Front Oncol. 2021;11:700407.
373. Becerra C, Paulson AS, Cavaness KM, Celinski SA. Gemcitabine, nab-paclitaxel, cisplatin, and anakinra (AGAP) treatment in patients with localized pancreatic ductal adenocarcinoma (PDAC). J Clin Oncol. 2018;36:449-449.
374. Lythgoe MP, Prasad V. Repositioning canakinumab for non-small cell lung cancer—important lessons for drug repurposing in oncology. Br J Cancer. 2022;127:785-7.
375. Benner B, Good L, Quiroga D, Schultz TE, Kassem M, Carson WE, et al. Pexidartinib, a Novel Small Molecule CSF-1R Inhibitor in Use for Tenosynovial Giant Cell Tumor: A Systematic Review of Pre-Clinical and Clinical Development. Drug Des Devel Ther. 2020;14:1693-704.
376. Hodi FS, O'Day SJ, McDermott DF, Weber RW, Sosman JA, Haanen JB, et al. Improved survival with ipilimumab in patients with metastatic melanoma. N Engl J Med. 2010;363:711-23.
377. Meindl-Beinker NM, Betge J, Gutting T, Burgermeister E, Belle S, Zhan T, et al. A multicenter open-label phase II trial to evaluate nivolumab and ipilimumab for 2nd line therapy in elderly patients with advanced esophageal squamous cell cancer (RAMONA). BMC Cancer. 2019;19:231.
378. Dang TO, Ogunniyi A, Barbee MS, Drilon A. Pembrolizumab for the treatment of PD-L1 positive advanced or metastatic non-small cell lung cancer. Expert Rev Anticancer Ther. 2016;16:13-20.
379. Motzer RJ, Penkov K, Haanen J, Rini B, Albiges L, Campbell MT, et al. Avelumab plus Axitinib versus Sunitinib for Advanced Renal-Cell Carcinoma. N Engl J Med. 2019;380:1103-15.
380. Fujiwara Y, Iguchi H, Yamamoto N, Hayama M, Nii M, Ueda S, et al. Tolerability and efficacy of durvalumab in Japanese patients with advanced solid tumors. Cancer Sci. 2019;110:1715-23.
381. Sullivan RJ, Hamid O, Gonzalez R, Infante JR, Patel MR, Hodi FS, et al. Atezolizumab plus cobimetinib and vemurafenib in BRAF-mutated melanoma patients. Nat Med. 2019;25:929-35.
382. Alnefaie A, Albogami S, Asiri Y, Ahmad T, Alotaibi SS, Al-Sanea MM, et al. Chimeric Antigen Receptor T-Cells: An Overview of Concepts, Applications, Limitations, and Proposed Solutions. Front Bioeng Biotechnol. 2022;10:797440.
383. Su Z, Dong S, Zhao SC, Liu K, Tan Y, Jiang X, et al. Novel nanomedicines to overcome cancer multidrug resistance. Drug Resist Updat. 2021;58:100777.
384. Ali ES, Sharker SM, Islam MT, Khan IN, Shaw S, Rahman MA, et al. Targeting cancer cells with nanotherapeutics and nanodiagnostics: Current status and future perspectives. Semin Cancer Biol. 2021;69:52-68.
385. Yue M, Guo T, Nie DY, Zhu YX, Lin M. Advances of nanotechnology applied to cancer stem cells. World J Stem Cells. 2023;15:514-29.
386. Hamers-Casterman C, Atarhouch T, Muyldermans S, Robinson G, Hamers C, Songa EB, et al. Naturally occurring antibodies devoid of light chains. Nature. 1993;363:446-8.
387. Romão E, Krasniqi A, Maes L, Vandenbrande C, Sterckx YGJ, Stijlemans B, et al. Identification of Nanobodies against the Acute Myeloid Leukemia Marker CD33. Int J Mol Sci. 2020;21:310.

388. Huet HA, Growney JD, Johnson JA, Li J, Bilic S, Ostrom L, et al. Multivalent nanobodies targeting death receptor 5 elicit superior tumor cell killing through efficient caspase induction. MAbs. 2014;6:1560-70.
389. Wang H, Wang Y, Xiao Z, Li W, Dimitrov DS, Chen W. Human Domain Antibodies to Conserved Epitopes on HER2 Potently Inhibit Growth of HER2-Overexpressing Human Breast Cancer Cells In Vitro. Antibodies (Basel). 2019;8:25.
390. Oliveira S, Schiffelers RM, van der Veeken J, van der Meel R, Vongpromek R, van Bergen En Henegouwen PMP, et al. Downregulation of EGFR by a novel multivalent nanobody-liposome platform. J Control Release. 2010;145:165-75.
391. Talelli M, Oliveira S, Rijcken CJF, Pieters EHE, Etrych T, Ulbrich K, et al. Intrinsically active nanobody-modified polymeric micelles for tumor-targeted combination therapy. Biomaterials. 2013;34:1255-60.

13

CHAPTER

Approach to the Classification of Papillary Lesions of Breast

Nishtha Ahuja

INTRODUCTION

Papillary lesions of the breast encompass a broad spectrum of lesions ranging from intraductal papilloma (IDP) to invasive papillary carcinoma. A good understanding of their morphology and accurate interpretation of the immunohistochemistry (IHC) panel is required to diagnose them. When we read these lesions, they appear quite interesting and easy to approach. The real trouble arises in practical scenarios when we are given biopsy specimens for interpretation or when there are morphological variations or a lack of appropriate IHCs. World Health Organization (WHO) 5th edition of Breast Tumors classifies these lesions into IDP, IDP with atypical ductal hyperplasia/ductal carcinoma in situ (ADH/DCIS), papillary DCIS, encapsulated papillary carcinoma (EPC), solid papillary carcinoma (SPC), and invasive papillary carcinoma.

In this chapter, we are going to discuss these lesions along with their salient features, differential diagnosis, morphological variations, associated pathologies and advances in the molecular pathology of papillary lesions of breast. Before we discuss the individual entities, let us understand the concept of the distribution of myoepithelial cells (MECs) in these lesions.

How important are myoepithelial cells?

Intraductal papillomas show MECs both in the periphery and the papillary fronds of the lesion. When there is the presence of ADH or DCIS within the IDP (also known as atypical papilloma), that atypical proliferation shows the absence of MECs. In cases of papillary DCIS, MECs are present only at the periphery of the lesion. Whereas in majority of the cases of EPC and SPC, MECs are absent both in the periphery and papillae. **Figure 1** shows the distribution of MECs (orange dots) in the papillary lesions.

The MECs can show various cytomorphology which at times makes it difficult to recognize them on H&E stained sections. They can have plasmacytoid or spindle or clear cell morphology **(Fig. 2)**. Sometimes it becomes difficult to identify them in the routine H&E stained section. Thus, to highlight immunohistochemical stains for P63, calponin, smooth muscle actin (SMA) or smooth

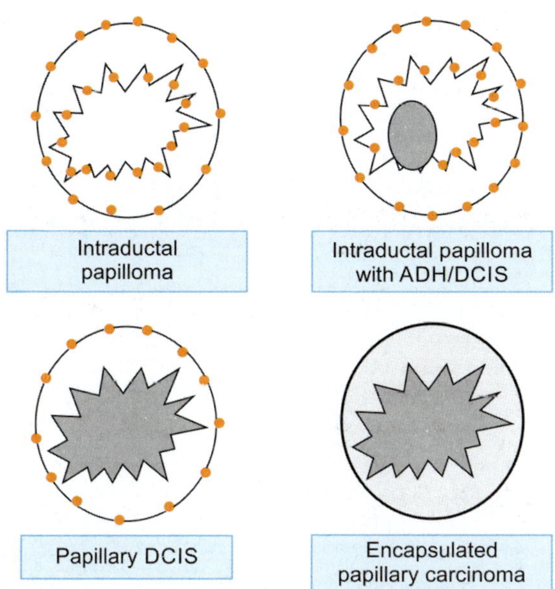

FIG. 1: A diagram to highlight the distribution of myoepithelial cells in papillary lesions of breast (myoepithelial cells are shown with orange dots).

(ADH/DCIS: atypical ductal hyperplasia/ductal carcinoma in situ)

muscle myosin heavy chain (SMMHC) can be used. These antibodies differ in their sensitivity and specificity. Caveat: Be cautious in interpreting these IHCs. SMA, SMMHC, and calponin can be expressed by pericytes of capillaries of fibrovascular cores or in the periphery. SMA and calponin can be expressed by reactive myofibroblasts in the periphery of the lesion. P63 can sometimes be expressed by scattered tumor cells in papillary carcinoma **(Figs. 2A to F)**. Therefore, when in doubt use a combination of P63 and calponin.[1]

What about high molecular weight cytokeratins?

Apart from luminal epithelial and abluminal MECs, breast glandular components also contain multipotent mammary stem cells (MaSCs) which can differentiate into either epithelial or MECs. These stem cells express basal cell markers such as CK5, CK6, and CK14. On differentiation, epithelial cells lose expression of basal markers. However, MECs retain the expression of basal markers, and in addition, gain expression of MECs markers, i.e., p63, SMA, and SMMHC.[2]

This concept is used in the diagnosis of papillary lesions of breast.

High molecular weight cytokeratin (HMWCK) (CK5/6 and CK14) highlights the MECs in IDP and shows mosaic pattern of positivity in the areas of usual ductal hyperplasia (UDH) while it is negative in cases of apocrine metaplasia, ADH, DCIS, neoplastic cell population of papillary DCIS, EPC, and SPC.

Now, we will read about individual entities, their immunoprofile and differential diagnosis. A Summary of every entity is given in the STAT PEARLS boxes.

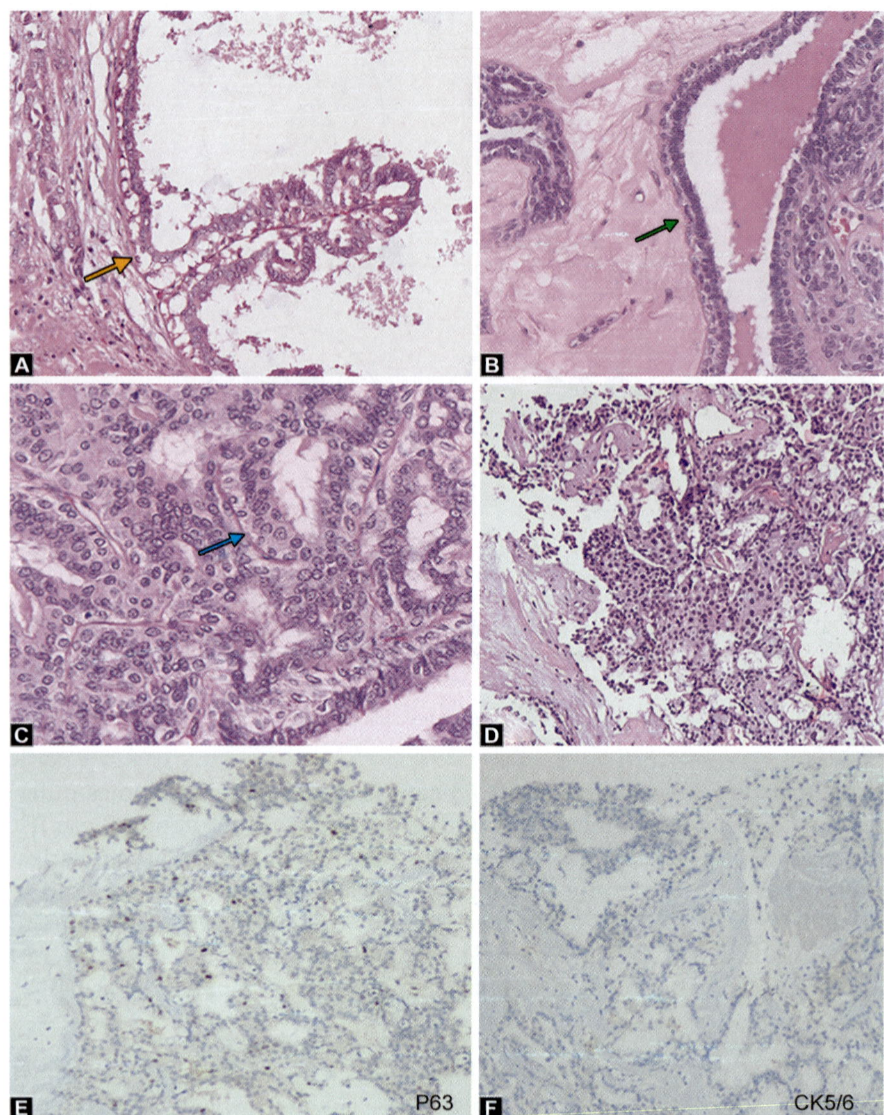

FIGS. 2A TO F: Microphotographs to show different morphologies of myoepithelial cells: Clear cell in (A) (orange arrow), spindle-shaped in (B) (green arrow) and plasmacytoid in (C) (blue arrow). (D and E) Biopsy from a papillary lesion, where the neoplastic epithelial cells show aberrant positivity for p63. (F) This case showed lack of myoepithelial cells on smooth muscle actin (SMA) (not shown here) and were negative for CK5/6.

INTRADUCTAL PAPILLOMA

Intraductal papillomas are benign breast papillary lesions characterized by presence of papillary proliferation within dilated ducts. Lewis et al.[3] evaluated >9,000 biopsies with benign breast diseases and found that 5.3% of those cases were reported as IDP. These can be central or peripheral. Central IDPs are more common and present as a solitary papilloma of central ducts whereas peripheral IDPs present as multiple papillomas of smaller ducts. The term papillomatosis is not recommended in the current WHO.

Clinically, IDPs can present at any age, however more common in 30–50 years of age.[3] Central IDP usually presents with clear to serosanguinous nipple discharge and less commonly as a palpable mass. Peripheral IDPs are usually clinically occult, rarely can present with nipple discharge, more seldom as a palpable mass especially in case when small clusters of papillomas are present.

On breast imaging, central papillomas are seen as benign looking circumscribed retroareolar mass or as a solitary retroareolar dilated duct or rarely with microcalcification. Peripheral papillomas are occult even on imaging. However, they may be seen as microcalcifications.[4]

On gross examination, central IDP is identified as a well-circumscribed tumor with papillary fronds within a dilated duct. The papillary fronds can be seen attached to the duct wall by one or more pedicles. Their size can vary from a few millimeters to >5 cm. You may find focal areas of necrosis or hemorrhage, especially when there is history of prior needling. Peripheral IDPs are usually occult unless associated with some other pathology.

On histopathology, IDPs are seen as dilated ducts containing cohesive arborizing papillae with fibrovascular cores. These papillae and the duct wall are lined by both epithelial and MEC layers. In cases, when MECs are not easily visible, IHC markers for MEC can be used to highlight them. The epithelial cells are usually cuboidal to columnar in shape with almost no mitosis **(Figs. 3A to F)**. Sometimes only a part of the duct wall is visible, especially on biopsy. There may be presence of coexisting UDH or apocrine metaplasia. In rare circumstances, mucinous change, clear cell change, squamous metaplasia (commonly seen in association with areas of infarction), or collagenous spherules may be seen.[5,6]

On immunohistochemistry, MECs are present, both in the papillary fronds and periphery of the lesion. The neoplastic cell population shows heterogeneous positivity for estrogen receptor (ER), progesterone receptor (PR), and HMWCK. UDH shows heterogeneous positivity for ER, PR, and HMWCK. Apocrine metaplasia or hyperplasia shows lack of expression of ER, PR, and HMWCK; and diminished presence of MECs **(Figs. 3A to F)**.[7]

INTRADUCTAL PAPILLOMA WITH ATYPICAL DUCTAL HYPERPLASIA/DUCTAL CARCINOMA IN SITU

Atypical ductal hyperplasia/ductal carcinoma in situ can be seen in the IDP (previously named as atypical papillomas). These are more commonly seen in the peripheral IDP than the central IDP. One must understand here that we are talking about atypia inside papillary proliferation of IDP, not in the surrounding breast parenchyma. The distinction between ADH and DCIS is done based either on the size (<3 mm: ADH and >3 mm: DCIS) or the proportion of neoplastic cells showing atypia (<30%: ADH and >30%: DCIS).[8] The current WHO accepts both these criteria.[7] The area with ADH/DCIS shows a monotonous population

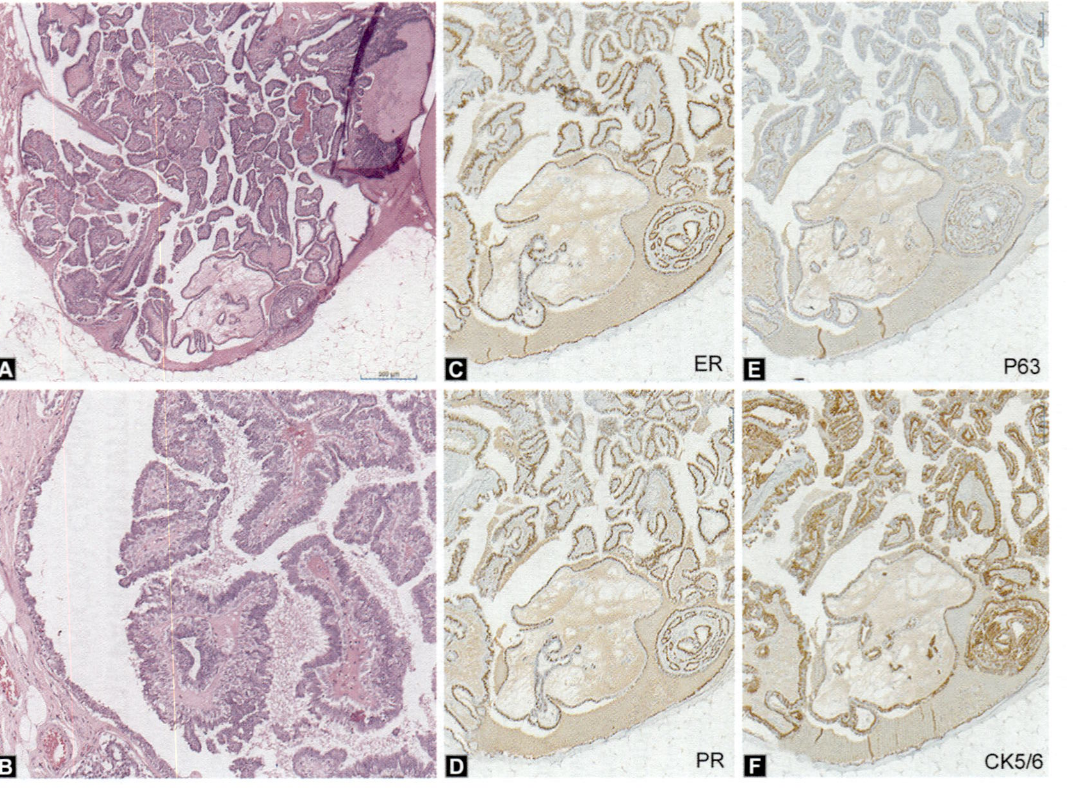

FIGS. 3A TO F: Intraductal papilloma. This is the case of a 77-year-old female who presented with a left breast lump with bloody nipple discharge. Mammography revealed a 1.4 × 1.8 × 1.7 cm hypoechoic mass with micro margins and intraductal extension with a 1.1 × 0.8 cm sized solid cystic lesion at 3 o'clock position. H&E sections of the microdochectomy specimen received show dilated ducts with papillary proliferation (A and B). (C and D) ER and PR show heterogeneous nuclear expression. (E) P63 highlights myoepithelial cells in the periphery as well as papillary fronds. (F) CK5/6 shows heterogeneous positivity.

(ER: estrogen receptor; PR: progesterone receptor)

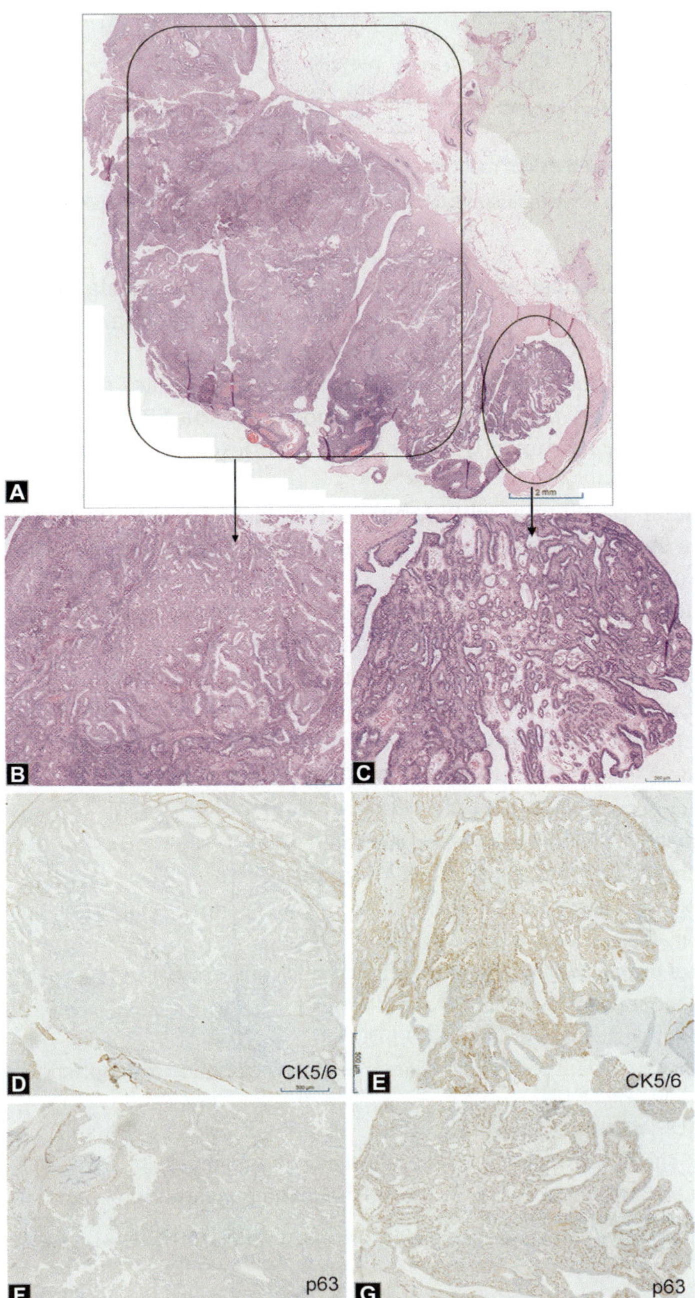

FIGS. 4A TO G: Intraductal papilloma (IDP) with DCIS. This is the case of a 69-year-old female who presented with a left breast lump for 2 years. Mammography revealed 6.8 × 9.7 × 7.6 cm (AP × TR × CC), round high density solid—cystic mass with circumscribed margins (BIRADS—4B). Histopathology shows dilated duct with IDP [right hand side of image (A) and image (C)] and atypical proliferation of monotonous population of cells (rest of the image 4A and image 4B). (D and F) The DCIS area shows complete loss of CK5/6 and p63 whereas; (E and G) The background IDP shows retained expression of both CK5/6 and p63.

(AP: anteroposterior; BIRADS: breast imaging-reporting and data system; CC: craniocaudal; DCIS: ductal carcinoma in situ; TR: transverse)

Single IDP without atypia
<
Multiple IDPs without atypia
<
ADH/DCIS without associated IDP
<
Single IDP with atypia
<
Multiple IDPs with atypia

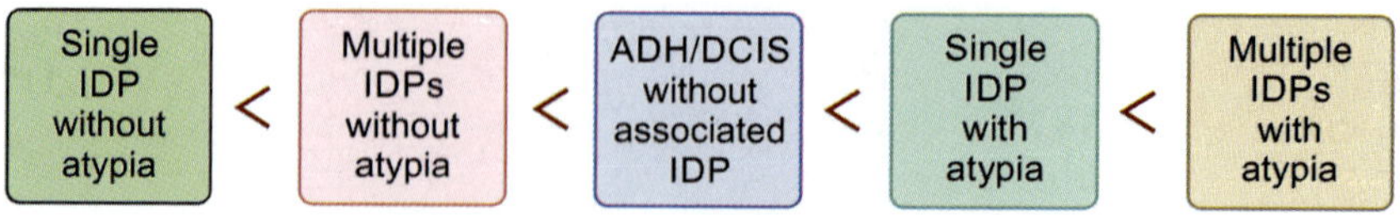

FLOWCHART 1: Derived risk of malignant potential.

(ADH/DCIS: atypical ductal hyperplasia/ductal carcinoma in situ; IDPs: intraductal papillomas)

of cells with cytological atypia of low-grade ductal neoplasia **(Figs. 4A to G)**. Whenever, there is intermediate to high-grade nuclear atypia, then the diagnosis is always IDP with DCIS irrespective of size/extent.[9]

On immunohistochemistry, these atypical cells show lack of MEC with absent HMWCK expression and diffuse strong positivity for ER and PR **(Figs. 4A to G)**. Background IDP shows IHC expression as described in *section Intraductal Papilloma.*

Intraductal papilloma with lobular neoplasia in situ or atypical lobular hyperplasia should be reported as IDP and these findings should be mentioned in the microscopic description.

Intraductal papillomas are also clonal neoplastic proliferation and they increase the risk of developing malignancy. Central IDP increases the risk by twofold, peripheral IDPs by threefold, and atypical papillomas by 5- to 7.5-fold. Lewis et al. evaluated >9,000 cases and derived the risk of malignant potential which is depicted in the **Flowchart 1**.

Stat Pearls: Intraductal papilloma

- Dilated ducts with cohesive arborizing papillae
- Papillae are lined by both epithelial and myoepithelial cells
- Usually involves central ducts (solitary) and sometimes peripheral ducts (multiple)
- No nuclear atypia or mitosis in the epithelial cells
- Presence of myoepithelial cells in the periphery and cores of papillae
- Heterogeneous positivity for ER, PR, and HMWCK

Stat Pearls: Intraductal papilloma with ADH/DCIS

- IDP showing areas with proliferation of monotonous population of neoplastic epithelial cells exhibiting nuclear atypia
- <3 mm: ADH; >3 mm: DCIS
- ADH/DCIS shows strong and uniform positivity for ER and negativity for HMWCK
- MEC markers highlight lack of MEC in the ADH/DCIS component and presence of myoepithelial cells in the background IDP

PAPILLARY DUCTAL CARCINOMA IN SITU

Papillary DCIS is a subtype of DCIS which accounts to around 3% of DCIS.[10] It can be peripheral or central in location. It usually occurs along with other types of DCIS or near EPC (especially when subareolar in location). Rarely, papillary DCIS occurs alone. Clinically, it presents in postmenopausal women and is the most common type of DCIS in males.[11] *On radiology,* peripherally located ones are usually occult or may present with microcalcifications. The centrally located ones are difficult to distinguish from EPC.

On histopathology, papillary DCIS shows dilated ducts with papillary proliferation consisting of filiform arborizing fibrovascular cores which are lined by neoplastic epithelial cells. Sometimes, these epithelial cells proliferate and fill the spaces between papillae giving rise to solid or cribriform patterns. Presence of comedo necrosis is uncommon. The grading is performed based on nuclear grade for DCIS.[12]

In most cases, papillary DCIS shows a uniform population of neoplastic cells with low-to-intermediate nuclear grade. However, cases of high nuclear grade have also been reported in literature. In some cases, a dimorphic population is seen additionally of globoid cells mimicking MEC because of vacuolated cytoplasm. These globoid cells show similar nuclear atypia as the other neoplastic epithelial cells.[13]

On immunohistochemistry, MEC markers highlight the lack of MEC in the papillary fronds with presence at the periphery of the involved ducts. The neoplastic epithelial cells show strong and uniform positivity for ER and negativity for HMWCK (in case of low-to-intermediate grade). Papillary DCIS with high nuclear grade may show different patterns of positivity for ER.[7]

Differential Diagnosis

Intraductal papilloma with DCIS/ADH: MEC markers can be used to differentiate as the MECs of the background IDP will be highlighted. EPC and SPC can be differentiated from papillary DCIS on the basis of the fact that papillary DCIS shows intact MEC in the periphery of the involved duct which is either absent (majority) or incomplete (minority) in the cases of EPC and SPC.

Stat Pearls: Papillary DCIS

- Dilated ducts with filiform arborizing papillae lined by neoplastic epithelial cells
- Low-to-intermediate nuclear grade in most cases
- Usually associated with (a/w) DCIS of other patterns or EPC
- Strong and uniform positivity for ER and negativity for HMWCK (in case of low-to-intermediate grade)
- High nuclear grade shows different patterns of positivity for ER
- MEC markers highlight lack of MEC in the papillary fronds with presence at the periphery of the involved ducts

ENCAPSULATED PAPILLARY CARCINOMA

Encapsulated papillary carcinoma, previously known as intracystic papillary carcinoma or encysted papillary carcinoma are rare papillary neoplasms of breast accounting to 0.5–1% of all breast carcinomas. In 2012, WHO incorporated this entity under papillary breast lesions and classified it as a type of papillary carcinoma.[14] It was earlier believed that EPC are noninvasive tumors, but recently many authors have talked about its invasive nature as there is lack of MECs at tumor-stromal interface.[14] In the 5th edition of the WHO, EPC is classified as EPC and EPC with invasion.

Encapsulated papillary carcinoma, *clinically*, presents in postmenopausal women mostly in their seventh decade as palpable mass with/without nipple discharge or an asymmetry. Majority of the cases are central/subareolar in location (WHO).

Mammography reveals a solitary, round, circumscribed lobulated, solid cystic mass in the central, or subareolar region in the majority of cases. The lesion may contain areas of microcalcification or satellite lesions. Ultrasound is preferred over mammography for the detection.[14] In the cases of invasion, the borders become irregular.

On gross examination, EPC can vary in size from 1 to 10 cm.[15] Cut surface shows a friable growth within a cystic cavity.

On histopathology, there is a cystic cavity with a rounded pushing border, surrounded by fibrous capsule of varying thickness. Sometimes, you can find aggregates of close nodules. The cystic cavity shows papillary proliferation with delicate fibrovascular cores. These papillae are lined by one to multiple layers of neoplastic cells which are monomorphic with low-to-intermediate nuclear grade **(Figs. 5A to G)**.[7] Sometimes, EPC gives a solid appearance with neoplastic cells forming micropapillary and cribriform structures filling the space in-between papillae.[16]

On immunohistochemistry, MECs are absent in the papillary fronds and periphery of the lesion. However, rare incidence of presence of incomplete MEC layer in the periphery has been reported.[17] The neoplastic cell population is negative for basal markers and HER2/ERBB2 nonamplified and show diffuse uniform positivity for ER and PR (usually). Ki-67 proliferation index is low to occasionally moderate.

For the diagnosis of EPC with invasion, there has to be evidence of definite invasion. Definite invasion is characterized by permeation of the fibrous capsule by neoplastic cells giving an irregular infiltrative appearance. One has to take care not to overcall entrapment of tumor cells within the capsule **(Figs. 6A and B)**[7] or displaced neoplastic cells due to a prior biopsy or fine needle aspiration cytology (FNAC) as invasion. The most common type of invasive carcinoma is invasive breast carcinoma (IBC), no special type (NST). However, occasional cases of special types of IBC have also been reported.[18]

Encapsulated papillary carcinomas without invasion have a prognosis similar to DCIS and are staged as Tis. In case of EPC with invasion, staging is done as per the size of the invasive component and interpretation of hormonal markers is done only on the invasive component.[7]

Rarely, the neoplastic cells in EPC show high-grade nuclear features and inconsistent ER staining, such cases should be staged/managed as IBC.[19]

Encapsulated papillary carcinomas frequently show PIK3CA mutations.[20] PAM50—majority luminal A and minority luminal B different from SPC—downregulation of genes related to cell migration.[21]

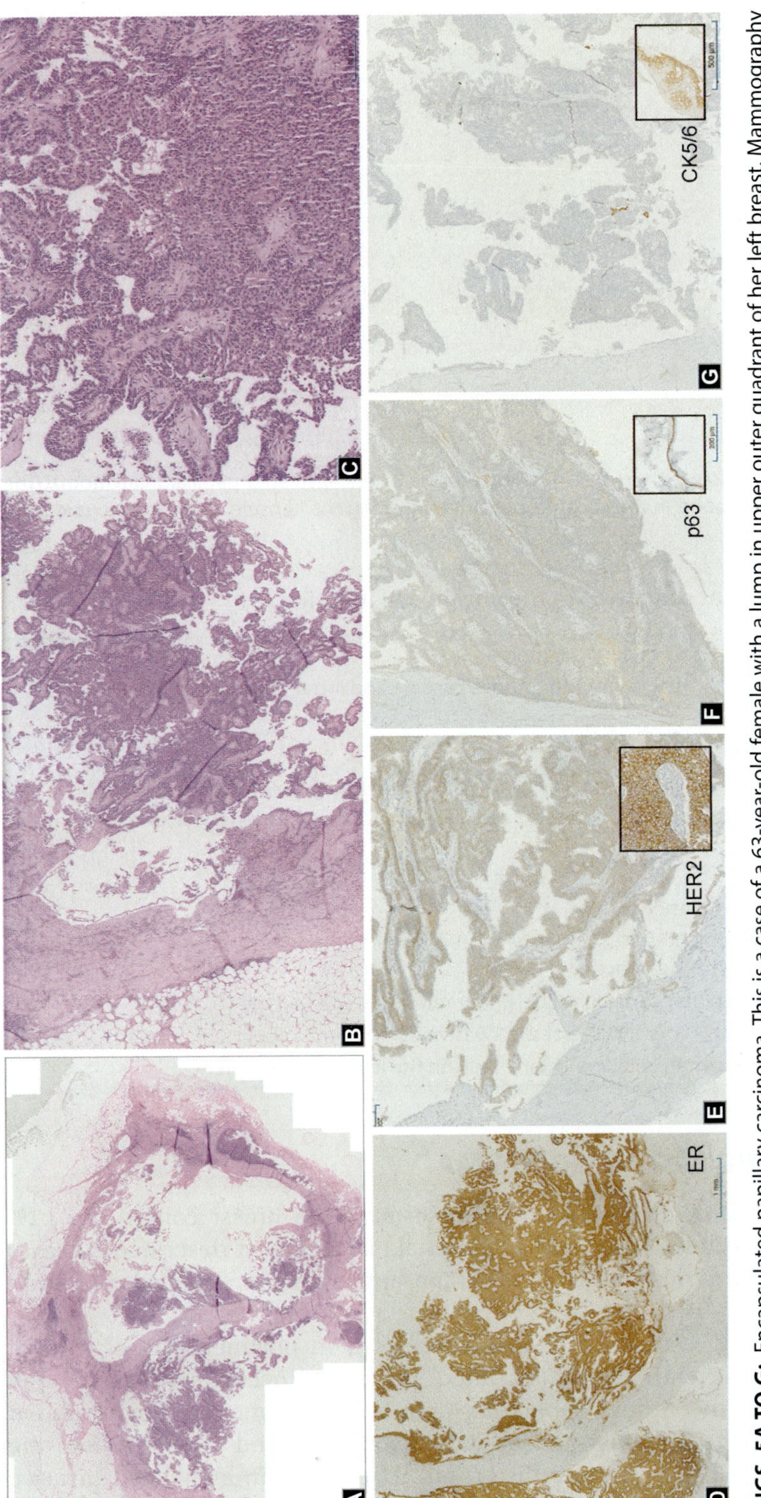

FIGS. 5A TO G: Encapsulated papillary carcinoma. This is a case of a 63-year-old female with a lump in upper outer quadrant of her left breast. Mammography revealed a 21 × 16 mm hypoechoic lesion with internal vascularity within at 10 o'clock position (BIRADS—4A). Scanner view shows an encapsulated tumor with papillary proliferation within the fibrous capsule (A and B). The tumor cells lining the papillae show monomorphic cells with mild nuclear atypia and moderate amount of cytoplasm (C). (D to G) The tumor cells show diffuse and strong nuclear positivity for ER and PR (not shown here) and are negative for HER2, p63 (negative both in periphery of the tumor and papillary fronds) and CK5/6 (insets show external controls on the slides).

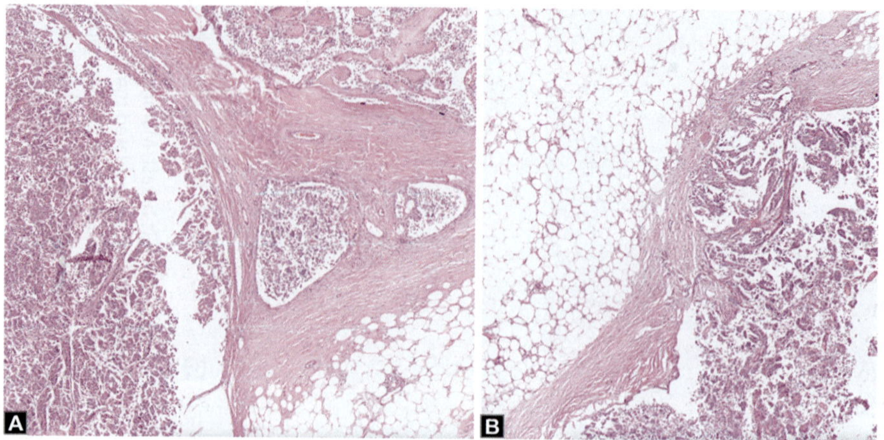

FIGS. 6A AND B: Microphotographs showing a case of encapsulated papillary carcinoma. The tumor cells are entrapped in the capsule, but not infiltrating the capsule. This is not regarded as invasion.

Prognosis: Excellent prognosis in the absence of invasion.[22]

Stat Pearls: Encapsulated papillary carcinoma

- Well-circumscribed cystic cavity with fibrous capsule and intracystic papillary proliferation
- Usually mild-to-moderate nuclear atypia
- Graded as per Nottingham nuclear grade
- CK5/6 and HER2 negative, ER positive (strong and uniform), and PR variable expression
- Myoepithelial cells absent in the cores of papillae (all cases) and periphery of lesions (majority of cases)
- Staged as Tis

Stat Pearls (EPC with invasion):

- Invasive component presents as permeation of the capsule by neoplastic cells giving an irregular infiltrative appearance
- The invasive component is usually IBC, NST, or rarely any special type
- The staging is done as per the size of the invasive component
- Hormone receptor interpretation is done only on the invasive component

SOLID PAPILLARY CARCINOMA

Solid papillary carcinoma is a rare neoplasm of the breast comprising <1% of breast neoplastic lesions.[23] HM Maluf et al., in 1995 first described 20 cases of SPC as papillary neoplasms with benign appearance on clinical and gross examination.[24]

Solid papillary carcinoma, *clinically*, presents in postmenopausal women mostly in their seventh decade or later. These can occur anywhere in the breast. However, the central/subareolar area is most commonly involved. *On mammography*, these appear as well circumscribed round masses. When the mass is associated with stromal distortion, it suggests an associated invasive component.

On gross examination, SPC appears as a soft, circumscribed, and tan-pink mass. They are usually unifocal[16] and 95% of the cases have unilateral presentation with size varying from 1 to 15 cm in maximum dimension.[14] The WHO 5th edition on Breast Tumors classifies SPC into SPC without invasion and SPC with invasion.

On histopathology, SPC (without invasion) appears as expansile solid nodules on low power with distribution pattern as an in situ disease. On higher power, the nodules show papillae with delicate fibrovascular cores and neoplastic cells proliferation filling the intervening areas giving a solid appearance. These nodules lack a fibrotic capsule as we see in EPC. The fibrovascular cores are so delicate that sometimes it is difficult to identify them.[25] Nuclear palisading may be present at the stromal epithelial interface. The tumor cells may be arranged in rosette and pseudorosette architecture.[24] The individual tumor cells are monotonous, round to spindle in shape with mild-to-moderate nuclear atypia, and eosinophilic granular cytoplasm. Mitosis is variable but is usually low **(Figs. 7A to G)**. The tumor cells frequently show neuroendocrine differentiation, especially when associated with mucinous carcinoma **(Figs. 8A and B)**.[26] The tumor cells may sometimes show prominent signet ring cell morphology.

On immunohistochemistry, MECs are absent in the papillary fronds and may be present in the periphery of lesions (in around 20% of cases). The neoplastic cell population is negative for basal markers and HER2/ERBB2 nonamplified and shows diffuse uniform positivity for ER and variable positivity for PR.

In SPC with invasion, the invasive component lacks MECs and shows geographic jigsaw pattern with ragged and irregular margins within a desmoplastic stroma. Staging of these carcinomas is done based on the size of the invasive component. Hormonal markers are also interpreted only in the invasive component. The invasive component is usually the luminal molecular subtype. SPC may be associated with intracellular and/or extracellular mucin. The extracellular mucin is considered as the invasive component only when clusters or strands or singly scattered tumor cells are identified in that mucin **(Figs. 8A and B)**. The invasive component of SPC with invasion can be mucinous carcinoma type B or IBC, NST, or rarely special types of IBC like lobular, tubular, cribriform, etc.[7]

These tumors are biologically indolent and have excellent prognosis.[23] Shyangping Guo et al. studied 11 cases of SPC and reviewed 253 cases described previously in literature and found that out of the total 264 cases, axillary lymph node metastasis could be only found in 3% of the cases with rare local recurrence and distant metastasis. Rare deaths (3 out of 264 cases) were reported because of the disease. This study then suggested avoiding overtreatment of the disease.[23]

Differential Diagnosis

- *Intraductal papilloma with florid UDH or IDP with florid lobular carcinoma in situ (LCIS):* Intraductal papilloma when associated with UDH or LCIS may show cellular proliferation filling the spaces intervening the papillary fronds, giving a solid appearance. This solid look can mimic SPC. Points for differentiation: The papillary fronds of IDP are usually broad and may show

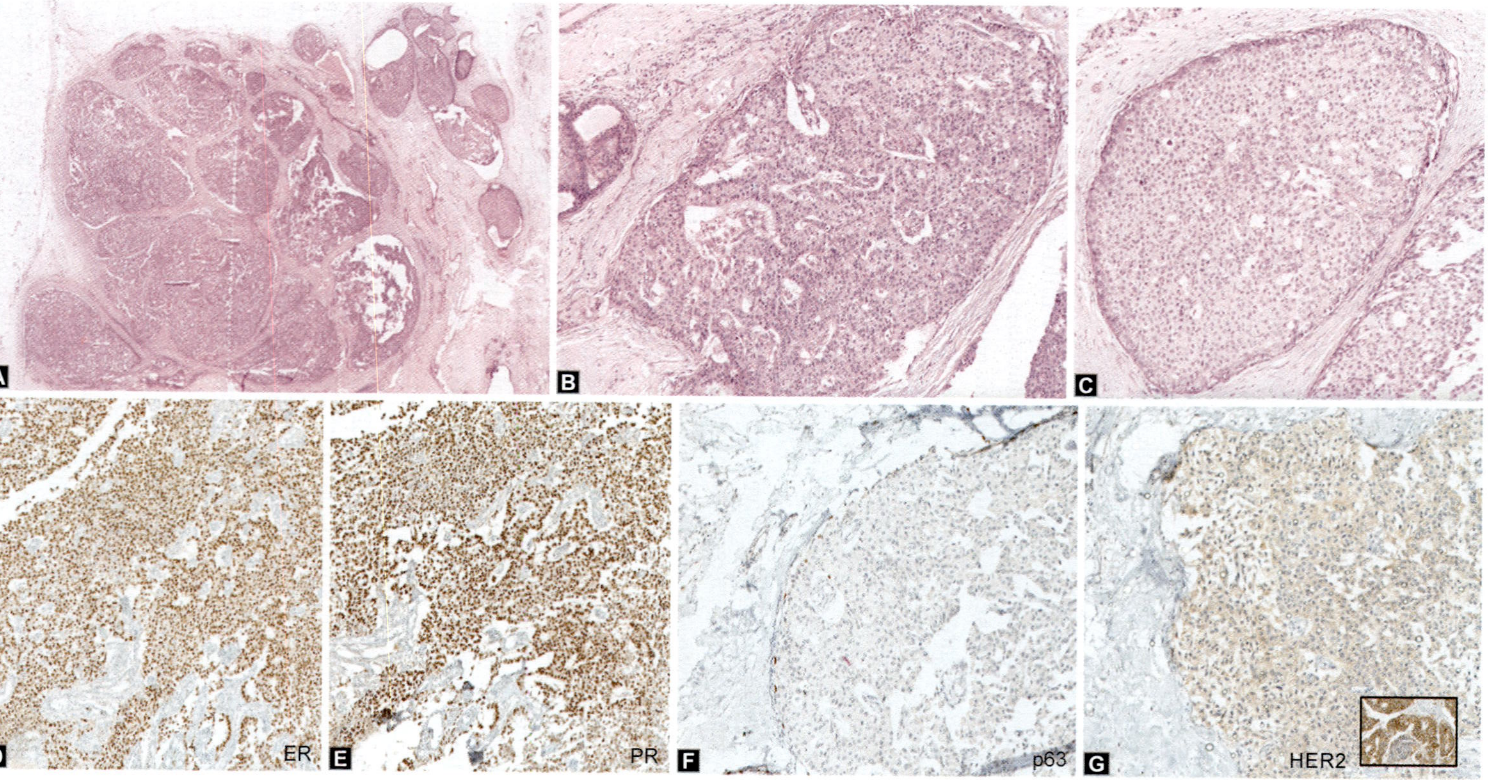

FIGS. 7A TO G: Solid papillary carcinoma. This is a case of a 76-year-old female. Mammography shows a well-defined round lobulated high density lesion measuring 2 × 1.8 × 1.8 cm seen in inner lower central region of left breast. Microphotographs show multiple nodules which appear solid on scanner view (A). These nodules show fine fibrovascular cores and monomorphic nuclei with fine chromatin (B and C). The tumor cells show diffuse and strong positivity for ER and PR (D and E). (F) P63 shows patchy positivity in the periphery of the nodules and is negative in the papillary fronds. (G) HER2 is negative in the tumor cells (inset—external control on the slide).

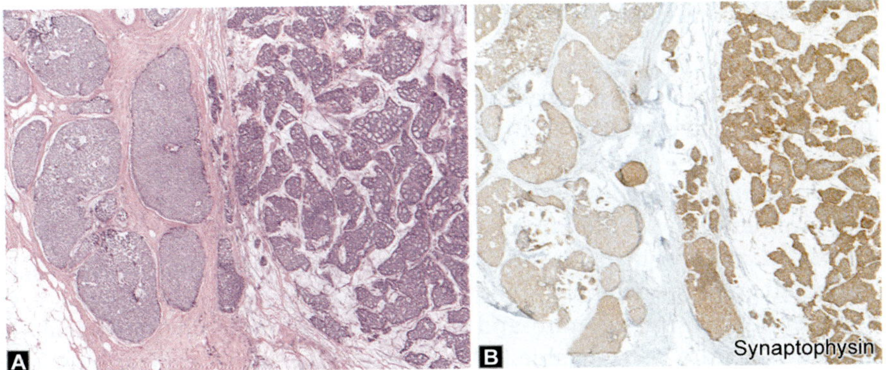

FIGS. 8 AND B: Microphotograph showing solid nodules of SPC (in the left) with an associated mucinous carcinoma (in the right). The tumor cells, both in the in situ component and invasive component, show positivity for synaptophysin and chromogranin (not shown here).

(SPC: solid papillary carcinoma)

prominent stromal components. The proliferating cells are not monotonous such as SPC, express HMWCK, and ER (heterogeneous). MEC markers highlight the MEC in the papillary fronds of background IDP. The LCIS component can mimic SPC in cellular morphology as they both may show intracytoplasmic mucin. The LCIS cells do not show expression of E-cadherin and β-catenin and show diffuse cytoplasmic expression for p120.[27] The associated UDH will show heterogeneous cellular proliferation. The nuclei may show nuclear grooves or intranuclear cytoplasmic inclusions. Nuclear atypia is not seen as in SPC (mild-to-moderate nuclear atypia). The UDH shows mosaic (checkerboard) pattern positivity for HMWCK, heterogeneous expression of ER, and MEC.[27]

- *Encapsulated papillary carcinoma:* SPCs lack the fibrous capsule of EPC. The architecture of SPC is like solid nodules of neoplastic cells, whereas EPC has the appearance of a cystic cavity filled with papillary proliferation.

Stat Pearls (SPC in situ):

- Solid well-circumscribed nodules with delicate fibrovascular cores
- Frequent neuroendocrine differentiation
- Usually mild-to-moderate nuclear atypia
- Graded as per Nottingham nuclear grade
- CK5/6 and HER2 negative, ER positive (strong and uniform), and PR variable expression
- Myoepithelial cells absent in the cores of papillae (all cases) and periphery of lesions (majority of cases)
- Staged as Tis

Stat Pearls (SPC with invasion):

- Invasive component presents as geographical jigsaw and irregular pattern with an associated desmoplastic response
- The invasive component may be IBC, NST, or any special type (mostly type B mucinous carcinoma)
- The staging is done as per the size of the invasive component
- Hormone receptor interpretation is done only on the invasive component

INVASIVE PAPILLARY CARCINOMA

Invasive papillary carcinomas are invasive carcinomas characterized by papillae with fibrovascular cores covered by neoplastic epithelium. In addition, there is presence of dilated ducts and microcysts with papillary proliferation within them.

On immunohistochemistry, MEC markers are negative in both the papillary fronds and periphery of the tumor. Tumor cells are negative for high molecular cytokeratins and positive for ER and PR. These tumors are graded as per Nottingham grading system.

This entity is extremely rare and thus much clinical, epidemiological, and prognostic data are not available.[7] These are usually single lesions. Most cases diagnosed as invasive papillary carcinoma are actually EPC or SPC or a metastasis from another organ. Care should be taken while diagnosing this entity. The nonpapillary invasive carcinoma arising in association with EPC or SPC should not be diagnosed as invasive papillary carcinoma.[28,29] A metastasis from ovarian serous carcinoma, papillary thyroid carcinoma, and pulmonary papillary adenocarcinoma must be ruled out on the basis of morphology and appropriate immunophenotypic markers. Micropapillary carcinoma of breast should not be misdiagnosed as invasive papillary carcinoma as the former shows characteristic morphology of presence of micropapillae within clear stromal spaces.

APPLICATIONS AND FUTURE PROSPECTS OF MOLECULAR PATHOLOGY IN PAPILLARY NEOPLASMS OF BREAST

We have understood that IDPs confer a risk for developing invasive breast malignancy. Therefore, they do share molecular genetic features. PIK3CA mutations have been identified in IDP, atypical IDP as well as in breast carcinomas. Around 37% of core biopsies diagnosed as atypical IDP on core biopsies turn out to be DCIS or IDC on surgical excision.[30] A recent study showed that IDP without any copy number alteration (CNA) lack the potential for malignant transformation.[31] Presence of copy number events—16q loss, 1q gain, and 11q loss has been identified in atypical papillomas as well as papillary carcinomas and IBCs. Thus, molecular testing done on core biopsies diagnosed as IDP can aid in taking appropriate decisions for disease management. For example, surgical excision can be avoided in cases of IDP with presence of PIK3CA mutations and absence of CNA.[30]

CONCLUSION

The concept of Papillary Lesions of the Breast has been evolving over many years. The current 5th edition of WHO Blue Books provides a spectrum of these lesions with a better understanding. This chapter has tried to simplify the approach to their diagnosis. From the point of view of a Histopathologist, a holistic approach is needed taking into consideration clinical, radiological, histopathological and appropriate immunohistochemistry of the case. Papillary lesions in biopsy samples may not provide the complete picture of the lesion. In such cases, it is recommended to discuss at the multidisciplinary meeting and give appropriate differential diagnoses.

REFERENCES

1. Troxell ML, Masek M, Sibley RK. Immunohistochemical staining of papillary breast lesions. Appl Immunohistochem Mol Morphol. 2007;15(2):145-53.
2. Wang Y, Zhu JF, Liu YY, Han GP. An analysis of cyclin D1, cytokeratin 5/6 and cytokeratin 8/18 expression in breast papillomas and papillary carcinomas. Diagn Pathol. 2013;8:8.
3. Lewis JT, Hartmann LC, Vierkant RA, Maloney SD, Shane Pankratz V, Allers TM, et al. An analysis of breast cancer risk in women with single, multiple, and atypical papilloma. Am J Surg Pathol. 2006;30(6):665-72.
4. Brookes MJ, Bourke AG. Radiological appearances of papillary breast lesions. Clin Radiol. 2008;63(11):1265-73.
5. Flint A, Oberman HA. Infarction and squamous metaplasia of intraductal papilloma: a benign breast lesion that may simulate carcinoma. Hum Pathol. 1984;15(8):764-7.
6. Jiao YF, Nakamura S, Oikawa T, Sugai T, Uesugi N. Sebaceous gland metaplasia in intraductal papilloma of the breast. Virchows Arch. 2001;438(5):505-8.
7. International Agency for Research on Cancer. (2024). Breast Tumours: WHO classification of tumours, 5th edition, volume 2. [online] Available from https://publications.iarc.fr/Book-And-Report-Series/Who-Classification-Of-Tumours/Breast-Tumours-2019 [Last accessed November, 2024].
8. Moritani S, Ichihara S, Hasegawa M, Endo T, Oiwa M, Shiraiwa M, et al. Uniqueness of ductal carcinoma in situ of the breast concurrent with papilloma: implications from a detailed topographical and histopathological study of 50 cases treated by mastectomy and wide local excision. Histopathology. 2013;63(3):407-17.
9. Ali-Fehmi R, Carolin K, Wallis T, Visscher DW. Clinicopathologic analysis of breast lesions associated with multiple papillomas. Hum Pathol. 2003;34(3):234-9.
10. Perez AA, Balabram D, Salles M de A, Gobbi H. Ductal carcinoma in situ of the breast: correlation between histopathological features and age of patients. Diagn Pathol. 2014: 227.
11. Hittmair AP, Lininger RA, Tavassoli FA. Ductal carcinoma in situ (DCIS) in the male breast: a morphologic study of 84 cases of pure DCIS and 30 cases of DCIS associated with invasive carcinoma—a preliminary report. Cancer. 1998;83(10):2139-49.
12. Consensus Conference on the classification of ductal carcinoma in situ. The Consensus Conference Committee. Cancer. 1997;80(9):1798-802.
13. Lefkowitz M, Lefkowitz W, Wargotz ES. Intraductal (intracystic) papillary carcinoma of the breast and its variants: a clinicopathological study of 77 cases. Hum Pathol. 1994;25(8): 802-9.
14. Mulligan AM, O'Malley FP. Papillary lesions of the breast: a review. Adv Anat Pathol. 2007;14(2):108-19.
15. Farrokh D, Abedi M, Fallah Rastegar Y. An Intracystic Papillary Carcinoma of the Breast. Iran J Cancer Prevt]. 2013;6(2):11821.
16. Kulka J, Madaras L, Floris G, Lax SF. Papillary lesions of the breast. Virchows Arch. 2022;480(1):65-84.
17. Wynveen CA, Nehhozina T, Akram M, Hassan M, Norton L, Van Zee KJ, et al. Intracystic papillary carcinoma of the breast: An in situ or invasive tumor? Results of immunohistochemical analysis and clinical follow-up. Am J Surg Pathol. 2011;35(1):1-14.
18. Wang Y, Song EC. Papillary neoplasm of the breast—A review and update. Hum Pathol Rep. 2021;26:300581.
19. Rakha EA, Varga Z, Elsheik S, Ellis IO. High-grade encapsulated papillary carcinoma of the breast: an under-recognized entity. Histopathology. 2015;66(5):740-6.

20. Duprez R, Wilkerson PM, Lacroix-Triki M, Lambros MB, MacKay A, A'Hern R, et al. Immunophenotypic and genomic characterization of papillary carcinomas of the breast. J Pathol. 2012;226(3):427-41.
21. Piscuoglio S, Ng CKY, Martelotto LG, Eberle CA, Cowell CF, Natrajan R, et al. Integrative genomic and transcriptomic characterization of papillary carcinomas of the breast. Mol Oncol. 2014;8(8):1588-602.
22. George K, Anna Z, Evanthia K, Vassilios K. Encapsulated papillary carcinoma of the breast: An overview. J Cancer Res Ther. 2013;9(4):564-70.
23. Guo S, Wang Y, Rohr J, Fan C, Li Q, Li X, et al. Solid papillary carcinoma of the breast: A special entity needs to be distinguished from conventional invasive carcinoma avoiding over-treatment. Breast. 2016;26:67-72.
24. Maluf HM, Koerner FC. Solid papillary carcinoma of the breast. A form of intraductal carcinoma with endocrine differentiation frequently associated with mucinous carcinoma. Am J Surg Pathol. 1995;19(11):1237-44.
25. Jorns JM. Papillary Lesions of the Breast: A Practical Approach to Diagnosis. Arch Pathol Lab Med. 2016;140(10):1052-9.
26. Otsuki Y, Yamada M, Shimizu S ichi, Suwa K, Yoshida M, Tanioka F, et al. Solid-papillary carcinoma of the breast: clinicopathological study of 20 cases. Pathol Int. 2007;57(7):421-9.
27. Brogi E, Krystel-Whittemore M. Papillary neoplasms of the breast including upgrade rates and management of intraductal papilloma without atypia diagnosed at core needle biopsy. Mod Pathol. 2021;34(Suppl 1):78-93.
28. Ueng SH, Mezzetti T, Tavassoli FA. Papillary neoplasms of the breast: a review. Arch Pathol Lab Med. 2009;133(6):893-907.
29. Wei S. Papillary Lesions of the Breast: An Update. Arch Pathol Lab Med. 2016;140(7): 628-43.
30. Nuñez DL, González FC, Ibargüengoitia MC, Fuentes Corona RE, Hernández Villegas AC, Zubiate ML, et al. Papillary Lesions of the Breast: A Review. Breast Cancer Manag. 2020; 9(4).
31. Kader T, Elder K, Zethoven M, Semple T, Hill P, Goode DL, et al. The genetic architecture of breast papillary lesions as a predictor of progression to carcinoma. NPJ Breast Cancer. 2020;6:9.

14

CHAPTER

The Role of Pathology in Precision Medicine

Dipanwita Biswas, Suvradeep Mitra

INTRODUCTION

Precision medicine is a specialized form of medicine where the prevention, diagnosis, prognosis, and management of a disease is tailored according to a subpopulation depending upon its common genetic susceptibility, response to treatment, and social, environmental, ethnic, and demographic factors. The disease manifestations of an individual and his/her response to the therapy depend upon the genetic makeup. Still, it is also affected by the transcriptome, epigenome, and metabolome of the individual. Besides, the social, behavioral, environmental, and demographic factors also influence the individual. Thus, treatment of a disease does not require any drug directed toward the disease, but needs to be tailored according to the necessity of an individual belonging to a subpopulation with similar genome, epigenome, metabolome, and preferably similar sociodemographic factors. This holistic and combinatorial management approach toward a disease belonging to a subpopulation along with preventive and public health policies make precision medicine a futuristic goal of medicine practice.

DEFINITION

The United States National Cancer Institute (USNCI) defined personalized medicine, an archaic name for precision medicine, as "a form of medicine that uses information about a person's genes, proteins, and environment to prevent, diagnose, and treat disease".[1] It does not indicate the development of unique drugs for individual patients, but rather the ability to classify a unique subpopulation that will behave similarly to the occurrence of a disease and respond similarly to the same standard treatment implemented for the disease. Thus, the concept of precision medicine distinguishes the individuals who tend to benefit from a therapy before implementing the same therapy to every individual after the occurrence of a disease.[1] **Table 1** compares the precision medicine with the traditional medicine.

TABLE 1: A comparison and contrast between the traditional and precision medicine.

Parameters	Traditional medicine	Precision medicine
Use of the drugs	Disease-specific	Patient-specific
Drug response	Only a certain percentage of these patients would respond to the particular drug	All patients would respond to the particular drug
Genetic variations, age, gender, addictions, race, ethnicity, concomitant drugs, comorbidities, and environmental factors	Causes interindividual differences	Does not affect the drug response
Wastage of drugs	More	Less

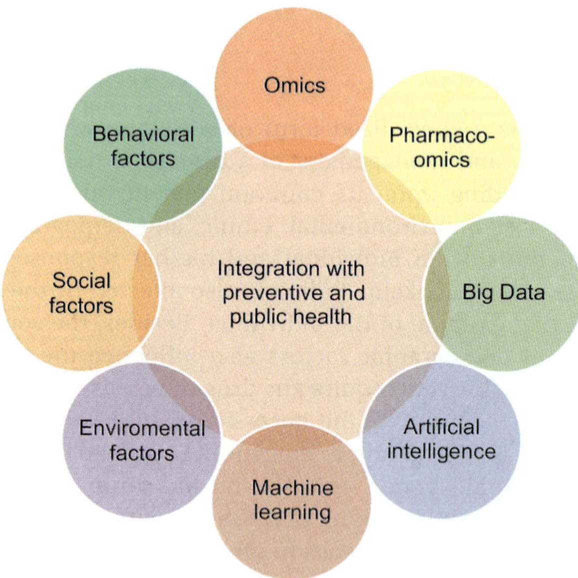

FIG. 1: Different components/tools of precision medicine.

COMPONENTS/TOOLS OF PRECISION MEDICINE

Different tools of precision medicine are depicted in **Figure 1**. These components encompass:

- Omics
- Pharmaco-omics
- Big Data
- Artificial intelligence (AI) and machine learning (ML)
- Environmental, demographic, ethnic, social, and behavioral factors
- Preventive and public health

Omics

The human as an organism functions through the complex interaction between various chemical compounds, especially proteins. The generation of these proteins occurs from the messenger ribonucleic acid (mRNA) via a process known as translation. mRNA is formed from the deoxyribonucleic acid (DNA), coded within a gene through a process called transcription. Therefore, the human DNA contains all the coded information relevant to health and disease. Central dogma indicates the generation of mRNA from DNA via transcription and protein from mRNA via translation in the same sequence. The complete set of human DNA is called the human *genome*. The subject dealing with the human genome is called *genomics*. The completion of the human genome project (HGP) required more than two decades of time, more than a few thousand dedicated and skilled scientists, and more than a few million dollars fund speaking volumes of the complexity, intricacy, and volume of the work.[2]

The DNA generates both coding and noncoding RNA material. The coding RNA (mRNA) is responsible for protein formation, whereas the noncoding RNA is responsible for various other functions. This includes the stability of the mRNA, modification of the coding, transfer of the RNA to its designated site, etc. The function of these noncoding RNA is equally important to coding RNA and thus, often dictates/modifies a disease occurrence. Therefore, the generation of coding RNA is not a linear equivalent of genomic DNA. The complete set of human RNA is called the human *transcriptome*. The subject dealing with the human transcriptome is called *transcriptomics*. Similarly, a complete set of human proteins is called the human *proteome* and the subject dealing with the human proteome is called *proteomics*. The proteome also does not maintain a linear relation with the human transcriptome and is modified before and after translation. The expression and transcription of the genetic DNA are further affected by various chemical modifications of the DNA. These chemical modifications promote/inhibit the transcription of the DNA sequence via mechanical/electrostatic interactions. The two most common chemical modifications include modifications of the histone proteins, involved in the coiling of the DNA, and DNA methylation characterized by covalent bonding of the DNA base with acetyl/methyl group(s). Special forms of RNAs known as microRNA (miRNA) and small interfering RNA (siRNA) also regulate the stability of the mRNA modifying the genomic expression at the supragenomic level/nongenomic level. These chemical alterations of the genome by DNA methylation, histone modifications, and/or miRNA expression are known under the rubric of epigenetics. The complete set of epigenetic modifications is called *epigenome*, while the subject dealing with the human epigenome is called *epigenomics*.[2]

Proteins are one of the major functional molecules of the human body though there are various other molecules including carbohydrates, lipids, lipoproteins, glycoproteins, glycolipids, etc. Besides, numerous other molecules generated by the metabolism of endogenous and exogenous products including organic anions, nucleic acids, aldehydes, alcohols, acids, bases, amines, toxins, gases, pollutants, and drug metabolites are also found in the human body, which directly/indirectly affect the individual system irrespective of the individual's genome, epigenome, transcriptome, and proteome. The whole set of these metabolites is known as *metabolome* and the subject dealing with the metabolome is called *metabolomics*.[2]

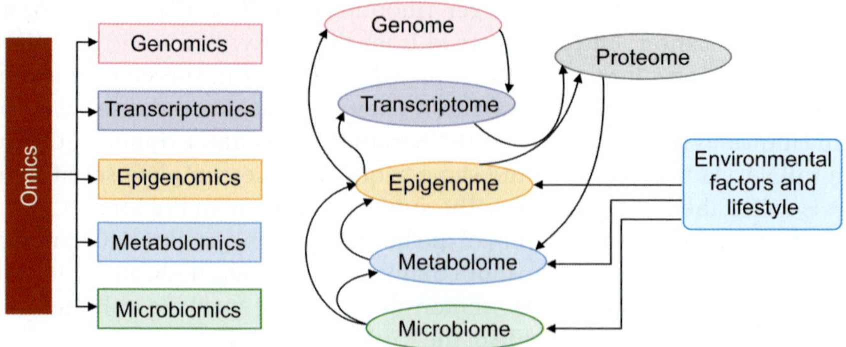

FIG. 2: The interrelation between different types of omics.

An individual human being is a complex organism that constantly maintains a dynamic homeostasis with other species on earth. This interaction varies from individual to individual and depends on social status, behavioral status, ethnicity, regional status, lifestyle, occupation, dietary habits, and miscellaneous other factors. This interspecies interaction with various macroorganisms and microorganisms variably affects human health and diseases. Especially, the interactions of the human being with the microorganisms determine homeostasis and diseases of the gut and hepatobiliary system. The complete spectrum of the microorganisms interacting with the human individual is known as *microbiome*, while the study of the same is known as *microbiomics*. The alteration of the normal microbiome is known as dysbiosis and is related to various diseases of gastrointestinal and hepatobiliary systems.

The omics of an individual/a subpopulation are interrelated and not entirely different from each other **(Fig. 2)**.

Pharmaco-omics

The genetic makeup of an individual, epigenetic modifications, transcriptome, proteome, and metabolome dominantly predict the fate of the drug once administered within a human body. Thus, the detailed spectrum of human omics provides an insight into the drug response within an individual. Pharmaco-omics deals with the complex topic of pharmacotherapy and the spectrum of omics of an individual. Pharmaco-omics is divided into numerous branches including pharmaco-genomics, pharmaco-transcriptomics, pharmaco-proteomics, etc. The pharmaco-omics determines the pharmacodynamics and pharmacokinetics of a particular drug in a given individual. One of the most well-studied examples of pharmaco-omics is the genetic polymorphisms of the drug metabolizing cytochrome P450 enzymes giving rise to slow metabolizers and fast metabolizers of a drug. The metabolites following slow and fast metabolism can be different with different rates of clearance from the body and different adverse drug reaction profiles. Thus, the adverse drug reaction profile of the same drug with similar drug dosage can be different in two different individuals due to their different genomes determining different pharmaco-metabolomes.[2,3]

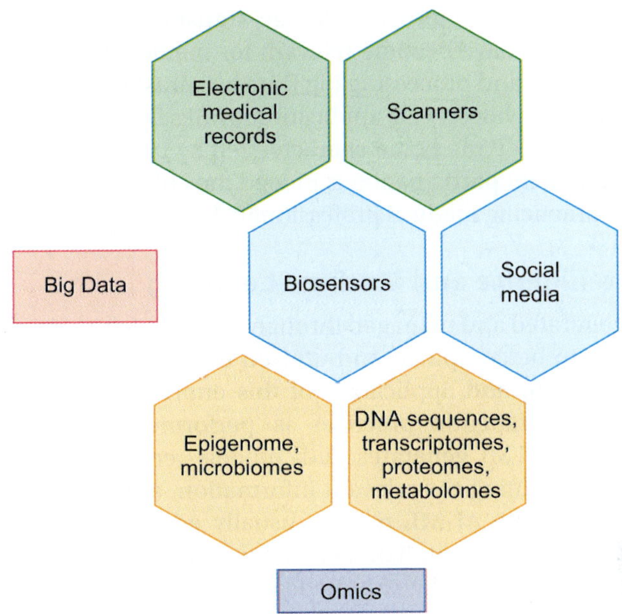

FIG. 3: Different components of Big Data.

Big Data

Big Data is the collective data of an individual and the subpopulation gathered from the detailed clinical features, socio-environmental features, omics data, and biochemical, radiological, and molecular assays. The data is also generated through social media, various sensors, medical records, and scanners **(Fig. 3)**. Therefore, Big Data provides a panoramic view of the health and disease of a subpopulation. As the dominant component of the Big Data is formed by multiple omics, "panoromic" terminology is used to denote the multiple omics.[2,3]

A culmination of the multiomics data is the generation of a *multiomics signature*, a complex biomolecular signature, peculiar for an individual and the subpopulation. A complex mathematical model is an integral part of the multiomics signature. The multiomics signature is generated through the omics data combined with the clinical phenotype, social, behavioral, lifestyle, and environmental factors. The integration of the multiomics signature in the Big Data is crucial.[2,3]

The advent of various new molecular techniques like next-generation sequencing and spatial transcriptomics is essential for the generation of Big Data. These techniques generate bulk data in gigabytes/terabytes corroborative with the term "Big" data. However, the true application of "Big data" in real-time disease management may be small. So, the large part of the data generated through multiomics and other socioenvironmental factors may not be relevant to the actual situation/problem/disease.[3]

The generation of Big Data becomes irrelevant without the ability to store, compute, and analyze it. Therefore, the enormous technical advances in the management of Big Data in terms of storage, transmission, internet bandwidth, and cloud computing have become relevant for medical professionals. Besides, the cost of generation and processing Big Data has drastically reduced in the past few years. It leads to widespread application of Big Data globally changing the medical practice. The 4P medicine characterized by *p*rediction, *p*ersonalization, *p*revention, and *p*atient participation is indeed the culmination of implementing Big Data in the practicing medical professionals.[4]

Artificial Intelligence and Machine Learning

The Big Data generated and managed through various high-throughput, new-age machines needs to be computed and utilized through an effective system. The handling, integration, and application of this enormous data into diagnostic, prognostic, and therapeutic practices is performed by AI and ML. The combination of AI and ML generates study models, reduces the disproportionate noise from the data sifting the relevant information, and makes rapid decision-making algorithms. The AI–ML models usually educate themselves from the previous errors in judgments/failures, continually updating, rectifying, and educating themselves from the experiences. The AI–ML models also generate flags to indicate human intervention. The application of AI–ML in telemedicine has been proven useful during various epidemics and pandemics where remote patient monitoring and management need to be performed with limited human resources.[2,5,6]

Behavioral, Lifestyle, Social, and Environmental Factors

The health and disease of an individual/a subpopulation is not only dependent upon its omics but also on different behavioral changes, dietary habits, lifestyle modifications, and socioenvironmental parameters. The true theragnostics of an individual/subpopulation are impossible without a detailed knowledge of these elements. For example, an individual with a genetic predisposition to develop type 2 diabetes mellitus can prevent its advent by regular exercise and a balanced diet while its advent can be accelerated through a sedentary life habit. These factors contribute to up to 70% of human diseases while only 30% of human diseases occur due to genetic alterations.[2,7] Thus, a knowledge of the accurate dietary habits, lifestyle, and socioenvironmental factors is critical for the diagnosis and management of the disease. This data needs intricate integration into the omics and Big Data for appropriate implementation of precision medicine. Furthermore, this is also critical for the preventive medicine and public health.

GOALS AND CONSTRAINTS OF PRECISION MEDICINE

The major goal of precision medicine is "The right drug, the right dose, for the right patient, at the right time".[8,9] The major bottlenecks of this approach are (1) the complexity of the biological details and its management and (2) the implication of this approach on the economy.

The tremendous amount of data generated through multiomics and Big Data is difficult to handle even by high-throughput machines and AI-generated models. Besides, only a small amount of data is practically relevant for day-to-day practice. The models of prediction also do not bear a linear relation with the individualistic disease manifestation. The biology of the individual, the maintenance of health, and the occurrence of a disease are multiparametric with numerous confounders and are more complex than imagined.

The generation of this data, its management, and implementation in real time are explosively expensive. However, the expense of the high-throughput tests has become cheaper over the last decade and has gradually become available to the plebeians. Yet, the cost is very high for universal acceptance and routine application. Thus, though the concepts of precision medicine are lucrative, the economic burden of the implementation of the same is an arduous task.[8]

PATHOLOGY IN PRECISION MEDICINE AND THE ROLE OF PATHOLOGISTS IN PRECISION MEDICINE

The pathologists have long served the role of diagnosticians in conjunction with the radiologists and the clinicians. The major role of pathologists in the past century has evolved from a morphologist to a molecular morphologist.[10] Thus, the role of pathologists in the era of precision medicine is not limited to rendering a diagnosis. A pathologist/oncopathologist is supposed to classify a disease, predict a prognosis, predict a response to therapy, and aid the clinician in deciding the therapy in some instances.

The addition of molecular pathology to various branches of surgical pathology is critical for the diagnosis and treatment. The availability of molecular-directed therapy to different tumors and nontumors has caused a major paradigm shift. As an example, the treatment and prognosis of adenocarcinoma of the lung were dismal a couple of decades back. However, the identification of molecular markers like *EGFR* mutation/*ALK* rearrangement and the availability of anti-EGFR/anti-ALK drugs has caused a radical shift in the scenario. Similarly, testing the breast carcinoma for *Her2/neu*, melanoma for *BRAFV*600E, and gastrointestinal stromal tumor for *c-KIT* use the same principle.[1-3,10,11]

It is important to note that the histomorphological changes are not the only changes that occur within a cell. The histomorphological changes are late to occur and are usually associated with molecular alterations. On the other hand, many early as well as a few late molecular alterations do not cause any clinical and/or histomorphological change. Thus, these alterations are subcellular, and only high-throughput, molecular techniques can detect them. While these changes do not have a histomorphological counterpart, they may be a potential and actionable target, making their detection relevant in clinical practice. The detection of these changes from the tissue/blood may act as an early method of disease detection or disease recurrence. Thus, "liquid biopsy", a minimally invasive form of detection of cancer cells/cellular DNA in the blood, may aid in finding the molecular signature of a cancer, thus predicting an early cancer/its recurrence.[1-3,10,11]

The concept of companion diagnostic/complementary diagnostics relies on the decision and principles of immunotherapy. Antitumor immunity is usually mediated by the cytotoxic T-lymphocytes as well as innate and humoral immunity. The tumor expresses several molecules that bind to the receptors expressed by the cytotoxic T-cells, downregulating/mitigating the expression of these cytotoxic molecules. This is one of the strategies employed by the tumor cells to evade the host immunity. Histologically, a higher number of tumor-infiltrating cytotoxic T-lymphocytes corroborates well with the prognosis. Therefore, abrogation of the expression of immune-evasive molecules expressed by the tumor cells can be therapeutically proven beneficial. This is the molecular basis of the programmed death 1 (PD-1)/programmed death ligand 1 (PDL-1) testing in various tumors including lung, head and neck, gastric/gastroesophageal, urothelial, etc. A particular PD-1/PD-L1 clone expressed by the viable tumor cells is measured by immunohistochemistry. An antibody directed against the same clone detects the tumor cells expressing the clone, and a companion drug raised against this molecule can be effective in treating the same tumor. 22c3 clone marketed by DAKO can be tested in lung carcinoma and gastric carcinoma and if positive, the patient is eligible to receive pembrolizumab, an anti-PD-L1 drug.[1-3,10,11]

Biomarker testing is also an important role played by the pathologist. The types of various biomarkers and their utilization in different cancers are depicted in **Table 2** and **Flowchart 1**.[12] These biomarkers have theragnostic and predictive roles and pathologists often employ them to aid clinicians. Different diagnostic methods used for biomarker detection are extraction-based, sequencing-based, polymerase chain reaction (PCR)-based, immunohistochemistry/immunofluorescence-based, mass spectroscopy-based, miscellaneous microscopy-based, and can be virtual too.

The advent of whole-slide imaging (WSI) and digital scanners has also radicalized the pathology practice in the era of precision medicine. WSI generates the complete histopathological data of a slide that can be stored, archived, shared, used for future diagnosis, and used for AI-generated models. Pathologists serve an essential role by generating enormous WSI data.

PROSPECTS OF PRECISION MEDICINE AND PRECISION PATHOLOGY

Precision medicine and precision pathology are the new-age branches of medicine and pathology. The role of the pathologists has changed in the last decade from only a histomorphologist to an individual who takes part in the prognostication of the disease and classification of the disease, aids in determining the therapy, judges the treatment response, archives the data for the generation of the Big Data, and forms an essential part of the multidisciplinary team. The widespread use of high-throughput techniques by both the medical and nonmedical fraternity has created a challenge for the survival of pathologists and at least partly forced the birth of molecular pathologists. Consequently, the classification of different tumor and nontumor entities see a radical

TABLE 2: List of the biomarkers and its association with the tumors.[12]

Name of the test/biomarker	Associated tumors
HER2/neu	Carcinoma (breast, stomach)
PD-L1	Melanoma, carcinoma (lung, kidney, head and neck, uterus, breast)
CTLA-4	Melanoma
CD20	B-non-Hodgin lymphoma
CD30	Anaplastic large cell lymphoma, Hodgkin lymphoma
ALK	Lung carcinoma, anaplastic large cell lymphoma
TOPO1	Carcinoma (urinary bladder, breast, colon, uterus, ovary)
MMR (MLH1, MSH2, MSH6, PMS2)	Carcinoma (colon, stomach)
EGFR	Carcinoma (colon, lung, pancreas, thyroid)
VEGF	Carcinoma (lung, kidney, colon), glioblastoma
TUBB3	Carcinoma (lung, bladder, uterus, kidney, prostate)
PTEN	Carcinoma (breast, uterus, head and neck, lung, prostate)
ER, PR	Carcinoma (breast, uterus, ovary)
K-RAS	Carcinoma (lung, colon)
Myc	Lymphoma
BCR-ABL1	Chronic myelogenous leukemia, Ph-positive acute lymphoblastic leukemia
BRCA1	Carcinoma (breast, ovary)
c-KIT protein	Gastrointestinal stromal tumor
BRAF	Melanoma, carcinoma (lung, colon)
EZH2	Follicular lymphoma
IDH1/2	Glioma, intrahepatic cholangiocarcinoma

(ER: estrogen receptor; PD-L1: programmed death ligand 1; PR: progesterone receptor; VEGF: vascular endothelial growth factor)

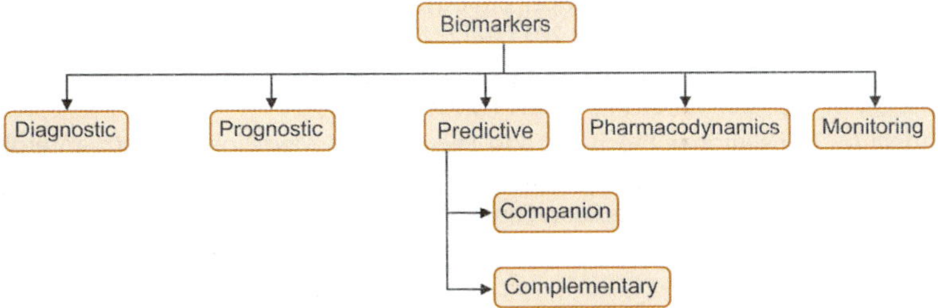

FLOWCHART 1: Different types of biomarkers in precision cancer medicine.

change and incorporation of molecular markers in the diagnosis, confirmation of the diagnosis, and at times the complete nomenclature dictated by the molecular alteration. The recognition of these molecular alterations has forced pharmaceutical companies to test drugs against the disease-defining molecular alterations, creating scope and hope for the tumors with dismal prognosis. Thus, the pathologists are supposed to take the lead in the era of precision medicine and provide the diagnosis, diagnostic clues, background pathophysiology, genomics, and theragnostics.

CONCLUSION

The concept of precision medicine has evolved in the last couple of decades from merely a concept to a new-age branch of medicine. The evolution has occurred parallel to technological advances, advances in the field of pharmacotherapy, economic growth, and slow but gradual changes in societal status. This evolution has also unraveled the complexity of human health and disease, the variability, and the economic burden of such evolution. Despite many limitations, this evolution is a beacon in the history of mankind marking a giant leap toward the achievement of immortality and AI.

REFERENCES

1. Vranic S, Gatalica Z. The Role of Pathology in the Era of Personalized (Precision) Medicine: A Brief Review. Acta Med Acad. 2021;50(1):47-57.
2. Naithani N, Sinha S, Misra P, Vasudevan B, Sahu R. Precision medicine: Concept and tools. Med J Armed Forces India. 2021;77(3):249-57.
3. Gu J, Taylor CR. Practicing pathology in the era of big data and personalized medicine. Appl Immunohistochem Mol Morphol. 2014;22(1):1-9.
4. Hood L, Friend SH. Predictive, personalized, preventive, participatory (P4) cancer medicine. Nat Rev Clin Oncol. 2011;8(3):184-7.
5. Dey P, Dey R. Artificial neural network--mechanism and application in pathology. Indian J Pathol Microbiol. 2002;45(3):371-4.
6. Dey P. The emerging role of deep learning in cytology. Cytopathology. 2021;32(2):154-60.
7. Mackenbach JP. Genetics and health inequalities: hypotheses and controversies. J Epidemiol Community Health. 2005;59(4):268-73.
8. Moch H, Blank PR, Dietel M, Elmberger G, Kerr KM, Palacios J, et al. Personalized cancer medicine and the future of pathology. Virchows Arch. 2012;460(1):3-8.
9. Stricker T, Catenacci DV, Seiwert TY. Molecular profiling of cancer—the future of personalized cancer medicine: a primer on cancer biology and the tools necessary to bring molecular testing to the clinic. Semin Oncol. 2011;38(2):173-85.
10. Masood S. The changing role of pathologists from morphologists to molecular pathologists in the era of precision medicine. Breast J. 2020;26(1):27-34.
11. Candelli M. Translational, Precision, and Personalized Medicine in Gastroenterology. Int J Mol Sci. 2022;23(15):8201.
12. Jasani B, Huss R, Taylor CR. Precision Cancer Medicine. Switzerland: Springer Cham; 2021.

15

CHAPTER

Updates in Pancreaticobiliary Cytopathology

Parikshaa Gupta

INTRODUCTION

The pancreaticobiliary (PB) tree, constituted by a network of ducts and glands essential for digestion and bile secretion, lies intricately snuggled within the human gastrointestinal (GI) tract. The PB tract, like all other body organs, may be affected by various pathologies spanning from benign cystic lesions to highly aggressive malignancies. PB cytology is one of the most pivotal diagnostic tools available for studying the pathological mysteries within this critical anatomic region. A variety of techniques can be employed for obtaining optimum tissue samples from these lesions, although the diagnostic yield and accuracy vary with the technique used. Nonetheless, a vast majority of PB lesions can be reliably diagnosed on cytologic examination.

Pancreaticobiliary cytology not only aids in distinguishing benign from malignant conditions but also plays a crucial role in disease staging, treatment planning, as well as prognostication. The diagnostic accuracy has further improved with the use of various ancillary techniques that can be readily employed on the cytologic samples.

This chapter will cover the major advances in PB cytology, including the advances in sampling techniques, cytologic reporting systems, and the ancillary techniques for the diagnosis of lesions affecting this vital anatomical tract.

SAMPLING TECHNIQUES FOR PANCREATICOBILIARY LESIONS

Owing to their minimally invasive nature and no/minimal procedure-related complications, the cytologic sampling methods are often used as the first-line diagnostic modality for the evaluation of PB lesions. Traditionally, transabdominal image-guided fine-needle aspiration (FNA) was the most used method; however, nowadays, a variety of techniques are available for sampling these lesions.

- *Transabdominal FNA*: FNA serves as the cornerstone of cytologic evaluation and facilitates the procurement of cellular material for microscopic examination. In the case of large pancreatic masses that are easily palpable, palpation-guided transabdominal FNA can be performed. However, it is always preferred to perform an image-guided FNA under either ultrasonographic (USG) or computerized tomography (CT) guidance. USG-guided FNA helps in direct visualization of the lesion in real-time, thereby allowing more representative sampling. CT-guided FNA ensures better visualization with high resolution; however, does not allow for real-time localization of the needle tip during sampling.

- *Endoscopic retrograde cholangiopancreatography (ERCP)-guided biliary brushings*: This cytologic sampling technique is often used for evaluating biliary strictures. Brush cytology is often preferred over biopsy, mainly owing to the higher complication rate associated with the latter. Furthermore, the brush can sample more surface area as compared to a biopsy and hence is associated with higher diagnostic accuracy.[1,2]

  Biliary brushing involves the systematic collection of the lining ductal epithelial cells by using a specialized brush, typically guided over a wire via an endoscopic intervention. The brush is positioned across the stricture, scrapes the lesional mucosa, and is then retracted into its sheath and withdrawn. The scraped material is then used to make smears for microscopic examination. The brush head can also be removed and put in a fixative solution for obtaining liquid-based cytologic preparations. Its minimally invasive nature, low complication rate, rapid turnover time, and high specificity make its use pivotal in the early diagnosis of biliary malignancies.[1]

- *Endoscopic ultrasound (EUS)-guided FNA*: EUS is a highly effective diagnostic modality for detecting PB lesions with sensitivity ranging from 90 to 100%.[3] Owing to the proximity of the echoendoscope to the pancreas, EUS allows for much clearer visualization of the pancreatic lesions compared to other imaging modalities, thereby allowing for more accurate disease localization and staging. In contrast to radial echoendoscopes, the use of linear array echoendoscopes permits performing simultaneous FNA, through the same instrument, in real time. EUS-FNA, thus, integrates endoscopy with ultrasound imaging and needle aspiration, allowing for precise localization and sampling of both luminal as well as intramural lesions that are generally inaccessible by conventional methods.

  This approach is currently used as the standard of care for obtaining representative tissue samples from the PB tract. It can be effectively used for diagnosing solid, solid-cystic, as well as purely cystic PB lesions. It is minimally invasive, safe, and has higher diagnostic accuracy, especially for small and inaccessible PB lesions compared to transabdominal image-guided FNA.[4,5]

  The echoendoscope features an ultrasound probe tip and an aspiration needle portal. Needle size varies based on approach and lesion type, with 19, 22, and 25 gauge being common. The needle is inserted through a separate channel, locked in place, and adjusted to target the lesion. Under real-time visualization, the needle is advanced to the lesion, aspiration is performed from multiple sites, and the aspirate is used to prepare both air-dried and alcohol-fixed smears.[6]

For cystic lesions, wherein the fluid is aspirated, the sample can be collected in an anticoagulant solution for preparing sediment smears or in specialized fixatives for liquid-based cytologic preparations. It is preferable to perform rapid on-site evaluation (ROSE) to ensure the adequacy of the sample. The use of ROSE in the endoscopy suite has been found to improve the diagnostic yield by significantly decreasing the inadequacy rates and ensuring more representative sampling in the same sitting.[7] Additional passes may be taken to obtain samples for various ancillary tests including, cell block preparation and immunocytochemistry (ICC), flow cytometry, biochemical analysis, microbiological cultures, and molecular studies, depending on the clinicoradiologic suspicion.

REPORTING AND NOMENCLATURE IN PANCREATICOBILIARY CYTOPATHOLOGY

As cytologic sampling methods are often used as the first-line diagnostic modality for evaluation of the PB lesions, it is essential to use standardized reporting systems and nomenclature that ensure uniformity in reporting and are easily interpretable by the treating clinicians, thereby aiding in triaging the patients and guiding the therapeutic management.

The Papanicolaou Society of Cytopathology System for Reporting Pancreaticobiliary Cytology

In 2014, the Papanicolaou Society of Cytopathology (PSC) proposed guidelines encompassing various aspects of PB cytology including the indications, techniques, reporting terminologies, nomenclature, ancillary studies, and postprocedure management. These guidelines highlight a multidisciplinary approach for diagnosing PB lesions and emphasize assessment of all relevant clinical, imaging, biochemical, and serological details to ensure an accurate cytologic diagnosis.[8,9] **Table 1** lists all the PSC system diagnostic categories along with the common lesions and risk of malignancy (ROM) for each category.

TABLE 1: The PSC system diagnostic categories along with the common lesions and risk of malignancy in each category.

Diagnostic category	Included entities	Estimated risk of malignancy (%)	Recommended management
Nondiagnostic	• Cellular artifact, obscuring hemorrhage, or necrosis • Pure gastrointestinal contamination • Nonmucinous cyst acellular aspirate • Benign pancreatic parenchyma (with a mass on imaging)	8–50%	Reassess/repeat

Continued

Continued

Diagnostic category	Included entities	Estimated risk of malignancy (%)	Recommended management
Negative	• Pancreatitis • Pseudocyst • Lymphoepithelial cyst • Accessory spleen • Benign pancreatic tissue (no mass)	0–40%	Conservative
Atypical	• Ductal cells with indeterminate atypia (reactive vs. low-grade dysplasia, vs. scant lesional tissue) • Abundant intracytoplasmic mucin in the epithelium	28–100%	Repeat/ conservative/ surgery
Neoplastic-benign	• Serous cystadenoma (SCA) • Lymphangioma • Cystic teratoma • Schwannoma	0%	Conservative
Neoplastic-other	• GIST • Extra-adrenal paraganglioma • Pancreatic solitary fibrous tumor • IPMN with dysplasia • IPNB • MCN with dysplasia • PanNET • Solid pseudopapillary neoplasm (SPN)	0–31%	Surgery/ conservative in some cases
Suspicious for malignancy	Aspirates with cytologic features indicative of malignancy but qualitatively or quantitatively insufficient for an unequivocal diagnosis of malignancy	82–100%	Surgery
Positive/ malignant	• PDAC and variants • Cholangiocarcinoma • Acinar cell carcinoma • Small and large cell neuroendocrine carcinoma • Pancreatoblastoma • Lymphomas • Sarcomas • Metastases to the pancreas	97–100%	Surgery with/ without chemotherapy

(GIST: gastrointestinal stromal tumor; IPNB: intraductal papillary neoplasm of the bile duct; IPMN: intraductal papillary mucinous neoplasm; MCN: mucinous cystic neoplasm; PanNET: pancreatic neuroendocrine tumor; PDAC: pancreatic ductal adenocarcinoma; PSC: Papanicolaou Society of Cytopathology)

The salient features of the recommended cytologic diagnostic categories include:

- *Nondiagnostic*: A cytologic sample that provides no diagnostic information about the lesion sampled is categorized as nondiagnostic (ND). A classic example is an acellular aspirate in a nonmucinous cystic lesion. However, the mere absence of "epithelial cells" in the sample does not necessarily make it ND. Aspiration from a pancreatic pseudocyst would not show epithelial cells; however, the radiologic features would favor a benign lesion. Similarly, aspirate from a mucinous cyst may show thick colloid-like mucin without epithelial cells; however, in such a case an elevated carcinoembryonic antigen (CEA) level in the cyst fluid would support the cytologic diagnosis of a neoplastic mucinous cyst. Thus, all relevant clinical, biochemical, and imaging details should be correlated before labeling a sample as ND. Additionally, a sample demonstrating cellular atypia should never be labeled as ND regardless of its cellularity.
- *Negative (for malignancy)*: An adequately cellular cytologic sample not demonstrating any cellular atypia is categorized as negative. This category would include cytologic samples from normal PB tract, chronic pancreatitis, cholangitis, pseudocyst, or other non-neoplastic lesions. It is recommended that whenever possible, a specific cytologic diagnosis should also be offered for the sample.
- *Atypical*: A cytologic sample demonstrating cytoplasmic, nuclear, or architectural atypia more than that attributable to reactive cellular changes, but not sufficient, either quantitatively or qualitatively, to qualify for a neoplasm or suspicious for malignancy, is labeled as atypical. This is the most heterogeneous diagnostic category and often includes paucicellular samples with reactive changes or premalignant changes.
- *Neoplastic*:
    - Neoplastic-benign: This category includes cytologic samples showing representative cellular features that are diagnostic of a benign neoplasm, with or without supporting clinical, imaging, and ancillary studies. The benign neoplasms in the PB tract may include serous cystadenoma (SCA), cystic teratoma, schwannoma, and leiomyoma.
    - Neoplastic-other: This is yet another heterogeneous category in the PSC system. It includes samples demonstrating features either of a premalignant neoplasm such as intraductal papillary mucinous neoplasm (IPMN) or mucinous cystic neoplasm (MCN) with low, intermediate, or high-grade cytological dysplasia, or a low-grade malignant neoplasm such as well-differentiated pancreatic neuroendocrine tumors (PanNETs) or solid pseudopapillary neoplasm (SPN). This was in line with the 2010 World Health Organization (WHO) classification that categorizes both PanNET and SPN as "neoplasms" rather than carcinomas.
- *Suspicious for malignancy*: A cytologic sample is labeled as suspicious for malignancy when some but an insufficient number of the typical features of a specific malignant neoplasm, generally adenocarcinoma, are present. The cytological features raise a strong suspicion of malignancy, but the findings

are qualitatively and/or quantitatively insufficient for a conclusive diagnosis, or tissue is not adequate for ancillary studies to confirm a specific diagnosis. This category is associated with a very high positive predictive value and ROM.

- *Positive/malignant*: This category includes samples that unequivocally demonstrate malignant cytologic features. It includes samples from pancreatic ductal adenocarcinoma (PDAC) and its variants, cholangiocarcinoma (CC), high-grade neuroendocrine carcinoma, acinar cell carcinoma, pancreatoblastoma (PBL), lymphomas, sarcomas, and other tumors metastatic to the pancreas.

The WHO Reporting System for Pancreaticobiliary Pathology

Recently, the WHO, the International Academy of Cytology, and the International Agency for Research on Cancer, with expert contributors from around the world, have developed an international approach for standardized reporting of PB cytopathology. The WHO Reporting System for Pancreaticobiliary Cytopathology revises and replaces the six-tiered PSC system with a seven-tiered system and reiterates clinicoradiologic correlation supplemented by ancillary tests including biochemical and molecular tests.[10]

The primary difference is related to the classification of PB tumors. The PSC system used a single category for neoplastic lesions that includes two groups, one for *"benign neoplasms"* and the *"other"*, which included premalignant intraductal neoplasms and low-grade malignant neoplasms, including IPMN, PanNETs, and SPN. In contrast, the WHO system categorizes benign neoplasms with almost no ROM in the *"benign"* category (category 2), and the low-grade malignancies including PanNET and SPN are included in the "malignant" category (category 7), in line with the new WHO Classification of Digestive System Tumours.[8-13] In the WHO system, the *"neoplasm"* category of the PSC system has been replaced by two categories of *"low-risk/low-grade"* and *"high-risk/high-grade"* pancreatic neoplasms. **Table 2** lists all the WHO system diagnostic categories along with the common lesions and their management recommendations.

The recommended diagnostic categories include:

- *Insufficient/Inadequate/ND*: A cytologic sample that qualitatively and/or quantitatively does not allow a diagnosis of the targeted lesion should be labeled by any of these three terms. In PB cytopathology, to date, there are no defined criteria to define adequate cellularity. Around 12% of EUS-FNA samples fall in this category.[14] Mostly, the solid lesions or duct strictures with acellular to paucicellular or nonrepresentative samples are included in this category. However, cystic lesions with acellular/paucicellular smears but diagnostic clinicoradiologic features should not be included in this category.[11] The presence of any cellular atypia in the sample precludes this categorization. The ROM for this category for pancreatic samples ranges from 5 to 25%. For biliary brushings, the ROM ranges from 28 to 69%.[11,13,15-17]

TABLE 2: The WHO system diagnostic categories along with the common lesions and their management recommendations.

Diagnostic category	Included entities	Estimated risk of malignancy (%)	Recommended management
Nondiagnostic	• Cellular artifact, obscuring hemorrhage, or necrosis • Pure gastrointestinal contamination • Nonmucinous cyst acellular aspirate • Benign pancreatic parenchyma (with a mass on imaging)	• 5–25%: Pancreas • 28–69%: Biliary brushings	Reassess/repeat
Benign/negative for malignancy	• Pancreatitis • Pseudocyst • Lymphoepithelial cyst • Accessory spleen • Benign pancreatic tissue (no mass) • Serous cystadenoma (SCA) • Lymphangioma • Cystic teratoma • Schwannoma	• 0–15%: Pancreas • 26–55%: Biliary brushings	Conservative with clinical correlation
Atypical	• Ductal cells with indeterminate atypia (reactive vs. low-grade dysplasia, vs. scant lesional tissue) • Abundant intracytoplasmic mucin in the epithelium	• 30–40%: Pancreas • 25–77%: Biliary brushings	Repeat/ conservative
Pancreaticobiliary neoplasm: low-risk/grade (PaN-low)	• IPMN with low and intermediate-grade dysplasia • IPNB with low and intermediate-grade dysplasia • MCN with low and intermediate-grade dysplasia	• 5–20%: Pancreas • NA: Biliary brushings	Conservative with clinical correlation
Pancreaticobiliary neoplasm: high-risk/grade (PaN-high)	• IPMN with high-grade dysplasia • IPNB with high-grade dysplasia • MCN with high-grade dysplasia	• 60–95%: Pancreas • NA: Biliary brushings	Surgery/ conservative in some cases

Continued

Continued

Diagnostic category	Included entities	Estimated risk of malignancy (%)	Recommended management
Suspicious for malignancy	Aspirates with cytologic features indicative of malignancy but qualitatively or quantitatively insufficient for an unequivocal diagnosis of malignancy	• 80–100%: Pancreas • 74–100%: Biliary brushings	Surgery/repeat sampling with ancillary studies
Positive for malignancy	• PDAC and variants • Cholangiocarcinoma • Acinar cell carcinoma • PanNET • Solid pseudopapillary neoplasm (SPN) • Small and large cell neuroendocrine carcinoma • Pancreatoblastoma • Lymphomas • Sarcomas • Metastases to the pancreas	• 99–100%: Pancreas • 96–100%: Biliary brushings	Surgery with/without chemotherapy according to the disease stage

(IPNB: intraductal papillary neoplasm of the bile duct; IPMN: intraductal papillary mucinous neoplasm; MCN: mucinous cystic neoplasm; PanNET: pancreatic neuroendocrine tumor; PDAC: pancreatic ductal adenocarcinoma)

- *Benign/negative for malignancy*: A sample is categorized as "benign/negative for malignancy" if it is adequate, representative, and displays unequivocal benign cytologic features (no cytologic atypia), which may/may not be diagnostic of a specific pathology. If a specific pathology can be identified, it should be added to the report. This category, in contrast to the PSC system, incorporates both non-neoplastic and neoplastic entities, including acute pancreatitis, chronic pancreatitis, cholangitis, autoimmune pancreatitis, pseudocyst, lymphoepithelial cyst, accessory spleen, SCA, lymphangioma, and schwannoma. The ROM for pancreatic lesions in this category ranges from 0 to 15% while it is much higher, around 55% for biliary brushings.[11,17,18]
- *Atypical*: A sample is categorized as "*atypical*" if it demonstrates predominantly benign cytomorphologic features but also exhibits some features that raise the possibility of malignancy; however, overall these are insufficient either qualitatively or quantitatively to diagnose a lesion as benign, premalignant, or malignant. For biliary brushings, the "*atypical*" category is applied to samples wherein the degree of atypia is beyond that seen with reactive and inflammatory changes but is still quantitatively and/or qualitatively insufficient for categorization as "*suspicious for malignancy*". Subsequent histopathology in this category may reveals benign, premalignant, or malignant diagnoses in these cases.[11,13,18,19] It is important to use this category judiciously and as less commonly as possible, as its indiscriminate use might

lead to patients being subjected to unnecessary additional investigations and procedures. Around 5.5% of the pancreatic cytologic samples are diagnosed as "atypical", the range being 0–14%.[11,20] This frequency is higher for biliary brushings, ranging from 11 to 40%.[17,21,22] The recommended management includes multidisciplinary discussion, expert and consensus review, repeat sampling with ROSE, and use of ancillary tests including fluorescence in situ hybridization (FISH) and other molecular studies.[11]

- *Pancreatic neoplasm: Low risk/low-grade (PaN-low)*: A sample is categorized as PaN-low if it demonstrates features of an intraductal and/or cystic neoplasm with low-grade atypia. The lesions included in this category include IPMN and MCN with low-grade atypia. Accurate grading of the epithelial atypia as low-risk/low-grade, which includes low- and intermediate-grade dysplasia, and distinguishing it from high-risk/high-grade atypia, is challenging requiring well-preserved epithelium and diagnostic experience.[11,23-25] These characteristic features are herein described along with the specific pancreatic cystic neoplasms. The recommended management includes surveillance.[26,27]
- *Pancreatic neoplasm: High risk/high-grade (PaN-high)*: A sample is categorized as PaN-high if it demonstrates features of an intraductal and/or cystic neoplasm with high-grade cytologic atypia. This category encompasses all intraductal and cystic PB lesions with high-grade atypia often including invasive carcinoma as these generally cannot be distinguished in aspirates. High-grade atypia is typically defined as a cell with high nuclear-to-cytoplasmic (N/C) ratio, nuclear membrane irregularity, abnormal chromatin distribution, and prominent nucleoli, with or without background necrosis.[23,28] PaN-high has a ROM of around 60–95%.[11,17,18] Primary management option for PaN-high is surgical resection. However, conservative observation may be opted in poor surgical candidates.[11]
- *Suspicious for malignancy*: A PB cytology sample is categorized as suspicious for malignancy when it demonstrates some cytologic features suggestive of malignancy but these are qualitatively or quantitatively insufficient for an unequivocal diagnosis of malignancy. It accounts for around 5–16% of all PB cytologic diagnoses.[11,21] Similar to the atypical category, the interobserver variability is high for this category, thereby attributing to the variable ROM (74–100%).[11,17,18,21,22] In these cases, the cytologic report should have a detailed mention of the suspicious as well as the compromising features with emphasis on clinicoradiologic correlation as a guide to further management.
- *Malignant*: A sample categorized as malignant when it demonstrates unequivocal cytologic features of malignancy. This category includes both primary and secondary malignancies (including well-differentiated PanNET and SPN), with PDAC and CC being the most common.[11] The ROM ranges from 97 to 100%.[11,17,18] Surgical resection is generally the first-line treatment for PB malignancies with or without neoadjuvant chemotherapy depending upon the extent of the disease. Chemoradiation is the recommended option for patients with unresectable disease.[29,30]

CYTOLOGY OF NORMAL PANCREATICOBILIARY TRACT

A complete knowledge of normal PB cytology is quintessential before attempting to diagnose the complex pathologies of this anatomical corridor. Pancreas is a mixed exocrine-endocrine gland having three anatomical parts, the head, body, and tail. Around 80–85% of the pancreas is exocrine, being composed of acini, ducts, and the supporting connective tissue with blood vessels. The endocrine part of the pancreas is composed mainly of the islets of Langerhans, which are mostly localized in the tail of the pancreas.

Fine-needle aspiration from the normal pancreas mainly show acinar cells with few scattered ductal epithelial cells, while the pancreatic and bile duct brushings mostly show sheets of ductal epithelial cells.[6]

CONTAMINANTS IN PANCREATICOBILIARY CYTOLOGY

Besides the normal cellular constituents, aspirates from the PB tract may show a variety of other cell types as *"contaminants"*. These may include mesothelial cells, benign hepatocytes, normal gastric or duodenal epithelium, renal, or stromal tissues.[31,32] Many of these cells are seen because of the needle traversing via and sampling the adjacent organs. Pathologists should be aware of the sampling approach, as the types of contaminant cells can vary depending on the method used.

CYTOLOGY OF NON-NEOPLASTIC SOLID PANCREATIC LESIONS

Non-neoplastic solid lesions that mimic pancreatic neoplasms are frequently identified incidentally. Common non-neoplastic lesions presenting as solid masses on imaging include acute, chronic and autoimmune pancreatitis, heterotopic spleen, sarcoidosis, and certain rare infections **(Table 3)**.[6,33,34] Accurate diagnosis in these cases can be obtained by a careful correlation of clinical, radiologic, and cytomorphologic features.

CYTOLOGY OF MALIGNANT SOLID PANCREATIC LESIONS

Pancreatic carcinomas are very aggressive malignancies associated with a high mortality rate. Most patients present with advanced disease with poor 5-year survival rates. Early diagnosis of the disease and prompt management can improve patient outcomes. Cytology plays an important role in the diagnosis of these pancreatic malignancies.

The most common pancreatic tumors are exocrine tumors, constituting >95% of tumors, of which PDAC is the most common (>90%).[35] Other malignant neoplasms of the pancreas are neuroendocrine tumors, SPN, acinar cell carcinoma, and PBL. The characteristic cytomorphologic features of various pancreatic malignancies are presented along with their immunochemical and key molecular features.

TABLE 3: Key cytomorphologic features of common non-neoplastic solid pancreatic lesions.

Non-neoplastic solid pancreatic lesions	Key cytomorphologic features
Acute pancreatitis	• Variable numbers of acute inflammatory cells • Fat necrosis • Granular necrotic debris • Pancreatic acinar and ductal cells with moderate reactive cytologic atypia
Chronic pancreatitis	• Low cellularity (mainly due to fibrosis) • Cohesive sheets of ductal epithelial cells with focal crowding • Ductal epithelial cells show mild nuclear enlargement; however, the nuclear-to-cytoplasmic (N/C) ratio remains low • Round nuclei with smooth nuclear membranes • Variably conspicuous nucleoli • Fibroinflammatory tissue fragments • Background shows stromal cells, lymphocytes, and calcific debris • Cell block sections can reveal typical periductal fibrosis and inflammation
Autoimmune pancreatitis	• Variable cellularity • Ductal cells showing mild cytologic atypia, nuclear crowding, high N/C ratio, and irregular nuclear membranes • Scattered fibroinflammatory fragments • Background shows lymphoplasmacytic infiltrate with an increased immunoglobulin G4 (IgG4)/IgG positive plasma cells
Intrapancreatic accessory spleen	• Polymorphous population of lymphocytes admixed with eosinophils, macrophages, plasmacytoid cells, neutrophils, and hemosiderin-laden macrophages • Scattered endothelial cells and small vascular fragments • Multiple platelet aggregates • No tingible body macrophages
Intrapancreatic reactive lymph node	• Polymorphous population of lymphocytes • Scattered tingible body macrophages • Background shows numerous lymphoglandular bodies
Sarcoidosis	• Compact epithelioid cell granulomas • No/minimal necrosis • Scattered multinucleate giant cells

Pancreatic Ductal Adenocarcinoma and its Variants

Pancreatic ductal adenocarcinoma is the most common neoplasm of the pancreas, comprising around 90% of all pancreatic malignancies.[36] Although radiology plays an important role in assessment of pancreatic masses, a reliable diagnosis of PDAC mandates radiology in conjunction with EUS-FNA.[37,38]

The WHO reporting system for PB cytopathology has refined the diagnostic criteria for these tumors.[11] The classical cytomorphologic features of PDAC are presented here.

Key Cytomorphologic Features[39]

- *Well-differentiated PDAC*:
  - Variable cellularity
  - Cohesive clusters of ductal epithelial cells
  - Crowding and overlapping in the cell clusters *"drunken honeycomb"* appearance
  - Moderate anisonucleosis with at least fourfold variation in the nuclear size
  - Enlarged nuclei with high N/C ratio, irregular nuclear membranes, chromatin clearing, and moderate amount of mucinous cytoplasm
  - Background is often clean or hemorrhagic
- *High-grade PDAC*:
  - Cellular smears
  - Singly dispersed tumor cells or loosely cohesive clusters with nuclear crowding or overlapping
  - Marked anisonucleosis
  - Large cells with high N/C ratio, irregular nuclei, coarse chromatin, prominent nucleoli, and moderate cytoplasm with cytoplasmic vacuolations
  - Multiple mitotic figures
  - Dirty necrotic background

Common Cytologic Mimics

- Chronic pancreatitis
- Lymphoplasmacytic sclerosing pancreatitis
- PBL
- Acinar cell carcinoma
- Islet cell hyperplasia

Special Stains and Immunocytochemistry

- Mucicarmine highlights the intracytoplasmic mucin
- The tumor cells are positive for epithelial markers including EMA, CA-19-9, CK7, CK8, CK18, CK19, and CK20 (patchy)
- Positive for mucin proteins including MUC1, MUC3, MUC4, and MUC5AC
- Tumor cells may show loss of SMAD4 or mutant-type p53 immunoexpression
- These are negative for vimentin and show retained E-cadherin expression

Molecular Genetics

- Both the well-differentiated and high-grade PDCA share a similar molecular profile
- Most cases demonstrate mutations in *KRAS* (90%), *TP53* (50%), *SMAD4* (55%), and *CDKN2A*

TABLE. 4: Grading of the pancreatic neuroendocrine tumors.

Pancreatic neuroendocrine tumor	Mitotic count	Ki-67 labeling index
Grade 1	<2 per 10 high-power field (HPF)	<2%
Grade 2	2–20 per 10 HPF	3–20%
Grade 3	>20 per 10 HPF	>20%

Pancreatic Neuroendocrine Tumors

Pancreatic neuroendocrine neoplasia (PNEN) includes both well-differentiated PanNETs and poorly differentiated pancreatic neuroendocrine carcinomas (PanNECs). The distinction is important due to significant prognostic and therapeutic differences. PanNETs are much more common and follow a less aggressive course than the rare PanNECs. Based on the Ki-67 index assessed on cell bock sections, PanNETs can be divided into three grades: G1, G2, and G3, using cytologic aspirates **(Table 4).**[40]

Clinical Features

Clinically, a majority of PanNETs are incidentally detected and nonfunctioning tumors. Among the functioning ones, insulinomas and gastrinomas are the most common.[41,42]

Radiologic Features

Radiologically, these are seen as hypervascular and hyperenhancing masses.[43]

Gross Pathology

Grossly, PanNETs are generally solid, well-circumscribed masses, common in the body and tail of pancreas; however, larger lesions may present as cystic masses.[41]

Key Cytomorphologic Features[41,44-46]

- Cellular smears
- Predominantly dispersed tumor cells with some pseudorosettes
- Tumor cells are relatively monomorphic, round to polygonal in shape; rarely spindle morphology may also be seen.
- Nuclei are round, may be central or eccentrically placed with smooth nuclear borders, "*salt and pepper*" chromatin, inconspicuous nucleoli, and moderate amount of finely granular cytoplasm with occasional vacuoles.
- Scattered binucleate and occasional bizarre (endocrine atypia) tumor cells
- Higher mitotic activity and background necrosis common in higher grade tumors
- PanNECs show cellular smears with dyscohesive tumor cells having high N/C ratio, round nuclei, stippled chromatin, inconspicuous nucleoli, and scant cytoplasm. Nuclear threading and crushing are common. Mitosis is brisk and the background shows numerous apoptotic bodies.

Common Cytologic Mimics

- Pancreatic acinar cell carcinoma (PACC)
- Chronic pancreatitis with islet cell hyperplasia

Immunocytochemistry[47]

- The tumor cells in PanNETs are positive for neuroendocrine markers including chromogranin, synaptophysin, INSM1, and CD56.
- PanNETs may show focal positivity for CD10 and progesterone receptors in some cases.
- PanNECs may lack positivity for chromogranin and may show aberrant p53 expression.

Molecular Genetics

- Various genetic alterations noted in PanNETs include mutations in *MEN1*, *ATRX* (α-thalassemia/intellectual X-linked disability syndrome), *DAXX* (death domain associated), *mTOR* (mammalian target of rapamycin), *PTEN* (phosphatase and tensin homolog), *PIK3CA* (phosphatidylinositol-4,5-bisphosphate 3-kinase catalytic subunit alpha), and *TSC2* (tuberous sclerosis complex 2) genes.[48]
- PanNECs are generally associated with mutations in *TP53* and *RB* genes.[49]

Pancreatic Acinar Cell Carcinoma

These are rare pancreatic malignancies that account for around 1–2% of all adult pancreatic tumors.

Clinical Features

They commonly involve the head of the pancreas in elderly males, however, also be seen in children and alone account for around 15% of the pediatric pancreatic tumors.[10,40,50] Although the tumor is associated with frequent distant metastasis; the 5-year survival rates are better than PDAC.

Radiologic Features

Radiologically, PACC presents as a large predominantly solid tumor in the head of the pancreas.[43]

Gross Pathology

Grossly, PACCs are seen as large, well-circumscribed tumors with areas of necrosis and cystic degeneration.[10,50,51]

Key Cytomorphologic Features[52-54]

- Cellular aspirate
- Predominantly dispersed tumor cells, scattered loose acini-like clusters, and few large aggregates of tumor cells with transgressing capillary channels
- Granulovacuolar background, with many naked nuclei

- Tumor cells are round to polygonal with variably pleomorphic, round nuclei, smooth nuclear membrane, coarse chromatin, conspicuous nucleoli, and moderate amount of granulovacuolar cytoplasm.
- Increased mitotic activity and necrosis may be seen in poorly differentiated tumors.

Common Cytologic Mimics[51]

- Benign pancreatic acini
- Pancreatic mixed acinar carcinomas (>30% of each cellular component): Mixed acinar-neuroendocrine carcinoma (MANEC), mixed acinar-ductal carcinoma, and mixed acinar-neuroendocrine-ductal carcinoma

Immunocytochemistry[52,55]

- Tumor cells are positive for markers of acinar differentiation: trypsin, chymotrypsin, Bcl-10, and carboxypeptidase A1.
- These show variable positivity for β-catenin, lipase, and amylase.
- Synaptophysin and chromogranin are generally negative.

Molecular Genetics[54]

- Around 50% PACCs demonstrate loss of chromosome 11p.
- Germline pathogenic variants in homologous recombination or deoxyribonucleic acid (DNA) damage-response genes have been noted in around 50% cases.
- Around 20% of these cases exhibit mutations in *BRCA1/2* genes and the APC/β-catenin pathway.
- *KRAS*, *TP53,* and *CDKN2A* mutations are generally not seen in PACC.

Pancreatoblastoma

Clinical Features

Pancreatoblastoma (PBL), although extremely rare, is the most common malignant pediatric pancreatic tumor in children <10 years of age. Adult PBLs are very rare. Unlike PDAC, the 5-year survival rates are higher (50%) in PBL.[10]

Radiologic Features

Radiologically, PBLs present as large, well-circumscribed heterogeneous masses with internal septations and peripheral calcification.[43]

Gross Pathology

Grossly, PBLs are seen as large, well circumscribed but lobulated masses, with areas of necrosis.

Key Cytomorphologic Features[56,57]

- Highly cellular aspirate
- Tumor cells arranged in large loosely cohesive aggregates, solid sheets, and singly dispersed.
- The smears may show both epithelial and mesenchymal components.

- Epithelial tumor cells commonly show acinar differentiation but can also show ductal or neuroendocrine differentiation.
- The presence of squamoid nests, with or without keratinization, is a characteristic feature of PBL and can be best appreciated on cell block sections.
- The mesenchymal component is seen as hypercellular stromal fragments composed of pleomorphic spindle cells.

Common Cytologic Mimics

- Wilms tumor
- Hepatoblastoma
- Neuroblastoma

Immunocytochemistry

- The acinar tumor cells show positivity for trypsin, chymotrypsin, and lipase.
- The neuroendocrine tumor cells show positivity for chromogranin and synaptophysin.
- The squamoid nests show nuclear expression of β-catenin.

Molecular Genetics[51]

- Loss of chromosome 11p is the most common genetic abnormality in PBL.
- Somatic mutations in the APC/β-catenin pathway can also be seen in >50% PBLs.
- *KRAS*, *TP53*, and *CDKN2A/p16* mutations are not seen in PBL.

Solid Pseudopapillary Neoplasms

Clinical Features

Solid pseudopapillary neoplasm is a rare, often incidentally detected malignant tumor, occurring in adolescent and middle-aged women.[58,59]

Radiologic Features

Radiologically, these are seen as well circumscribed, solid-cystic lesions with calcification and internal septations.[43]

Gross Pathology

Solid pseudopapillary neoplasm is seen as a solitary, well-circumscribed solid or solid-cystic lesion in the body and tail of the pancreas.

Key Cytomorphologic Features[60]

- Variable cellularity (depending upon the area sampled)
- Predominantly singly scattered tumor cells with many pseudopapillary structures composed of a central hyalinized capillary, surrounded by tumor cells
- The tumor cells are round to polygonal with mild nuclear pleomorphism, round to indented nuclei, bland granular chromatin, indistinct nucleoli, and longitudinal nuclear grooves.

- Cytoplasm is clear to eosinophilic with vacuolations.
- The background may show hyaline globules, foamy macrophages, cholesterol crystals, and necrotic debris.

Common Cytologic Mimics

- Pancreatic NETs
- PACC
- PBL
- IPMN

Special Stains and Immunocytochemistry[61]

- Periodic acid–Schiff (PAS)-positive hyaline globules are often noted in the background.
- The tumor cells characteristically demonstrate diffuse nuclear staining with β-catenin and strong and lymphoid enhancer-binding factor 1 (LEF1).
- Tumor cells show diffuse positivity for CD10 and progesterone receptors.
- There is loss of E-cadherin expression.
- SPNs may show focal and weak positivity for CK, CD56, and synaptophysin.

Molecular Genetics[51]

- Activating mutations in the *CTNNB1*/β-*catenin* gene are seen in almost all the cases.
- Occasional cases associated with germline *APC* mutations.
- *KRAS*, *TP53*, *SMAD4*, and *CDKN2A/p16* mutations are not seen in SPNs.

CYTOLOGY OF CYSTIC PANCREATIC LESIONS

Pancreatic cystic lesions encompass a wide variety of entities including both non-neoplastic and neoplastic lesions **(Table 5)**.[6] Cytologic assessment along with biochemical analysis of the cyst fluid often plays a pivotal role in the preoperative characterization of these lesions.[6]

TABLE 5: Various cystic lesions seen in the pancreas.

Non-neoplastic cystic lesions	Neoplastic cystic lesions
Pseudocyst	Serous cystadenoma
Lymphoepithelial cyst	Intraductal papillary mucinous neoplasm
Dermoid cyst	Mucinous cystic neoplasm
Squamoid cyst of the pancreatic ducts	Solid pseudopapillary neoplasm with cystic degeneration
Retention cyst	Pancreatic neuroendocrine tumor with cystic degeneration
Enterogenous duplication cyst	Pancreatic ductal adenocarcinoma with cystic degeneration
Acinar cell cystadenoma (cystic acinar transformation)	Pancreatic acinar cell carcinoma with cystic degeneration

CYTOLOGY OF NEOPLASTIC CYSTIC PANCREATIC LESIONS

Recently, major advancements have been made in the understanding of neoplastic cystic lesions of the pancreas. Following the development of PSC and the WHO reporting systems for standardized terminologies, estimated ROM, and management recommendations, multiple validation studies have been performed leading to refinement of the diagnostic criteria for cystic pancreatic neoplasms.[8,9,11,12]

The most common neoplastic cystic pancreatic lesions include SCAs, IPMNs, and MCNs. Other neoplastic cystic pancreatic lesions have been listed in **Table 5**. The characteristic cytomorphologic, immunocytochemical, and molecular genetic features of the common lesions are presented here.

Serous Cystadenoma

Serous cystadenomas are one of the most common benign cystic neoplasms of the pancreas, commonly occurring in body and tail of the pancreas, in elderly women. SCA follows a benign clinical course, with negligible risk of malignant transformation.

Clinical Features

- Most cases are asymptomatic and discovered incidentally.
- Symptomatic patients may present with abdominal pain, palpable mass, nausea, vomiting, and weight loss.

Radiologic Features[62]

- SCAs may have a multicystic or lobulated contour with or without septations.
- Location in the pancreatic head, lobulated contours, and lack of wall enhancement favor a SCA.
- These may be microcystic, macrocystic, oligocystic (2 cm in diameter), mixed, or solid type.
- The macrocystic SCAs are difficult to distinguish from MCNs and branch duct (BD)-IPMNs. The mixed micro- and macrocystic SCAs show combination of features of both microcystic and macrocystic types. The solid SCAs show small cysts separated by multiple, thick fibrous septa.

Key Cytologic Features[63]

- Paucicellular aspirate
- Few sheets of cuboidal tumor cells with round, regular nuclei with fine chromatin, moderate to abundant amount of clear to granular, and non-mucinous cytoplasm may be seen.
- The background is generally hemorrhagic and may show hemosiderin-laden macrophages.

Common Cytologic Mimics[63]

- Cystic PanNET
- Pancreatic pseudocyst
- Neoplastic mucinous cysts (aspirates with contaminating GI epithelium and mucin)[6,7]

Special Stains and Immunocytochemistry

- PAS and PAS/diastase stains can help highlight the glycogen present in SCA cells.
- ICC for inhibin can help in diagnosis.[64]

Cyst Fluid Biochemistry

- SCAs typically have low cyst fluid CEA (<5 ng/mL) and amylase (<250 IU/L) levels.[65]

Molecular Genetics

- Mutations in the *VHL* gene has been identified in around 65% of SCAs.[66]

Intraductal Papillary Mucinous Neoplasm

Intraductal papillary mucinous neoplasms are premalignant lesions, commonly detected incidentally in elderly males.[67,68]

Clinical Features

- Most IPMNs are asymptomatic; however, some may present with abdominal pain, weight loss, and jaundice.
- Around one-third of these cases may be associated with diabetes mellitus.[69]

Radiologic Features[70,71]

- Upper GI endoscopy may demonstrate a *"fish mouth"* papilla extruding mucin, which is a characteristic finding in an IPMN with main duct involvement.
- IPMNs can be BD-IPMN with cystic dilatation of one or more BDs, or *main duct IPMN* (MD-IPMN) with main duct involvement only and *combined-type IPMN* with involvement of both the main duct and the BDs.
- Radiologically, MD-IPMNs show segmental or diffuse dilation of the main duct >5 mm without any other obstruction cause. BD-IPMNs are seen as cysts >5 mm in size, mostly in the uncinate process, without dilation of main duct but have a communication with it. Some may show thick enhancing wall, septae, and mural nodules. Combined-type IPMNs show features of both MD-IPMN and BD-IPMN.

Gross Pathology

- IPMNs are characterized by a grossly visible (≥1 cm) lesion in the main pancreatic duct and/or the BDs.
- MD-IPMNs show diffuse or segmental dilatation of the main duct. BD-IPMNs are seen as multicystic grape-like structures.
- IPMNs associated with an invasive carcinoma may show irregular thick cyst walls, mural nodules, or gelatinous stromal masses. In all cases, extensive gross sampling is essential to exclude an invasive component.[35]

Key Cytologic Features[28,72-74]

The main role of the cytologic examination in these cases is to assess the degree of the epithelial atypia.

- Variably cellular smears

- Thick extracellular mucin; diagnostic characteristic of a neoplastic mucinous cyst, irrespective of the presence/absence of mucinous epithelium. This may be difficult to discern in liquid-based cytologic preparations.
- Papillae, micropapillae, or sheets of variably pleomorphic cuboidal to columnar mucinous epithelial cells.
- Scattered degenerated epithelial cells within the mucin
- The lining epithelium may exhibit varying degrees of dysplasia and the cytology sample may not be representative of the severity of dysplasia in the lesion. The concept of cytology as a predictor of the grade of dysplasia and/or invasive carcinoma for pancreatic mucinous neoplasms has developed over time.
- *Low-grade epithelial atypia* on cytology includes both low-grade and intermediate-grade dysplasia cases. It is seen as mucinous cells with low nuclear-cytoplasmic ratio, fine nuclear chromatin, and inconspicuous nucleoli. Contaminant gastric foveolar epithelium is a close mimicker; presence of intranuclear pseudoinclusions favors neoplastic epithelium in such cases.[75]
- *High-grade epithelial atypia* includes cases with high-grade dysplasia and is seen as cohesive clusters or scattered epithelial cells with high N/C ratio, coarse chromatin, and irregular nuclear membranes. Necrotic background is also a diagnostic clue.[23]

Immunocytochemistry

Aberrant p53 and loss of p16, and SMAD4 expression are common in high-grade IPMNs and associated invasive carcinoma.

Cyst Fluid Biochemistry

Carcinoembryonic antigen is the most common cyst fluid marker to differentiate between mucinous and nonmucinous cysts. A CEA cutoff value of 109.9 ng/mL has high accuracy for the diagnosis of a mucinous cyst with a specificity of 98%; however, it cannot differentiate an IPMN from a MCN.[76,77]

Molecular Genetics[66,78,79]

- Somatic mutations of *KRAS, GNAS,* and *RNF43* genes are seen in 30–80% IPMNs.
- A combination of *KRAS* and *GNAS* mutation testing is highly sensitive for diagnosing IPMNs.
- *TP53, BRAF,* and *CDKN2A* mutations are common in cases with high-grade dysplasia.
- *SMAD4* mutations are seen in IPMNs with an invasive carcinoma.

Mucinous Cystic Neoplasm

Mucinous cystic neoplasm is an uncommon tumor of the pancreas, almost exclusively occurring in middle-aged females. It is characterized by the presence of subepithelial ovarian-type stroma. Although most of these tumors are benign, they are considered premalignant as they have a predilection to develop dysplasia and invasive carcinoma.[80]

Clinical Features

- Most cases are asymptomatic and detected incidentally on imaging.
- Some patients may present with abdominal pain, abdominal mass, pancreatitis, or weight loss.

Radiologic Features

- Majority of MCNs are located in the body or tail of the pancreas.[81]
- Radiologically, they appear as smooth-contoured macrocystic lesions without any communication with the main pancreatic duct.[82]
- The presence of large size, thick wall, septation, and mural nodules or calcifications indicate a high-grade lesion or an associated malignancy.[83]

Key Cytologic Features

Mucinous cystic neoplasms and IPMNs cannot be distinguished reliably based on cytologic features alone as the subepithelial ovarian-type stroma, a diagnostic prerequisite for MCN, is not readily identifiable on smears.[6,9] However, the useful cytologic features of MCNs include:

- Paucicellular aspirates
- Abundant thick extracellular mucin with or without neoplastic mucinous epithelium
- The epithelial cells can display variable nuclear pleomorphism.
- The cytologic criteria for low and high-grade epithelial atypia are same as for IPMNs.
- Background necrosis and cellular debris are common in high-grade cases, while macrophages are more commonly seen in low-grade cases.
- Cell block sections may demonstrate the characteristic subepithelial ovarian-type stroma.

Immunocytochemistry[84]

- The neoplastic epithelial cells in MCN are positive for MUC5AC and negative for MUC1. MUC2 expression is seen only in interspersed goblet cells.[85]
- The stromal cells typically show positivity for estrogen and progesterone receptors; the luteinized cells are positive for inhibin, and calretinin.
- Aberrant p53 and loss of SMAD4 expression is noted in cases with high-grade dysplasia and invasive carcinoma.

Cyst Fluid Biochemistry

- CEA levels in MCNs are high, similar to IPMNs.
- Amylase levels are variable in MCNs; not useful in differentiation from IPMNs.[77]

Molecular Genetics[86,87]

- Mutations in *KRAS* gene have been identified as an early event in MCNs.
- Mutations in *RNF43, TP53, SMAD4, PIK3CA,* and *CDKN2A* are common in MCNs with high-grade dysplasia or associated invasive carcinomas.
- Typically, *GNAS* mutations are not common in MCNs, unlike IPMNs.[78]

ANCILLARY TECHNIQUES IN PANCREATICOBILIARY TRACT CYTOLOGY

A variety of ancillary techniques, including immunocytochemistry, cyst fluid analysis, ploidy analysis, and molecular tests can be performed on the PB cytology samples to supplement and/or confirm the cytomorphologic diagnoses.

Special Stains

These can be performed on direct smears, sediment smears, liquid-based preparations, as well as cell block sections.

- Histochemical stains for mucin can be used for demonstration of the intracellular mucin as well as the extracellular mucin in various PB cytologic aspirates. The most commonly used ones include alcian blue, mucicarmine, and PAS. These highlight the intracellular mucin in IPMNs and MCNs.
- PAS stain can be used to highlight the glycogen present in the epithelial cells in SCAs.

Cyst Fluid Analysis

In context of the cystic lesions of pancreas, the cyst fluid constitutes a vital resource and can be used for performing multiple analyses.[88]

- *Visual inspection*: This is an indispensable method for differentiating mucinous from nonmucinous cysts. Thick, viscid fluid, and difficult to expel from the needle indicates the presence of mucin. A *"string"* test can be performed by placing the fluid between the thumb and index finger and gently pulling apart, formation of a "string" longer than of 3.5 mm indicates mucin. Although not diagnostic on its own, a combination of string sign, cyst fluid biochemistry, and cytomorphology is highly reliable in distinguishing mucinous from nonmucinous cysts.[89]
- *Cyst fluid biochemistry:* Biochemical testing is one of the most accurate methods to distinguish between pancreatic mucinous and nonmucinous cysts.[90] Various biochemical parameters that can be analyzed include:
    - Cyst fluid amylase: Amylase activity is elevated in IPMNs, and markedly elevated in pseudocysts. Colorimetric assays can be used for the assessment. Amylase activity may also be elevated in MCNs and hence is not useful in distinguishing IPMN from MCN.
    - Cyst fluid CEA: CEA is a highly reliable marker for mucinous differentiation with high sensitivity and specificity.[91,92] However, these levels cannot be reliably used to diagnose dysplasia or malignancy. Major limitation is the availability of sufficient cyst fluid (0.2–1 mL) for analysis, which is often not possible, especially in very small cysts or those with very viscous fluid.[6]
    - Cyst fluid mucin expression patterns: MUC1 is expressed in normal pancreatic ductal epithelium. MUC5AC is expressed in MCNs. MUC2 is expressed in lesions with intestinal differentiation.

- Other biochemical markers: Biochemical testing for many other markers including, CA-19-9, lipase, pancreatitis-associated protein, CA-72-4, CA-15-3, granulocyte-macrophage colony-stimulating factor, hepatocyte growth factor, vascular endothelial growth factor, interleukin (IL)-1β, IL-5, IL-8, prostaglandin E2, Brg1, and glucose, can also be performed in cyst fluids.[6]

- *Cyst fluid genetic sequencing*: Next-generation sequencing (NGS) can successfully be used for genetic sequencing of cyst fluids to ascertain the nature of the pancreatic cystic neoplasms. The presence of *KRAS* mutation ascertains mucinous nature independent of cytomorphology and CEA level. Testing for *GNAS* and *KRAS* mutations in pancreatic cyst fluid is useful for accurately diagnosing IPMN. Such testing, in combination with cytomorphology, and cyst fluid biochemistry can aid in reliable characterization of cystic pancreatic lesions. It has been seen that it is easier to obtain sufficient fluid for genetic testing than for biochemical testing or cytomorphologic analysis.[93,94]
- *Cyst fluid microRNA analysis:* Differences in microRNA expression in pancreatic cyst fluid samples may aid in predicting high-grade cystic neoplasms, especially as an adjunct to other diagnostic procedures, from patients with cysts.[95]
- *Cyst fluid telomerase activity*: A higher telomerase activity in pancreatic cyst fluid samples can help predict cystic neoplasms with high-grade dysplasia, in combination with other tests.[96]
- *Cyst fluid DNA methylation profiling*: Methylation of specific genes, evaluated using methylation-specific droplet digital polymerase chain reaction (ddPCR), can help in accurately identifying high-grade cystic neoplasms. Among these, methylation of SOX17 has been noted to be the most accurate single marker.[97]

Immunocytochemistry

Immunocytochemistry serves as a vital complementary tool to further characterize the PB cytologic specimens. It not only helps in diagnosis of the specific lesions but also plays a significant role in prognostication and therapeutic decision making. **Table 6** lists the specific immunocytochemical panels can be used to diagnose various PB neoplasms.[98]

Deoxyribonucleic Acid Ploidy Analysis

Quantifying nuclear DNA can help identify malignant biliary tract lesions, using methods including DNA flow cytometry and digital image analysis.[99] By staining the tumor cells with Feulgen dye and measuring optical density at specific wavelengths, one can assess nucleic acid levels, which is especially useful for specimens with limited cellularity. The results indicate whether cells are diploid, aneuploid, or tetraploid; with aneuploidy and tetraploidy favoring malignancy. While DNA quantification alone shows variable accuracy for

TABLE 6: Specific immunocytochemical panels used to diagnose various pancreaticobiliary neoplasms.

Pancreatic tumor	Immunocytochemistry
Pancreatic ductal adenocarcinoma (PDAC)	• Positive for CK7, CK20, CK19, CK8, CK18, pVHL, maspin, S100, and IMP3 • Loss of SMAD4 and p16 expression • Aberrant p53 and mesothelin overexpression
Pancreatic neuroendocrine tumor (PanNET)	• Positive for chromogranin, synaptophysin, CD56, CD57, insulinoma-associated protein 1 (INSM1), and neuron-specific enolase • Also express CK8, CK18, and CA 19-9 with retained E-cadherin expression • Ki-67 is used for grading
Pancreatic neuroendocrine carcinoma (PanNEC)	• Positive for synaptophysin, CD56, CD57, insulinoma-associated protein 1 (INSM1), and neuron-specific enolase • Also, express CK8, CK18, and CA-19-9 with retained E-cadherin expression • Absent to patchy chromogranin positivity
Pancreatic acinar cell carcinoma (PACC)	Positive for amylase, lipase, trypsin, and chymotrypsin; also express BCL-10, claudin-7, and p120
Pancreatoblastoma (PBL)	• Positive for panCK • Acinar cells are positive for trypsin, chymotrypsin, BCL10, and lipase • Ductal cells are positive for CEA, CK7, and CK19 • Neuroendocrine cells are positive for synaptophysin, chromogranin, INSM1, and CD56
Solid pseudopapillary neoplasm (SPN)	• Strong, diffuse nuclear positivity for β-catenin • Positive for vimentin, α-1-antitrypsin (hyaline globules), synaptophysin, CD56, CD10, progesterone receptor, and lymphoid enhancer-binding factor 1 (LEF-1) • Show paranuclear, dot-like positivity with CD99
Intrahepatic cholangiocarcinoma (iCCA)	• Positive for CK7, CK19, CK17, MOC31, EMA, claudin4, and pVHL • Negative for CK20, ER, PR, GATA3, HepPar1, and glypican 3
Extrahepatic cholangiocarcinoma	• Positive for CK7, CK19, CK20, MOC31, EMA, claudin4, MUC1, MUC5AC, and CA 19-9 • Negative for ER, PR, GATA3, HepPar1, and glypican 3

detecting malignancy in PB cytologic samples, combining it with traditional cytomorphologic techniques improves the diagnostic accuracy.

Fluorescence in Situ Hybridization

Fluorescence in situ hybridization is a promising adjunct in improving the sensitivity of cytomorphology for diagnosing malignancy in PB samples including biliary washings, brushings, and EUS-FNAs. The UroVysion probe set (Abbott Molecular Inc., Des Plaines, IL), which consists of a specific probe for the *CDKN2A* locus on chromosome 9p21, as well as centromeric enumeration

TABLE 7: Common genetic alterations noted in various pancreaticobiliary neoplasms.

Pancreatic tumor	Common genetic alterations
Pancreatic ductal adenocarcinoma (PDAC)	• Somatic: *KRAS*, *TP53*, *SMAD4*, *CDKN2A*, and *GNAS* • Germline: *BRCA1*, *BRCA2*, *ATM*, and *PALB2*
Pancreatic neuroendocrine tumor (PanNET)	*MEN1*, *VHL*, *ATRX*, *DAXX*, and *PHLDA3*. Less commonly, *PIK3CA*, *PTEN*, or *TSC2*
Pancreatic neuroendocrine carcinoma (PanNEC)	Loss-of-function mutations in *TP53* and *RB1*
Pancreatic acinar cell carcinoma (PACC)	Loss of chromosome 11p, microsatellite instability (10%)
Pancreatoblastoma (PBL)	Loss of chromosome 11p, alterations in *CTNNB1*, *APC*, and *BRAF*
Solid pseudopapillary neoplasm (SPN)	Gain of function mutations in *CTNNB1*
Intrahepatic cholangiocarcinoma (iCCA)	Mutations in *IDH1*, *IDH2*, *FGFR2*, *PBRM1*, *BAP1*, *CDKN2A*, *KRAS*, *BRAF*, *or EGFR* genes

probes (CEPs) for chromosomes 3, 7, and 17, is commonly used for PB samples. The presence of polysomy, defined as the presence of more than two signals in at least two of the three CEPs, and 9p21 loss constitute reliable indicators of malignancy in PB cytology.[100]

Sanger Sequencing

Sanger sequencing can be used for evaluating various oncogenes including KRAS, GNAS, IDH1, and IDH2 oncogenes in PB cytology samples. However, NGS is preferred, since it can detect mutations at a lower allele frequency and can also be used for multiple gene sequencing.

Next-generation Sequencing

Next-generation sequencing can be used for diagnostic, prognostic, and predictive purposes in PB tumors, primarily for their genetic profiling. Depending on the needs, either a limited or extended gene panel can be selected, with considerations for both sequencing depth and breadth. Greater sequencing depth can detect copy number changes as well as mutations, which is especially useful for samples with low cellularity. Furthermore, detection of specific genetic alterations by sequencing can help in accurately diagnosing various PB neoplasms, especially in cases with indeterminate cytomorphology and ICC. **Table 7** lists the common genetic alterations found in various PB tumors.[22]

MicroRNA Profiling

MicroRNA profiling is a novel method for identifying malignancy in PB cytology samples. Extracellular vesicles, found in biologic fluids like bile, play a key role in cell communication and are rich in microRNA and long noncoding RNA, can be used for microRNA profiling. Specific microRNA profiles can be used as promising diagnostic markers for pancreatic tumors.[101] Quantification through allele-specific real-time polymerase chain reaction allows detection of differential microRNA expression between benign and malignant tissues.

DNA Methylation Profiling

Aberrant DNA methylation can be used to detect the presence of high-grade dysplasia and invasive carcinoma in PB cytology samples. Methylation of *TFPI2*, *NPTX2*, and *CCND2* can help distinguish benign from malignant lesions, especially in biliary and pancreatic brushings.[102]

Pancreatic Juice and Bile Analysis

Both bile and pancreatic juice can also serve as useful samples for performing various analyses for early detection of malignancy.[103] Molecular testing for various mutations can also be performed using these samples. Mass spectrometry-based proteomic studies can also be performed on bile for a variety of biomarkers including, acrylonitrile, insulin-like growth factor-1, carcinoembryonic cell adhesion molecule-6, and other proteins.

CONCLUSION

Cytology plays a pivotal role in the diagnosis of pancreaticobiliary lesions, with its accuracy significantly enhanced when combined with clinical and radiologic findings. The adoption of standardized reporting nomenclature has improved the clarity of pathologic interpretations, fostering better communication between pathologists and clinicians, and ultimately improving patient management. The use of various ancillary techniques including advanced molecular tests on the cytologic samples has further enhanced the efficacy of this minimally-invasive diagnostic tool. Molecular testing on the pancreaticobiliary cytology samples not only allows for precise diagnosis, but also allows prognostication and aids in therapeutic decision-making. Nonetheless, it is important to be aware of the limitations of pancreaticobiliary cytology, including the potential for false negatives and challenges in diagnosing certain benign conditions.

REFERENCES

1. Rösch T, Hofrichter K, Frimberger E, Meining A, Born P, Weigert N, et al. ERCP or EUS for tissue diagnosis of biliary strictures? A prospective comparative study. Gastrointest Endosc. 2004;60:390-6.
2. Moff SL, Clark DP, Maitra A, Pandey A, Thuluvath PJ. Utility of bile duct brushings for the early detection of cholangiocarcinoma in patients with primary sclerosing cholangitis. J Clin Gastroenterol. 2006;40:336-41.
3. Gress FG, Hawes RH, Savides TJ, Ikenberry SO, Cummings O, Kopecky K, et al. Role of EUS in the preoperative staging of pancreatic cancer: a large single-center experience. Gastrointest Endosc. 1999;50:786-91.
4. Horwhat JD, Paulson EK, McGrath K, Branch MS, Baillie J, Tyler D, et al. A randomized comparison of EUS-guided FNA versus CT or US-guided FNA for the evaluation of pancreatic mass lesions. Gastrointest Endosc. 2006;63:966-75.
5. Banafea O, Mghanga FP, Zhao J, Zhao R, Zhu L. Endoscopic ultrasonography with fine-needle aspiration for histological diagnosis of solid pancreatic masses: a meta-analysis of diagnostic accuracy studies. BMC Gastroenterol. 2016;16(1):108.
6. Goyal A, Siddiqui MT, Rao R. Pancreas and Biliary Tract Cytohistology. Germany: Springer International Publishing; 2019.

7. Hébert-Magee S, Bae S, Varadarajulu S, Ramesh J, Frost AR, Eloubeidi MA, et al. The presence of a cytopathologist increases the diagnostic accuracy of endoscopic ultrasound-guided fine needle aspiration cytology for pancreatic adenocarcinoma: a meta-analysis. Cytopathology. 2013;24(3):159-71.
8. Pitman MB, Centeno BA, Ali SZ, Genevay M, Stelow E, Mino-Kenudson M, et al. Standardized terminology and nomenclature for pancreatobiliary cytology: the Papanicolaou Society of Cytopathology guidelines. Diagn Cytopathol. 2014;42:338-50.
9. Pitman MB, Layfield LJ. Guidelines for pancreaticobiliary cytology from the Papanicolaou Society of Cytopathology: a review. Cancer Cytopathol. 2014;122:399-411.
10. Bosman FT, Carneiro F, Hruban RH, Theise ND. WHO Classification of Tumours of the Digestive System. Lyon: International Agency for Research on Cancer; 2010.
11. Pitman MB, Centeno BA, Reid MD, Siddiqui MT, Layfield LJ, Perez-Machado M, et al. The World Health Organization Reporting System for Pancreaticobiliary Cytopathology. Acta Cytol. 2023;67(3):304-20.
12. Jones VM, Allison D. WHO Reporting System for Pancreaticobiliary Cytopathology, 1st edition. Lyon: International Agency for Research on Cancer; 2022.
13. Saieg M, Pitman MB. Experience and future perspectives on the use of the Papanicolaou Society of Cytopathology Terminology System for reporting pancreaticobiliary cytology. Diagn Cytopathol. 2020;48(5):494-8.
14. Hewitt MJ, McPhail MJ, Possamai L, Dhar A, Vlavianos P, Monahan KJ. EUS-guided FNA for diagnosis of solid pancreatic neoplasms: a meta-analysis. Gastrointest Endosc. 2012;75(2):319-31.
15. Layfield LJ, Zhang T, Esebua M. Diagnostic sensitivity and risk of malignancy for bile duct brushings categorized by the Papanicolaou Society of Cytopathology System for reporting pancreaticobiliary cytopathology. Diagn Cytopathol. 2022;50(1):24-7.
16. Nikas IP, Proctor T, Seide S, Chatziioannou SS, Reynolds JP, Ntourakis D. Diagnostic performance of pancreatic cytology with the Papanicolaou society of cytopathology system: a systematic review, before shifting into the upcoming WHO international system. Int J Mol Sci. 2022;23(3):1650.
17. Hoda RS, Arpin RN 3rd, Rosenbaum MW, Pitman MB. Risk of malignancy associated with diagnostic categories of the proposed world Health organization international system for reporting pancreaticobiliary cytopathology. Cancer Cytopathol. 2022;130(3):195-201.
18. Sung S, Del Portillo A, Gonda TA, Kluger MD, Tiscornia-Wasserman PG. Update on risk stratification in the Papanicolaou society of cytopathology system for reporting pancreaticobiliary cytology categories: 3-year, prospective, single-institution experience. Cancer Cytopathol. 2020;128(1):29-35.
19. Choi WT, Swanson PE, Grieco VS, Wang D, Westerhoff M. The outcomes of "atypical" and "suspicious" bile duct brushings in the identification of pancreaticobiliary tumors: follow-up analysis of surgical resection specimens. Diagn Cytopathol. 2015;43(11):885-91.
20. Abdelgawwad MS, Alston E, Eltoum IA. The frequency and cancer risk associated with the atypical cytologic diagnostic category in endoscopic ultrasound-guided fine-needle aspiration specimens of solid pancreatic lesions: a meta-analysis and argument for a Bethesda System for Reporting Cytopathology of the Pancreas. Cancer Cytopathol. 2013;121(11):620-8.
21. Chadwick BE, Layfield LJ, Witt BL, Schmidt RL, Cox RNK, Adler DG. Significance of atypia in pancreatic and bile duct brushings: follow-up analysis of the categories atypical and suspicious for malignancy. Diagn Cytopathol. 2014;42(4):285-91.
22. Dudley JC, Zheng Z, McDonald T, Le LP, Dias-Santagata D, Borger D, et al. Next-generation sequencing and fluorescence in situ hybridization have comparable performance characteristics in the analysis of pancreaticobiliary brushings for malignancy. J Mol Diagn. 2016;18(1):124-30.
23. Pitman MB, Centeno BA, Daglilar ES, Brugge WR, Mino-Kenudson M. Cytological criteria of high-grade epithelial atypia in the cyst fluid of pancreatic intraductal papillary mucinous neoplasms. Cancer Cytopathol. 2014;122(1):40-7.

24. The European Study Group on Cystic Tumours of the Pancreas. European evidence-based guidelines on pancreatic cystic neoplasms. Gut. 2018;67(5):789-804.
25. Hoda RS, Lu R, Arpin RN 3rd, Rosenbaum MW, Pitman MB. Risk of malignancy in pancreatic cysts with cytology of high-grade epithelial atypia. Cancer Cytopathol. 2018;126(9):773-81.
26. Elta GH, Enestvedt BK, Sauer BG, Lennon AM. ACG clinical guideline: diagnosis and management of pancreatic cysts. Am J Gastroenterol. 2018;113(4):464-79.
27. Pitman MB, Yaeger KA, Brugge WR, Mino-Kenudson M. Prospective analysis of atypical epithelial cells as a high-risk cytologic feature for malignancy in pancreatic cysts. Cancer Cytopathol. 2013;121(1):29-36.
28. Pitman MB, Centeno BA, Genevay M, Fonseca R, Mino-Kenudson M. Grading epithelial atypia in endoscopic ultrasound-guided fine-needle aspiration of intraductal papillary mucinous neoplasms: an international interobserver concordance study. Cancer Cytopathol. 2013;121(12):729-36.
29. McGuigan A, Kelly P, Turkington RC, Jones C, Coleman HG, McCain RS. Pancreatic cancer: a review of clinical diagnosis, epidemiology, treatment and outcomes. World J Gastroenterol. 2018;24(43):4846-61.
30. Khorana AA, Mangu PB, Berlin J, Engebretson A, Hong TS, Maitra A, et al. Potentially curable pancreatic cancer: American society of clinical oncology clinical practice guideline. J Clin Oncol. 2016;34(21):2541-56.
31. Hoda RS, Pitman MB. Pancreatic cytology. Surg Pathol Clin. 2018;11(3):563-88.
32. Stelow EB, Bardales RH, Stanley MW. Pitfalls in endoscopic ultrasound-guided fine-needle aspiration and how to avoid them. Adv Anat Pathol. 2005;12(2):62-73.
33. Okun SD, Lewin DN. Non-neoplastic pancreatic lesions that may mimic malignancy. Semin Diagn Pathol. 2016;33(1):31-42.
34. Frampas E, Morla O, Regenet N, Eugene T, Dupas B, Meurette G. A solid pancreatic mass: tumour or inflammation? Diagn Interv Imaging. 2013;94(7–8):741-55.
35. Nagtegaal ID, Odze RD, Klimstra D, Paradis V, Rugge M, Schirmacher P, et al; the WHO Classification of Tumours Editorial Board. The 2019 WHO Classification of Tumors of Digestive System. Histopathology. 2019;76(2):182-8.
36. De La Cruz MS, Young AP, Ruffin MT. Diagnosis and management of pancreatic cancer. Am Fam Physician. 2014;89(8):626-32.
37. Centeno BA, Stelow EB, Pitman MB. Pancreatic Cytohistology. Cambridge: Cambridge University Press; 2015.
38. Jang DK, Lee SH, Lee JK, Paik WH, Chung KH, Lee BS, et al. Comparison of cytological and histological preparations in the diagnosis of pancreatic malignancies using endoscopic ultrasound guided fine needle aspiration. Hepatob Pancreat Dis. 2017;16(4):418-23.
39. Lin F, Staerkel G. Cytologic criteria for well differentiated adenocarcinoma of the pancreas in fine-needle aspiration biopsy specimens. Cancer Cytopathol. 2003;99(1):44-50.
40. Sigel CS. Advances in the cytologic diagnosis of gastroenteropancreatic neuroendocrine neoplasms. Cancer Cytopathol. 2018;126:980-91.
41. Bellizzi AM, Stelow EB. Pancreatic cytopathology: a practical approach and review. Arch Pathol Lab Med. 2009;133(3):388-404.
42. Milan SA, Yeo CJ. Neuroendocrine tumors of the pancreas. Curr Opin Oncol. 2012;24(1):46-55.
43. Shah S, Mortele KJ. Uncommon solid pancreatic neoplasms: ultrasound, computed tomography, and magnetic resonance imaging features. Semin Ultrasound CT MR. 2007;28(5):357-70.
44. Jahan A, Yusuf MA, Loya A. Fine-needle aspiration cytology in the diagnosis of pancreatic neuroendocrine tumors: a single-center experience of 25 cases. Acta Cytol. 2015;48(3):163-8.
45. Gu M, Ghafari S, Lin F, Ramzy I. Cytological diagnosis of endocrine tumors of the pancreas by endoscopic ultrasound-guided fine-needle aspiration biopsy. Diagn Cytopathol. 2005;32(4):204-10.

46. Paschalis C, Charitini S, Panagiotis K, Ioannis K, Stratigoula S, Irini D. Endoscopic ultrasound-guided fine-needle aspiration cytology of pancreatic neuroendocrine tumors: a study of 48 cases. Cancer Cytopathol. 2008;114(4):255-62.
47. Burford H, Baloch Z, Liu X, Jhala D, Siegal GP, Jhala N. E-cadherin/beta-catenin and CD10: a limited immunohistochemical panel to distinguish pancreatic endocrine neoplasm from solid pseudopapillary neoplasm of the pancreas on endoscopic ultrasound-guided fine-needle aspirates of the pancreas. Am J Clin Pathol. 2009;132(6):831-9.
48. Jiao Y, Shi C, Edil BH, de Wilde RF, Klimstra DS, Maitra A, et al. DAXX/ATRX, MEN1, and mTOR pathway genes are frequently altered in pancreatic neuroendocrine tumors. Science. 2011;331(6021):1199-203.
49. Yachida S, Vakiani E, White CM, Zhong Y, Saunders T, Morgan R, et al. Small cell and large cell neuroendocrine carcinomas of the pancreas are genetically similar and distinct from well-differentiated pancreatic neuroendocrine tumors. Am J Surg Pathol. 2012;36(2):173-84.
50. Chhieng DC, Stelow EB. Pancreatic cytopathology. New York: Springer; 2007.
51. Odze RD, Goldblum JR. Surgical pathology of the GI tract, liver, biliary tract, and pancreas. Philadelphia: Saunders/Elsevier; 2015.
52. Simmons S, Eltoum IA. Acinar cell carcinoma of the pancreas: cytologic, immunohistochemical, and ultrastructural features. Pathol Case Rev. 2015;20(4):192-5.
53. Wood LD, Klimstra DS. Pathology and genetics of pancreatic neoplasms with acinar differentiation. Semin Diagn Pathol. 2014;31(6):491-7.
54. La Rosa S, Sessa F, Capella C. Acinar cell carcinoma of the pancreas: overview of clinicopathologic features and insights into the molecular pathology. Front Med (Lausanne). 2015;2:41.
55. Serra S, Chetty R. Revision 2: an immunohistochemical approach and evaluation of solid pseudopapillary tumour of the pancreas. J Clin Pathol. 2008;61(11):1153-9.
56. Pitman MB, Faquin WC. The fine-needle aspiration biopsy cytology of pancreatoblastoma. Diagn Cytopathol. 2004;31(6):402-6.
57. Henke AC, Kelley CM, Jensen CS, Timmerman TG. Fine-needle aspiration cytology of pancreatoblastoma. Diagn Cytopathol. 2001;25(2):118-21.
58. Huang HL, Shih SC, Chang WH, Wang TE, Chen MJ, Chan YJ. Solid-pseudopapillary tumor of the pancreas: clinical experience and literature review. World J Gastroenterol. 2005;11(9):1403-9.
59. Ersen A, Agalar AA, Ozer E, Agalar C, Unek T, Egeli T, et al. Solid-Pseudopapillary neoplasm of the pancreas: a clinicopathological review of 20 cases including rare examples. Pathol Res Pract. 2016;212(11):1052-8.
60. Bardales RH, Centeno B, Mallery JS, Lai R, Pochapin M, Guiter G, et al. Endoscopic ultrasound-guided fine-needle aspiration cytology diagnosis of solid-pseudopapillary tumor of the pancreas: a rare neoplasm of elusive origin but characteristic cytomorphologic features. Am J Clin Pathol. 2004;121(5):654-62.
61. Ohara Y, Oda T, Hashimoto S, Akashi Y, Miyamoto R, Enomoto T, et al. Pancreatic neuroendocrine tumor and solid-pseudopapillary neoplasm: key immunohistochemical profiles for differential diagnosis. World J Gastroenterol. 2016;22(38):8596-604.
62. Choi JY, Kim MJ, Lee JY, Lim JS, Chung JJ, Kim KW, et al. Typical and atypical manifestations of serous cystadenoma of the pancreas: imaging findings with pathologic correlation. AJR Am J Roentgenol. 2009;193:136-42.
63. Lilo MT, VandenBussche CJ, Allison DB, Lennon AM, Younes BK, Hruban RH, et al. Serous cystadenoma of the pancreas: potentials and pitfalls of a preoperative cytopathologic diagnosis. Acta Cytol. 2017;61:27-33.
64. Salomao M, Remotti H, Allendorf JD, Poneros JM, Sethi A, Gonda TA, et al. Fine-needle aspirations of pancreatic serous cystadenomas: improving diagnostic yield with cell blocks and α-inhibin immunohistochemistry. Cancer Cytopathol. 2014;122:33-9.
65. Belsley NA, Pitman MB, Lauwers GY, Brugge WR, Deshpande V. Serous cystadenoma of the pancreas: limitations and pitfalls of endoscopic ultrasound-guided fine-needle aspiration biopsy. Cancer. 2008;114:102-10.

66. Reid MD, Saka B, Balci S, Goldblum AS, Adsay NV. Molecular genetics of pancreatic neoplasms and their morphologic correlates: an update on recent advances and potential diagnostic applications. Am J Clin Pathol. 2014;141:168-80.
67. Pergolini I, Sahora K, Ferrone CR, Morales-Oyarvide V, Wolpin BM, Mucci LA, et al. Long-term risk of pancreatic malignancy in patients with BD intraductal papillary mucinous neoplasm in a Referral Center. Gastroenterology. 2017;153:1284-94.
68. Morales-Oyarvide V, Fong ZV, Fernández-Del Castillo C, Warshaw AL. Intraductal papillary mucinous neoplasms of the pancreas: strategic considerations. Visc Med. 2017;33:466-76.
69. Morales-Oyarvide V, Mino-Kenudson M, Ferrone CR, Sahani DV, Pergolini I, Negreros-Osuna AA, et al. Diabetes mellitus in intraductal papillary mucinous neoplasm of the pancreas is associated with high-grade dysplasia and invasive carcinoma. Pancreatology. 2017;17: 920-6.
70. Efthymiou A, Podas T, Zacharakis E. Endoscopic ultrasound in the diagnosis of pancreatic intraductal papillary mucinous neoplasms. World J Gastroenterol. 2014;20:7785-93.
71. Tanaka M, Fernández-Del Castillo C, Kamisawa T, Jang JY, Levy P, et al, et al. Revisions of international consensus Fukuoka guidelines for the management of IPMN of the pancreas. Pancreatology. 2017;17:738-53.
72. Layfield LJ, Cramer H. Fine-needle aspiration cytology of intraductal papillary-mucinous tumors: a retrospective analysis. Diagn Cytopathol. 2005;32:16-20.
73. Michaels PJ, Brachtel EF, Bounds BC, Brugge WR, Pitman MB. Intraductal papillary mucinous neoplasm of the pancreas: cytologic features predict histologic grade. Cancer. 2006;108: 163-73.
74. Pitman MB, Genevay M, Yaeger K, Chebib I, Turner BG, Mino-Kenudson M, et al. High-grade atypical epithelial cells in pancreatic mucinous cysts are a more accurate predictor of malignancy than "positive" cytology. Cancer Cytopathol. 2010;118:434-40.
75. Lee PJ, Fischer AH, Owens CL, Hutchinson L. Intranuclear cytoplasmic inclusions are a specific diagnostic feature distinguishing low-grade pancreatic intraductal papillary mucinous neoplasms from contaminating gastric epithelium. J Am Soc Cytopathol. 2013;2:S66-7.
76. Cizginer S, Turner BG, Bilge AR, Karaca C, Pitman MB, Brugge WR. Cyst fluid carcinoembryonic antigen is an accurate diagnostic marker of pancreatic mucinous cysts. Pancreas. 2011;40:1024-8.
77. Oh HC, Kang H, Brugge WR. Cyst fluid amylase and CEA levels in the differential diagnosis of pancreatic cysts: a single-center experience with histologically proven cysts. Dig Dis Sci. 2014;59:3111-6.
78. Singhi AD, Nikiforova MN, Fasanella KE, McGrath KM, Pai RK, Ohori NP, et al. Preoperative GNAS and KRAS testing in the diagnosis of pancreatic mucinous cysts. Clin Cancer Res. 2014;20:4381-9.
79. Jones M, Zheng Z, Wang J, Dudley J, Albanese E, Kadayifci A, et al. Impact of next-generation sequencing on the clinical diagnosis of 7 Intraductal Papillary Mucinous Neoplasms 202 pancreatic cysts. Gastrointest Endosc. 2016;83:140-8.
80. Fukushima N, Zamboni G. Mucinous cystic neoplasms of the pancreas: update on the surgical pathology and molecular genetics. Semin Diagn Pathol. 2014;31:467-74.
81. Thompson LD, Becker RC, Przygodzki RM, Adair CF, Heffess CS. Mucinous cystic neoplasm (mucinous cystadenocarcinoma of low-grade malignant potential) of the pancreas: a clinicopathologic study of 130 cases. Am J Surg Pathol. 1999;23:1-16.
82. Kim SY, Lee JM, Kim SH, Shin KS, Kim YJ, An SK, et al. Macrocystic neoplasms of the pancreas: CT differentiation of serous oligocystic adenoma from mucinous cystadenoma and intraductal papillary mucinous tumor. AJR Am J Roentgenol. 2006;187:1192-8.
83. Procacci C, Carbognin G, Accordini S, Biasiutti C, Guarise A, Lombardo F, et al. CT features of malignant mucinous cystic tumors of the pancreas. Eur Radiol. 2001;11:1626-30.
84. Zamboni G, Scarpa A, Bogina G, Iacono C, Bassi C, Talamini G, et al. Mucinous cystic tumors of the pancreas: clinicopathological features, prognosis, and relationship to other mucinous cystic tumors. Am J Surg Pathol. 1999;23:410-22.

85. Lüttges J, Feyerabend B, Buchelt T, Pacena M, Klöppel G. The mucin profile of noninvasive and invasive mucinous cystic neoplasms of the pancreas. Am J Surg Pathol. 2002;26: 466-71.
86. Wu J, Jiao Y, Dal Molin M, Maitra A, de Wilde RF, Wood LD, et al. Whole-exome sequencing of neoplastic cysts of the pancreas reveals recurrent mutations in components of ubiquitin-dependent pathways. Proc Natl Acad Sci U S A. 2011;108:21188-93.
87. Wood LD, Hruban HR. Genomic landscapes of pancreatic neoplasia. J Pathol Transl Med. 2015;49:13-22.
88. van der Waaij LA, van Dullemen HM, Porte RJ. Cyst fluid analysis in the differential diagnosis of pancreatic cystic lesions: a pooled analysis. Gastrointest Endosc. 2005;62(3):383-9.
89. Oh SH, Lee JK, Lee KT, Lee KH, Woo YS, Noh DH. The combination of cyst fluid carcinoembryonic antigen, cytology and viscosity increases the diagnostic accuracy of mucinous pancreatic cysts. Gut Liver. 2017;11(2):283-9.
90. Soyer OM, Baran B, Ormeci AC, Sahin D, Gokturk S, Evirgen S, et al. Role of biochemistry and cytological analysis of cyst fluid for the differential diagnosis of pancreatic cysts: a retrospective cohort study. Medicine (Baltimore). 2017;96(1):e5513.
91. Rockacy M, Khalid A. Update on pancreatic cyst fluid analysis. Ann Gastroenterol. 2013;26(2):122-7.
92. Ngamruengphong S, Lennon AM. Analysis of pancreatic cyst fluid. Surg Pathol Clin. 2016;9(4):677-84.
93. Maker AV, Carrara S, Jamieson NB, Pelaez-Luna M, Lennon AM, Dal Molin M, et al. Cyst fluid biomarkers for intraductal papillary mucinous neoplasms of the pancreas: a critical review from the international expert meeting on pancreatic branch-duct-intraductal papillary mucinous neoplasms. J Am Coll Surg. 2015;220(2):243-53.
94. Khalid A, McGrath KM, Zahid M, Wilson M, Brody D, Swalsky P, et al. The role of pancreatic cyst fluid molecular analysis in predicting cyst pathology. Clin Gastroenterol Hepatol. 2005;3(10):967-73.
95. Wang J, Paris PL, Chen J, Ngo V, Yao H, Frazier ML, et al. Next generation sequencing of pancreatic cyst fluid microRNAs from low grade benign and high grade-invasive lesions. Cancer Lett. 2015;356(2 Pt B):404-9.
96. Hata T, Dal Molin M, Suenaga M, Yu J, Pittman M, Weiss M, et al. Cyst fluid telomerase activity predicts the histologic grade of cystic neoplasms of the pancreas. Clin Cancer Res. 2016;22(20):5141-51.
97. Vincent A, Omura N, Hong SM, Jaffe A, Eshleman J, Goggins M. Genome-wide analysis of promoter methylation associated with gene expression profile in pancreatic adenocarcinoma. Clin Cancer Res. 2011;17(13):4341-54.
98. Hart J, Parab M, Mandich D, Cartun RW, Ligato S. IMP3 immunocytochemical staining increases sensitivity in the routine cytologic evaluation of biliary brush specimens. Diagn Cytopathol. 2012;40(4):321-6.
99. Ryan ME, Baldauf MC. Comparison of flow cytometry for DNA content and brush cytology for detection of malignancy in pancreaticobiliary strictures. Gastrointest Endosc. 1994; 40(2 Pt 1):133-9.
100. Kipp BR, Barr Fritcher EG, Pettengill JE, Halling KC, Clayton AC. Improving the accuracy of pancreatobiliary tract cytology with fluorescence in situ hybridization: a molecular test with proven clinical success. Cancer Cytopathol. 2013;121(11):610-9.
101. Rizvi S, Khan SA, Hallemeier CL, Kelley RK, Gores GJ. Cholangiocarcinoma—evolving concepts and therapeutic strategies. Nat Rev Clin Oncol. 2018;15(2):95-111.
102. Parsi MA, Li A, Li CP, Goggins M. DNA methylation alterations in endoscopic retrograde cholangiopancreatography brush samples of patients with suspected pancreaticobiliary disease. Clin Gastroenterol Hepatol. 2008;6(11):1270-8.
103. Young MR, Wagner PD, Ghosh S, Rinaudo JA, Baker SG, Zaret KS, et al. Validation of biomarkers for early detection of pancreatic cancer: summary of the alliance of pancreatic cancer consortia for biomarkers for early detection workshop. Pancreas. 2018;47(2):135-41.

16

CHAPTER

Dual-Color Dual-Hapten In Situ Hybridization: Basic Principles and Applications

Sankalp Sancheti

INTRODUCTION

In situ hybridization (ISH) is a powerful technique for localizing specific nucleic acid sequences within fixed tissues or cells, enabling us to study gene expression patterns and cellular localization of deoxyribonucleic acid DNA or ribonucleic acid (RNA). The dual-color dual-hapten in situ hybridization (D-DISH) method expands upon traditional ISH by employing dual-color and dual-hapten strategies to enhance the resolution and multiplexing capability of the assay. This chapter delves into the basic principles, procedure, applications, advantages, and limitations of D-DISH, providing a comprehensive overview for this advanced technique.

TECHNIQUE OVERVIEW

The D-DISH is a sophisticated ISH method designed to simultaneously detect and visualize two different targets within the same tissue section or cell preparation. This is achieved through the use of dual-hapten labeling and dual-color detection systems. The technique leverages the specificity of hapten-antibody interactions and the sensitivity of colorimetric or fluorescent detection methods to allow for the spatial and quantitative analysis of gene expression.[1]

BASIC PRINCIPLES

- *Dual-hapten system*: D-DISH utilizes two distinct hapten molecules, each conjugated to a different nucleic acid probe. Haptens are small molecules that are not immunogenic on their own but can be recognized by specific antibodies. In D-DISH, these haptens enable the differentiation of the two targets through distinct antibody binding and detection.
- *Dual-color detection*: The system employs two separate detection systems for visualizing the targets. This is typically achieved using colorimetric methods with chromogenic substrates or fluorescent dyes, allowing for the simultaneous visualization of two different targets in the same sample.

TYPE OF SPECIMEN

The D-DISH can be applied to a variety of specimen types,[2] including:

- *Tissue sections*: Formalin-fixed paraffin-embedded (FFPE) tissues are commonly used. These specimens are well-preserved and allow for detailed spatial resolution of gene expression.
- *Cell preparations*: Cultured cells or isolated cell populations can also be utilized, providing insights into gene expression at a cellular level.
- *Embryos*: Whole-mount ISH in embryos can provide information on gene expression patterns during development.

BASIC PROCEDURE

The D-DISH procedure involves several key steps:

- *Sample preparation*: Tissue or cell samples are fixed, embedded (if necessary), and sectioned onto slides. For whole-mount specimens, the tissue or embryo is prepared accordingly.
- *Probe design and labeling*: Two probes are designed, each targeting a distinct sequence. These probes are conjugated with different hapten molecules.
- *Hybridization*: The labeled probes are hybridized to the target nucleic acid within the specimen. This step is typically performed at an elevated temperature to ensure specific binding.
- *Washing*: Excess unbound probes are removed through a series of washes, which helps reduce background noise and increase specificity.
- *Detection*: The hybridized probes are detected using hapten-specific antibodies conjugated with colorimetric or fluorescent reporters. For dual-color detection, distinct substrates or dyes are used to visualize the two targets.
- *Imaging and analysis*: The specimen is examined under a light microscope, and the dual-color signals are analyzed to assess the expression patterns of the target.

APPLICATIONS

The D-DISH offers several applications in molecular and cell biology to study gene expression studies.[3] It is most widely used for analyzing the hormone receptor status in breast cancer. Assessment of HER2/neu protein over expression or amplification status is the standard of care for the pathologic evaluation of breast carcinoma specimens.[4] Traditionally, assessment of HER2/neu status has been performed by either immunohistochemistry (IHC) or fluorescence in situ hybridization (FISH).[5] However, both have their limitations and disadvantages which can be overcome by D-DISH. Various images related to interpretation of HER2 amplification by D-DISH are shown in **Figures 1 and 2**.

ADVANTAGES

- *Simultaneous detection*: The dual-color and dual-hapten approach allows for the simultaneous visualization of two RNA targets, enhancing the amount of information obtained from a single sample.

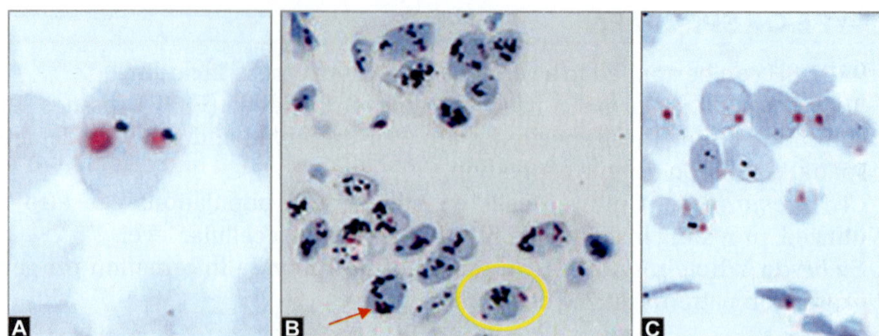

FIGS. 1A TO C: The images mentioned represent the tumor cells. (A) The typical pattern for a normal cell or nonamplified tumor cell. The black spot represents the *HER2/neu* gene and red depicts the CEN17. The stromal cells and other in situ carcinoma show the particular pattern of signals. (B) Shows the *HER2* gene amplified black clusters. The analysis of this cluster is done by the arbitrary determination of the cluster's size. For instance, the cell marked by the circle, which have been at least 12 black signals and the cells marked by an arrow have 6 black signals in the cluster, because the size of the cluster is comparatively less than the cluster representing 12 signals. (C) there are some evident signals; however, it is shown as a nonuniform pattern. Since signals are absent in (C), this case should not be considered for counting.

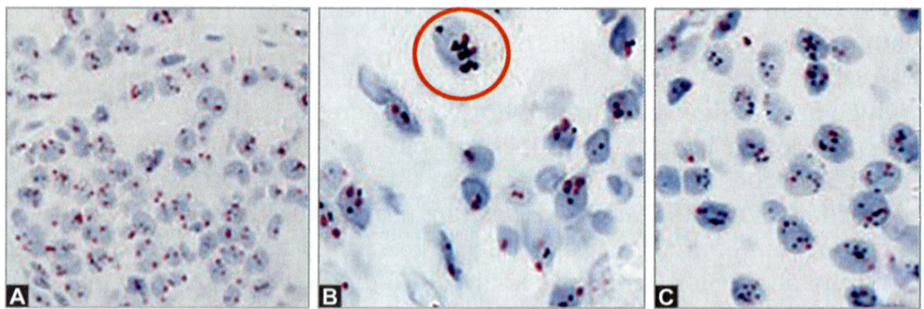

FIGS. 2A TO C: These images which represent the classic patterns of HER2 (black) and CEN17 (red) signals. The image (A) which shows polysomy of chromosome 17 which is identified by the uniform proportion of black and red signals. A heterogeneously amplified cell is evident in image (B) (circled), that detects the intermixed population. The percentage of heterogeneity also should be reported, as well as validated twice if required. The image (C) is also an amplified case of HER2-immunohistochemistry expression. The HER2/CEN17 ratio is ≥2; it is considered as amplified. Apart from gene amplification, gene duplication, extra chromosomal circular deoxyribonucleic acid (DNA), and so on will also leads to this appearance. This should be count if there is no obscureness and overlapping of cells.

- *High sensitivity and specificity*: The use of hapten-based detection systems provides high sensitivity and specificity, reducing background noise and increasing the accuracy of the results.
- *Spatial resolution*: D-DISH maintains high spatial resolution, allowing for precise localization of gene expression within tissues or cells. The technique is useful for light microscopy obviating the need for fluorescent microscope set up.
- *Versatility*: The method can be adapted for various specimen types and research questions, making it a versatile tool in molecular biology.

DISADVANTAGES

- *Complexity*: The D-DISH technique is more complex than traditional ISH methods, requiring careful optimization of probe design, hybridization conditions, and detection systems. Automatic platforms are required for performing the assay adding to cost.
- *Cost*: The dual-hapten and dual-color systems may be more expensive due to the need for specialized reagents and equipment.
- *Technical expertise*: The procedure requires a high level of technical skill and expertise to ensure successful implementation and accurate interpretation of results.
- *Potential for overlap*: In cases where the two RNA targets are expressed at very high levels or are very close in proximity, there may be issues with signal overlap or interference.

CONCLUSION

Dual-color dual-hapten in situ hybridization represents a significant advancement in the field of ISH, offering the ability to simultaneously detect and analyze multiple targets within a single specimen. Its high sensitivity, specificity, and spatial resolution make it a valuable tool for a range of applications in molecular and cell biology. As of today routine use is limited to enumeration of HER2 signals in breast and other cancers. Despite its complexity and cost, the benefits of D-DISH make it an important technique for researchers seeking detailed insights into gene expression patterns and interactions.

REFERENCES

1. Bauer A, Callaghan A. Dual-Color In Situ Hybridization: Methodology and Applications. J Mol Biol. 2018;430(10):1637-51.
2. Eberwine J, Hargreaves R. Advanced In Situ Hybridization Techniques. Methods Mol Biol. 2019;1920:55-71.
3. Liu J, Shen X. (2021). Dual-color in situ hybridization: from theory to application. Front Cell Dev Biol. 2021;9:724560.
4. Williams R, Brown D. The Use of Dual-Hapten Systems in Molecular Research. Curr Protoc Mol Biol. 2020;130(1):e109.
5. Layfield LJ, Wallander ML, Tripp SR, Redpath S, Banks PM. Comparison of Dual-ISH (DISH) With Fluorescence In Situ Hybridization (FISH) and Correlation With Immunohistochemical Findings for HER2/Neu Status in Breast Carcinoma. Appl Immunohistochem Mol Morphol. 2017;25(4):231-6.

17

CHAPTER

Updates in Glial Tumors

Debajyoti Chatterjee, Nivetha Ambalavanan

INTRODUCTION

The gliomas encompass a wide range of tumors arising from the neuroepithelial tissue involving the brain and spinal cord. The age range is broad, including individuals from infancy to old age without any age restrictions. The histological spectrum is also as diverse as the nomenclature, with varied morphology described through the years for diagnosis of the same. Gliomas are the most prevalent central nervous system (CNS) tumors encountered in adults in routine practice.

The classification took a radical shift in nomenclature, and the way we look at our bread-and-butter gliomas underwent a radical shift when they were classified into whole new categories and subtypes which either essentially or desirably needed to fulfill molecular alteration for their diagnosis.

A brief overview of the changes and their implications on the further treatment protocol of patients will be discussed.

GLIAL NEOPLASMS: THE PARADIGM SHIFT IN NOMENCLATURE

Since the introduction of the World Health Organization (WHO) Blue Books, gliomas, the nomenclature and classification of tumors originating from neuroepithelial tissue have undergone numerous changes. Histomorphology played a key role in classification in the year 2007.[1] They were classified into astrocytic, oligodendroglial, and pligoastrocytic tumors decided mainly by their morphological appearance into consideration. The WHO classification emphasized the importance of histological grading which was solely altered by the presence of certain morphological features, viz., cytological atypia, anaplasia, mitotic activity, microvascular proliferation, and necrosis.

The 2016 update of the WHO Blue Books incorporated well-established molecular parameters into the classification and that brought in a whole lot of changes with itself. The diffuse gliomas were histologically classified into three compartments (oligodendroglioma, astrocytoma, and oligoastrocytoma phenotype) based on histology, immunohistochemistry (IHC), and molecular alterations.[2] Isocitrate dehydrogenase (IDH) 1 and 2 mutations were identified as the cornerstone of the pathogenesis of adult type diffuse gliomas. In addition to the morphology, IHC for IDH, ATRX, and p53 along with 1p/19q codeletion status became part of routine evaluation for typifying diffuse adult glioma into astrocytoma/oligodendroglioma, IDH-mutant, or wildtype. The concept of molecular integrated diagnosis was proposed and histomorphology slowly started to take a backseat from then.

The current WHO classification of CNS tumors (WHO CNS5) 2021 has included many new entities and revolutionized the classification from a different perspective.[3] This version has tried to build onto the integrated diagnosis established in 2016 along with the recommendations of the Consortium to Inform Molecular and Practical Approaches to CNS Tumor Taxonomy (cIMPACT-NOW).[4] WHO CNS5 has gone into the next step with advanced molecular diagnostics with their strong anchor to established characterization for the years.

The new WHO CNS5 puts neuroepithelial tumors into six different groups as following:

1. Adult-type diffuse gliomas
2. Pediatric-type diffuse low-grade gliomas (LGG)
3. Pediatric-type diffuse high-grade gliomas
4. Circumscribed astrocytic gliomas
5. Glioneuronal and neuronal tumors
6. Ependymal tumors

Notably, the choroid plexus tumors have been removed from this subgroup due to the marked epithelial properties possessed by them and separated from the "gliomas, glioneuronal, and neuronal tumors" heading.

The gliomas are classified as "diffuse" and "circumscribed" by the growth-pattern. The diffuse tumors are the ones which show diffuse infiltrative pattern of growth while circumscribed ones are referred to the ones with more contained circumscribed pattern of growth. This is defined mostly by neuroimaging. The diffuse gliomas are now classified into "adult-type" and "pediatric-type" primarily based on the age of occurrence, pattern of growth, and underlying molecular mechanisms. They are classified primarily in broader sense, and adult-type can occur in pediatric age group while pediatric-type can occur in adult patients as well. This separation was brought in for the prognostication and difference of tumor behavior observed in these set of tumors over the years, despite their morphological similarities. This was established mainly through the better understanding of pathogenesis and molecular alterations in these tumors.

Adult-type diffuse gliomas according to WHO CNS5 encompass only three entities, viz., astrocytoma, IDH-mutant; oligodendroglioma, IDH-mutant and 1p/19q codeleted; and glioblastoma, IDH-wildtype in comparison to WHO CNS4 2016 which were previously spread out into 15 entities mainly due to the presence of different grade assigned to them. The term "glioblastoma, IDH-wildtype" is exclusively reserved to the IDH-wildtype high-grade gliomas with histomorphological features of microvascular proliferation and necrosis. However, in the absence of these histomorphological features, a IDH-wildtype glioma can be classified as glioblastoma if there are molecular defined events such as presence of either TERT promoter mutation or *EGFR* gene amplification or gain of 7/loss of 10 chromosome with copy number alterations, and provided the tumor is IDH-wildtype as well as H3-wildtype or possessing the DNA methylation profile of glioblastoma in methylation classifier incorporated from CIMPACT-NOW.[4]

Pediatric-type diffuse gliomas were classified as high- and low-grade based on their outcome and prognosis. The high-grade gliomas are the ones with proven dismal prognosis while low-grade gliomas had a favorable outcome.

WHO CNS5 standardized the use of "type" instead of "entity" and "subtype" instead of "variant" with subtypes described in the histopathology section with no change in nomenclature. For example, epithelioid glioblastoma, gliosarcoma, giant cell glioblastoma, glioblastoma—NOS are clubbed under a single entity as "glioblastoma—IDH wildtype" where in the tumor fitting with essential criteria of an IDH-wildtype, H3-wildtype with diffuse astrocytic pattern and one or more following features (microvascular proliferation, necrosis, TERT promoter mutation, *EGFR* gene amplification, +7/–10 chromosome copy number alterations). The presence of certain histopathological features can be mentioned in the final report. However, these features do not confer significant prognostic information in IDH-wildtype glioblastoma.

Other major changes in nomenclature based on the 2019 cIMPACT-NOW Utrecht meeting to make it consistent and simple.[5] Anatomic site modifiers were removed from certain entities (e.g., chordoid glioma of the third ventricle). Genetic modifiers were added to certain entities [e.g., glioblastoma, IDH-wildtype; diffuse low-grade glioma, mitogen-activated protein kinase (MAPK) pathway-altered]. The grade indicating modifiers in the nomenclature was removed and described in the same term (e.g., "anaplastic" and "diffuse" are removed from astrocytoma and oligodendroglioma). **Box 1** shows the list of tumors with updated nomenclature in WHO CNS5.

UPDATES IN THE TUMOR GRADING

The major change is the segregation of CNS and non-CNS tumors by introducing the CNS WHO grade status along with the removal of Roman numerals to Arabic to ease neuro-oncology clinical practice. The traditionally used Roman numerals had the danger of typographical errors, and major clinical mistreatments of "II" treated as "III" or "IV" being treated as "I". Hence, using Arabic numbers (1, 2, 3, and 4) instead of Roman numbers (I, II, III, and IV) reduces the margin of error. Another major change in the nomenclature is grading within the tumor types. This was adopted from non-CNS tumors primarily in the case of breast carcinoma or prostate carcinoma. This also helps in the inference of grade III anaplastic meningioma and grade III anaplastic astrocytoma carry a different connotation altogether. This provides fluidity to assign grades based on

BOX 1 **Tumor types with revised nomenclature as per recent (2021) World Health Organization of central nervous system tumors (glial neoplasms in bold entries).**

- **Astrocytoma, IDH-mutant**
- **Diffuse midline glioma, H3K27-altered**
- **Chordoid glioma**
- **Astroblastoma, MN-altered**
- **Supratentorial ependymoma, ZFTA fusion-positive**
- Embryonal tumor with multilayered rosettes
- Malignant melanotic nerve sheath tumor
- Solitary fibrous tumor
- Mesenchymal chondrosarcoma (formerly a subtype)
- Adamantinomatous craniopharyngioma (formerly a subtype)
- Papillary craniopharyngioma (formerly a subtype)
- Pituicytoma, granular cell tumor of the sellar region, and spindle cell oncocytoma (now grouped rather than separate)
- Pituitary adenoma/pituitary neuroendocrine tumor (pitNET)

(IDH: isocitrate dehydrogenase; ZFTA: zinc finger translocation associated)

the presence or absence of features in each tumor type instead of following the rigid categorization being followed in updated WHO CNS4 (2016).

NEWLY RECOGNIZED TUMORS

There are multiple new entities included in this WHO CNS5 and beyond. Various changes were introduced in the classification of glial neoplasms along with new entities based on their molecular signatures for diagnosis. The newly added entities are enlisted in **Box 2**.

Apart from the entities described in the WHO CNS5 **(Box 2)**, there are a few other entities that are slowly barking their way such as high-grade glioma with pleomorphic and pseudopapillary features (HPAP), hemispheric pilocytic astrocytoma, adult-type IDH-wildtype astrocytoma, oligosarcoma, neuroepithelial tumor with PATZ1 fusion, glial tumor with BCOR fusion (a separate condition distinct from a CNS tumor with BCOR-ITD), etc.[6-8] A detailed discussion about these entities is beyond the scope of this chapter. However, we will briefly discuss about some of these entities in the subsequent sections.

ROLE OF MOLECULAR DIAGNOSTICS IN DIAGNOSIS

Despite the role of histology in the classification of tumors morphologically, molecular diagnostic techniques have taken priority by being incorporated as the major diagnostic criteria for many entities. This was achieved majorly by the advent of methylation classification of the tumors and observation of clustering of the tumors with similar methylome data. The data analyzed strongly correlates with distinct prognoses and responses to therapy in major instances. Data on the clustering of the tumors, based on analysis of >50,000 CNS tumors in the largest

BOX 2 Newly recognized entities in the current World Health Organization (WHO) classification of central nervous system tumors.

- Diffuse astrocytoma, MYB- or MYBL1-altered
- Polymorphous low-grade neuroepithelial tumor of the young (PLNTY)
- Diffuse low-grade glioma, mitogen-activated protein kinase (MAPK) pathway-altered
- Diffuse hemispheric glioma, H3 G34-mutant
- Diffuse pediatric-type high-grade glioma, H3-wildtype, and isocitrate dehydrogenase (IDH)-wildtype
- Infant-type hemispheric glioma
- High-grade astrocytoma with piloid features
- Diffuse glioneuronal tumor with oligodendroglioma-like features and nuclear clusters (DGONC)—provisional entity
- Myxoid glioneuronal tumor
- Multinodular and vacuolating neuronal tumor
- Supratentorial ependymoma, YAP1 fusion-positive
- Posterior fossa group A, ependymoma
- Posterior fossa group B, ependymoma
- Cribriform neuroepithelial tumor (CRINET)—provisional entity

database using a classifier available at http://www.molecularneuropathology.org. (*Source:* WHO CNS5).[3]

Methylation-based classification has shown that despite the presence of similar histomorphological features, many tumors tend to behave individually due to their distinct molecular signature while tumors that are completely unrecognizable from each other based on morphology might tend to behave similarly.

Hence, the importance of performing molecular analysis before classifying gliomas was established clearly in this WHO CNS5. Not only the presence of the mutation is important for diagnosis, but certain grade-modifying mutations have also been put forth in the diagnostic criteria under a few glial neoplasms. Various methods can be used for detecting the molecular alterations, including surrogate IHC, fluorescence in situ hybridization (FISH), Sanger sequencing, next-generation sequencing, methylation profiling, etc. among these, methylation profiling is being used as an upcoming tool for classification of CNS tumors.

The new CNS WHO5 classification introduced several molecularly defined entities that necessitate the use of one or more diagnostic methods to establish a comprehensive diagnosis incorporating molecular characteristics. This can be challenging as it requires multiple diagnostic modalities to be routinely implemented. **Table 1** outlines the gliomas that either need molecular techniques for diagnosis or prognosis, along with the preferred methods used. The presence of various IHC surrogates can aid in diagnosis. For instance, H3G34R/V IHC is robust for diagnosing hemispheric gliomas. Similarly, H3K27M and H3K27me3 immunostains help diagnose diffuse midline gliomas. P16 in being a good surrogate for the CDKN2A/B helps in upgrading the tumor to molecular IDH-mutant astrocytomas.

TABLE 1: List of molecularly defined glial tumors and their preferred molecular diagnostic techniques.

Tumor type	Gene to be assessed	Preferred technique
Astrocytoma, IDH-mutant	*IDH1, IDH2, ATRX, and p53*	IHC
	CDKN2A/B	FISH
Oligodendroglioma	*1p/19q codeletion*	FISH
GBM, IDH-wildtype	*TERT promoter, chromosome 7,10,* and *EGFR*	FISH and PCR
Pediatric diffuse gliomas	*MYB and MYBL1*	qPCR and methylation classifier
Diffuse midline glioma	*EZHIP, H3K27M*, and *H3K27me3*	IHC
	EGFR	FISH and PCR
Infant-type hemispheric glioma	*NTRK, ALK, ROS*, and *MET*	
Pilocytic astrocytoma	KIAA::BRAF fusion	FISH
	BRAFV600E	IHC
High-grade astrocytoma with piloid features	*BRAF, NF1, ATRX*, and *CDKN2A/B*	Methylation classifier
Subependymal giant cell astrocytoma	*TSC1* and *TSC2*	IHC
Astroblastoma, MN1 altered	*MN1*	FISH

(FISH: fluorescence in situ hybridization; GBM: glioblastoma; IDH: isocitrate dehydrogenase; IHC: immunohistochemistry; PCR: polymerase chain reaction)

Methylation Classifier

Methylation serves as a key molecular regulatory mechanism influencing gene expression, in addition to genetic, transcriptomic, and proteomic changes.[9] Methylation analysis involves identifying whether specific DNA regions have methyl groups (CH3) attached to them. The importance of the methylation status is that it is diverse and unique for each tumor subtype, unlike the genetic alterations which are quite overlapping through the spectrum of entities. The diverse neoplasms are organized into methylome-based classifications, aiding clinicians in deciding the next course of action for treatment. For example, in a diagnostically challenging case with varied histomorphology, it is important to be classified further because tumors like pilocytic astrocytoma require only surgical resection while high-grade glioma with piloid features requires additional assistance from radiotherapy. This classification also addresses the interobserver variability in a few tumor subgroups.[10,11]

Role of methylation-based classification in day-to-day practice:
- Establish the subtyping of medulloblastoma
- Methylation-based classification of meningioma helps in risk stratification. Some meningiomas with grade 1 morphology can show high-grade features on methylation classifier, which correlates with their aggressive clinical behavior.
- Discover or confirm diagnosis of rare tumor entities

GLIOMAS: IN A NUTSHELL

Adult-type Diffuse Gliomas

Astrocytoma, IDH-mutant

A diffusely infiltrating glioma with astrocytic morphology, possessing mutation of IDH1 codon 132 or IDH2 codon 172 missense mutation, and loss of nuclear ATRX expression or ATRX mutation or excluding of whole-arm deletions of 1p and 19q with desirable TP53 mutation is diagnostic of astrocytoma, IDH-mutant. They have been previously classified as "diffuse astrocytoma", "anaplastic astrocytoma" and "glioblastoma" based on morphology and assigned grades, whereas current classification recommends the presence of microvascular proliferation, necrosis, and homozygous deletion of CDKN2A, and CDKN2B (molecular analysis) as part of grading. An IDH-mutant astrocytoma, with either necrosis or microvascular proliferation or homozygous deletion of CDKN2A and CDKN2B, is now classified as astrocytoma, IDH-mutant, grade 4 **(Fig. 1)**. Hence, the mere histological grading might be underdiagnosing a higher-grade glioma molecularly. Emphasis on diagnostic molecular pathology with the presence of IDH1 R132H mutation can be established using IHC which is described in 90% of the supratentorial IDH-mutant astrocytomas.

Oligodendroglioma, IDH-mutant, and 1p/19q Codeleted

A diffusely infiltrating glioma with morphology ranging from oligodendroglial, oligoastrocytic, astrocytic, or ambiguous features on histology but detection

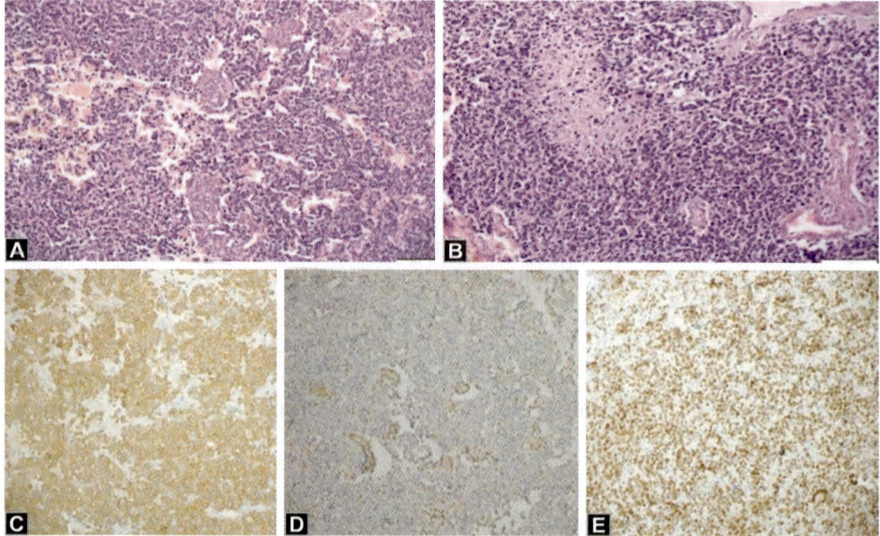

FIGS. 1A TO E: Histopathological features of IDH-mutant astrocytoma grade 4. This grade 4 IDH-mutant astrocytoma is characterized by a highly cellular tumor with a monomorphic population of cells. High-grade histological features include palisading necrosis (B—H&E, 200×) and microvascular proliferation (A—H&E, 200×). The tumor cells are immunopositive for IDH1 R132H (C), exhibit loss of ATRX expression (D), and show mutant expression of p53 (E).

of combined presence of IDH1R132H or IDH2R172H missense mutation and whole-arm deletions of 1p and 19q with desirable ATRX retained expression, TERT promoter mutation or a DNA-methylome profile of oligodendroglioma. This diagnosis is relatively straightforward when considering its basic histomorphology and immunohistochemical profile. However, it can sometimes present with ambiguous morphology, becoming a pathologist's nightmare. The commonly mistaken tumors are pilocytic astrocytomas with oligodendroglial morphology and pediatric gliomas (MYB and MYBL1 altered) can assume oligodendroglioma morphology, polymorphous low-grade neuroepithelial tumor of the young (PLNTY), diffuse leptomeningeal tumor or H3 G34-mutant hemispheric gliomas, among others. Hence, the importance here is to establish the IDH mutation status using IHC or sequencing analysis and presence of 1p/19q codeletion using FISH.

Pediatric-type Diffuse Gliomas

Two new families of tumor types have been included in the WHO CNS5, viz., pediatric-type low-grade gliomas and pediatric-type high-grade gliomas. An important thing to note is that these tumors are reserved for the pediatric age group. A dictum to be noted is that pediatric-type diffuse gliomas can be rarely seen in adult age groups and pediatric age groups are not immune to present with adult-type gliomas.

Pediatric-type Diffuse Low-grade Gliomas

Diffuse Astrocytoma, MYB- or MYBL1 Altered

Diffuse astrocytoma, MYB- or MYBL1-altered, is a diffusely infiltrating astroglial neoplasm composed of monomorphic cells with genetic alterations in *MYB* or *MYBL1* gene. It is assigned CNS WHO grade 1. These tumors were first incorporated in CNS WHO5. They commonly present as refractory seizures in the pediatric age-group or often present since childhood, hence referred to as long-term epilepsy-associated tumors (LEATs). The median age of presentation being 10 years. There is a mild temporal lobe predilection noted with rare brain stem cases as well reported in literature.[12] These tumors on histology assume a bland monomorphic glial cell in a fibrillary matrix. The sequencing demonstrates structural variation for fusion in *MYB* and *MYBL1* and a partner gene (PCDHGA1, MMP16, MAML2, QKI, etc.).[13] They have benign clinical behavior with 90% becoming seizure free postresection of the tumor.[14]

Angiocentric Glioma

Angiocentric glioma is a diffusely infiltrating glioma located in cerebral cortex commonly presenting in temporal or frontal lobe causing gray-white junction blurring. This is composed of cytologically uniform, bland bipolar spindle cells radially arranged in perivascular pattern. They express glial fibrillary acidic protein (GFAP) and epithelial membrane antigen (EMA) in perinuclear dot-like pattern. The molecular diagnostic criteria are alteration of MYB with fusions of *MYB* and *QKI* genes. They typically lack mutations in *TP53, ATRX, IDH1, IDH2,* and *Histone H3* genes. These tumors have indolent behavior and radiologically stable.[15]

Polymorphous Low-grade Neuroepithelial Tumor of the Young

This is an indolent LEATs commonly presenting in young individuals, diffuse growth patterns, with frequently present oligodendroglioma-like components, presence of microcalcifications, CD34 immunoreactivity, and presence of MAPK pathway-activating genetic abnormalities **(Fig. 2)**.[9] These tumors can show both infiltrative and compact growth patterns. The differentials considered are diffuse astrocytomas and oligodendrogliomas. Molecular diagnosis of BRAF p V600E mutations and *FGFR2* or *FGFR3* gene fusions needs to be established. The presence of *FGFR3::TACC3* gene fusions is associated with aggressive behavior.[16]

Diffuse Low-grade Glioma, MAPK Pathway-altered

Diffuse low-grade glioma with diffuse astrocytic or oligodendroglial morphology presenting in childhood with MAPK-alterations. They typically lack minimal mitotic activity, microvascular proliferation, and necrosis. They should show MAPK pathway alteration, IDH-wildtype, H3-wildtype phenotype, and absence of homozygous deletion of CDKN2A. There are three subtypes: (1) FGFR1 tyrosine kinase domain duplication, (2) FGFR1-mutant, and (3) BRAFV600E-mutant.[17] They rarely undergo anaplastic progression and respond to MEK inhibitors and BRAF inhibitors.[18]

Pediatric-type Diffuse High-grade Gliomas

Diffuse Midline Glioma, H3K27-altered

The important change in this particular entity is that nomenclature has been changed to H3 K27-altered instead of H3 K27-mutant due to presence of newer mutations associated with H3 alterations. These are infiltrative gliomas with

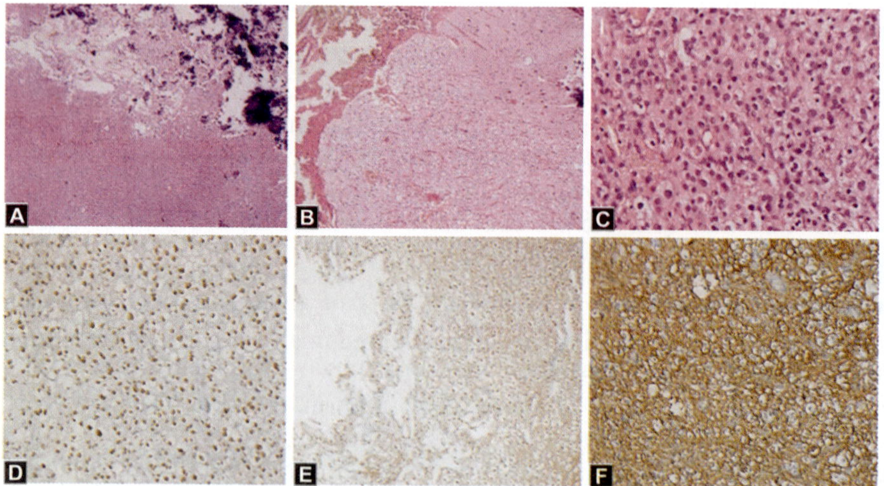

FIGS. 2A TO F: Histopathological features of polymorphous low-grade neuroepithelial tumor of the young (PLNTY). PLNTY exhibits (A) diffuse surface microcalcifications with a surface pattern of growth, and (B) and (C) an oligodendroglioma-like appearance (H&E, ×200). The tumor cells are immunopositive for OLIG2 (D), show retained ATRX expression (E), and show diffuse immunoreactivity for CD34 (F).

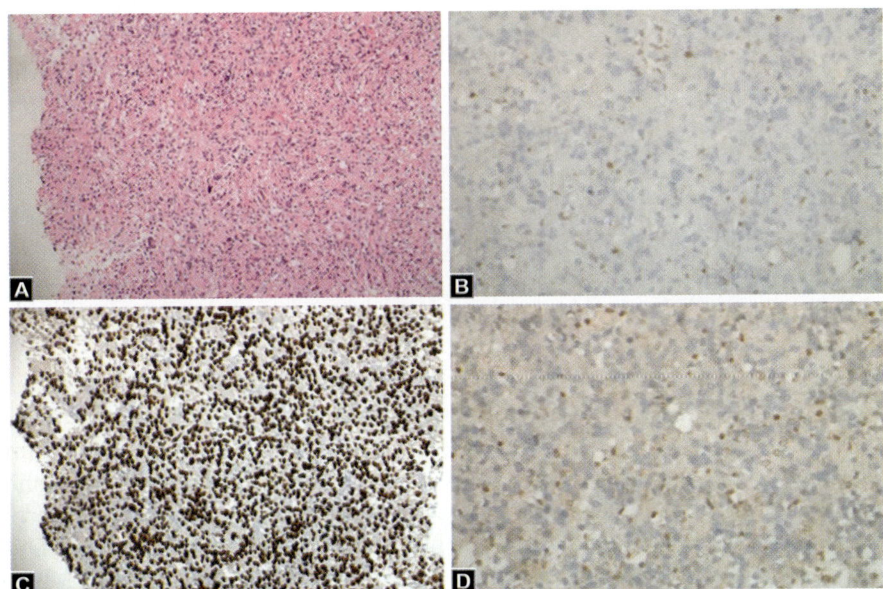

FIGS. 3A TO D: Histopathological features of diffuse midline glioma with H3K27M alteration. This high-grade glial neoplasm is characterized by high cellularity and scattered pleomorphic cells (A—H&E, 200× magnification). The tumor shows loss of ATRX expression (B—400× magnification) and diffuse, strong nuclear expression of the H3K27M protein (C), along with loss of H3K27me3 protein (D).

loss of H3K27me3 usually associated with H3 isoforms, aberrant expression of EZHIP, or EGFR mutation. They do not have a classical histomorphology as such and ranges from astrocytic, piloid, oligodendroglial, giant cell, undifferentiated, or epithelioid morphology **(Fig. 3)**.[19] Irrespective of histological appearance, it is considered as grade 4. Despite it being labeled as midline, rare nonmidline, cortical, or hemispheric locations have been described in literature.[12,20] They carry a poor prognosis with a 2-year survival rate of <10%.[20]

Diffuse Hemispheric Glioma, H3 G34-mutant

An infiltrative glioma in pediatric age group involving the cerebral hemispheres with missense mutation of *H3-3A* gene. Histologically, a glioblastoma-like pattern is observed characterized by highly cellular and infiltrative pattern of growth with brisk mitotic activity or may resemble embryonal tumors in hemispheric locations **(Fig. 4)**. The typical IHC pattern of these tumors (ATRX loss, p53-mutant, and FOXG1 and MAP2 positivity with OLIG2 negativity) can indicate toward the diagnosis; however, it is important to demonstrate H3G34R/V-mutant proteins. This can be done using IHC or sequencing.[21]

Diffuse Pediatric-type High-grade Glioma, H3-wildtype, and IDH-wildtype

These infiltrating high-grade gliomas are rare and many are related to previous cranial irradiation and in context of congenital mismatch repair deficiency syndrome (CMMRD), Lynch syndrome, or Li-Fraumeni syndrome. These are not well known since pediatric glioblastomas are diverse in their molecular natures. They are further subdivided into three subgroups based on the underlying

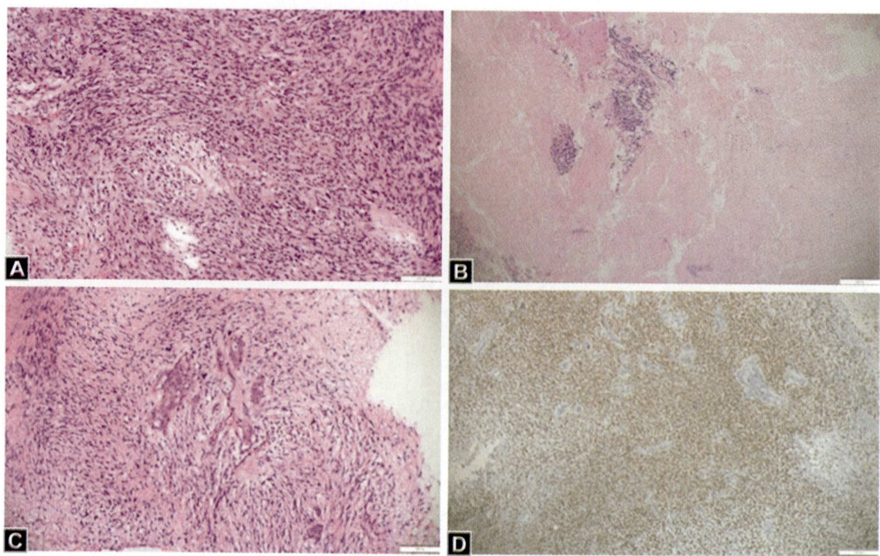

FIGS. 4A TO D: Histopathological features of diffuse hemispheric glioma with H3G34 mutation. This infiltrative glioma displays spindled to pleomorphic morphology (A—H&E, 200× magnification) and high-grade features, including geographic areas of necrosis (B—H&E, 200× magnification) and microvascular proliferation (C—H&E, 200× magnification). The tumor shows positivity for H3G34R/V immunostaining (D).

genetic alterations. Not much epidemiological data exist for this subtype because of its rarity. They are clinically aggressive tumors and assigned CNS WHO grade 4 and outcome was worse with MYCN subtype tumors in comparison to RTK1 and RTK2.[22]

Infant Type Hemispheric Glioma

A diffusely infiltrative cerebral based high-grade glioma arising in early childhood as early as infancy with tyrosine kinase fusions (ROS1, ALK, and MET). These tumors show highly cellularity with high-grade features, viz., microvascular proliferation, necrosis, and areas of primitive appearance. They are subclassified into (1) Infant-type hemispheric glioma, NTRK-altered; (2) Infant-type hemispheric glioma, ROS1-altered; (3) Infant-type hemispheric glioma, ALK-altered; and (4) Infant-type hemispheric glioma, MET-altered. They do not respond well to the conventional therapy, and targeted therapies are being explored. The ALK-rearranged tumors show best overall outcome compared to the rest.[23]

Circumscribed Astrocytic Gliomas

High-grade Astrocytoma with Piloid Features

The newly described entity in CNS WHO5 is an astrocytoma with distinct DNA methylation profile with high-grade piloid and or GBM-like histological features. These tumors typically show MAPK pathway gene alteration, homozygous deletion of CDKN2A and/or CDKN2B, and/or amplification of CDK4 with loss of ATRX expression or mutation of ATRX. They do possess varied histomorphological spectrum, with morphological resemblance to IDH-wildtype GBM, PXA, and pilocytic astrocytoma. Thus, these mimickers need to be excluded.[24] Varied MAPK alterations have been described in literature, viz., NF1 mutation, NF1 heterozygous deletion, KIAA1549::BRAF fusion, BRAFV600E mutation, FGFR1, and KRAS1 mutation.[24] The prognosis data available for this entity is based on a single retrospective study alone; however, it appears to be better than IDH-wildtype glioblastoma, despite high-grade morphology.

Astroblastoma, MN1 Altered

This is a circumscribed neoplasm with *MN1* gene alteration. Histologically, it is composed of round, cuboidal, or columnar cells with variable pseudopapillary or perivascular growth patterns. They are often located in frontal and parietal lobes. The common fusion partners of MN1 are BEND2 and CXXC5, resulting in increased expression of MN1; however, pathogenesis still remains unclear. The histological hallmark of this tumor is presence of astroblastic pseudorosette which is a perivascular structuring of neoplastic cells radially arranged around vessels. The molecular demonstration of MN1 alteration is important in this tumor since they can be misdiagnosed as ependymoma, e-glioblastomas, PXA, embryonal neoplasm, or any circumscribed gliomas. ZFTA fusion and BRAF mutation are somehow mutually exclusive with MN1 alteration; hence, presence of these alterations negate the diagnosis.[25]

Glioneuronal and Neuronal Tumors

A newly added entity in this subset of tumors is diffuse glioneuronal tumor with oligodendroglioma-like features and nuclear clusters (DGONC). This is as of now a provisional tumor type proposed as a neuroepithelial tumor characterized by variably differentiated cells frequently showing perinuclear halos, scattered multinucleated cells, and nuclear clusters with a distinct DNA methylation profile and frequent monosomy of chromosome 14. Till now only 21 cases have been described in literature. Methylation profiling is necessary for confirming the diagnosis.[9,11]

Ependymomas

Ependymomas are now classified based on a combination of histological, anatomical location, and molecular features. They are thus divided into 10 molecular subgroups spanning across supratentorial, infratentorial, and spinal locations. Myxopapillary ependymomas (MPE) and subependymomas have lost their tumor type status and are classified as tumor subtypes instead based on location. The MPE have been upgraded to CNS WHO grade 2 instead of previous grade 1 status due to likelihood of recurrence.[26]

Beyond CNS WHO5 2021

Additional proposed gliomas have been proposed by tumor methylation profiling and presented in the literature since the publication of WHO CNS 2021 classification.[10,27] These have been shown in **Box 3**.

BOX 3 List of proposed glial tumors beyond 2021 classification.

- High-grade glioma with pleomorphic and pseudopapillary features (HPAP)
- Neuroepithelial tumor with PATZ1 fusion
- Glial tumor with BCOR fusion
- Cerebellar high-grade glioma
- Early ependymal tumor with MN1-BEND2 fusion
- Isocitrate dehydrogenase (IDH)-wildtype glioma with low-grade morphology
- Hemispheric pilocytic astrocytoma

The list is endless and beyond the advent of the methylation classifier, the need to subtype and classify the morphologically ambiguous, not-so-fitting into a box diagnosis. The key feature to note is that some entities are still being under scrutiny to be part of an existing tumor and not an individual entity as such. For instance, the IDH-wildtype gliomas with low-grade morphology can be fit into a rare mutation-positive glioma on whole-exome sequencing. The existing CNS WHO5 2021 is not so perfect in itself. It needs further clarification for overlapping desirable criteria mentioned under certain entities. For example, TERT promoter mutation in itself upgrades a tumor as molecular glioblastoma; however, the presence of TERT has been linked to better prognosis in recent studies.[28] The hereditary predisposition tumor syndromes have not been included in this WHO5 clearly.

CONCLUSION

Gliomas encompass a highly diverse range of tumors with much still to be discovered. The current WHO classification of glial tumors includes a large number of molecularly defined entities, though the role of histological analysis still remains relevant. The current level of understanding might be insufficient to fully grasp their tumor pathobiology and natural behavior. Regardless of the molecular entities presented, the essential task is to recognize the histomorphology and accompanying subtle indicators to guide the selection of the appropriate tests in cases of diagnostic uncertainty. Further understanding about targetable molecular alterations in glial tumors will pave in the pathway for better individualization of treatment.

REFERENCES

1. Louis DN, Ohgaki H, Wiestler OD, Cavenee WK, Burger PC, Jouvet A, et al. The 2007 WHO Classification of Tumours of the Central Nervous System. Acta Neuropathol. 2007;114(2):97-109.
2. Louis DN, Perry A, Reifenberger G, von Deimling A, Figarella-Branger D, Cavenee WK, et al. The 2016 World Health Organization Classification of Tumors of the Central Nervous System: a summary. Acta Neuropathol. 2016;131(6):803-20.
3. International Agency for Research on Cancer. Central Nervous System Tumours: WHO Classification of Tumours, 5th edition, volume 6. [online] Available from https://publications.iarc.fr/Book-And-Report-Series/Who-Classification-Of-Tumours/Central-Nervous-System-Tumours-2021 [Last accessed November 2024].

4. Gonzalez Castro LN, Wesseling P. The cIMPACT-NOW updates and their significance to current neuro-oncology practice. Neurooncol Pract. 2020;8(1):4-10.
5. Louis DN, Wesseling P, Aldape K, Brat DJ, Capper D, Cree IA, et al. cIMPACT-NOW update 6: new entity and diagnostic principle recommendations of the cIMPACT-Utrecht meeting on future CNS tumor classification and grading. Brain Pathol. 2020;30(4):844-56.
6. Pratt D, Abdullaev Z, Papanicolau-Sengos A, Ketchum C, Panneer Selvam P, Chung HJ, et al. High-grade glioma with pleomorphic and pseudopapillary features (HPAP): a proposed type of circumscribed glioma in adults harboring frequent TP53 mutations and recurrent monosomy 13. Acta Neuropathol. 2022;143(3):403-14.
7. Pizzimenti C, Fiorentino V, Germanò A, Martini M, Ieni A, Tuccari G. Pilocytic astrocytoma: The paradigmatic entity in low-grade gliomas (Review). Oncol Lett. 2024;27(4):146.
8. Liu L, Liu Y, Chen J, Jiang T, Liu X, Zhang KN. Methylation class oligosarcoma, IDH-mutant could exhibit astrocytoma-like molecular features. Acta Neuropathol. 2024;147(1):49.
9. Capper D, Jones DTW, Sill M, Hovestadt V, Schrimpf D, Sturm D, et al. DNA methylation-based classification of central nervous system tumours. Nature. 2018;555(7697):469-74.
10. Jaunmuktane Z, Capper D, Jones DTW, Schrimpf D, Sill M, Dutt M, et al. Methylation array profiling of adult brain tumours: diagnostic outcomes in a large, single centre. Acta Neuropathol Commun. 2019;7(1):24.
11. Park JW, Lee K, Kim EE, Kim SI, Park SH. Brain Tumor Classification by Methylation Profile. J Korean Med Sci. 2023;38(43):e356.
12. Ryall S, Zapotocky M, Fukuoka K, Nobre L, Guerreiro Stucklin A, Bennett J, et al. Integrated Molecular and Clinical Analysis of 1,000 Pediatric Low-Grade Gliomas. Cancer Cell. 2020;37(4):569-83.e5.
13. Ellison DW, Hawkins C, Jones DTW, Onar-Thomas A, Pfister SM, Reifenberger G, et al. cIMPACT-NOW update 4: diffuse gliomas characterized by MYB, MYBL1, or FGFR1 alterations or BRAFV600E mutation. Acta Neuropathol. 2019;137(4):683-7.
14. Chiang J, Harreld JH, Tinkle CL, Moreira DC, Li X, Acharya S, et al. A single-center study of the clinicopathologic correlates of gliomas with a MYB or MYBL1 alteration. Acta Neuropathol. 2019;138(6):1091-2.
15. Shakur SF, McGirt MJ, Johnson MW, Burger PC, Ahn E, Carson BS, et al. Angiocentric glioma: a case series. J Neurosurg Pediatr. 2009;3(3):197-202.
16. Bielle F, Di Stefano AL, Meyronet D, Picca A, Villa C, Bernier M, et al. Diffuse gliomas with FGFR3-TACC3 fusion have characteristic histopathological and molecular features. Brain Pathol. 2018;28(5):674-83.
17. Zhang J, Wu G, Miller CP, Tatevossian RG, Dalton JD, Tang B, et al. Whole-genome sequencing identifies genetic alterations in pediatric low-grade gliomas. Nat Genet. 2013;45(6):602-12.
18. Hargrave DR, Bouffet E, Tabori U, Broniscer A, Cohen KJ, Hansford JR, et al. Efficacy and Safety of Dabrafenib in Pediatric Patients with *BRAF* V600 Mutation-Positive Relapsed or Refractory Low-Grade Glioma: Results from a Phase I/IIa Study. Clin Cancer Res. 2019;25(24):7303-11.
19. Solomon DA, Wood MD, Tihan T, Bollen AW, Gupta N, Phillips JJ, et al. Diffuse Midline Gliomas with Histone H3-K27M Mutation: A Series of 47 Cases Assessing the Spectrum of Morphologic Variation and Associated Genetic Alterations. Brain Pathol. 2016;26(5):569-80.
20. Mackay A, Burford A, Carvalho D, Izquierdo E, Fazal-Salom J, Taylor KR, et al. Integrated Molecular Meta-Analysis of 1,000 Pediatric High-Grade and Diffuse Intrinsic Pontine Glioma. Cancer Cell. 2017;32(4):520-37.e5.
21. Sturm D, Witt H, Hovestadt V, Khuong-Quang DA, Jones DTW, Konermann C, et al. Hotspot mutations in H3F3A and IDH1 define distinct epigenetic and biological subgroups of glioblastoma. Cancer Cell. 2012;22(4):425-37.
22. Korshunov A, Schrimpf D, Ryzhova M, Sturm D, Chavez L, Hovestadt V, et al. H3-/IDH-wild type pediatric glioblastoma is comprised of molecularly and prognostically distinct subtypes with associated oncogenic drivers. Acta Neuropathol. 2017;134(3):507-16.

23. Guerreiro Stucklin AS, Ryall S, Fukuoka K, Zapotocky M, Lassaletta A, Li C, et al. Alterations in ALK/ROS1/NTRK/MET drive a group of infantile hemispheric gliomas. Nat Commun. 2019;10(1):4343.
24. Reinhardt A, Stichel D, Schrimpf D, Sahm F, Korshunov A, Reuss DE, et al. Anaplastic astrocytoma with piloid features, a novel molecular class of IDH wildtype glioma with recurrent MAPK pathway, CDKN2A/B and ATRX alterations. Acta Neuropathol. 2018; 136(2):273-91.
25. Wood MD, Tihan T, Perry A, Chacko G, Turner C, Pu C, et al. Multimodal molecular analysis of astroblastoma enables reclassification of most cases into more specific molecular entities. Brain Pathol. 2018;28(2):192-202.
26. Ellison DW, Aldape KD, Capper D, Fouladi M, Gilbert MR, Gilbertson RJ, et al. cIMPACT-NOW update 7: advancing the molecular classification of ependymal tumors. Brain Pathol. 2020;30(5):863-6.
27. Komori T. Beyond the WHO 2021 classification of the tumors of the central nervous system: transitioning from the 5th edition to the next. Brain Tumor Pathol. 2024;41(1):1-3.
28. Fujimoto K, Arita H, Satomi K, Yamasaki K, Matsushita Y, Nakamura T, et al. TERT promoter mutation status is necessary and sufficient to diagnose IDH-wildtype diffuse astrocytic glioma with molecular features of glioblastoma. Acta Neuropathol. 2021;142(2):323-38.

18
CHAPTER

Updates in Kidney Transplant Disease

Nupur Pradhan

INTRODUCTION

The XVII meeting for allograft pathology by Banff, Alberta, Canada as a combined gathering with the Canadian Society of Transplantation was held from September 19 to September 23, 2022. The effect of microvascular inflammation (MVI) was the main point of discussion, in addition to other features of kidney transplant pathology such as T cell-mediated rejection (TCMR), antibody-mediated rejection (AMR), biopsy-based transcript analysis, activity and chronicity scores, digital pathology, xenotransplantation, clinical trials, and surrogate endpoints. The classification of Banff remains unchanged and the main agenda of the recent Banff working groups was to pose unsolved queries. This chapter further describes each of the following points in a conceptualized manner.

TCMR AND PIVOTAL ROLE OF INFLAMMATION IN TUBULAR ATROPHY AND INTERSTITIAL FIBROSIS (I-IFTA) REGIONS

Two troublesome diagnoses in the Banff classification were rigorously evaluated: Chronic active T cell-mediated rejection (caTCMR) and borderline (BL) (suspicious) for acute TCMR (aTCMR).

Chronic Active T Cell-mediated Rejection

There has been a strong association between inflammation present in vicinity of the area with interstitial fibrosis and tubular atrophy (i-IFTA) and graft loss. However, i-IFTA can also be observed in association with pyelonephritis, recurrent or de novo kidney disease, and polyomavirus nephropathy. Therefore, the definition of i-IFTA now includes (1) a prerequisite for ruling out other diseases and (2) a prerequisite for a minimal level of concomitant ti lesion and tubulitis. The ti score must be considered in addition to the i-IFTA score so that too much weightage is not given to extremely focal areas rich in inflammatory infiltrate in the scarred cortex.

The high frequency of i-IFTA (about 50% of biopsies taken more than a year after transplant)[1] and its correlation with the progression of *cv* and *cg* lesions scores over time were emphasized at a special Banff 2022 session.[2]

There has been a difference in molecular profile noted in inflammation in caTCMR as opposed to inflammation in acute TCMR. There is an interferon gamma activation seen with acute cases while chronic active cases show mast cell activation and signals pertaining to injury repair.[3,4]

In summary, i-IFTA is nonspecific in its molecular profile as well as in its clinical association, but is associated with a poorer prognosis, and is worse when compared to areas of fibrosis without inflammation.

Borderline (Suspicious) for Acute T Cell-mediated Rejection

The cutoff set as active infiltrates present in <25% of the nonscarred interstitium, leads to a large proportion of cases being classified as BL for TCMR; however, recent data indicates that a sizable fraction of BL behaves as TCMR. The aTCMR and BL definitions and criteria need to be re-evaluated for the present era of immunosuppression, as was stated in the Banff 2022 summit.

ANTIBODY-MEDIATED REJECTION

The latest Banff states that there should be an interdisciplinary viewpoint on the use of AMR diagnoses. The key priority was for the patients that showed MVI which were negative for both donor-specific antibody (DSA) and C4d or MVI less than what is required to diagnose AMR **(Flowchart 1)**. The results to date were that there is room for interpretation error in the Banff AMR definition, which might have consequences for patient care and made suggestions for a uniform set of factors that had to be disclosed in order to identify immunological hazards.

BIOPSY-BASED TRANSCRIPT DIAGNOSTICS

The classification's language was changed to "if thoroughly validated for this context of use and available" instead of previously used "if thoroughly validated" for the use of transcript analysis for making a definite diagnosis of rejection. This was done given the fact that transcript-based diagnosis needs more confirmation and is not generally accessible. It was decided that consensus thresholds for molecular classifiers and gene sets linked to Banff lesions and diagnosis need to be created and confirmed for particular clinical contexts of usage because no transcript possesses diagnostic specificity (similar to Banff histologic lesions).[2]

BANFF ACTIVE/CHRONIC LESION SCORES/INDICES

Data regarding the stage of the disease and the reversibility of disease processes are obtained from the histological and molecular analyses of kidney transplant biopsies. The report should include "active Banff Lesion Scores" (i, t, v, g, ptc, and C4d), "chronic Banff lesions" (ci, ct, cv, cg, and ptcml) and active and "chronic

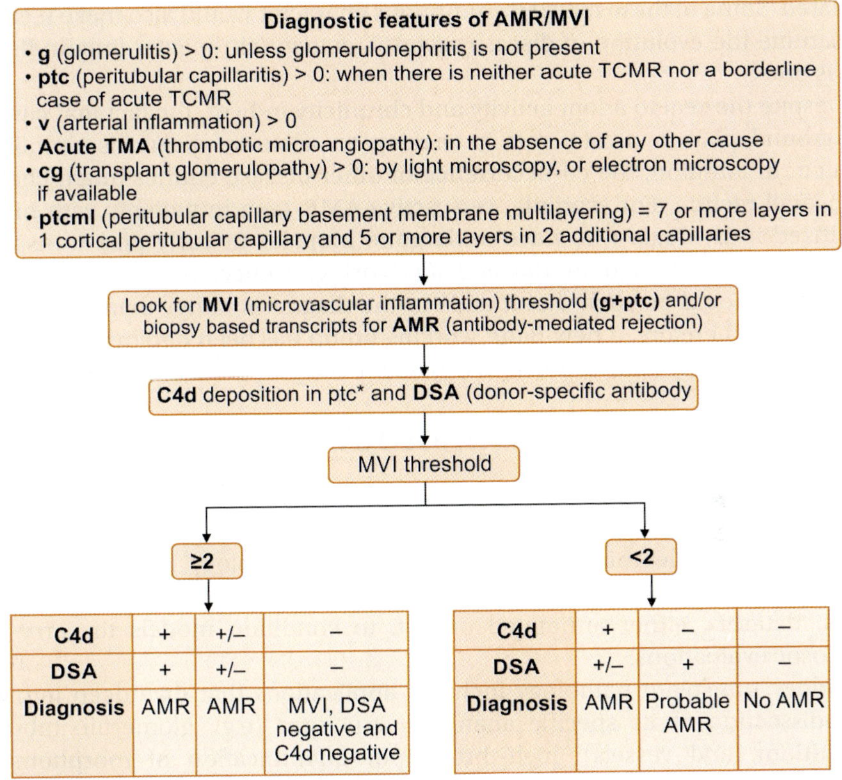

*C4d deposition in the peritubular capillaries by immunofluorescence or by immunohistochemistry.

FLOWCHART 1: The Banff 2022 classification scheme for microvascular injury and antibody-mediated rejection (AMR/MVI).

(TCMR: T cell-mediated rejection)

Banff scores" (ti, i-IFTA, t-IFTA, and pvl).[2] Temporal association has been proposed as there will be active matrix remodeling due to inflammation in due course of time. For example, *v* is later associated with *cv*, *i* is associated with later *ci*, *t* and *t-IFTA* are associated with later *ct*, and *g* is associated with *cg*.

Based on arbitrary standards, the several stages of the disease (active, chronic/active, and chronic disease) are distinguished; however, there is no specific well-defined cutoff. These have been a constant topic of debate, because of which it was proposed that a scoring system could be used in cases of AMR, as that used in cases of lupus nephritis.

Different scoring systems were proposed by studies carried out across the globe. These indices were seen as strong predictors for graft failure and therefore also had a clinical implication. Furthermore, these indices may offer medical professionals a better understanding of the extent and reversibility of an injury. In comparison to a biopsy with low activity and high chronicity, one with high activity and low chronicity in a sufficient biopsy sample could be more reversible.[2] Therefore, activity and chronicity indices might indicate which medicines would be more effective than others, but this fact is yet to be validated. Some of these metrics' continuous character would also make it easier to examine the evolution of disease severity (activity/chronicity) longitudinally across time.

Despite the zeal to adopt activity and chronicity indices, the fact that clinical background plays a pivotal role in making an accurate diagnosis cannot be negated. In addition, the co-occurrence of other disease entities might change the overall picture. For example, very active AMR seen in patients with highly sensitized individuals who have undergone biopsies in early post-transplant might not be recorded in the activity scoring. Hence, the scoring system developed should be such that it adds to the diagnosis rather than completely replacing it. Therefore, a new Banff working group has been deployed to further validate the activity and chronicity assessment in a proper medical background.

DIGITAL TRANSPLANT PATHOLOGY AND MACHINE LEARNING

The Banff 2022 session featured many presentations that examined developments in machine learning as they relate to digital pathology. A surging number of kidney transplant pathologists are beginning to compile whole slide images (WSIs) datasets, either annotated or not, to condition models to carry out diagnostic evaluations.

Kidney transplant pathology includes applications that dive deep into the microdissection of its specific anatomic structures (e.g., glomeruli, tubules, interstitium, and vessels), high-throughput quantification of morphometry (e.g., diameter of tubules)[5] and object detection (e.g., cell of interest). Research has demonstrated a substantial correlation between digital features and Banff Lesion Scores. Additionally, digital features are more responsive to modest pathological alterations that fall below the Banff grading system's criteria.[6]

One of the biggest obstacles to creating deep learning models is still gaining access to large WSI datasets that have been annotated for both clinical and pathological characteristics, including outcomes. Techniques like the human artificial intelligence loop (H-AI-L) have made it easier to train algorithms algorithmically while minimizing human annotations.[7]

XENOTRANSPLANT PATHOLOGY

The developments in genetically engineered pig-to-human xenotransplantation were discussed at a joint meeting with the Canadian Society of Transplantation (CST). When comparing laboratory models with first human data, certain pathological parallels were observed, including the presence of glomerular fibrin and platelet thrombi as well as other endothelial damage signs in some (but not all) patients. However, none of the characteristics of a Banff rejection were present. It is hypothesized that in due course of graft survival, there is a chance for the development of antibody-mediated pathology to occur over a while due to differences in the antigenicity of primates and pigs.

By examining gene homology, the Banff Human Organ Transplant (B-HOT) NanoString transcript panel was evaluated for its ability to function as a Banff

Pig Organ Transplant panel.[2] Preliminary findings indicated a rise in AMR-associated gene expression.[8] Nevertheless, it remains necessary to establish a comprehensive panel that combines both pig-selective and human-selective genes. A suggestion for a Banff working group for xenotransplantation was proposed in addition to considerations for reporting pathology in xenotransplantation. The recommendations include assessing of lesions of thrombotic microangiopathy and C4d, a complement degradation product, immunostaining for immunoglobulin and complement, along with ribonucleic acid (RNA) and ultrastructural analysis.

BANFF GUIDELINES FOR CLINICAL TRIALS

Histological Endpoints

Taking into consideration inputs from the "Surrogate Endpoints Working Group", a session was entirely committed to implementing the Banff classification in clinical trials. The conclusion was that clinical use categorization should be completely consistent with definitions agreed upon for clinical studies. As recently stated by a committee of the European Society of Organ Transplantation, there is agreement that when using histological endpoints as clinical trial endpoints, it is important to differentiate between AMR and TCMR and to refrain from using "biopsy-proven acute rejection".

Furthermore, discontinuous/semiquantitative histologic grading was shown to make repeatability challenging in clinical studies. This reiterates the fact there is a need for larger study groups aided by better resources. The implication of this requires a well-formed set diagnostic definition in conjunction with the latest Banff classification, panels of three (central) pathologists, which is ideal to prevent ties, auditable evaluations, WSI for centralized slide review, and adjudication procedures in the event of disputes. Furthermore, it is envisaged that automated digital image analysis would contribute to improving the repeatability and severity of kidney transplant damage assessment.

While biopsy-based transcript diagnostics may be a valuable tool for repeatable and quantitative evaluation of biopsies, additional studies are required to establish their added value, use, and acceptance by regulatory bodies as a therapeutic registration trial outcome.

Surrogate Endpoints

The topic of discussion also included the fact that complex and varied factors contributing to late graft failure, the short-term results that are often employed for kidney transplantation studies do not always translate into long-term success. Therefore, it is crucial to have multidimensional (surrogate) endpoints that can identify the multiple reasons for graft failure early in the course of the disease.

The iBox Scoring System, therapeutically significant elements of which include proteinuria, estimated glomerular filtration rate (eGFR), the existence of anti-human leukocyte antigen (HLA) DSA, and the Banff Lesion Scores (IFTA grade, g + ptc, cg, and i + t scores).[2] For the composite biomarker to be a reliable predictor, these histological lesion scores may not necessarily be included. In a few of the scenarios, the use of an abbreviated iBox Scoring System which has inclusion of only graft functional parameters and DSA could be adequate.[2] However, the application of the full iBox Scoring System increases prediction accuracy in other particular scenarios, such as sensitized patients and AMR trials.

CONCLUSION

According to a recent study, the Banff classification for renal allograft pathology has demonstrated flexibility in responding to new diagnostic methods, evolving clinical and regulatory settings, and growing pathophysiological understanding over the past 30 years. This flexibility is still essential. In this chapter, the major updates in the kidney transplant have been highlighted. The next Banff 2024 summit, scheduled for September 16–20, 2024, in Paris, France, will discuss the progress of the current changes made in the year 2022.

REFERENCES

1. Nankivell BJ, Shingde M, Keung KL, Fung CLS, Borrows RJ, O'Connell PJ, et al. The causes, significance and consequences of inflammatory fibrosis in kidney transplantation: The Banff i-IFTA lesion. Am J Transplant. 2018;18(2):364-76.
2. Roufosse C, Naesens M, Haas M, Lefaucheur C, Mannon RB, Afrouzian M, et al. The Banff 2022 Kidney Meeting Work Plan: Data-driven refinement of the Banff Classification for renal allografts. Am J Transplant. 2024;24(3):350-61.
3. Kung VL, Sandhu R, Haas M, Huang E. Chronic active T cell–mediated rejection is variably responsive to immunosuppressive therapy. Kidney Int. 2021;100(2):391-400.
4. Halloran PF, Matas A, Kasiske BL, Madill-Thomsen KS, Mackova M, Famulski KS. Molecular phenotype of kidney transplant indication biopsies with inflammation in scarred areas. Am J Transplant. 2019;19(5):1356-70.
5. Bouteldja N, Klinkhammer BM, Bülow RD, Droste P, Otten SW, Freifrau von Stillfried S, et al. Deep Learning–Based Segmentation and Quantification in Experimental Kidney Histopathology. J Am Soc Nephrol. 2021;32(1):52.
6. Yi Z, Salem F, Menon MC, Keung K, Xi C, Hultin S, et al. Deep learning identified pathological abnormalities predictive of graft loss in kidney transplant biopsies. Kidney Int. 2022;101(2):288-98.
7. Lutnick B, Ginley B, Govind D, McGarry SD, LaViolette PS, Yacoub R, et al. An integrated iterative annotation technique for easing neural network training in medical image analysis. Nat Mach Intell. 2019;1(2):112-9.
8. Loupy A, Giarraputo A, Goutaudier V, Robin B, Mezine F, Mangiola M, et al. 414.2: Histological and Molecular Characterization of Kidney Xenografts Transplanted to Decedent Humans. Transplantation. 2022;106(9S):S419.

19

CHAPTER

An Introduction to Spatial Transcriptomics

Suvendu Purkait

INTRODUCTION

Cells are considered the structural and functional unit of any living organism. The deoxyribonucleic acid (DNA) present in the cells houses several genes. Depending upon the cellular requirement, the genes are transcribed into messenger ribonucleic acid (mRNA), which ultimately translates into proteins. The structural differentiation and functional efficiency of a cell are critically determined by its mRNA and protein expression profile. For example, all cells of the human body essentially have the same DNA, but they differ in structure and function because of their ribonucleic acid (RNA) expression profile, and thus, protein content is different. A comprehensive evaluation of this process is essential for the understanding of developmental biology, various physiological processes, and pathobiology of diseases, including infective, degenerative, autoimmune, neoplastic, etc.[1] Transcriptomics deals with the analysis of the RNA expression profile. Initially, the analysis was limited to the assessment of bulk RNA extracted from the tissue, which is a relatively crude method and mostly representative of the major cellular component of the tissue. It does not address tissue heterogeneity and cannot also assesses the expression status of the minor cellular components. For example, bulk RNA analysis of the tumor will not be helpful in ascertaining the differential expression profile of various subpopulations of tumor cells or tumor microenvironments such as endothelial cells, stromal cells, immune cells, etc. This issue was addressed by single-cell RNA sequencing (scRNA-seq), allowing the analysis of a large number of gene expressions, even whole transcriptomes, at a single-cell resolution. However, for the scRNA-seq, the viable single cells need to be isolated from the tissue, which leads to a loss of spatial information. Further, the release of a single cell from all the organs is not always easy. Isolating neuronal cells from the brain may be technically more demanding than isolating lymphocytes from the lymph node.[2-6] It is pretty evident that most of the biological systems (physiological and pathological) constitute different cell types, and their spatial organization and cell-to-cell interaction are critical for appropriate functionality. For example, tumor cells in various niches are exposed to different microenvironments depending upon vascular supply, interaction with stroma, exposure to other signaling molecules, etc., ultimately determining their biological behavior. Similarly, during embryogenesis or in developmental biology, the relative position of cells and cell-to-cell interaction is critical for normalcy. Hence, spatially resolved information on gene expression is of immense importance. Various forms of in situ hybridization (ISH) techniques were developed during the 1970s and 1980s, which was implied in the tissue sections to retain the spatial information. However, only a limited number of genes could be assessed at a time with these methods. For example, Epstein–Barr encoding region ISH is a commonly performed test in a pathology laboratory that gives specific information about the target RNA.

Spatial transcriptomics (ST) or spatially resolved transcriptomics enables the systematic assessment of the expression profile of a significantly large number of genes within an intact tissue with preserved spatial information of the cells.[7-10] It was considered the "method of the year" in 2020 by *"nature method"*.[11]

BASIC PRINCIPLE OF DIFFERENT SPATIAL TRANSCRIPTOMICS TECHNOLOGIES

The different ST platforms available work on few basic principles. They are discussed under the following subheading:

- In situ hybridization (ISH)
- In situ sequencing (ISS)
- In situ capture (ISC) followed by sequencing/analysis
- Others

ISH and ISS require high-resolution imaging and are hence also classified under imaging-based technology. On the other hand, ISC is considered to be under the broad heading of sequencing-based technology. Technological evolution is a continuous process, and a few newer methods do not strictly fall under either of them. Further, there is a constant evolution of the basic techniques to address the shortcomings associated with a particular technology; hence, a strict classification appears difficult.

In Situ Hybridization Based Methods

This technique allows direct visualization of the target RNA with the help of a complementary probe labeled with a fluorescent detection system. The probe hybridizes with the target present in the tissue, and the intensity of the signal is used for the quantification of the RNA. There are several technical modifications to this fundamental principle for the detection of an increased number of targets with high efficiency.[7-9]

Sequential fluorescence in situ hybridization (seqFISH) is based on the ISH principle, in which sequential rounds of hybridization are followed by the digestion of the probes with deoxyribonuclease (DNase) enzyme. The probes used are for the same targets but are attached to different color fluorophores in different rounds. Hence, single target RNA is hybridized multiple times with different color-coded probes to increase specificity. The hybridized probes are assessed in each round by imaging, the colocalization of the fluorescent signal in the different rounds is analyzed further, and the abundance of the signal is considered for the measurement **(Fig. 1A)**. In seqFISH+ techniques, the primary probes have multiple binding sites for the secondary fluorophore-labeled probes.[7,8,12] The spatial resolution of this technique is excellent with high-resolution imaging. However, in techniques with sequential hybridization, there is always a risk of error due to nonspecific hybridization, which may increase exponentially with subsequent rounds.

Another technique known as multiplexed error-robust fluorescence in situ hybridization (MERFISH) uses secondary labeled and unlabeled probes instead of the different fluorophores sequentially like earlier mentioned. In each round of imaging, a binary answer can be obtained in the form of 0 (negative signal) or 1 (positive signal). A set of RNA will give a positive signal, and the other set will provide a negative signal. For example, if an experiment is targeted to detect mRNA of gene "A", "B", "C", "D", and "E", it may use the positive probe combination as follows: First round—A, B, and C; in the second round—B, C, and D; third round—A, C, and D, fourth round—A, D, and E... and so on. It is easily understandable that after the fourth round the code 1, 0, 1, 1 is indicative of A, similarly 1, 1, 0, 0 is indicative of B, and 1, 1, 1, 0 indicative of C **(Fig. 1B)**. Now, with permutation and combination, the number of the target transcript can be increased significantly at an exponential rate. More importantly, the hybridization error of one round can be corrected based on the results of other rounds.[13]

As imaging is the mainstay of ISH techniques, there may be problems with resolution pertaining to the thickness of the tissue (z-axis). A relatively newer technique known as enhanced electric FISH electrophoretically moves the RNA from the tissue to the glass slide before hybridization, which helps in the two-dimensional visualization of the signals. This increases the clarity of imaging and reduces the imaging time.[14] Even three-dimensional resolution on thicker tissue sections can be achieved by the more recently developed expansion-assisted iterative fluorescence in situ hybridization (EASI-FISH) or expansion-assisted interactive fluorescence ISH technique.[15]

The ISH methods usually provide a high resolution up to the subcellular level but are often technically demanding apart from the chance of error as described earlier. The requirement of high-resolution and high-magnification microscopy usually increases the imaging time.[7,8]

In Situ Sequencing Based Methods

In situ sequencing method uses the basic principle of sequencing by synthesis in situ with the help of a unique probe called a "padlock probe". The tissue RNA is initially fixed and then converted to complementary DNA (cDNA) using reverse transcriptase, followed by RNA digestion. Some of the methods skip the reverse transcription step. A padlock probe is then added, which is hybridized to the cDNA/mRNA. The padlock probe is a specially designed linear oligonucleotide probe in which the two ends contain the sequence that is complementary

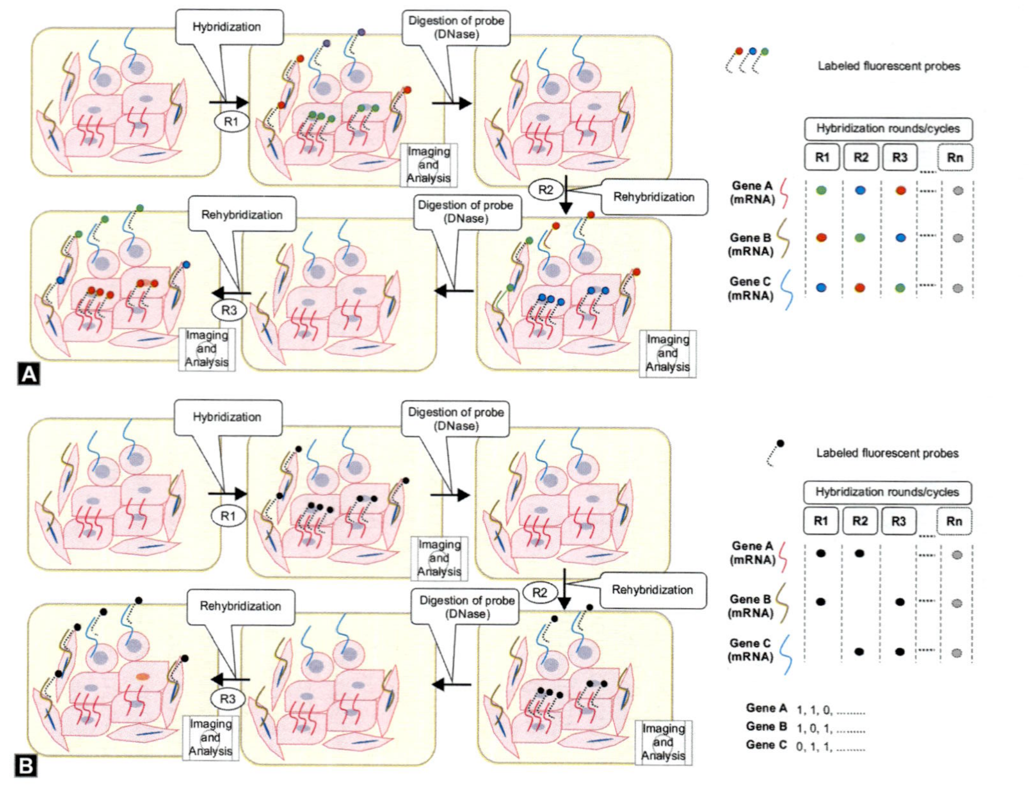

FIGS. 1A AND B: Simplified flow diagram showing the basic principle and workflow of in situ hybridization based spatial transcriptomics platforms including sequential fluorescence in situ hybridization (A) and multiplexed error-robust fluorescence in situ hybridization (B).

(mRNA: messenger ribonucleic acid)

to the target sequence. In the middle, there is an anchor sequence, primarily common for all probes, along with an identification sequence (barcode), which is unique for each target transcript. When the padlock probe is attached to the specific target by its two ends, it forms a circular DNA structure **(Fig. 2)**. The two ends of the probe are ligated by using thermostable DNA ligase derived from *Thermus thermophilus*. DNA ligase has high discriminatory power to detect even single base mismatch, imparting high specificity. Then, the circular DNA formed from the probe is amplified by rolling cycle amplification to form a single-stranded DNA product containing multiple repeats of the padlock probe sequence in a small area, which is often called a DNA nanoball. This DNA nanoball is then subjected to sequencing by ligation with the use of fluorescence-conjugated anchor primer, which is common, and an interrogation oligonucleotide probe for the identification of target-specific barcode sequence. The presence of a significant number of anchor and identification (barcode) sequences at a particular point led to a highly amplified signal, which can be detected by lower magnification imaging and significantly reduces imaging time. After one imaging cycle, the probe can be stripped off, and the next cycle can be targeted to detect the following barcode[16,17] **(Fig. 2)**. The most significant advantage of

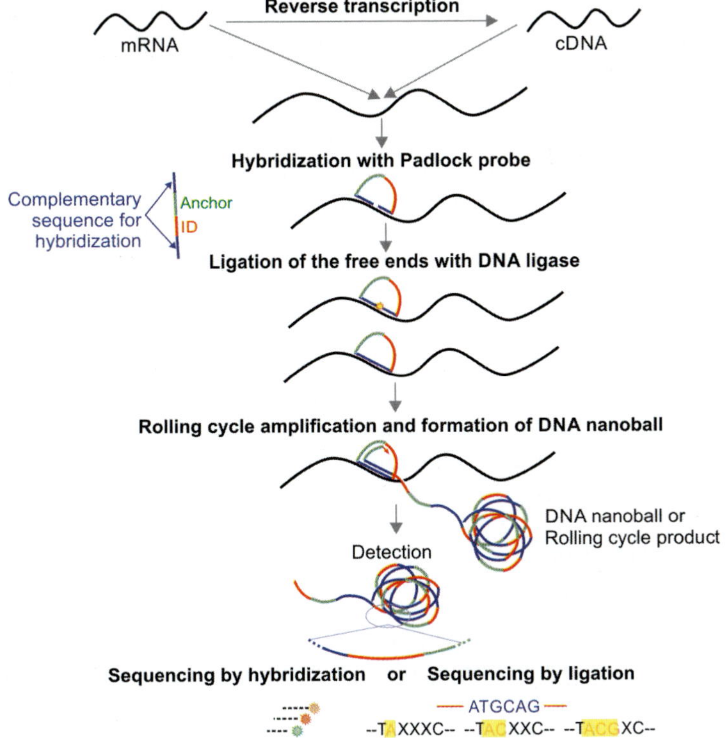

FIG. 2: Simplified flow diagram showing the basic principle and workflow of in situ sequencing based spatial transcriptomics.

(cDNA: complementary deoxyribonucleic acid; mRNA: messenger ribonucleic acid) the technique is that it uses the discriminatory power of DNA ligase to detect mismatch even up to a single base.

Methods like Cartana were developed based on this principle but without the reverse transcription and fixation steps described earlier, which led to relatively low specificity. There is one base quarry per round. Methods developed later, like fluorescent in situ RNA sequencing (FISSEQ) or expansion sequencing (ExSeq), use cDNA conversion, fixation, and ISS. More recent techniques like STARmap enable additional three-dimensional localization of the transcript with the use of hydrogel.[18-20]

In Situ Capture Based Methods

These techniques capture the RNA from the tissue, and the spatial information regarding the position of capture is retained. Then, the mRNA is converted to cDNA and quantitated based on the gene-specific sequence on next-generation sequencing (NGS)-based platforms.

The earliest example of this application is laser capture microdissection (LCM), in which an area of interest is captured, followed by microarray-based analysis of the mRNA profile. The modification of this technique is discussed later.[7,10]

Spatially encoded RNA sequencing technology, such as Visium, Slide-seq, Slide-seqV2, and high-definition ST, uses spatially barcoded probes to capture the RNA from the tissue. These barcodes are responsible for preserving the spatial information. All these techniques have their unique features and resolution.[21-23] The basic principle here is described in a simplified form. The tissue section is usually mounted over an array for the transfer of the RNA, which is followed by cDNA conversion, library preparation, and sequencing base analysis **(Fig. 3)**. The probes used in this process are primarily not gene-specific, instead for capturing the poly-A tail of mRNA. The resolution of this technique depends upon the area containing the same positional barcode, which one can compare with a pixel of a photograph.[24] The technologies mentioned earlier have different resolutions, starting from 55 to 0.5 μm. Most of these techniques are designed for fresh frozen tissue with well-preserved RNA. However, Visium formalin-fixed paraffin-embedded (FFPE) claimed to work on paraffin-embedded tissue as well.[7,8]

The major advantage of these technologies is that they do not require high-resolution imaging, which is often technically demanding and requires complex instruments and expertise.

Other Technologies

Digital Spatial Profiling

This technology has some components of imaging, probe-based hybridization, and ISC. It uses a complementary oligonucleotide probe attached to an oligonucleotide barcode tag by a photocleavable linkage. After the hybridization process, the probe is photocleaved by ultraviolet (UV) illumination from the region of interest and collected by the spatial profiler instrument for analysis. The region of interest is user-defined and can be modified based on the histology of the tissue or additional ancillary techniques like immunofluorescence.[25,26]

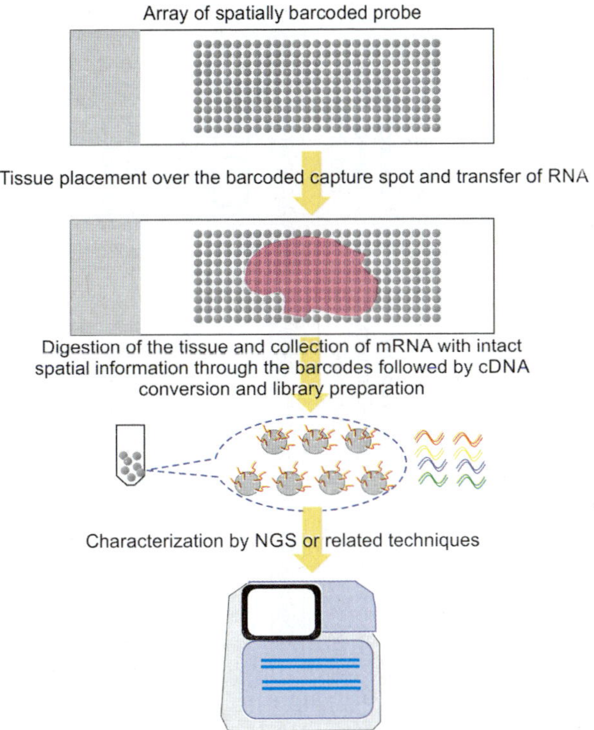

FIG. 3: The basic principle and workflow of in situ capture-based spatial transcriptomics.

(cDNA: complementary deoxyribonucleic acid; mRNA: messenger ribonucleic acid; NGS: next-generation sequencing; RNA: ribonucleic acid)

For example, if the investigator wants to assess the expression profile of endothelial cells, he/she can use specific endothelial cell markers like CD31 to mark these cells and evaluate the expression profile by selective collection. Similarly, other cell types may be targeted from the same tissue, and the expression of different subpopulations or cell types may be compared. This technique may be regarded as a complex version of the LCM and can be applied easily on the FFPE tissue sections **(Fig. 4)**. Although this technique has a high sensitivity, the throughput may be relatively low, and there is a chance of RNA damage by the UV ray.[8,9]

Image-guided Spatially Resolved Single Cell Transcriptomics

This newer technique combined scRNA-seq with microscopy or image-based techniques. Thus, it provides the desired depth of whole single-cell transcriptomics profiling in a spatial context. Different technologies that follow this principle include Geo-seq, NICHE-seq, FUN-seq, etc. These techniques use various modifications and combinations of microscopy, LCM, photocleavable probes, fluorescence-activated cell sorting, and scRNA-seq **(Fig. 4)**. Techniques like Geo-seq combine LCM and scRNA-seq to provide spatial information along

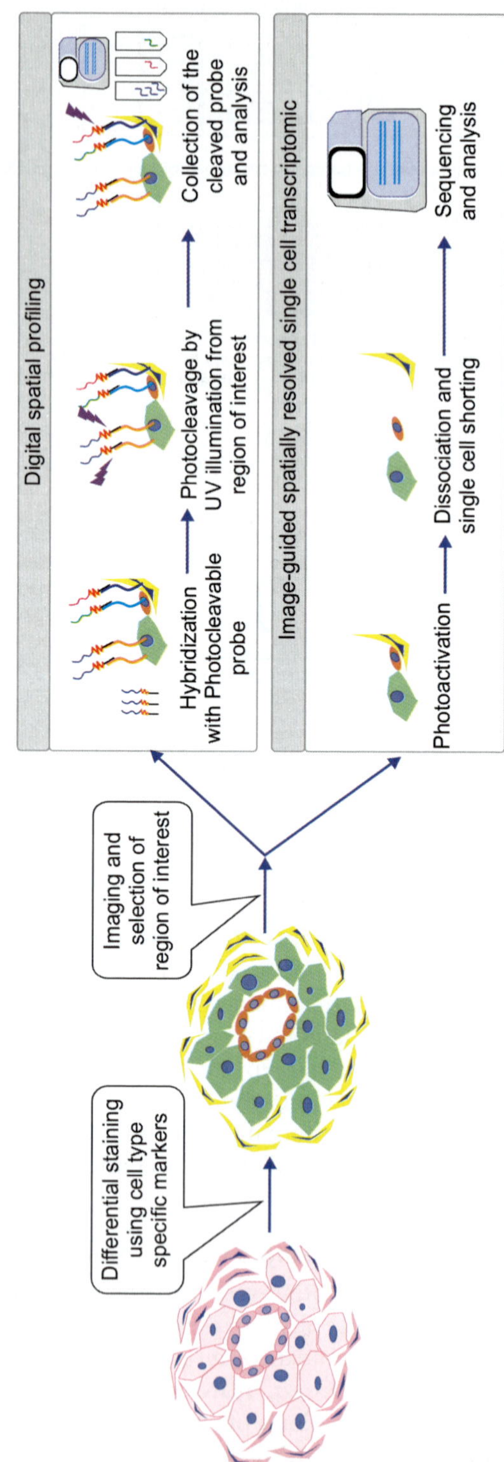

FIG. 4: The basic principle and workflow of digital spatial profiling and image-guided spatially resolved single cell transcriptomics.

with the whole transcriptomics profile.[27] On the other hand, NICHE-seq and FUN-seq use fluorescent dye and microscopy for spatial labeling of the cells, followed by fluorescent-assisted cell sorting and analysis.[28,29]

All these techniques provide a single-cell spatial resolution with a significant sequencing depth; however, they can assess only a limited proportion of the cell population.

BRIEF OUTLINE OF DATA PROCESSING AND DOWNSTREAM ANALYSIS

The analysis should be done using the appropriate toolkit and software. The basic steps in data processing include quality checks, normalization, and dimensionality reduction. The quality check indicates the depth of the data, which, in simplified terms, indicates the number of genes detected per spot. The normalization process deals with the variability of the depth across the tissue and differences in sequencing. The dimensionality reduction compresses the massive gene expression data into fewer dimensions to produce a path for informative analysis. It includes summarization methods and visualization methods.

The downstream analysis is achieved by processes such as clustering, mapping, deconvolution, and ligand-receptor matching. Clustering allows the analysis of cells in a particular organization or niche. In mapping and deconvolution, transcriptional data is integrated with the spatial profile. Mapping helps to give a cell type to its spatial counterpart based on the transcriptomics data. At the same time, deconvolution predicts the presence of a single cell type and its proportion from a mixture of transcripts in a particular area. The ligand-receptor matching helps to identify the cell-to-cell interaction.[7,8,30,31]

COMPARISON BETWEEN DIFFERENT TECHNIQUES

The comparison among different techniques can be done based on the following major points: (1) spatial resolution, (2) transcriptomics coverage and detection efficiency, (3) tissue area coverage, and (4) types of tissue required. There has been continuous technological improvement in all different methods of ST over the years to diminish the shortcomings associated with them. Most importantly, the user/researcher should select the best pertinent technology that is suitable for the research question.

Spatial Resolution

Spatial resolution practically indicates the minimum distance between two detection points. It varies from <10 μm to >50 μm with different techniques. Low-resolution methods allow detection of transcripts at single cell or even subcellular level. Mostly, image-guided methods such as ISH and ISS have a very high resolution, almost reaching the subcellular level. On the other hand, the resolution of ISC-based spatial barcoded capture methods depends upon the size of the barcode and is relatively lower than the imaging-based methods. However, more recently developed methods claimed to provide comparable spatial resolution.[7,8,10]

Transcriptomics Coverage and Detection Efficiency

Transcriptomics coverage indicates the proportion of the whole transcriptomics profile that can be detected by a method, in simplified terms, the average number of target genes whose expression profile can be detected by a method. On the other hand, detection efficiency indicates the percentage of the existing transcripts of different genes that can be detected. Methods such as ISS and ISH usually follow a probe based targeted approach; hence, the detection efficiency is relatively better. However, the number of target genes is often limited. ISC methods capture the transcripts in an unbiased manner and, hence, have better coverage but at the cost of relatively lower efficiency.[7,8,10]

Area of a Tissue Section Covered

Usually, the techniques with lower detection efficiency or spatial resolution cover a relatively larger tissue area. The imaging-based techniques are usually confined to a smaller area. Nevertheless, the tissue area can be increased by the selection of additional regions of interest, or the depth of the coverage can be increased with additional costs.[7,8,10]

Types of Tissue Required

Most of the methods are applicable to the fresh frozen tissue but some are also claimed to produce good results in the FFPE tissue. The user should be well learned about the applicability before selecting a particular platform.[7,8,10]

APPLICATION OF SPATIAL TRANSCRIPTOMICS

To date, ST technology has mostly been used as one of the research tools to explore cellular heterogeneity, cellular connectome, regulatory networks of various cell types, and microenvironmental influences. In neurological research, ST provided important insight into the expression profile of different neuron subtypes and their axonal projection and interaction. The role of the astrocytic cells in diseases like amyotrophic lateral sclerosis, primarily thought to be a neuronal disease, has also been highlighted recently.[32,33] The techniques also gave newer insight into the pathobiology of Alzheimer's disease and cerebral vascular malformation.[34-36] The embryonic development largely depends upon stem cell differentiation, lineage commitment, cellular organization or migration, and cell-to-cell interaction. Two recent studies documented the transcriptional landscape of the human embryonic heart and intestinal developmental process.[37,38] In cancer biology, ST-based research is focused predominantly on the tumor heterogeneity and tumor microenvironment, including immune cells and stromal cells. Few studies have documented the ST profile of malignancies, including melanoma, breast carcinoma, prostatic carcinoma, central nervous system (CNS) malignancies, pancreatic carcinoma, etc. It provides a more detailed understanding of the pathobiology of tumor progression and metastasis. The combination of ST and scRNA-seq is thought to help detect newer spatial biomarkers and therapeutic efficiency by identifying therapy-resistant tumor subclones.[39,40]

CONCLUSION

The ST is a powerful research tool and provides a novel dimension to understand cell biology by exploring the dynamics of several physiological and pathological processes in situ. A number of technologies have been developed and are also in the process of evolution in the field of ST. Each of these techniques is unique and has certain advantages and shortcomings. The user should be well acquainted with these and choose the ST technology most pertinent to the research question. Newer technologies provide higher resolution, depth, coverage, throughput, sensitivity, and compatibility with paraffin embed tissue section. Some of the methods are even able to provide three-dimensional resolution. However, most ST technology is technically demanding. The tissue processing, customized standardization, and data acquisition are often laborious and require significant expertise. The processing of the large amount of data generated also requires high computational ability. The ST platforms, especially the newer ones, are not easily accessible to all researchers worldwide and are not very cost-effective. Hopefully, with the rapid and continuous development in the field of technology, ST may contribute significantly in the field of basic research as well as clinical decision-making in the near future.

REFERENCES

1. Garcia HG, Berrocal A, Kim YJ, Martini G, Zhao J. Lighting up the central dogma for predictive developmental biology. Curr Top Dev Biol. 2020;137:1-35.
2. Wu X, Yang B, Udo-Inyang I, Ji S, Ozog D, Zhou L, et al. Research Techniques Made Simple: Single-Cell RNA Sequencing and its Applications in Dermatology. J Invest Dermatol. 2018;138(5):1004-9.
3. Kolodziejczyk AA, Kim JK, Svensson V, Marioni JC, Teichmann SA. The technology and biology of single-cell RNA sequencing. Mol Cell. 2015;58(4):610-20.
4. Patel AP, Tirosh I, Trombetta JJ, Shalek AK, Gillespie SM, Wakimoto H, et al. Single-cell RNA-seq highlights intratumoral heterogeneity in primary glioblastoma. Science. 2014;344(6190):1396-401.
5. Haque A, Engel J, Teichmann SA, Lönnberg T. A practical guide to single-cell RNA-sequencing for biomedical research and clinical applications. Genome Med. 2017;9(1):75.
6. Tang F, Barbacioru C, Wang Y, Nordman E, Lee C, Xu N, et al. mRNA-Seq whole-transcriptome analysis of a single cell. Nat Methods. 2009;6(5):377-82.
7. Williams CG, Lee HJ, Asatsuma T, Vento-Tormo R, Haque A. An introduction to spatial transcriptomics for biomedical research. Genome Med. 2022;14(1):68.
8. Piñeiro AJ, Houser AE, Ji AL. Research Techniques Made Simple: Spatial Transcriptomics. J Invest Dermatol. 2022;142(4):993-1001.e1.
9. Chen TY, You L, Hardillo JAU, Chien MP. Spatial Transcriptomic Technologies. Cells. 2023; 12(16):2042.
10. Moses L, Pachter L. Museum of spatial transcriptomics. Nat Methods. 2022;19(5):534-46. Erratum in: Nat Methods. 2022;19(5):628.
11. Marx V. Method of the Year: spatially resolved transcriptomics. Nat Methods. 2021;18(1): 9-14. Erratum in: Nat Methods. 2021;18(2):219.
12. Lubeck E, Coskun AF, Zhiyentayev T, Ahmad M, Cai L. Single-cell in situ RNA profiling by sequential hybridization. Nat Methods. 2014;11(4):360-1.
13. Chen KH, Boettiger AN, Moffitt JR, Wang S, Zhuang X. RNA imaging. Spatially resolved, highly multiplexed RNA profiling in single cells. Science. 2015;348(6233):aaa6090.

14. Borm LE, Mossi Albiach A, Mannens CCA, Janusauskas J, Özgün C, Fernández-García D, et al. Scalable in situ single-cell profiling by electrophoretic capture of mRNA using EEL FISH. Nat Biotechnol. 2023;41(2):222-31.
15. Wang Y, Eddison M, Fleishman G, Weigert M, Xu S, Wang T, et al. EASI-FISH for thick tissue defines lateral hypothalamus spatio-molecular organization. Cell. 2021;184(26): 6361-77.e24.
16. Magoulopoulou A, Salas SM, Tiklová K, Samuelsson ER, Hilscher MM, Nilsson M. Padlock Probe-Based Targeted In Situ Sequencing: Overview of Methods and Applications. Annu Rev Genomics Hum Genet. 2023;24:133-50.
17. Hilscher MM, Gyllborg D, Yokota C, Nilsson M. In Situ Sequencing: A High-Throughput, Multi-Targeted Gene Expression Profiling Technique for Cell Typing in Tissue Sections. Methods Mol Biol. 2020;2148:313-29.
18. Lee JH, Daugharthy ER, Scheiman J, Kalhor R, Ferrante TC, Terry R, et al. Fluorescent in situ sequencing (FISSEQ) of RNA for gene expression profiling in intact cells and tissues. Nat Protoc. 2015;10(3):442-58.
19. Alon S, Goodwin DR, Sinha A, Wassie AT, Chen F, Daugharthy ER, et al. Expansion sequencing: Spatially precise in situ transcriptomics in intact biological systems. Science. 2021;371(6528):eaax2656.
20. Wang X, Allen WE, Wright MA, Sylwestrak EL, Samusik N, Vesuna S, et al. Three-dimensional intact-tissue sequencing of single-cell transcriptional states. Science. 2018;361(6400):eaat5691.
21. Rodriques SG, Stickels RR, Goeva A, Martin CA, Murray E, Vanderburg CR, et al. Slide-seq: A scalable technology for measuring genome-wide expression at high spatial resolution. Science. 2019;363(6434):1463-67.
22. Stickels RR, Murray E, Kumar P, Li J, Marshall JL, Di Bella DJ, et al. Highly sensitive spatial transcriptomics at near-cellular resolution with Slide-seqV2. Nat Biotechnol. 2021;39(3): 313-9.
23. Vickovic S, Eraslan G, Salmén F, Klughammer J, Stenbeck L, Schapiro D, et al. High-definition spatial transcriptomics for in situ tissue profiling. Nat Methods. 2019;16(10):987-90.
24. Ståhl PL, Salmén F, Vickovic S, Lundmark A, Navarro JF, Magnusson J, et al. Visualization and analysis of gene expression in tissue sections by spatial transcriptomics. Science. 2016;353(6294):78-82.
25. Merritt CR, Ong GT, Church SE, Barker K, Danaher P, Geiss G, et al. Multiplex digital spatial profiling of proteins and RNA in fixed tissue. Nat Biotechnol. 2020;38(5):586-99.
26. Zollinger DR, Lingle SE, Sorg K, Beechem JM, Merritt CR. GeoMx™ RNA Assay: High Multiplex, Digital, Spatial Analysis of RNA in FFPE Tissue. Methods Mol Biol. 2020;2148: 331-45.
27. Chen J, Suo S, Tam PP, Han JJ, Peng G, Jing N. Spatial transcriptomic analysis of cryosectioned tissue samples with Geo-seq. Nat Protoc. 2017;12(3):566-80.
28. Smit MM, Feller KJ, You L, Storteboom J, Begce Y, Beerens C, et al. Spatially Annotated Single Cell Sequencing for Unraveling Intratumor Heterogeneity. Front Bioeng Biotechnol. 2022;10:829509.
29. Medaglia C, Giladi A, Stoler-Barak L, De Giovanni M, Salame TM, Biram A, et al. Spatial reconstruction of immune niches by combining photoactivatable reporters and scRNA-seq. Science. 2017;358(6370):1622-6.
30. Lee J, Yoo M, Choi J. Recent advances in spatially resolved transcriptomics: challenges and opportunities. BMB Rep. 2022;55(3):113-24.
31. Hu J, Li X, Coleman K, Schroeder A, Ma N, Irwin DJ, et al. SpaGCN: Integrating gene expression, spatial location and histology to identify spatial domains and spatially variable genes by graph convolutional network. Nat Methods. 2021;18(11):1342-51.
32. Maynard KR, Collado-Torres L, Weber LM, Uytingco C, Barry BK, Williams SR, et al. Transcriptome-scale spatial gene expression in the human dorsolateral prefrontal cortex. Nat Neurosci. 2021;24(3):425-36.

33. Maniatis S, Äijö T, Vickovic S, Braine C, Kang K, Mollbrink A, et al. Spatiotemporal dynamics of molecular pathology in amyotrophic lateral sclerosis. Science. 2019;364(6435):89-93.
34. Orsenigo F, Conze LL, Jauhiainen S, Corada M, Lazzaroni F, Malinverno M, et al. Mapping endothelial-cell diversity in cerebral cavernous malformations at single-cell resolution. Elife. 2020;9:e61413.
35. Navarro JF, Croteau DL, Jurek A, Andrusivova Z, Yang B, Wang Y, et al. Spatial Transcriptomics Reveals Genes Associated with Dysregulated Mitochondrial Functions and Stress Signaling in Alzheimer Disease. iScience. 2020;23(10):101556.
36. Chen WT, Lu A, Craessaerts K, Pavie B, Sala Frigerio C, Corthout N, et al. Spatial Transcriptomics and In Situ Sequencing to Study Alzheimer's Disease. Cell. 2020;182(4):976-91.e19.
37. Asp M, Giacomello S, Larsson L, Wu C, Fürth D, Qian X, et al. A Spatiotemporal Organ-Wide Gene Expression and Cell Atlas of the Developing Human Heart. Cell. 2019;179(7):1647-60.e19.
38. Fawkner-Corbett D, Antanaviciute A, Parikh K, Jagielowicz M, Gerós AS, Gupta T, et al. Spatiotemporal analysis of human intestinal development at single-cell resolution. Cell. 2021;184(3):810-26.e23.
39. Yoosuf N, Navarro JF, Salmén F, Ståhl PL, Daub CO. Identification and transfer of spatial transcriptomics signatures for cancer diagnosis. Breast Cancer Res. 2020;22(1):6.
40. Zhang L, Chen D, Song D, Liu X, Zhang Y, Xu X, et al. Clinical and translational values of spatial transcriptomics. Signal Transduct Target Ther. 2022;7(1):111.

20

CHAPTER

Updates of 5th Edition of World Health Organization Classification of Lymphoid Neoplasm

Praveen Sharma, Sananda Kumar

INTRODUCTION

The foundation for *5th edition of World Health Organization classification of lymphoid neoplasms* (WHO-HAEM5) was laid by the International Agency for Research on Cancer (IARC) in 2018 and in 2021, the editorial board members and authors were invited to contribute to WHO-HAEM5.[1] The salient changes in the WHO-HEAM5 from the existing Revised 4th edition of WHO (WHO-HAEM4R) include:

- Reorganization of disease entities by a hierarchical system
- Modification of nomenclature of few entities
- Revision of diagnostic criteria—inclusion of "essential criteria" and "desirable criteria"
- Deletion as well as introduction of new entities
- Inclusion of tumor-like lesions and germline predisposition syndromes associated with the lymphoid neoplasms

Main text:

- The significant changes made in WHO-HAEM5 in the sections of lymphoid neoplasms (B- and T-cell) compared to WHO-HAEM4R are outlined in this chapter.
- It is to note that entities whose nomenclature/category/criteria have been unchanged/retained are not included in the text underneath.

SECTION A: WHO-HAEM5 UPDATES ON B-CELL LYMPHOID PROLIFERATIONS AND LYMPHOMAS

- This section includes four broad categories, i.e., tumor like-lesions, precursor B-cell neoplasms, mature B-cell neoplasms, and plasma cell neoplasms and other diseases with paraproteins.[2]
- These broad categories and the respective entities are summarized here.

Tumor-like Lesions with B-cell Predominance (Table 1)

- This new category has been introduced for the first time in WHO-HAEM5.
- It covers diseases characterized by the proliferation of B-cells, which can mimic a lymphomatous process but are not classified as lymphoid neoplasms.

B-cell Lymphoblastic Leukemias/Lymphomas (Table 2)

- The diagnosis of B-lymphoblastic leukemia/lymphoma (B-ALL/LBL) can be made based on morphology and immunophenotyping alone as B-ALL, not further classified (NFC).
- The classification based on recurrent genetic alterations remains largely consistent with WHO-HAEM4R; however, the nomenclature now emphasizes molecular events rather than cytogenetic alterations.

TABLE 1: New entities of tumor-like lesions with B-cell predominance.

New entities under the category:	
• Reactive B-cell-rich lymphoid proliferations that can mimic lymphoma • IgG4-related disease • Unicentric Castleman disease • Idiopathic multicentric Castleman disease	
Modification of nomenclature	
WHO-HAEM4R	**WHO-HAEM5**
Multicentric Castleman disease	KSHV/HHV8-associated multicentric Castleman disease

(IgG4: immunoglobulin G4)

TABLE 2: New entities of B-cell lymphoblastic lymphomas.

New entities under the category:	
• B-lymphoblastic leukemia/lymphoma with *ETV6::RUNX1*-like features • B-lymphoblastic leukemia/lymphoma with *TCF3::HLF* fusion	
Modification of nomenclature	
WHO-HAEM4R	**WHO-HAEM5**
B-lymphoblastic leukemia/lymphoma with hyperdiploidy	B-lymphoblastic leukemia/lymphoma with high hyperdiploidy
B-lymphoblastic leukemia/lymphoma with t(9;22)(q34;q11.2);*BCR-ABL1*	B-lymphoblastic leukemia/lymphoma with *BCR::ABL1* fusion
B-lymphoblastic leukemia/lymphoma, *BCR-ABL1-like*	B-lymphoblastic leukemia/lymphoma with *BCR::ABL1*-like features
B-lymphoblastic leukemia/lymphoma with t(v;11q23.3); *KMT2A*-rearranged	B-lymphoblastic leukemia/lymphoma with *KMT2A* rearrangement
B-lymphoblastic leukemia/lymphoma with t(12;21)(p13.2;q22.1); *ETV6-RUNX1*	B-lymphoblastic leukemia/lymphoma with *ETV6:: RUNX1* fusion
B-lymphoblastic leukemia/lymphoma with t(1;19)(q23;p13.3); *TCF3-PBX1*	B-lymphoblastic leukemia/lymphoma with *TCF3::PBX1* fusion
B-lymphoblastic leukemia/lymphoma with t(5;14)(q31.1;q32.1); *IGH/IL3*	B-lymphoblastic leukemia/lymphoma with *IGH::IL3* fusion

Mature B-cell Neoplasms

The hierarchical structure of mature B-cell neoplasms includes 12 families **(Tables 3 to 14 and Box 1)**.

TABLE 3: Preneoplastic and neoplastic small lymphocytic proliferations.

Entity/category	Major changes in WHO-HAEM5
Monoclonal B-cell lymphocytosis (MBL)	Three subtypes of MBL are recognized: Low count MBL, CLL/SLL-type MBL, non-CLL/SLL-type MBL
Chronic lymphocytic leukemia/small lymphocytic leukemia (CLL/SLL)	• More than 15% prolymphocytes in the peripheral blood of a patient with CLL/SLL is recognized and termed as "prolymphocytic progression" • In lymph nodes/ tissues, prominent proliferation centers or high Ki67 indexes is termed as aggressive form of CLL/SLL • "Richter transformation" is the term to be used over "Richter syndrome"
B-cell prolymphocytic leukemia (B-PLL)	• The entity B-PLL is no longer recognized • Some of these cases have been identified as "splenic B-cell lymphoma/leukemia with prominent nucleoli" (see **Table 4**), others as blastoid mantle cell lymphoma (harboring *IGH::CCND1*) or as prolymphocytic progression of CLL/SLL

TABLE 4: Splenic B-cell lymphomas and leukemias.

Entity/category	Major changes in WHO-HAEM5
Splenic diffuse red pulp small B-cell lymphoma (SDRPL)	• Now separately classified • On flow cytometry a mean fluorescence intensity (MFI) ratio of CD200/CD180 of less than 0.5 favors diagnosis of SDRPL over other entities in this category
Splenic B-cell lymphoma/ leukemia with prominent nucleoli (SBLPN)	• New entity biologically distinct from hairy cell leukemia (HCL) • Encompasses "HCL variant" and some cases of "CD5-negative B-cell prolymphocytic leukemia (B-PLL)" • Resistant to conventional HCL therapy

TABLE 5: Lymphoplasmacytic lymphoma.

Entity/category	Major changes in WHO-HAEM5
Lymphoplasmacytic lymphoma (LPL)	• Two subtypes of LPL are recognized: Immunoglobulin M (IgM)-LPL/ Waldenström macroglobulinemia (WM) type (most common) and the non-WM type LPL (5% of LPL cases) • Two molecular subsets of IgM-LPL/WM described based on detection of *MYD88* p.L265P mutation (present in >90% cases) • Desirable to perform CXCR4 mutation analysis, mainly for its therapeutic implications

TABLE 6: Marginal zone lymphoma.

Entity/category	Major changes in WHO-HAEM5
Marginal zone lymphoma	• Primary cutaneous marginal zone lymphoma is recognized as an independent distinct entity • Pediatric marginal zone lymphoma has been elevated from a subtype within nodal marginal lymphoma to a distinct entity • Cytogenetic and gene mutational profiles differing by anatomic site have been described

TABLE 7: Follicular lymphoma.

Entity/category	Major changes in WHO-HAEM5
In situ follicular neoplasia	Termed as "in situ follicular B-cell neoplasm"
Follicular lymphoma (FL)	• New way of subtyping of FL based on biology rather than classic grading • Three types: Classical FL (cFL), follicular large B-cell lymphoma (FLBL), and FL with uncommon features (uFL) • Grading of FL is no longer mandatory • FLBL is equivalent to FL grade 3B of WHO-HAEM4R • uFL has two subsets: (1) Blastoid or centrocyte variant and (2) diffuse variant

TABLE 8: Mantle cell lymphoma (MCL): This category includes in situ mantle cell neoplasm, MCL, and non-nodal MCL.

Entity/category	Major changes in WHO-HAEM5
In situ mantle cell neoplasia	Termed as "in situ mantle cell neoplasm"

MCL	• In occasional MCL cases:
	  ○ *CCND1* protein is strongly expressed but no *CCND1* rearrangement-cryptic rearrangements of *IGK* or *IGL* with *CCND1* identified
	• In few MCL cases:
	  ○ *CCND1* protein expression and rearrangement are negative-can have *CCND2, CCND3 or CCNE* rearrangements

Leukemic non-nodal MCL	• Chiefly peripheral blood, bone marrow or splenic involvement • Characterized by (1) absence of *SOX11* expression, (2) low proliferative index, and (3) lack of expression of CD5

TABLE 9: Transformations of indolent B-cell lymphomas.

Entity/category	Major changes in WHO-HAEM5
Transformations of indolent B-cell lymphomas	• This category is introduced for the first time in WHO-HAEM5 • When an aggressive lymphoma develops in a patient with a previously or concurrently diagnosed clonally related indolent B-cell lymphoma, it should be classified according to its aggressive lymphoma type • The report should also include the phrase "transformed from" along with the name of the indolent lymphoma from which it originated

Large B-cell Lymphomas (Box 1)

An algorithmic approach for classifying aggressive B-cell lymphomas in WHO-HAEM5, based on *MYC, BCL2, and BCL6* rearrangements as well as complex 11q gain/loss patterns, is described.

TABLE 10: High-grade B cell lymphoma.

Modification of nomenclature	
WHO-HAEM4R	**WHO-HAEM5**
High-grade B-cell lymphoma with *MYC* and *BCL2* and/or *BCL6* rearrangements	Diffuse large B-cell lymphoma (DLBCL)/high-grade B-cell lymphoma with *MYC* and *BCL2* rearrangements
Burkitt-like lymphoma with 11q aberration	High-grade B-cell lymphoma with 11q aberrations
Epstein–Barr virus (EBV)-positive DLBCL, not otherwise specified (NOS)	EBV-positive DLBCL
B-cell lymphoma, unclassifiable, with features intermediate between DLBCL and classic Hodgkin lymphoma	Mediastinal gray zone lymphoma

TABLE 11: Burkitt lymphoma (BL).

Entity/category	Major changes in WHO-HAEM5
BL	• Definition largely unchanged • Recent insights on BL biology suggest distinction into two types, (1) Epstein–Barr virus (EBV) positive BL and (2) EBV-negative BL

TABLE 12: KSHV/HHV8-associated B-cell lymphoid proliferations and lymphomas.

Modification of nomenclature	
WHO-HAEM4R	**WHO-HAEM5**
HHV8-positive diffuse large B-cell lymphoma, not otherwise specified (NOS)	KSHV/HHV8-positive diffuse large B-cell lymphoma
HHV8-positive germinotropic lymphoproliferative disorder	KSHV/HHV8-positive germinotropic lymphoproliferative disorder

TABLE 13: Lymphoid proliferations and lymphomas associated with immune deficiency.

New entities under the category:	
• Hyperplasias arising in immune deficiency/dysregulation • Polymorphic lymphoproliferative disorders arising in immune deficiency/dysregulation • Lymphomas arising in immune deficiency/dysregulation	
Modification of nomenclature	
WHO-HAEM4R	**WHO-HAEM5**
Lymphoproliferative diseases associated with primary immune disorders	Inborn error of immunity-associated lymphoid proliferations and lymphomas

TABLE 14: Hodgkin lymphoma.

Entity/category	Major changes in WHO-HAEM5
Hodgkin lymphoma	Nodular lymphocyte predominance Hodgkin lymphoma (NLPHL) may be more accurately labelled as "nodular lymphocyte predominant B-cell lymphoma (NLPBCL)", in view of B-cell origin, however, the existing terminology is still maintained

BOX 1 Large B-cell lymphomas.

New entities under the category:

- Fibrin-associated large B-cell lymphoma (LBCL) (previously under diffuse large B-cell lymphoma associated with chronic inflammation)
- Fluid overload-associated large B-cell lymphoma
- Primary large B-cell lymphoma of immune-privileged sites (includes primary diffuse LBCL of the central nervous system, vitreoretinal, and testis)

TABLE 15: Plasma cell neoplasm.

New entities under the category:	
• Cold agglutinin disease (CAD) • Monoclonal gammopathy of renal significance (MGRS) • Adenopathy and extensive skin patch overlying a plasmacytoma (AESOP) syndrome	
Modification of nomenclature	
WHO-HAEM4R	**WHO-HAEM5**
Primary amyloidosis	Immunoglobulin-related (AL) amyloidosis
Light chain and heavy chain deposition disease	Monoclonal immunoglobulin deposition disease

Lymphoid Proliferations and Lymphomas Associated with Immune Deficiency and Dysregulation

- Major changes on this category in WHO-HAEM5.
- In previous classifications, these disorders were categorized based on the underlying disease context in which they developed.
- The new standardized nomenclature integrates all relevant diagnostic data into a unified system, incorporating histological criteria, oncogenic virus status, and clinical context. This approach aims to resolve inconsistencies in terminology and diagnostic criteria across different immunodeficiency settings.

Plasma Cell Neoplasms

Plasma cell neoplasms and other diseases with paraproteins are given in **Tables 15 and 16**.

TABLE 16: Major changes in Plasma cell neoplasms and other diseases with paraproteins.

Entity/category	Major changes in WHO-HAEM5
Plasma cell neoplasms and other diseases with paraproteins	• Cold agglutinin disease, IgM and non-IgM monoclonal gammopathy of undetermined significance (MGUS), and monoclonal gammopathy of renal significance (MGRS) are clubbed as monoclonal gammopathies • Risk stratification model for IgM and non-IgM MGUS has been revised • In adenopathy and extensive skin patch overlying a plasmacytoma (AESOP) syndrome, there is diffuse hyperplasia of dermal vessels and dermal mucin deposition on skin biopsy and lymph node shows Castleman disease like features • In plasma cell myeloma, the genetics, particularly novel mutations, staging according to the revised International Staging System for Multiple Myeloma, the role of measurable residual disease testing using flow cytometry or next-generation testing have been emphasized

SECTION B: T-CELL AND NATURAL KILLER-CELL LYMPHOID PROLIFERATIONS AND LYMPHOMAS

- WHO-HAEM5 has restructured the entities previously classified as mature T- and natural killer (NK)-cell neoplasms in WHO-HAEM4R, now grouping them under the broader category of "T-cell and NK-cell lymphoid proliferations and lymphomas".
- In WHO-HAEM5, T- and NK-cell neoplasms are not divided into separate categories because many entities encompass a spectrum of tumors with NK, T, hybrid, or indeterminate phenotypes.
- This section includes three categories namely, tumor-like lesions with T-cell predominance, precursor T-cell neoplasms, and mature T-cell and NK-cell neoplasms.
- The broad categories and the respective entities are summarized here.

Tumor-like Lesions with T-cell Predominance

New class of tumor-like lesion included where the expansion of T-cells can be potentially mistaken for a lymphomatous process **(Box 2)**.

Precursor T-cell Neoplasms

Precursor T-cell neoplasms are given in **Table 17**.

Mature T-cell and Natural Killer-cell Neoplasms

The hierarchical structure of mature T-cell and NK-cell neoplasms includes families **(Tables 18 to 26)**.

Mature T-cell and Natural Killer-cell Leukemias

These are given in **Table 18**.

BOX 2 Tumor-like lesions with T-cell predominance.

New entities under the category:
- Kikuchi-Fujimoto disease
- Indolent T-lymphoblastic proliferation
- Autoimmune lymphoproliferative syndrome

TABLE 17: Precursor T-cell neoplasm.

Modification of nomenclature	
WHO-HAEM4R	**WHO-HAEM5**
T-lymphoblastic leukemia/lymphoma	T-lymphoblastic leukemia/lymphoma, not otherwise specified (NOS)
Early T-cell precursor lymphoblastic leukemia	Early T-precursor lymphoblastic leukemia/ lymphoma
Deleted entities under the category: • NK-lymphoblastic leukemia/lymphoma	

TABLE 18: Mature T-cell and natural killer (NK)-cell leukemias.

Modification of nomenclature	
WHO-HAEM4R	**WHO-HAEM5**
T-cell large granular lymphocytic leukemia	T-large granular lymphocytic leukemia
Chronic lymphoproliferative disorder of NK cells	NK-large granular lymphocytic leukemia

TABLE 19: Primary cutaneous lymphoma.

New entities under the category:	
• Primary cutaneous peripheral T-cell lymphoma, not otherwise specified (NOS)	
Modification of nomenclature	
WHO-HAEM4R	**WHO-HAEM5**
Primary cutaneous acral CD8-positive T-cell lymphoma	Primary cutaneous acral CD8-positive lymphoproliferative disorder

TABLE 20: Intestinal T-cell and natural killer (NK)-cell lymphoid proliferations and lymphomas.

New entities under the category:	
• Indolent NK-cell lymphoproliferative disorder of the gastrointestinal tract	
Modification of nomenclature	
WHO-HAEM4R	**WHO-HAEM5**
Indolent T-cell lymphoproliferative disorder of the gastrointestinal tract	Indolent T-cell lymphoma of the gastrointestinal tract

TABLE 21: Hepatosplenic T-cell lymphoma.

Entity/category	Major changes in WHO-HAEM5
Hepatosplenic T-cell lymphoma (HSTCL)	• HSTCL is not only confined to younger individuals; only 49% of patients are below 60 years of age • Dyshemopoiesis in bone marrow can be seen

TABLE 22: Anaplastic large cell lymphoma.

Modification of nomenclature	
WHO-HAEM4R	**WHO-HAEM5**
Anaplastic large cell lymphoma, anaplastic lymphoma kinase (ALK)-positive	ALK-positive anaplastic large cell lymphoma
Anaplastic large cell lymphoma, ALK-negative	ALK-negative anaplastic large cell lymphoma

TABLE 23: Major changes in anaplastic large cell lymphoma (ALCL).

Entity/category	Major changes in WHO-HAEM5
ALCL, anaplastic lymphoma kinase (ALK)-negative	• Specific molecular alterations in ALK-ALCL are associated with distinct morphological features • ALCLs with *DUSP22* rearrangement: neoplastic cells with a "doughnut cell" appearance with *LEF1* expression serving as a potential surrogate marker for this alteration • Hodgkin-like morphology may exhibit aberrant *ERBB4* protein expression • *JAK2* rearrangement is linked to a more anaplastic cell appearance

TABLE 24: Modification of nodal T-follicular helper (TFH) cell lymphoma.

Modification of nomenclature	
WHO-HAEM4R	**WHO-HAEM5**
Angioimmunoblastic T-cell lymphoma	Nodal TFH cell lymphoma, angioimmunoblastic type
Follicular T-cell lymphoma	Nodal TFH cell lymphoma, follicular-type
Nodal peripheral T-cell lymphoma with TFH phenotype	Nodal TFH cell lymphoma, not otherwise specified (NOS)

TABLE 25: Modification of Epstein–Barr virus (EBV)-positive natural killer (NK)/T-cell lymphoma.

New entities under the category:	
• EBV-positive nodal T- and NK-cell lymphoma	
Modification of nomenclature	
WHO-HAEM4R	**WHO-HAEM5**
Extranodal NK/T-cell lymphoma, nasal-type	Extranodal NK/T-cell lymphoma

TABLE 26: Epstein–Barr virus (EBV)-positive natural killer (NK)/T-cell lymphoma and lymphoma of childhood.

Modification of nomenclature	
WHO-HAEM4R	**WHO-HAEM5**
Hydroa vacciniforme-like lymphoproliferative disorder	Hydroa vacciniforme lymphoproliferative disorder
Chronic active EBV infection of T- and NK-cell type, systemic form	Systemic chronic active EBV disease

Primary Cutaneous T-cell Lymphomas

Primary cutaneous T-cell lymphomas are given in **Table 19**.

Nodal T-follicular Helper Cell Lymphoma (Table 24)

WHO-HAEM5 introduces a unified terminology for nodal T-follicular helper cell lymphomas (nTFHLs), grouping previously distinct entities under this family.

Epstein–Barr Virus-positive Natural Killer/T-cell Lymphomas

These are given in **Table 25**.

Epstein–Barr Virus-positive T- and Natural Killer-cell Lymphoid Proliferations and Lymphomas of Childhood

These are given in **Table 26**.

SECTION C: STROMA-DERIVED NEOPLASMS OF LYMPHOID TISSUES

- WHO-HAEM5 introduces a new category for stroma-derived neoplasms of lymphoid tissues.[3]
- This includes mesenchymal dendritic cell neoplasms, myofibroblastic tumor and spleen-specific vascular-stromal tumors.
- The broad categories and the respective entities are summarized here.

Mesenchymal Dendritic Cell Neoplasms (Table 27)

Follicular dendritic cell and fibroblastic reticular cell neoplasms have been moved from the "histiocytic and dendritic cell neoplasms" category (WHO-HEAM4R) to this category. This reclassification recognizes that follicular dendritic cells originate from mesenchymal tissue rather than hematopoietic stem cells.

Myofibroblastic Tumor

Myofibroblastic tumor is given in **Box 3**.

Spleen-specific Vascular-stromal Tumors

Spleen-specific vascular-stromal tumors are given in **Box 4**.

TABLE 27: Mesenchymal dendritic cell neoplasms.

Modification of nomenclature	
WHO-HAEM4R	**WHO-HAEM5**
Inflammatory pseudotumor-like follicular/ fibroblastic dendritic cell sarcoma	Epstein–Barr virus (EBV)-positive inflammatory follicular dendritic cell sarcoma

BOX 3 Myofibroblastic tumor.

New entities under the category:
- Intranodal palisaded myofibroblastoma

BOX 4 Vascular-stromal tumors.

New entities under the category:
- Littoral cell angioma
- Splenic hamartoma
- Sclerosing angiomatoid nodular transformation of spleen

CONCLUSION

The 5th Edition of the WHO Classification of Hematolymphoid Tumors introduces important updates to the categorization and understanding of lymphoid neoplasms. These revisions reflect advances in molecular genetics, diagnostics, and clinical management, offering a more precise and integrated framework. The changes enhance the accuracy of diagnosis, prognosis, and treatment strategies, improving patient outcomes in clinical practice.

REFERENCES

1. Swerdlow SH, Campo E, Harris NL, Jaffe ES, Pileri SA, Stein H, et al. World Health Organization classification of Tumours of Haematopoietic and Lymphoid Tissues. Revised 4th ed. Lyon: International Agency for Research on Cancer; 2017.
2. World Health Organization. WHO Classification of Hematolymphoid tumors. Lyon (France): International Agency for Research on Cancer; 2022.
3. Alaggio R, Amador C, Anagnostopoulos I, Attygalle AD, Araujo IBO, Berti E, et al. The 5th edition of the World Health Organization Classification of Haematolymphoid Tumours: Lymphoid Neoplasms. Leukemia. 2022;36(7):1720-48.

Index

Page numbers followed by *b* refer to box, *f* refer to figure, *fc* refer to flowchart, and *t* refer to table.

A

B

C

D

E

F

G

H

I

N

O

P

T

U

V

W

X

Z